HANDBOOK OF CHILD AND ADOLESCENT AGGRESSION

Also Available

Handbook of Peer Interactions, Relationships,
and Groups, Second Edition
Edited by William M. Bukowski,
Brett Laursen, and Kenneth H. Rubin

Socioemotional Development in Cultural Context
Edited by Xinyin Chen and Kenneth H. Rubin

The Development of Shyness and Social Withdrawal
Edited by Kenneth H. Rubin and Robert J. Coplan

HANDBOOK OF
CHILD AND ADOLESCENT AGGRESSION

Edited by
Tina Malti
Kenneth H. Rubin

Foreword by
Tracy Vaillancourt

THE GUILFORD PRESS
New York   London

To Wolfgang Edelstein and in memory of Tom Dishion

*With sincerest gratitude for being distinguished role models
for those who study aggression and its development*

Copyright © 2018 The Guilford Press
A Division of Guilford Publications, Inc.
370 Seventh Avenue, Suite 1200, New York, NY 10001
www.guilford.com

Printed in the United States of America

This book is printed on acid-free paper.

Last digit is print number: 9 8 7 6 5 4 3 2 1

The authors have checked with sources believed to be reliable in their efforts to provide information
that is complete and generally in accord with the standards of practice that are accepted at the time of
publication. However, in view of the possibility of human error or changes in behavioral, mental health,
or medical sciences, neither the authors, nor the editor and publisher, nor any other party who has
been involved in the preparation or publication of this work warrants that the information contained
herein is in every respect accurate or complete, and they are not responsible for any errors or omis-
sions or the results obtained from the use of such information. Readers are encouraged to confirm the
information contained in this book with other sources.

Library of Congress Cataloging-in-Publication Data

Names: Malti, Tina, editor. | Rubin, Kenneth H., editor.
Title: Handbook of child and adolescent aggression / edited by Tina Malti,
   Kenneth H. Rubin ; foreword by Tracy Vaillancourt.
Description: New York : The Guilford Press, 2018. | Includes bibliographical
   references and index.
Identifiers: LCCN 2018002528 | ISBN 9781462526208 (hardback)
Subjects: LCSH: Aggressiveness in children. | Aggressiveness in adolescence.
   | Developmental psychology. | BISAC: PSYCHOLOGY / Developmental / Child. |
   MEDICAL / Psychiatry / Child & Adolescent.
Classification: LCC BF723.A35 H36 2018 | DDC 155.4/18232—dc23
LC record available at *https://lccn.loc.gov/2018002528*

About the Editors

Tina Malti, PhD, is Professor of Psychology and Director of the Laboratory for Social–Emotional Development and Intervention at the University of Toronto. She serves as Associate Editor of *Child Development* and as Membership Secretary (2014–2020) of the International Society for the Study of Behavioural Development (ISSBD). She is a Fellow of the American Psychological Association and the Association for Psychological Science. Dr. Malti is a recipient of New Investigator awards from the Canadian Institutes of Health Research, the Ontario Ministry of Research and Innovation, the Society for Research on Adolescence, and the International Society for Research on Aggression. Her research interests include the origins, pathways, and consequences of aggression and kindness in childhood and adolescence. She creates and implements interventions to enhance social–emotional development and reduce aggression and exposure to violence in children facing multiple forms of adversity.

Kenneth H. Rubin, PhD, is Professor of Human Development and Quantitative Methodology and Founding Director of the Center for Children, Relationships, and Culture at the University of Maryland, College Park. He is a Fellow of the American and Canadian Psychological Associations, the Association for Psychological Science, and the ISSBD. Dr. Rubin is a recipient of Distinguished Contribution awards from the Society for Research in Child Development and the ISSBD, the Mentor Award in Developmental Psychology from the American Psychological Association, and the Pickering Award for Outstanding Contribution to Developmental Psychology in Canada from Carleton University. His research focuses on peer and parent–child relationships and the origins and developmental course of social and emotional adjustment and maladjustment in childhood and adolescence.

Contributors

Brendan Andrade, PhD, Child, Youth and Family Program, Centre for Addiction and Mental Health, Intergenerational Wellness Centre, Toronto, Ontario, Canada

Sheri A. Bauman, PhD, College of Education, Department of Disability and Psychoeducational Studies, University of Arizona, Tucson, Arizona

Sarah J. Blakely-McClure, MA, Department of Psychology, University at Buffalo, The State University of New York, Buffalo, New York

Michel Boivin, PhD, School of Psychology, Laval University, Quebec City, Quebec, Canada

Megan K. Bookhout, MA, Department of Psychological and Brain Sciences, University of Delaware, Newark, Delaware

Caroline L. Boxmeyer, PhD, Center for Prevention of Youth Behavior Problems, University of Alabama, Tuscaloosa, Alabama

Catherine P. Bradshaw, PhD, Curry School of Education, University of Virginia, Charlottesville, Virginia

Susan Branje, PhD, Department of Youth and Family, Utrecht University, Utrecht, The Netherlands

Mara Brendgen, PhD, Department of Psychology, University of Quebec at Montreal, Montreal, Quebec, Canada

William M. Bukowski, PhD, Department of Psychology, Concordia University, Montreal, Quebec, Canada

Connie Cheung, PhD, Department of Psychology, University of Toronto, Mississauga, Ontario, Canada

Tyler Colasante, PhD, Department of Psychology, University of Toronto, Mississauga, Ontario, Canada

Véronique Dupéré, PhD, School of Psychoeducation, University of Montreal, Montreal, Quebec, Canada

Margaret C. Elliott, PhD, Abt Associates, Cambridge, Massachusetts

Dorothy L. Espelage, PhD, Department of Psychology, University of Florida, Gainesville, Florida

Paul J. Frick, PhD, Department of Psychology, Louisiana State University, Baton Rouge, Louisiana

S. Andrew Garbacz, PhD, Department of School Psychology, University of Wisconsin–Madison, Madison, Wisconsin

Nancy G. Guerra, EdD, Department of Psychology and Social Behavior, University of California, Irvine, Irvine, California

Julie A. Hubbard, PhD, Department of Psychological and Brain Sciences, University of Delaware, Newark, Delaware

Shelley Hymel, PhD, Department of Educational and Counselling Psychology, University of British Columbia, Vancouver, British Columbia, Canada

Marc Jambon, PhD, Department of Psychology, University of Toronto, Mississauga, Ontario, Canada

Sarah Lindstrom Johnson, PhD, T. Denny Sanford School of Social and Family Dynamics, Arizona State University, Tempe, Arizona

Hans M. Koot, PhD, Department of Clinical, Neuro- and Developmental Psychology, Vrije University Amsterdam, Amsterdam, The Netherlands

Jennifer E. Lansford, PhD, Center for Child and Family Policy, Duke University, Durham, North Carolina

Tama Leventhal, PhD, Eliot-Pearson Department of Child Study and Human Development, Tufts University, Medford, Massachusetts

John E. Lochman, PhD, Center for Prevention of Youth Behavior Problems, University of Alabama, Tuscaloosa, Alabama

Sabina Low, PhD, T. Denny Sanford School of Social and Family Dynamics, Arizona State University, Tempe, Arizona

Tina Malti, PhD, Department of Psychology, University of Toronto, Mississauga, Ontario, Canada

Tatiana M. Matlasz, BA, Department of Psychology, Louisiana State University, Baton Rouge, Louisiana

Christina C. Moore, BA, Department of Psychological and Brain Sciences, University of Delaware, Newark, Delaware

Pietro Muratori, PhD, Department of Psychology, University of Pisa, Pisa, Italy

Tiina J. Ojanen, PhD, Department of Psychology, University of South Florida, Tampa, Florida

Jamie M. Ostrov, PhD, Department of Psychology, University at Buffalo, The State University of New York, Buffalo, New York

Kristin J. Perry, MA, Department of Psychology, University at Buffalo, The State University of New York, Buffalo, New York

K. Lee Raby, PhD, Department of Psychology, University of Utah, Salt Lake City, Utah

Glenn I. Roisman, PhD, Institute of Child Development, University of Minnesota, Minneapolis, Minnesota

Kenneth H. Rubin, PhD, Department of Human Development and Quantitative Methodology, University of Maryland, College Park, Maryland

Christina Salmivalli, PhD, Division of Psychology, University of Turku, Turku, Finland

Jelle Sijtsema, PhD, Department of Developmental Psychology, Tilburg University, Tilburg, The Netherlands

Ju-Hyun Song, PhD, Department of Child Development, California State University Dominguez Hills, Carson, California

Elizabeth A. Stormshak, PhD, Department of Counseling Psychology and Human Services, University of Oregon, Eugene, Oregon

Marion K. Underwood, PhD, Department of Psychological Sciences, Purdue University, West Lafayette, Indiana

Tracy Vaillancourt, PhD, Children's Mental Health and Violence Prevention; Department of Counselling Psychology, Faculty of Education; and School of Psychology, Faculty of Social Sciences, University of Ottawa, Ottawa, Ontario, Canada

Frank Vitaro, PhD, School of Psychoeducation, University of Montreal, Montreal, Quebec, Canada

Antonio Zuffianò, PhD, Department of Psychology, Liverpool Hope University, Liverpool, United Kingdom

Foreword

TRACY VAILLANCOURT

Aggression destroys individuals, communities, religions, and national economies. It creates physical and mental health problems and impacts achievement and productivity. Considering the destruction associated with aggression, it is important to document its etiology, developmental course, and consequences, and to start this inquiry at the beginning.

The beginning tells us that the use of physical aggression is pervasive in early childhood and that a notable number (one in six) of preschool children, mostly boys, continue to follow a trajectory of high physical aggression that extends into childhood (Côté, Vaillancourt, LeBlanc, Nagin, & Tremblay, 2006) and adolescence (Cleverley, Szatmari, Vaillancourt, Boyle, & Lipman, 2012). The beginning also tells us that during the early years another form of aggression is developing and that a notable number (one in three) of preschool children, mostly girls, follow a trajectory of increasing use of indirect aggression (e.g., peer group exclusion, rumor spreading) that extends into childhood (Vaillancourt, Miller, Fagbemi, Côté, & Tremblay, 2007) and adolescence (Cleverley et al., 2012). Importantly, high use of either form of aggression is associated with maladjustment concurrently and over time, which is acutely extended to targets (McDougall & Vaillancourt, 2015).

Because aggression is so detrimental to perpetrators and targets, a comprehensive review of the current state of knowledge about its development and treatment is warranted. The intricacies of the conditions that provoke aggression are such that no one viewpoint can be taken. Indeed, aggression is a complex issue that involves multiple systems like genetics, psychophysiology, temperament, social cognition, social–emotional competence, social inequality, family structure and functioning, and peer relationships and social networks, interacting with one another, and influencing its development and maintenance in nuanced ways. The involvement of these interacting systems is highlighted when considering heterogeneity in outcome: aggression does not always lead to the same pathological or nonpathological conclusion. Aggression can be adaptive and maladaptive. For example, some aggressive children are afforded high status and visibility within their peer group, while others are marginalized (Rodkin, Espelage, & Hanish, 2015). Knowing why some aggressors (or targets) fare poorly while others fare better provides important insight into processes and mechanisms, which in turn helps inform intervention and prevention efforts. That is, a better understanding of what moderates and/or mediates developmental pathways affords more therapeutic precision.

Few can dispute that aggression remains a pressing global issue. Children and adolescents are exposed to aggression in their families, their social networks, and their communities. They bully or are bullied. They are shot in their schools. They are exposed to chemical attacks within their country. This cruelty impairs their opportunities to develop relationship capacity by interfering with developmental pathways to adaptive outcomes (Vaillancourt, Sanderson, Arnold, & McDougall, 2017). The destructive nature of aggression demands a comprehensive and broad approach to advance our understanding and ultimately reduce its prevalence and caustic impact. This is the approach taken in the *Handbook of Child and Adolescent Aggression*.

REFERENCES

Cleverley, K., Szatmari, P., Vaillancourt, T., Boyle, M., & Lipman, E. (2012). Developmental trajectories of physical and indirect aggression from late childhood to adolescence: Sex differences and outcomes in emerging adulthood. *Journal of the American Academy of Child and Adolescent Psychiatry, 51*, 1037–1051.

Côté, S., Vaillancourt, T., LeBlanc, J. C., Nagin, D. S., & Tremblay, R. E. (2006). The development of physical aggression from toddlerhood to pre-adolescence: A nation-wide longitudinal study of Canadian children. *Journal of Abnormal Child Psychology, 34*, 68–82.

McDougall, P., & Vaillancourt, T. (2015). Long-term adult outcomes of peer victimization in childhood and adolescence: Pathways to adjustment and maladjustment. *American Psychologist, 70*, 300–310.

Rodkin, P. C., Espelage, D. L., & Hanish, L. D. (2015). A relational framework for understanding bullying: Developmental antecedents and outcomes. *American Psychologist, 70*, 311–321.

Vaillancourt, T., Miller, J. L., Fagbemi, J., Côté, S., & Tremblay, R. E. (2007). Trajectories and predictors of indirect aggression: Results from a nationally representative longitudinal study of Canadian children aged 2–10. *Aggressive Behavior, 33*, 314–326.

Vaillancourt, T., Sanderson, C., Arnold, P., & McDougall, P. (2017). The neurobiology of peer victimization: Longitudinal links to health, genetic risk, and epigenetic mechanisms. In C. P. Bradshaw (Ed,), *Handbook on bullying prevention: A life course perspective* (pp. 35–47). Washington, DC: National Association of Social Workers Press.

Preface

Aggression is harmful, hurtful, and destructive, comprising among the most notable and problematic behavioral challenges of humankind. Whether enacted directly and physically or indirectly, through such behaviors as verbal abuse, rumor, and exclusion, aggression is present from the early years of childhood through the adolescent and adult years. Aggression is also remarkably resistant to change and associated with a wide range of emotional and behavioral problems (Eisner & Malti, 2015). Truly, no one gains from interactions that violate, in one way or another, the perpetrator and the target. In so many ways, the enactment of aggression can destroy individuals, relationships, and groups; the young and the old; villages, cities, and countries.

Given the well-documented short- and long-term negative outcomes associated with aggression and aggressive interchanges, it is surprising that, until the publication of this handbook, there was not a comprehensive collection of reviews describing both major conceptualizations and theories, and the extant contemporary research pertaining to the origins, concomitants, and trajectories of child and adolescent aggression.

In addition, there has not heretofore existed, within a single handbook, an extensive collection describing the various intervention programs that have been developed to address the societal problem of preventing and/or intervening in the lives of youth who are at risk for, or who are already evidencing difficulties pertaining to, the production of aggressive behavior. The interventions are research based and address the display of child and adolescent aggressive behavior in multiple settings, including the family, school, and community. In sum, the primary goal of this handbook is to provide a broad-strokes review of what is known about the development and treatment of aggression in childhood and adolescence.

The target audience of this handbook includes researchers and practitioners who are interested in the development, prevention, and treatment of aggressive problem behaviors across childhood and adolescence, as well as advanced undergraduate and graduate students in developmental and clinical psychology, psychiatry, social work, education, and public health. Developmental and clinical psychologists may find the coverage of both basic research and its application particularly useful for the implementation of novel intervention strategies.

Research on the foundations and antecedents of aggression in childhood and adolescence was imbued by learning theories pertaining to social behavior, as well as theories emphasizing the inherent relational nature of aggression. More specifically, foundational experiments on the emergence and learning of aggression through observation and imitation (Bandura, Ross, & Ross, 1961) contributed to an increase in developmental research on aggression. In addition, psychoanalytic theorizing about attachment and its impact on aggressive and adaptive behaviors (Bowlby, 1969; Ainsworth, Blehar, Waters, & Wall, 1978), as well as interpersonal theories that stressed the genuine interpersonal character of aggression (Hinde, 1997; Sullivan, 1953), led to an investigation of how caregiver–child relationships and related factors in the family system contribute to aggression in childhood and adolescence. Indeed, in what may well be considered a precursor to the present volume, Pepler and Rubin edited *The Development and Treatment of Childhood Aggression* (1991), in which it was already acknowledged that aggression is the product of multiple individual and social factors and their complex interplay. Yet, recent methodological advances in genetics and biology, as well as foundational research on the significance of peer relationships, interactions, and groups (Bukowski, Laursen, & Rubin, 2018), along with more subtly nuanced analyses on how social inequality, poverty, or policies at the national and state levels (e.g., Dodge, 2008; Duncan, Magnuson, & Votruba-Drzal, 2015) shape child development and behavior, have initiated new approaches to the study of aggression.

The central notion underlying Part II of this handbook is that aggression always occurs within a social context. Therefore, in the *Handbook*, the significance of studying children's and adolescents' aggressive behaviors in the context of significant relationships, such as the family and peer group, is considered. While the idea of aggression as a contextualized behavior had been proposed earlier within an ecological systems theory perspective (Bronfenbrenner, 1977), recent approaches have examined such new contexts as cyberbullying and have investigated more systematically how potentially threatening social interactions, such as conflicts involving issues of fairness and the welfare of others, can affect the production of aggression and youth violence (Malti & Averdijk, 2017).

In Part III of the *Handbook*, we recognize that knowledge on the origins of and risk and protective factors for aggression can be utilized to improve existing strategies, as well as design novel strategies to prevent and treat it. When the Pepler and Rubin (1991) volume appeared, multiple means of preventing and treating aggression in childhood had already been developed. But it was noted at the time that the challenge for future researchers and practitioners was to identify varying developmental pathways of aggression; this would allow for the development of novel prevention and intervention programs. Among the most influential current topics discussed in the field of intervention are the processes through which sound practices are implemented, adapted, and sustained (Beelmann, Malti, Noam, & Sommer, 2018; Malti, Noam, Beelmann, & Sommer, 2016). For example, what are the most effective intervention delivery models? How can we tailor treatment to individual and developmental needs? How can we evaluate programs rigorously? These are topics addressed in the *Handbook*. Similarly, a current central topic is the identification of state-level policies required to be in place in countries/contexts to improve intervention. In addition, the field has moved from a primary focus on risk to the acknowledgment of the importance of protective factors and the promotion of prosocial dimensions of child and adolescent functioning, such as caring, benevolence, and kindness. If we are to reduce and prevent aggression sustainably, we must nurture socially responsible, engaged, and reflective citizens (Staub, 2011).

Organization of the Chapters

Each chapter in the *Handbook* is organized with an opening overview, a description of central issues, foundational theoretical approaches, research findings, implications, and future directions. The *Handbook* itself is organized topically and in three parts: Part I is focused on the foundations, trajectories, and antecedents of aggression in childhood and adolescence. It begins with a chapter outlining historical and theoretical underpinnings to research on aggression in childhood and adolescence. This is followed by two chapters on the clinical descriptions and taxonomies of aggressive behaviors in childhood and adolescence, aggression subtypes, and their differential trajectories. The next chapters outline the biological underpinnings of aggression, including behavioral genetics and psychophysiology. In the closing chapters of Part I, there are separate discussions pertaining to putative antecedents and concomitants of aggression, including temperament, social–emotional processes, and social-cognitive development.

Part II of the *Handbook* includes chapters on the central contextual dimensions influencing aggression. In the first chapter, the effects of parenting and parent–child relationships are discussed. The following chapters focus on the roles of peer relationships, moral conflicts, social networks, and cyberspace. In the last chapter of Part II, macrolevel effects on aggression, including poverty and social inequality, are described.

Part III of the *Handbook* is focused on prevention and intervention. The part begins with a chapter on assessment of social–emotional correlates of aggression. Subsequent chapters present intervention approaches across various contexts, including youth-focused interventions for severe aggression, family-based treatments for aggression, aggression in school contexts, international perspectives on bullying prevention, and positive youth development approaches to prevent aggression and related youth violence. We end with conclusions, challenges, and priorities for researchers, practitioners, and policymakers.

Taken together, the *Handbook of Child and Adolescent Aggression* marks a foundational step in the field of developmental psychopathology. A quarter century ago, the field was consumed by a focus on multiple risk factors for the development and treatment of aggressive behavior. Today, however, researchers and practitioners are more aware of the significance of both risk and protective characteristics in the emergence, pathways, and consequences of aggression in childhood and adolescence. Recent theoretical and methodological advances have contributed to an increased understanding of biological markers, as well as gene–environment interactions in aggression. Similarly, emerging attempts to integrate individual characteristics (e.g., emotional experiences associated with experiences of social change) and factors at the macrolevel, such as social inequality and discrimination, are extending current thoughts about the roles of experiences in the development of aggression in childhood and adolescence. Lastly, the field of intervention science has moved from outcome evaluation to an increased understanding of what works, for whom, and when. In conclusion, this handbook provides a comprehensive review of the origins, the dimensions, and prevention and intervention strategies of aggression.

Acknowledgments

We are grateful for the enormous aid we have received from the many people who have contributed to the *Handbook*. We are particularly indebted to C. Deborah Laughton of The Guilford Press for her support throughout the development of this compendium. We would also like to thank Tyler Colasante (University of Toronto) for his editorial assistance. And, of course, there would not be a *Handbook* without the masterful work of our contributors. Finally, we would like to thank our respective departments and universities (Psychology Department, University of Toronto, and Department of Human Development and Quantitative Methodology, University of Maryland, College Park) for making this collaborative effort possible. This volume could not have been produced without the aid of the Canadian Institutes of Health Research (Grant No. FDN-148389 to Tina Malti) and the National Institute of Mental Health (Grant No. R01 MH 103253 to Kenneth H. Rubin).

REFERENCES

Ainsworth, M. D. S., Blehar, M., Waters, E., & Wall, S. (1978). *Patterns of attachment.* Hillsdale, NJ: Erlbaum.

Bandura, A., Ross, D., & Ross, S. A. (1961). Transmission of aggression through imitation of aggressive models. *Journal of Abnormal and Social Psychology, 63,* 575–582.

Beelmann, A., Malti, T., Noam, G. G., & Sommer, S. (2018). Innovation and integrity: Desiderata and future directions for prevention and intervention science. *Prevention Science, 19*(3), 356–365.

Bowlby, J. (1969). *Attachment. Attachment and loss: Vol. 1. Loss.* New York: Basic Books.

Bronfenbrenner, U. (1977). Toward an experimental ecology of human development. *American Psychologist, 32,* 513–531.

Bukowski, W. M., Laursen, B., & Rubin, K. H. (Eds.). (2018). *Handbook of peer interactions, relationships, and groups* (2nd ed.). New York: Guilford Press.

Dodge, K. A. (2008). Framing public policy and prevention of chronic violence in American youths. *American Psychologist, 63*(7), 573–590.

Duncan, G. J., Magnuson, K., & Votruba-Drzal, E. (2015). Children and socioeconomic status. In M. H. Bornstein & T. Leventhal (Vol. Eds.) & R. M. Lerner (Series Ed.), *Handbook of child psychology and developmental science: Vol. 4. Ecological settings and processes* (7th ed., pp. 534–573). Hoboken, NJ: Wiley.

Eisner, M. P., & Malti, T. (2015). Aggressive and violent behavior. In M. E. Lamb (Vol. Ed.) & R. M. Lerner (Series Ed.), *Handbook of child psychology and developmental science: Vol. 3. Socioemotional processes* (7th ed., pp. 795–884). New York: Wiley.

Hinde, R. A. (1997). *Relationships. A dialectical perspective.* Hove, UK: Psychology Press.

Malti, T., & Averdijk, M. (Eds.). (2017). Severe youth violence: Developmental perspectives. Special section. *Child Development, 88*(1), 5–82.

Malti, T., Noam, G. G., Beelmann, A., & Sommer, S. (2016). Toward dynamic adaptation of psychological interventions for child and adolescent development and mental health. *Journal of Clinical Child and Adolescent Psychology, 45*(6), 827–836.

Pepler, D. J., & Rubin, K. H. (Eds.). (1991). *The development and treatment of childhood aggression.* Hillsdale, NJ: Erlbaum.

Staub, E. (2011). *Overcoming evil: Genocide, violent conflict, and terrorism.* New York: Oxford University Press.

Sullivan, H. S. (1953). *The interpersonal theory of psychiatry.* New York: Norton.

Contents

PART I

FOUNDATIONS OF AGGRESSION, TRAJECTORIES, AND ANTECEDENTS

CHAPTER 1

Aggression in Childhood and Adolescence
Definition, History, and Theory

TINA MALTI and KENNETH H. RUBIN

Brief Introduction

Aggression, in childhood and adolescence, is intolerable. Studies all over the world indicate that aggression among youth is associated concomitantly and predictively with all things negative—whether those "things" include peer rejection, bullying and victimization, gang participation, school failure, psychopathology, sociopathy, partner/spouse abuse, and so on (Eisner & Malti, 2015). Despite its intolerability, aggression is a rather prevalent social behavior. Furthermore, from an ethological perspective, it must be essential for humans' survival, given that it has continued to exist in the species for millennia. Indeed, if one reads a local newspaper, listens to a radio broadcast of the national news, or watches international reports on television or other visual media, one cannot escape the fact that aggression occurs within schools, homes, and neighborhoods; between groups that differ by ethnicity, race, social class, and religion; and between countries that maintain different ideologies that are unacceptable to those who wield the power to send young citizens to foreign destinations to basically search and destroy. Yes, aggression is intolerable.

It is also the case that there is great variability in the prevalence of aggression as it exists across the multiple contexts within which it occurs. By and large, most individuals refrain from exhibiting aggressive behavior on a regular basis. Moreover, the ways in which aggressive behavior is manifested varies, in prevalence and form, across the lifespan. With regard to the latter, physical acts of aggression appear to be more common during the early years of childhood; subtle and indirect forms of aggression become increasingly frequent as children become increasingly verbal and cognitively astute (Eisner & Malti, 2015; Tremblay, 2000). But one thing is for certain: The consequences of early, high, and intense levels of aggression are almost always detrimental to the social and emotional development and well-being of both the perpetrator of aggression and target of aggression and to the families, peer groups, and communities within which aggression occurs—whether the aggression is experienced directly or indirectly (e.g., Lereya, Copeland, Costello, & Wolke, 2015).

The emergence of aggression in early childhood is often associated with prolonged exposure to adversity, including stress, neglect, and maltreatment. These *within-family* experiences create additional risk factors that may place children on particularly maladaptive trajectories (Moffitt, 2003; Rubin & Burgess, 2002). When children enter school, it becomes quickly apparent that those who behave aggressively experience peer rejection by their nonaggressive schoolmates (Rubin, Bukowski, & Bowker, 2015), often become targets of peer exclusion because their disruptive behavior is frequently perceived as harmful (Killen & Malti, 2015), and provoke others to violate them (Salmivalli & Peets, 2018). In short, aggression harms both the antagonist and those within his or her circle of acquaintances. Thus, exposure to aggression is detrimental to the healthy development of those who regularly produce and receive it (Averdijk, Malti, Eisner, Ribeaud, & Farrington, 2016; Malti & Averdijk, 2017; Salmivalli, 2010; see Ostrov, Perry, & Blakely-McClure, Chapter 3, and Malti & Song, Chapter 7, this volume).

A primary goal of this chapter is to describe fundamental theories pertaining to the emergence of aggressive behavior and its development across childhood and adolescence. For purposes of this introductory chapter, we focus on aggression in peer relationships because it is within the peer context that interpersonal aggression among children and adolescents often takes place (for relevant reviews, see Bukowski & Vitaro, Chapter 10; Malti, Colasante, & Jambon, Chapter 11; Sijtsema & Ojanen, Chapter 12; and Underwood & Bauman, Chapter 13, this volume). As such, we begin by defining aggression. Then, we review fundamental theoretical accounts on aggression and its development. We focus on theories that have evolved from the perspectives of developmental science and psychopathology. Thereafter, we explore trends and turning points in early theories and research on children's and adolescents' aggressive behavior. Finally, we explicate implications from the theoretical accounts and historical viewpoints presented, followed by conclusions pertaining to gaps and advances.

Conceptualizing Aggression

Aggression is a broad and heterogeneous construct that includes, but is not limited to, behavior evaluated at the syndrome or symptom level (i.e., broadband externalizing behavior problems vs. specific expressions of externalizing behavior such as proactive aggression; Orobio de Castro, Veerman, Koops, Bosch, & Monshouwer, 2002). Aggressive behavior has generally been defined as behavior that is intentionally harmful, physically or psychologically, to others (Krahé, 2013).

Aggression encompasses behaviors that can be distinguished along two dimensions: form and function (Dodge & Coie, 1987; Little, Henrich, Jones, & Hawley, 2003). While *forms* of aggression describe *how* the behavior is enacted (e.g., physically, socially), *functions* refer to the question of *why* aggression is used (e.g., proactively to obtain a goal, reactively in response to others' behaviors).

From a clinical viewpoint, aggressive behavior is typically considered maladaptive because it causes harm to others and often, although not always, is harmful for the aggressor as well. For the purpose of clinical classification of aggressive symptoms in childhood and adolescence, there are two relevant diagnostic categories in the *Diagnostic and Statistical Manual of Mental Disorders* (DSM-5; American Psychiatric Association, 2013): (1) oppositional defiant disorder, which consists of symptoms that are grouped into three types: angry/irritable mood, argumentative/defiant behavior, and vindictiveness; and (2) conduct disorder, which comprises symptoms that entail a prolonged pattern of antisocial behavior, such as serious violations of norms. A specifier has been added to the classification of conduct disorder for children with limited prosocial emotions (i.e., for children who show callous and unemotional interpersonal traits across multiple settings and relationships). (See Frick & Matlasz, Chapter 2, this volume, for a more detailed description of clinical classifications of aggression in childhood and adolescence.)

In the field of developmental psychopathology, there are several terms that are related to aggression. First, *externalizing behaviors* typically refer to all antagonistic behaviors directed at the external environment, including aggressive, defiant, disruptive, hyperactive, and impulsive behaviors. Similarly, *antisocial behavior* refers to aggressive and nonaggressive behaviors that break social and/or legal norms but do not approach the spectrum of attention-deficit/hyperactivity disorder–related behaviors. Another frequently used term, *bullying*, refers to a specific type of aggression, repeated over time, that involves a power imbalance between the antagonist and his or her target (see Bukowski & Vitaro, Chapter 10, and Underwood & Bauman, Chapter 13, this volume) often within a group context (see Sijtsema & Ojanen, Chapter 12, this volume). *Violence* is often referred to in studies of aggression. According to the World Health Organization, violence involves the intentional use of physical force or power against oneself or another person, group, or community that results in—or has a high likelihood of resulting in—psychological harm, maladaptive development, injury, or death (Krug, Dahlberg, Mercy, Zwi, & Lozano, 2002). This definition encompasses three areas: *self-directed violence* such as suicide; *interpersonal violence,* such as aggression during peer interaction; and *collective violence* including war, genocide, torture, or terrorism. For purposes of this chapter, we limit the term *aggression* and the related phenomena of violence to the interpersonal domain—behaviors that involve the use or threat of use of physical force to hurt or damage other persons. We do so because our primary focus is on children's and adolescents' aggression in the peer group.

Historical Perspectives

Current psychological theorizing and research on the development of aggression in childhood and adolescence is historically rooted in a number of traditions. Three prominent accounts have substantially influenced contemporary theorizing pertaining to the development of aggressive behavior in childhood and adolescence: (1) psychoanalytic theory, (2) drive theory, and (3) social learning theory.

Psychoanalytic Theories of Aggression

Psychoanalytic theories of aggression and basic assumptions underlying the development of attachment relationships are the foundations for many contemporary studies of the origins and development of individual differences in aggressive behavior (see Raby & Roisman, Chapter 9, this volume). In Freud's (1920/1948) seminal writings pertaining to the origins of aggressive behavior (e.g., *thanatos* or the "death drive"), he argued that problematic aggression stemmed from child–caregiver conflicts at around the age of 6 years during the oedipal stage of development. Drawing on these seminal ideas, attachment theorists argued that aggression and anger are normal responses to a frustrated attachment relationship that originated earlier in development (i.e., in infancy; Bowlby, 1969).

The connection between attachment theory and the production of undercontrolled, aggressive behavior is best understood by referring to Bowlby's (1973) construct of "internal working models." For example, Bowlby (1969, 1973) proposed that the early mother–child relationship lays the groundwork for the development of internalized models of familial and extrafamilial relationships. These internal working models were thought to be the product of parental behavior—specifically, parental sensitivity and responsivity (Ainsworth & Bowlby, 1991; Cassidy & Shaver, 2016). Given an internal working model in which the parent is available and responsive, it was proposed that the young child would feel confident, secure, and self-assured when introduced to novel settings. Thus, *felt security* has been viewed as a highly significant developmental phenomenon that provides the child with sufficient emotional and cognitive sustenance to allow for active and positive interactions with the social environment. From this perspective, then, the association between security of attachment in infancy and the quality of children's social skills and behaviors is attributed, at least in part, to resources offered by the primary caregiver.

Alternatively, the development of an insecure infant–parent attachment relationship has been posited to result in an internal working model in which interpersonal relationships are perceived as rejecting and/or neglectful. In turn, the social world is perceived as a battleground that must be either attacked or escaped from (Bowlby, 1973). Thus, for the insecure and angry child, opportunities for peer play and interaction are nullified by displays of hostility and aggression in the peer group. Such behavior often results in the child missing out on opportunities to benefit from the communication, negotiation, and perspective-taking experiences that typically lead to normative development and adaptive childhood. Indeed, there has been substantial empirical support for connections between security of attachment and the display of aggressive behavior across development (Cassidy & Shaver, 2016; Doyle & Cicchetti, 2017).

Drive Theory and Aggression

One of the influential theories explaining the emergence of aggression in humans and animals is drive theory, also referred to as the frustration–aggression hypothesis. Originally proposed in 1939, the model states that thwarting an individual's efforts to reach a desired goal will induce frustration, which triggers an aggressive drive and behavioral response, such as harming the person who has caused the frustration. It remains one of the most prominent theories to explain the emergence of aggression in humans (Dollard, Doob, Miller, Mower, & Sears, 1939). The theory was later revised in order to explain instances during which frustration did not necessarily lead to aggressive behavior (Berkowitz, 1969). For instance, one proposed change of the 1939 model suggested that frustration generates aggressive inclinations to the degree that it arouses negative affect, such as anger, and depends on how situational cues are interpreted. Thus, frustration does not always lead to aggression but increases emotional arousal. This, in turn, can (and often does) create a condition for a readiness to cope with a social threat in an aggressive and hostile manner. For example, an individual's level of affective arousal and evaluation of social cues can determine if that individual responds aggressively to an ambiguous social cue. With this proposition, the revisited model includes essential assumptions of social learning theory of aggression, which is briefly reviewed below. An example would be that the level of affective arousal and evaluations of social cues can determine if an individual responds aggressively to an ambiguous social cue (e.g., Dodge, 1980). Despite various criticisms, drive theory continues to remain one of the most influential theoretical accounts that explains how individual characteristics, such as intense anger experiences, high emotional reactivity, or biased cognitive evaluations of various social cues, influence a child's unique propensity to engage in aggression and related hostile behaviors.

Social Learning Theory of Aggression

Another seminal account explaining aggressive behavior in children and adolescents is social learning theory. According to social learning models, aggression is learned through cycles of modeling, reinforcement, and punishment (Bandura, 1973). Accordingly, aggressive behavioral responses can be learned by observation, imitation, and modeling. More broadly, aggression is viewed as the result of the interplay between cognitive, behavioral, and contextual factors, wherein children learn aggression through observing others' behaviors and associated outcomes (e.g., vicariously experienced punishment). According to Bandura (1973), the environment and a child's behavior mutually effect each other. Children learn by observing others (i.e., a model) and either imitate the observed aggressive behavior or not, as a function of personal and contextual factors. Moving beyond strict behavioral theories, social learning theory assumes that the respective behavioral response is influenced by cognitive processes and the social context, such as attention allocation or anticipated rewards and costs associated with the displayed behavior (e.g., punishment; Bandura, 1986). The theory has been very influential in understanding the occurrence of children's aggressive behavior in peer relationships, as well as in explaining cycles of aggression in the family system (Patterson, 1982).

As an extension of social learning theory, a more recent approach in psychology that aims at explaining aggressive behavior is *moral disengagement theory* (Bandura, Barbaranelli, Caprara, & Pastorelli, 1996). This theory proposes that aggressive and violent behavior is often followed by/accompanied by post hoc, self-serving cognitive strategies. Similar to sociological and criminological theories that provide explanations linking self-serving cognitions to crime, delinquency, and aggression (e.g., Sykes & Matza, 1957), the theory of moral disengagement proposes that individuals feel the need to engage in some rationalizing/cognitive mechanisms to neutralize illegitimate actions, justify the violent behavior, and diffuse personal responsibility.

In sum, social learning theory offers fundamental insights into central learning mechanisms that can cause, stabilize, and exacerbate aggression in children and adolescents. Using self-serving cognitive strategies, individuals justify harmful acts and diffuse responsibility for their behavior (Hymel & Bonanno, 2014). More recent extensions of this approach have discussed such social–emotional processes as sympathy and guilt that can link cognitive processes and aggressive behavior more systematically (Thornberg, Pozzoli, Gini, & Jungert, 2015), and can explain how such links contribute to the stability or change in aggression over time.

Despite having received a wide variety of criticisms, all historical accounts that are briefly reviewed herein are foundational for modern approaches to the developmental study of aggression in childhood and adolescence. Each of the early theoretical accounts substantially influenced, and continue to shape, current conceptualizations of the origins, antecedents, and consequences of human aggression in the first two decades of life. More recent models address issues of causation, mechanisms, and long-term consequences in more nuanced ways than the early theories, specifically focusing on interactional processes between various genetic and environmental influences and examining psychological mechanisms with more depth, breadth, and methodological rigor than past research.

Theories of Aggression in Childhood and Adolescence

Developmental theories of aggression view the behavior as occurring through a complex interplay between the child, his or her socialization experiences, and his or her biological characteristics. Theorists have explained the emergence, pathways, and consequences of aggression in childhood and adolescence. Most of these models focus on the more proximal risk factors in the genesis of aggression. For example, research has supported the presence of developmental precursors of aggression as early as the toddler years. Examples include individual differences in the expression of dysregulated anger, hitting and biting, and conflict initiations (Hay et al., 2014; Rubin, Burgess, Dwyer, & Hastings, 2003; see Moore, Hubbard, & Bookhout, Chapter 6, this volume). A significant amount of work has also pointed to the early emotional precursors of aggressive problem behaviors, such as differences in young children's ability to show concern for others, feeling regret over wrongdoing, and regulating impulses and emotions. For example, recent research provides evidence for early signs of callous–unemotional traits in the prediction of later externalizing behavior problems, through children's autonomic functioning (e.g., Wagner, Hastings, & Rubin, 2017).

In addition, recent advances in the statistical modeling of trajectories help generate a richer understanding of normative trends in aggression over the first two decades of life (for a review of the trajectories of aggression subtypes, see Eisner &

Malti, 2015; Nagin, 2005; Tremblay, 2000, 2010; see also Ostrov et al., Chapter 3, this volume).

Several theoretical models have made central contributions to our understanding of the emergence, development, and consequences of aggression in childhood and adolescence. Here, we focus on three central theoretical accounts: (1) gene–environment interactions in children's aggressive behavior, (2) social-ecological frameworks of aggression in childhood and adolescence, and (3) individual characteristics and mechanistic models of aggression. Within the context of this broad conceptual framework, we now turn to more specific theories connecting biological factors, social conditions, and psychological characteristics with the development of aggression in childhood and adolescence. As it is beyond the scope of this chapter to provide an exhaustive overview of these frameworks, we focus on one specific theoretical account, acknowledging that other models have been proposed in the respective frameworks.

Gene–Environment Interactions in Children's Aggressive Behavior

Differences in social behaviors, such as aggression, are theorized to emerge due to gene–environment interactions. A prominent example is Moffitt's (1993, 2003) developmental theory of crime. Despite the known normative trend that many children "grow out" of their externalizing problems during the early years of childhood, there is a small but significant number of youth who show persistent aggression throughout development (Eisner & Malti, 2015). According to Moffitt (1993), two distinct types of aggressors can be distinguished by the timing of the onset of problem behavior: one limited to adolescence ("late starters") and one beginning in early childhood ("early starters"). The latter is characterized by high severity of aggression, and a high number of risk factors, including neurological dysfunctions, regulatory problems, and cognitive deficits (for the psychophysiological risk factors of aggression, see Branje & Koot, Chapter 5, this volume). This conglomerate of risk factors has been linked to the expression of aggressive behavior later in life (Huesmann, Dubow, & Boxer, 2009; Moffit & Caspi, 2001). The "early starter" group tends to show persistent aggression well beyond early childhood and appears to be responsible for the majority of adolescent crime, particularly violent offences that carry the most significant individual, familial, and societal costs (Cohen & Piquero, 2009; Moffitt, 2003). Additionally, these "early starters" are more likely to develop such behavioral difficulties as conduct disorder (Loeber, Green, Keenan, & Lahey, 1995), along with a host of related adjustment issues (Campbell, Spieker, Burchinal, Poe, & the NICHD Early Child Care Research Network, 2006).

A combination of biological risk factors and exposure to high adversity in socialization contexts, such as poverty or maltreatment, can cause an early onset of aggression. A meta-analytic review of the literature examining the interaction between variants of the monoamine oxidase A gene (*MAOA*) and childhood maltreatment in the prediction of aggression in males provides empirical support for the role of gene–environment interactions in the genesis of aggression (Byrd & Manuck, 2014; Caspi et al., 2002; Raine, 2002, 2013). Research findings have also disentangled the role of gene–environment interactions in child aggression in the peer versus family environment (for a review, see Brendgen, Vitaro, and Boivin, Chapter 4, this volume).

Research in this area has largely focused on antisocial behavior or externalizing problems broadly, and to a lesser extent on aggressive behavior specifically. While it is clear that aggressive behavior is related to gene–environment interactions, researchers have also acknowledged that these interactions are complex and that genes do not operate independently. Thus, genomewide association studies, which involve assessing a large set of genes and their association with expressed phenotypes, have been identified as a promising avenue to gain further insights into the risk factors for the development of aggression (Craig & Halton, 2009; Cicchetti, Hetzel, Rogosch, Handley, & Toth, 2016; Meaney, 2010).

In summary, gene–environment interaction models suggest that adverse environments, such as exposure to chronic early stress or abuse, combined with certain variants of genes related to neuroendocrine dopaminergic and serotonergic systems, increase the probability of aggressive behavior expression. As such, analyses of certain phenotype-associated alleles can generate more knowledge about the factors that cause and maintain aggression in childhood and adolescence (Waltes, Chiocchetti, & Freitag, 2016).

Social-Ecological Frameworks of Aggression in Childhood and Adolescence

Social-ecological frameworks of aggression propose that exposure to environmental risk and protective factors at various levels of the social ecology contribute to children's socially adaptive and maladaptive behaviors. Bronfenbrenner's (1977) seminal model describes how the microsystem (e.g., family, peers), mesosystem (e.g., interactions among microsystems), exosystem (e.g., neighborhood), and macrosystem (e.g. culture) all contribute to interindividual differences in human development. From this perspective, children's aggressive behavior is immersed in various interactions that occur within close relationships (see Sullivan, 1953); in turn, these close relationships are embedded in groups, networks, the sociocultural context of groups, and society at large.

The social-ecological model that has pervaded the literature is well supported by the dialectical framework of social complexity originally described by Hinde (e.g., 1987, 1995; Hinde & Stevenson-Hinde, 2014; Rubin et al., 2015). Hinde's model involves successive, interacting levels of social complexity that include transactions between levels of *individual* characteristics, interpersonal *interactions,* dyadic *relationships*, *groups,* and *society.*

In keeping with this latter perspective, researchers have explored whether such *individual* characteristics such as temperament (e.g., emotional reactivity and regulation) and gender are associated with, and predictive of, social initiations and *interactions* that express a "movement against the world." These agonistic behavioral expressions influence, and are influenced by, the quality of *relationships* that children come to develop within the family (e.g., attachment relationships) and the peer group (e.g., friendships). From this perspective, dispositional characteristics may be exacerbated or inhibited by the types of interactions and relationships developed in the social world. Furthermore, the peer *groups* within which children become members may contribute to the deescalation or escalation of aggressive behavior patterns; after all, it is not terribly surprising to note that homophily matters—children are attracted to, initiate relationships with, and become members of groups within which the cultural ethos comprises the expression of like-minded aggressive behavior (Dishion, 2014; Dishion & Tipsord, 2011; Eisner & Malti, 2015; Rubin et al., 2015).

Theories and research at the macro- or societal/cultural level emphasize the role of inequality, poverty, social disorganization, or governance structures on aggression (for a review on effects of poverty and social inequality on aggression, see Duncan, Magnuson, & Votruba-Drzal, 2015; Guerra, 2013; see also Leventhal, Dupéré, & Elliott, Chapter 14, this volume). While these traditions have predominantly developed in other disciplines, such as sociology, public health, and economics, increasing integration between these fields yields promise to gain a deeper understanding of how microlevel dynamics and macrolevel factors contribute to and help explain variations in aggression.

In summary, researchers who study the developmental course of aggression focus on the dialectical relations between children's individual characteristics, the interactions they have with others, their involvements in parent–child and peer relationships and groups, and the influences of culture on all the above. These factors reciprocally influence each other and contribute to aggression and its development in multifaceted ways. Linkages between developmental research on aggression and macrolevel variations in aggression, such as trends in aggression rates over time, can generate new knowledge on links between changes at the microlevel and macrolevel, and why such relations may (or may not) occur.

Individual Characteristics and Mechanistic Models of Aggression

Developmental approaches to the study of aggression have also focused on individual characteristics underlying the emergence and trajectories of aggression. Prominent models have focused, for example, on children's cognitive processing of social events. Such accounts have been complemented by theoretical models that explain how emotional experiences and regulation affect interindividual differences in children's aggression. More recently, attempts to explain aggression have also explored potential mechanisms that may underlie cognition–aggression and/or emotion–aggression links across development.

Social Information-Processing Models of Aggression

A prominent approach to explain the emergence and development of aggression is the social information-processing model (see Lansford, Chapter 8, this volume), which focuses on social-cognitive characteristics as a mechanism that can trigger aggression. According to the social information-processing theory proposed by Crick and Dodge (1994), children process information within challenging social situations in a series of steps, from encoding and interpreting social cues to enacting a response. The ways in which children process social information at each step may increase or decrease their proclivity to respond to these situations with aggressive behavior. The assumption that aggressive children show social-cognitive biases is supported by a large body of empirical research. For example, compared to children with low levels of aggression, highly aggressive children have been shown to display a hostile attribution bias—a phenomenon in which they atypically process situations that result in negative personal outcomes deriving from the hostile intentions of others (Burgess, Wojslawowicz, Rubin, Rose-Krasnor, & Booth-LaForce, 2006; Dodge, 1980; Orobio de Castro, Veerman, Koops, Bosch, & Monshouwer, 2002). These biases are thought to become part of children's latent knowledge structures and affect their perceptions of future social interactions (Crick & Dodge, 1994). Exposure to adversity, such as experiences of abuse and victimization, increase the probability of biased social information processing and often result in hostile attribution biases. These, in turn, are associated with increased levels of aggressive behavior (Dodge, Bates, & Pettit, 1990; Dodge et al., 2003, 2015). Peers will likely react negatively to children's aggression by rejecting or excluding them, confirming the hostile attributions that gave rise to their aggressive acts (i.e., the self-fulfilling prophecy effect; Lansford, Malone, Dodge, Pettit, & Bates, 2010). Ultimately, these aggressive children will likely attain poor academic achievement in the elementary and middle school years and become drawn to, and associated with, deviant peer groups who possess a higher probability of engaging in severe youth violence (Dodge, Greenberg, Malone, & the Conduct Problems Prevention Research Group, 2008).

Affective–Developmental Models of Aggression

The social information-processing model has been integrated with related accounts that aim at explaining emotional processes associated with aggression. For example, Lemerise and Arsenio (2000) proposed a revised model that integrates emotional responding into children's social information processing. Accordingly, social conflict situations are emotionally charged and typically entail a variety of emotional cues that influence each of the cognitive processing steps and result in adaptive (or maladaptive) behavioral outcomes. Because social conflict situations are multifaceted, developmental scientists have also recently emphasized the need to comprehensively understand the role of emotion regulation capacities and experiences of distinct emotions in both cognitive processing and behavioral outcomes (see Malti, 2016; Malti, Sette, & Dys, 2016; see also Malti & Song, Chapter 7, this volume). For instance, experiencing other-oriented emotions, such as empathy/sympathy, and/or self-evaluative emotions, such as guilt, can enhance adaptive behaviors, including prosocial orientations (Malti, 2016; Malti & Krettenauer, 2013). Alternately, a lack of empathy/sympathy and guilt can trigger aggression and violence, even in early childhood (Arsenio, 2014; Wagner et al., 2017; see Malti & Song, Chapter 7, and Malti, Zuffianò, & Cheung, Chapter 15, this volume). The capacity to regulate negative emotions, such as anger, can contribute to rational choices and adaptive behaviors consequently preventing aggression (Colasante, Zuffianò, & Malti, 2015, 2016; Malti et al., 2016). Recent longitudinal studies show that early differences in emotion regulation during toddlerhood explain a unique portion of variance in predicting whether or not male adolescents engage in serious violence (Sitnick et al., 2017).

A new extension of this emotional development framework emphasizes the dynamic nature of emotional processes. Using a real-time approach, the temporal unfolding of emotional experiences and underlying autonomic arousal can help understand how children process and respond to social conflict situations (Dys &

Malti, 2016; Malti, Dys, Colasante, & Peplak, 2018; Miller, Kahle, & Hastings, 2015). For example, Colasante, Zuffianò, Haley, and Malti (in press) showed that changes in 8-year-olds' respiratory sinus arrhythmia (RSA)—reflecting their parasympathetic regulation and corresponding sensitivity to environmental stimuli (Porges, 2011)—leading up to and during transgressions were uniquely associated with the intensity of guilt feelings after transgressions. Higher guilt, in turn, was related to lower parent reports of aggression. In this context, higher RSA leading up to transgressions was thought to reflect better regulation in response to the perceived gains of such acts (e.g., stealing a chocolate bar), whereas lower RSA and higher corresponding arousal during transgressions was thought to reflect greater concern for the morally relevant consequences of the acts. This microdynamic perspective can broaden our understanding of how emotions arise and fluctuate from moment to moment in the context of everyday conflict and explain why (or why not) children behave aggressively.

In sum, social information-processing theories emphasize that aggression in childhood and adolescence is perpetuated by atypical cognitive processing of challenging social situations wherein negative events that have ambiguous causes are interpreted as being intentionally and malevolently caused. While Dodge's social information-processing model elaborated on *reactions* to negative consequences of social interactions, Rubin and Krasnor's (1986) social problem-solving model also elaborated on *proactive* thinking about the ways in which various social goals may be achieved given the context and target.

Related models pertaining to emotional development show that affective cues trigger both cognitive and behavioral responses and reveal that the experience of distinct emotions and regulation capacities are associated with aggression. Finally, these theories highlight both age-related developmental differences and interindividual differences in real-time processing of social events, underscoring the need to explore how situational factors may be associated with the cognitive and affective processing of social events and aggressive behaviors at different points in development.

Recent theoretical advancements in the developmental study of aggression have shifted from focusing predominantly on stable individual characteristics to understanding psychological mechanisms underlying emotion–behavior and cognition–behavior links. One mechanism central to emotional development and the social-cognitive processing of conflict situations is attention. Since attention is largely responsible for what a person evaluates, it may strongly affect his or her subsequent emotions and behaviors (Scherer, 2009). To date, developmental research has focused on how aggressive children differ from nonaggressive children in the way they attend to hostile and ambiguous social cues (Horsley, de Castro, & Van der Schoot, 2010; Troop-Gordon, Gordon, Vogel-Ciernia, Ewing Lee, & Visconti, 2016). Examining attention to such cues, however, is far more important to some forms of aggression (e.g., reactive) than others (e.g., proactive), and represents only some types of cues that may motivate or mitigate children's aggressive behavior.

Summary

The reviewed theories help to understand why it is that some individuals may develop tendencies to become aggressive. The theories also explicate how biological factors and contextual conditions may interact to predict distinct pathways leading to the expression of aggression during the first two decades of life. Finally, the theories explain how individual characteristics, such as temperament (emotion reactivity and regulation) and social information processing, may underlie interindividual and intraindividual differences in aggressive behavior. Within the context of these theoretical approaches, we turn to implications that have influenced contemporary research on aggression and its development in childhood and adolescence.

Implications and Conclusions

Aggression in childhood and adolescence is a prevailing concern for children, families, and society at large. In this chapter, we attempted to provide a brief overview of fundamental conceptualizations of aggression and related phenomena, including externalizing behaviors, bullying, and violence, as well as taxonomies to distinguish subtypes of aggression (such as the form and function of aggression). We then reviewed major theoretical accounts on the emergence, correlates, and consequences of aggression across childhood and adolescence. The focus of this review was on theories rooted in the traditions of developmental psychology and developmental psychopathology. We briefly discussed historical accounts that have been foundational in contemporary theorizing on human aggression and its development from a psychopathology perspective. In summary, this selected review illustrates that there have been significant theoretical advances and a good deal of empirical progress that provide current researchers with a deeper understanding of aggression in childhood and youth (Lansford, 2018).

What seems clear from the theories reviewed in this chapter is that both environmental factors and genetic/biological dispositions, as well as their complex interplay, account for interindividual differences in aggression and distinct trajectories across the first two decades of life. There is also concrete evidence that psychological mechanisms can cause and trigger aggression (e.g., biased cognitions in peer social interactions; see Bukowski & Vitaro, Chapter 10, this volume). Recent perspectives emphasize the role of protective factors and mechanisms that can prevent and reduce aggression in children and adolescents. For example, social–emotional accounts of aggression argue that the presence of other-oriented emotions (such as empathic concern) and self-evaluative emotions (such as guilt) following one's own wrongdoing protect children and adolescents from behaving aggressively (Malti, 2016; see Malti et al., Chapter 11, this volume). These accounts are important because they point to the direct and indirect psychological processes and mechanisms through which environmental adversity and/or biological predispositions may exacerbate or prevent aggression. Similarly, research has pointed to the substantial role of peer relationships, parenting, and the parent–child relationship as protective or exacerbating factors in the emergence and development of aggression in childhood and adolescence (see Raby & Roisman, Chapter 9, this volume).

Many theoretical advances have been made in the developmental study of human aggression in the first two decades of life, and deeper and broader knowledge has been gained to understand the causes and mechanisms of aggression.

Likewise, the field of aggression has gained substantial knowledge on the risk factors associated with increases in aggression, related consequences, and associated long-term negative outcomes.

ACKNOWLEDGMENTS

This research was supported in part by a Canadian Institutes of Health Research Foundation Scheme Grant awarded to Tina Malti (No. FDN-148389) and by a National Institute of Mental Health Grant awarded to Kenneth H. Rubin (No. R01 MH 103253).

REFERENCES

Ainsworth, M. D. S., & Bowlby, J. (1991). An ethological approach to personality development. *American Psychologist, 46,* 331–341.

American Psychiatric Association. (2013). *Diagnostic and statistical manual of mental disorders* (5th ed.). Arlington, VA: Author.

Arsenio, W. (2014). Moral emotion attributions and aggression. In M. Killen & J. Smetana (Eds.), *Handbook of moral development* (2nd ed., pp. 235–256). New York: Psychology Press.

Averdijk, M., Malti, T., Eisner, M., Ribeaud, D., & Farrington, D. (2016). A vicious circle of peer victimization?: Problem behavior mediates stability in peer victimization over time. *Journal of Developmental and Life-Course Criminology, 2*(2), 162–181.

Bandura, A. (1973). *Aggression: A social learning analysis.* Englewood Cliffs, NJ: Prentice-Hall.

Bandura, A. (1986). *Social foundations of thought and action: A social cognitive theory.* Englewood Cliffs, NJ: Prentice-Hall.

Bandura, A., Barbaranelli, C., Caprara, G. V., & Pastorelli, C. (1996). Mechanisms of moral disengagement in the exercise of moral agency. *Journal of Personality and Social Psychology, 71*(12), 364–374.

Berkowitz, L. (1969). The frustration–aggression hypothesis revisited. In L. Berkowitz (Ed.), *Roots of aggression* (pp. 1–28). New York: Atherton Press.

Bowlby, J. (1969). *Attachment and loss: Vol. 1. Attachment.* New York: Basic Books.

Bowlby, J. (1973). *Attachment and loss: Vol. 2. Separation.* New York: Basic Books.

Bronfenbrenner, U. (1977). Toward an experimental ecology of human development. *American Psychologist, 32*(7), 513–531.

Burgess, K. B., Wojslawowicz, J. C., Rubin, K. H., Rose-Krasnor, L., & Booth-LaForce, C. (2006). Social information processing and coping styles of shy/withdrawn and aggressive children: Does friendship matter? *Child Development, 77,* 371–383.

Byrd, A. L., & Manuck, S. B. (2014). MAOA, childhood maltreatment, and antisocial behavior: Meta-analysis of a gene–environment interaction. *Biological Psychiatry, 75,* 9–17.

Campbell, S. B., Spieker, S., Burchinal, M., Poe, M. D., & the NICHD Early Child Care Research Network. (2006). Trajectories of aggression from toddlerhood to age 9 predict academic and social functioning through age 12. *Journal of Child Psychology and Psychiatry, 47*(8), 791–800.

Caspi, A., McClay, J., Moffitt, T. E., Mill, J., Martin, J., Craig I. W., et al. (2002). Role of genotype in the cycle of violence in maltreated children. *Science, 297,* 851–854.

Cassidy, J., & Shaver, P. R. (Eds.). (2016). *Handbook of attachment: Theory, research, and clinical applications* (3rd ed.). New York: Guilford Press.

Cicchetti, D., Hetzel, S., Rogosch, F. A., Handley, E. D., & Toth, S. L. (2016). An investigation of child maltreatment and epigenetic mechanisms of mental and physical health risk. *Development and Psychopathology, 28*(4), 1305–1317.

Cohen, M., & Piquero, A. (2009). New evidence on the monetary value of saving a high risk youth. *Journal of Quantitative Criminology, 25,* 25–49.

Colasante, T., Zuffianò, A., Haley, D., & Malti, T. (in press). Children's autonomic nervous system activity while transgressing: Relations to guilt feelings and aggression. *Developmental Psychology.*

Colasante, T., Zuffianò, A., & Malti, T. (2015). Do moral emotions buffer the anger–aggression link in children and adolescents? *Journal of Applied Developmental Psychology, 41,* 1–7.

Colasante, T., Zuffianò, A., & Malti, T. (2016). Daily deviations in anger, guilt, and sympathy: A developmental diary study of aggression. *Journal of Abnormal Child Psychology, 44*(8), 1515–1526.

Craig, I. W., & Halton, K. E. (2009). Genetics of human aggressive behavior. *Human Genetics, 126,* 101–113.

Crick, N. R., & Dodge, K. A. (1994). A review and reformulation of social information-processing mechanisms in children's social adjustment. *Psychological Bulletin, 115,* 74–101.

Dishion, T. J. (2014). A developmental model of aggression and violence: Microsocial and macrosocial dynamics within an ecological framework. In M. Lewis & K. Rudolph (Eds.), *Handbook of developmental psychopathology* (pp. 449–465). Boston: Springer.

Dishion, T. J., & Tipsord, J. M. (2011). Peer contagion in child and adolescent development. *Annual Review of Psychology, 62,* 189–214.

Dodge, K. A. (1980). Social cognition and children's aggressive behavior. *Child Development, 51,* 162–170.

Dodge, K. A., Bates J. E., & Pettit, G. S. (1990). Mechanisms in the cycle of violence. *Science, 250,* 1678–1683.

Dodge, K. A., & Coie, J. D. (1987). Social-information-processing factors in reactive and proactive aggression in children's peer groups. *Journal of Personality and Social Psychology, 53*(6), 1146–1158.

Dodge, K. A., Greenberg, M. T., Malone, P. S., & the Conduct Problems Prevention Research Group. (2008). Testing an idealized dynamic cascade model of the development of serious violence in adolescence. *Child Development, 79*(6), 1907–1927.

Dodge, K. A., Lansford, J. E., Burks, V. S., Bates, J. E., Pettit, G. S., Fontaine, R., et al. (2003). Peer rejection and social information-processing factors in the development of aggressive behavior problems in children. *Child Development, 74*(2), 374–393.

Dodge, K. A., Malone, P. S., Lansford, J. E., Sorbring, E., Skinner, A. T., Tapanya, S., et al. (2015). Hostile attributional bias and aggressive behavior in global context. *Proceedings of the National Academy of Sciences, 112*(30), 9310–9315.

Dollard, J., Doob, L., Miller, N., Mowrer, O., & Sears, R. (1939). *Frustration and aggression.* New Haven, CT: Yale University Press.

Doyle, C., & Cicchetti, D. (2017). From the cradle to the grave: The effect of adverse caregiving environments on attachment and relationships throughout the lifespan. *Clinical Psychology: Science and Practice, 24*(2), 203–217.

Duncan, G. J., Magnuson, K., & Votruba-Drzal, E. (2015). Children and socioeconomic status. In M. H. Bornstein & T. Leventhal (Vol. Eds.) & R. M. Lerner (Series Ed.), *Handbook of child psychology and developmental science: Vol. 4. Ecological settings and processes* (pp. 534–573). Hoboken, NJ: Wiley.

Dys, S. P., & Malti, T. (2016). It's a two-way street: Automated and controlled processes in children's emotional responses to moral transgressions. *Journal of Experimental Child Psychology, 152,* 31–40.

Eisner, M. P., & Malti, T. (2015). Aggressive and violent behavior. In M. E. Lamb (Vol. Ed.) & R. M. Lerner (Series Ed.), *Handbook of child psychology and developmental science: Vol. 3. Socioemotional processes* (pp. 794–841). New York: Wiley.

Freud, S. (1948). *Beyond the pleasure principle.* London: Hogarth Press. (Original work published 1920)

Guerra, N. (2013). Macroeconomic factors, youth violence, and the developing child. In R. Rosenfeld, M. Edberg, X. Fang, & C. S. Florence (Eds.), *Economics and youth violence: Crime, disadvantage, and community* (pp. 255–277). New York: New York University Press.

Hay, D. F., Waters, C. S., Perra, O., Swift, N., Kairis, V., Phillips, R., et al. (2014). Precursors to aggression are evident by 6 months of age. *Developmental Science, 17*(3), 471–480.

Hinde, R. A. (1987). *Individuals, relationships and culture.* Cambridge, UK: Cambridge University Press.

Hinde, R. A. (1995). A suggested structure for a science of relationships. *Personal Relationships, 2,* 1–15.

Hinde, R. A., & Stevenson-Hinde, J. (2014). Framing our analysis: A dialectical perspective. In L. F. Leckman, C. Panter-Brick, & R. Salah (Eds.), *Pathways to peace: The transformative power of children and families* (pp. 19–26). Cambridge, MA: MIT Press.

Horsley, T. A., de Castro, B. O., & Van der Schoot, M. (2010). In the eye of the beholder: Eye-tracking assessment of social information processing in aggressive behavior. *Journal of Abnormal Child Psychology, 38,* 587–599.

Huesmann, L. R., Dubow, E. F., & Boxer, P. (2009). Continuity of aggression from childhood to early adulthood as a predictor of life outcomes: Implications for the adolescent-limited and life-course-persistent models. *Aggressive Behavior, 35*(2), 136–149.

Hymel, S., & Bonanno, R. A. (2014). Moral disengagement processes in bullying. *Theory into Practice, 53*(4), 278–285.

Killen, M., & Malti, T. (2015). Moral judgments and emotions in contexts of peer exclusion and victimization. *Advances in Child Development and Behavior, 48,* 249–276.

Krahé, B. (2013). *The social psychology of aggression.* Hove, UK: Psychology Press.

Krug, E. G., Dahlberg, L. L., Mercy, J. A., Zwi, A. B., & Lozano, R. (2002). *World report on violence and health.* Geneva: World Health Organization.

Lansford, J. E. (2018). Development of aggression. *Current Opinion in Psychology, 19,* 17–21.

Lansford, J. E., Malone, P. S., Dodge, K. A., Pettit, G. S., & Bates, J. E. (2010). Developmental cascades of peer rejection, social information processing biases, and aggression during middle childhood. *Development and Psychopathology, 22,* 593–602.

Lemerise, E. A., & Arsenio, W. F. (2000). An integrated model of emotion processes and cognition in social information processing. *Child Development, 71,* 107–118.

Lereya, S., Copeland, W. E., Costello, E. J., & Wolke, D. (2015). Adult mental health consequences of peer bullying and maltreatment in childhood: Two cohorts in two countries. *Lancet Psychiatry, 2*(6), 524–531.

Little, T. D., Henrich, C. C., Jones, S. M., & Hawley, P. H. (2003). Disentangling the "whys" from the "whats" of aggressive behavior. *International Journal of Behavioral Development, 27*(2), 122–133.

Loeber, R., Green, S. M., Keenan, K., & Lahey, B. B. (1995). Which boys will fare worse?: Early predictors of the onset of conduct disorder in a six-year longitudinal study. *Journal of the American Academy of Child and Adolescent Psychiatry, 34*(4), 499–509.

Malti, T. (2016). Toward an integrated clinical–developmental model of guilt. *Developmental Review, 39,* 16–36.

Malti, T., & Averdijk, M. (2017). Severe youth violence: Developmental perspectives: Introduction to the special section. *Child Development, 88,* 5–15.

Malti, T., Dys, S. P., Colasante, T., & Peplak, J. (2018). Emotions and morality: New developmental perspectives. In C. Helwig (Vol. Ed.) & M. Harris (Series Ed.), *Current issues in developmental psychology: New perspectives on moral development* (pp. 55–72). New York: Psychology Press.

Malti, T., & Krettenauer, T. (2013). The relation of moral emotion attributions to prosocial and antisocial behavior: A meta-analysis. *Child Development, 84*(2), 397–412.

Malti, T., Sette, S., & Dys, S. P. (2016). Social–emotional responding: A perspective from developmental psychology. In R. A. Scott, M. Buchmann, & S. M. Kosslyn (Eds.), *Emerging trends in the social and behavioral sciences* (pp. 1–15). Hoboken, NJ: Wiley.

Meaney, M. J. (2010). Epigenetics and the biological definition of gene x environment interactions. *Child Development, 81,* 41–79.

Miller, J. G., Kahle, S., & Hastings, P. D. (2015). Roots and benefits of costly giving: Young children's altruism is related to having less family wealth and more autonomic flexibility. *Psychological Science, 26*(7), 1038–1045.

Moffitt, T. E. (1993). Adolescence-limited and life-course persistent antisocial behavior: A developmental taxonomy. *Psychological Review, 100*(4), 674–701.

Moffitt, T. E. (2003). Life-course persistent and adolescent-limited antisocial behaviour: A 10-year research review and a research agenda. In B. B. Lahey, T. E. Moffitt, & A. Caspi (Eds.), *Causes of conduct disorder and juvenile delinquency* (pp. 49–75). New York: Guilford Press.

Moffitt, T. E., & Caspi, A. (2001). Childhood predictors differentiate life-course-persistent and adolescence-limited antisocial pathways among males and females. *Development and Psychopathology, 13*(2), 355–375.

Nagin, D. (2005). *Group-based modeling of development.* Cambridge, MA: Harvard University Press.

Orobio de Castro, B., Veerman, J. W., Koops, W., Bosch, J. D., & Monshouwer, H. J. (2002). Hostile attribution of intent and aggressive behavior: A meta-analysis. *Child Development, 73*(3), 916–934.

Patterson, G. R. (1982). *A social learning approach: III. Coercive family process.* Eugene, OR: Castalia.

Porges, S. W. (2011). *The polyvagal theory: Neurophysiological foundations of emotions, attachment, communication, and self-regulation.* New York: Norton.

Raine, A. (2002). Biosocial studies of antisocial and violent behavior in children and adults: A review. *Journal of Abnormal Child Psychology, 30*(4), 311–326.

Raine, A. (2013). *The anatomy of violence: The biological roots of crime.* New York: Pantheon/Random House.

Rubin, K. H., Bukowski, W. M., & Bowker, J. C. (2015). Children in peer groups. In R. M. Lerner, M. H. Bornstein, & T. Leventhal (Eds.), *Handbook of child psychology and developmental science* (pp. 175–222). Hoboken, NJ: Wiley.

Rubin, K. H., & Burgess, K. (2002). Parents of aggressive and withdrawn children. In M. Bornstein (Ed.), *Handbook of parenting* (2nd ed., Vol. 1, pp. 383–418). Hillsdale, NJ: Erlbaum.

Rubin, K. H., Burgess, K. B., Dwyer, K. M., & Hastings, P. D. (2003). Predicting preschoolers' externalizing behaviors from toddler temperament, conflict, and maternal negativity. *Developmental Psychology, 39,* 164–176.

Rubin, K. H., & Krasnor, L. R. (1986). Social-cognitive and social behavioral perspectives on problem solving. In M. Perlmutter (Ed.), *Minnesota Symposia on Child Psychology: Cognitive perspectives on children's social and behavioral development* (Vol. 18, pp. 1–68). Hillsdale, NJ: Erlbaum.

Salmivalli, C. (2010). Bullying and the peer group: A review. *Aggression and Violent Behavior, 15*(2), 112–120.

Salmivalli, C., & Peets, K. (2018). Bullying and victimization. In W. M. Bukowski, B. Laursen, & K. H. Rubin (Eds.), *Handbook of peer interactions, relationships, and groups* (2nd ed., pp. 302–321). New York: Guilford Press.

Scherer, K. R. (2009). The dynamic architecture of emotion: Evidence for the component process model. *Cognition and Emotion, 23*(7), 1307–1351.

Sitnick, S. L., Shaw, D., Weaver, C. M., Shelleby, E. C., Choe, D. E., Reuben, J. D., et al. (2017). Early childhood predictors of severe youth violence in low-income male adolescents. *Child Development, 88,* 27–40.

Sullivan, H. S. (1953). *The interpersonal theory of psychiatry.* New York: Norton.

Sykes, G. M., & Matza, D. (1957). Techniques of neutralization: A theory of delinquency. *American Sociological Review, 22*(6), 664–670.

Thornberg, R., Pozzoli, T., Gini, G., & Jungert, T. (2015). Unique and interactive effects of moral emotions and moral disengagement on bullying and school defending among school children. *Elementary School Journal, 116*(2), 322–337.

Tremblay, R. E. (2000). The development of aggressive behavior during childhood: What have we learned in the past century? *International Journal of Behavior Development, 24*(2), 129–141.

Tremblay, R. E. (2010). Developmental origins of disruptive behaviour problems: The "original sin" hypothesis, epigenetics and their consequences for prevention. *Journal of Child Psychology and Psychiatry, 51*(4), 341–367.

Troop-Gordon, W., Gordon, R. D., Vogel-Ciernia, L., Ewing Lee, E., & Visconti, K. J. (2016). Visual attention to dynamic scenes of ambiguous provocation and children's aggressive behavior. *Journal of Clinical Child and Adolescent Psychology,* 1–16. [Epub ahead of print]

Wagner, N. J., Hastings, P. D., & Rubin, K. H. (2017). Callous–unemotional features and autonomic functioning in toddlerhood interact to predict externalizing behaviors in preschool. *Journal of Abnormal Child Psychology.* [Epub ahead of print]

Waltes, R., Chiocchetti, A. G., & Freitag, C. M. (2016). The neuroiological basis of human aggression: A review on genetic and epigenetic mechanisms. *American Journal of Medical Genetics, Part B: Neuropsychiatric Genetics, 171*(5), 660–675.

CHAPTER 2

Clinical Classifications of Aggression in Childhood and Adolescence

PAUL J. FRICK and TATIANA M. MATLASZ

Brief Introduction

···

Since 1980, the primary clinical classifications for children with serious behavior problems have been the diagnoses of oppositional defiant disorder (ODD) and conduct disorder (CD; American Psychiatric Association, 1980). Furthermore, the defining features of these two disorders have not changed greatly over this time period (Frick & Nigg, 2012). That is, ODD is defined as a frequent and persistent pattern of angry, irritable, argumentative, defiant, and vindictive behavior. CD is defined as a persistent pattern of behavior in which the basic rights of others or major age-appropriate norms or rules are violated.

One change in the most recent edition of the *Diagnostic and Statistical Manual of Mental Disorders* (DSM-5; American Psychiatric Association, 2013) is that these disorders are no longer grouped together within a class of disorders labeled "disorders usually first diagnosed in infancy, childhood, or adolescence," as in previous editions of the manual (American Psychiatric Association, 1980, 1987, 1994, 2000). Instead, they are now classified in a chapter of disorders labeled the "disruptive, impulse control, and conduct disorders," which include "conditions involving problems in the self-control of emotions and/or behaviors" (American Psychiatric Association, 2013, p. 461). This change was made to reflect the goal of promoting a lifespan view of mental disorders in which continuities and changes in manifestations across development are considered (Kupfer, Kuhl, & Regier, 2013). A chapter grouping disorders based on timing of onset was not consistent with such a goal. Furthermore, this change was made to foster a more dimensional approach to diagnosis by organizing disorders according to shared risk factors and etiology (Kupfer et al., 2013).

The most recent criteria for the diagnosis of ODD and CD also reflect how the symptoms are clustered. For example, in DSM-5, the symptoms of ODD are now grouped into three dimensions:

1. Angry/irritable mood
2. Argumentative/defiant behavior
3. Vindictiveness

This grouping was designed to reflect the results of factor analyses that have supported the presence of these distinct dimensions (Burke, Hipwell, & Loeber, 2010; Rowe, Costello, Angold, Copeland, & Maughan, 2010). Furthermore, research has indicated that these dimensions have different predictive associations with certain outcomes. That is, all three dimensions seem to predict risk for later CD, but the argumentative–defiant dimension is related to attention-deficit/hyperactivity disorder (ADHD), and the angry–irritable dimension predicts risk for later emotional disorders (i.e., anxiety and depression; Burke et al., 2010; Rowe et al., 2010; Stringaris & Goodman, 2009). Similarly, in the two most recent editions of DSM (American Psychiatric Association, 1994, 2013), the symptoms of CD are grouped into four dimensions:

1. Aggression to people and animals
2. Destruction of property
3. Deceitfulness or theft
4. Serious violations of rules

These dimensions were also based on factor analyses supporting the covariation of these symptoms into distinct clusters of behaviors (Frick et al., 1993).

Although the primary symptoms for CD have not changed greatly over the most recent versions of the DSM, there have been substantial changes in the subtypes that are recognized in the manual. In DSM-III (American Psychiatric Association, 1980), persons with CD could be differentiated into those who were (1) aggressive or not aggressive and (2) those who were considered "socialized" (e.g., had lasting friendships, felt guilt/remorse) or undersocialized. Due to confusion about the best indicators of whether a person was socialized or undersocialized (Lahey, Loeber, Quay, Frick, & Grimm, 1992), this distinction was changed in the revised third edition of the manual to whether the person committed antisocial behavior alone (i.e., solitary–aggressive type) or with other antisocial individuals (i.e., group type; American Psychiatric Association, 1987). The method of subtyping CD was changed yet again in the fourth edition of the manual. In DSM-IV, subtypes of CD were largely based on when the severe conduct problems first onset, with a childhood-onset group showing onset before adolescence (i.e., before age 10) and an adolescent-onset group showing onset of severe conduct problems at age 10 or later (American Psychiatric Association, 1994).

Based on supporting research, (Moffitt et al., 2008), this distinction was retained in the most recent DSM-5. However, an additional specifier was added for those persons with CD who also show impairments in their development of empathy, guilt, and other prosocial emotions, as indicated by elevated rates of callous–unemotional (CU) traits (American Psychiatric Association, 2013). The specifier of "with limited prosocial emotions" (LPE) was added and can be used if the individual with CD shows two more of the following CU traits persistently over 12 months in more than one relationship or setting:

- Lack of remorse or guilt
- Callous–lack of empathy
- Unconcern about performance at school, work, or in other important activities
- Shallow or deficient affect

Main Issues

From this brief review of major changes in the clinical classification of behavioral problems over the past several decades, two critical issues are evident in how aggressive behavior fits within these clinical conceptualizations. First, throughout these various changes (and even prior to these recent revisions; see Pardini, Frick, & Moffitt, 2010), aggression has been considered as one part of a broader pattern of antisocial behavior. That is, rather than being a separate clinical entity, aggressive behavior has been viewed as one of many possible indicators of a failure to appropriately regulate emotions and behavior that can lead to conflict with authority figures or to the violation of rights of others. The emotional component of aggressive behavior (i.e., anger) has been part of the criteria for ODD, whereas the behavioral component of aggression (i.e., physical aggression) has been part of the criteria for CD. Second, it is evident that, from the various subtypes of CD that have been included within the recent criteria, persons within this diagnostic category can vary greatly in terms of the severity and stability of their behavior and in terms of the most important causal processes leading to their behavior problems (Frick & Viding, 2009). The presence or absence of aggressive behavior has been one common method for parsing this heterogeneity into meaningful subtypes.

The goal of this chapter is to critically examine research related to the role of aggressive behavior in clinical classification of disorders of conduct in children and adolescents. The focus on youth is important because, as noted later in the chapter, although normative levels of aggression vary across different developmental stages, there seems to be a rather substantial level of rank-order stability in aggressive behavior. Thus the most aggressive adults tend to have histories of aggressive behavior starting in childhood or adolescence (Tremblay, 2010). Furthermore, the treatment of disorders of conduct, including interventions that target a reduction in aggressive behavior, is more effective when implemented early in development (Frick, 2012). Thus early intervention is critical for any comprehensive approach to reducing the level of aggression and violence in society.

In critically examining aggression in relation to clinical diagnosis of CD, we focus on several critical issues. First, we highlight important theoretical and conceptual considerations on how aggression relates to other forms of antisocial behavior. That is, we review research on the behavioral covariation among the different types of antisocial behavior, including aggression, to determine how these behaviors tend to covary within individuals and whether such covariation supports aggression as being one part of a broader construct of antisocial behavior. We also highlight the related conceptual issue of whether aggressive behavior itself should be used to define clinically and etiologically important subgroups of antisocial individuals or whether differences in the level, severity, and type of aggressive behavior should be viewed as an important way to validate other methods of defining meaningful subgroups of antisocial youth. We then review available empirical research comparing these different approaches for including aggression in clinical conceptualizations of antisocial youth. Specifically, we review research comparing (1) aggressive versus nonaggressive antisocial youth, (2) childhood-onset versus adolescent-onset antisocial youth, and (3) antisocial youth with elevated CU traits and those with developmentally normative levels of these traits. We compare these approaches in their ability to define clinically and etiologically important groups of children with severe behavior problems. Finally, we discuss the implications of this research for guiding causal theories of aggression and antisocial behavior and treatment of children and adolescents with severe behavior problems. We highlight important directions for future research that attempts to advance knowledge on how aggression is best integrated into clinical conceptualizations of antisocial behavior.

Theoretical Considerations

Aggressive behavior, defined as behavior that intentionally harms another person, fits into the overall conceptualization of CD because it is one way that a person's behavior can violate the rights of others (Frick & Nigg, 2012). However, in addition to the conceptual consistency of including aggression within this broader category of antisocial behavior, there is a wealth of research suggesting that aggressive behavior is highly correlated with other forms of conduct problems. For example, in a comprehensive review of research, Burt (2012) reported that the average correlation between aggressive and nonaggressive conduct problems is .43 in nonreferred samples and .51 in clinical samples. Furthermore, when examining the same list of conduct problems across multiple large samples ($n = 27,861$) and using different informants, the correlations did not differ based on age of the child but were found to be somewhat higher in boys (.68) than girls (.63) and for parent report of conduct problems (.67) than for self-report (.64; Burt et al., 2015). However, these differences were fairly minimal in magnitude, albeit statistically significant. Given this high degree of association between aggressive and nonaggressive conduct problems, it is not surprising that factor analyses of broad indicators of children's emotional and behavioral problems generally find that aggressive behavior tends to load with other behavior problems on a higher order externalizing dimension (Lahey, van Hulle, Singh, Waldman, & Rathouz, 2011). Thus there are both conceptual and empirical reasons for grouping aggressive behavior as part of a larger symptom list of behavior problems, as they seem to covary to a high degree within individuals.

However, there is also evidence that some distinctions can be made within the broad dimension of conduct problems, even in terms of behavioral covariation. For example, Frick and colleagues (1993) conducted a meta-analytic summary of 60 factor analyses from 44 published studies of more than 28,401 children and adolescents (ages 5–18) that examined the patterns of covariation just within conduct problems (i.e., they did not include other dimensions of emotions or behavior). To be included, the studies had to contain factor analyses of conduct problems using either parents' or teachers' reports and objective assessment methods (e.g., rating scales or structured interviews). The results of the meta-analysis suggested that the covariation among conduct problems could be summarized by two bipolar dimensions. One dimension distinguished between overt (i.e., involving direct confrontation of others) and covert types of conduct problems, and a second dimension distinguished between destructive (i.e., involving harm to victims and/or their property) and nondestructive types of conduct problems. Thus the behaviors clustered into an overt–destructive cluster (physical aggression), an overt–nondestructive cluster (oppositional defiant behaviors), a covert–destructive cluster (property violations such as stealing and vandalism), and a covert–nondestructive cluster (status violations such as running away from home and truancy).

Thus research clearly suggests that aggressive behavior covaries highly with other forms of behavior problems but that, within behavior problems, aggression seems to form a distinct cluster of behaviors. This would seem to suggest that physical aggression can be appropriately conceptualized as part of a broader pattern of conduct problems. However, it also leaves open the possibility that physical aggression could be important for designating an important subgroup of antisocial youth that involves direct confrontation of others and that is destructive (i.e., violates the rights of others). This possibility is important because, as noted previously, there has been a general consensus that clinical classifications of children and adolescents with serious conduct problems result in very heterogeneous groups of individuals that vary greatly in severity, outcome, and etiology. Also, as noted earlier, many previous attempts to define more homogenous subtypes of antisocial individuals have used the level of aggression displayed by the child. However, subtyping approaches have also used other methods, such as the age of onset of severe behavior problems and the level of CU traits. These latter distinctions have resulted in groups that differ on their levels of aggression. Thus all of these methods could be important for understanding how aggressive behavior fits within clinical conceptualizations of antisocial behavior. The critical question is which approach provides the best way to define clinically important subgroups of antisocial youth (i.e., differing in severity of behavior, impairment, and outcome) or etiologically important subgroups of antisocial youth (i.e., differing on important causal factors).

Central Research Findings

Clinical and Etiological Importance of Aggression

By definition, the presence of aggression is a clinically important specifier for CD. That is, the presence of behavior that intentionally harms others is itself an indicator of a high level of impairment because it involves conflict with others and it indicates the need for treatment to reduce behavior that results in harm to others. To reflect this clinical importance, recent definitions of CD in DSM (American Psychiatric Association, 1994, 2013) have included a severity specifier based on both number of symptoms present beyond the diagnostic threshold and the degree of harm to others that is caused by the symptoms of diagnosis. It includes three levels:

1. *Mild:* with few symptoms beyond the diagnostic threshold and behavior that causes relative minor harm to others (e.g., lying, truancy).
2. *Moderate:* the number of symptoms and amount of harm to others is intermediate to those specified as "mild" or "severe."
3. *Severe:* with many symptoms beyond the diagnostic threshold that cause considerable harm to others (e.g., rape, use of a weapon).

Research also supports the importance of aggression as a severity indicator by suggesting that aggressive behaviors often start early in life and show a relatively high level of rank-order stability. That is, the peak frequency of physical aggression is typically observed between the ages of 2 and 4, when over half of preschoolers display at least moderate levels of physical aggression (Côté, Vaillancourt, Barker, Nagin, & Tremblay, 2007; Tremblay, 2010); but the overall level of aggressive behavior decreases through childhood and adolescence (Eisner & Malti, 2015; Stanger, Achenbach, & Verhulst, 1997; Tremblay, 2003). Thus there appears to be a normative decline in physical aggression across childhood. However, there also appears to be a high degree of rank-order stability in aggression, despite this normative decline. That is, the most aggressive preschoolers are likely to be the most aggressive adolescents and the most aggressive adults (Broidy et al., 2003; Maughan, Pickles, Rowe, Costello, & Angold, 2000; Moffitt, 2006; Tremblay, 2003). For example, in a large community sample (n = 856) followed over 40 years (ages 8–48 years), peer-rated aggression at age 8 was correlated with self-report of aggression at age 19 (r = .37, p < .001), age 30 (r = .35, p < .001), and age 48 (r = .29, p < .001) for males (Huesmann, Dubow, & Boxer, 2009). The three stability coefficients were still significant (all p < .05) but lower for females (r = .23, .15, and .13, respectively). Furthermore, those children who showed persistent high aggression were more likely to show a host of problematic outcomes in adulthood, such as being arrested, being divorced, showing depression, and abusing alcohol.

Thus research suggests that aggressive behavior is relatively stable across the lifespan and predicts important legal, social, and mental health outcomes. However, a critical question is whether the presence of aggressive behavior within children and adolescents with broader patterns of behavior problems designates a clinically important subgroup of antisocial youth. As noted previously, early definitions of CD included an "undersocialized aggressive" subtype that was defined based on (1) an inability to form lasting social relationships and an absence of prosocial emotions such as empathy and guilt (i.e., undersocialization) and (2) the presence of aggressive behavior. Reviews of research on this subgroup suggested that they had poorer adjustment in juvenile institutions and were more likely to continue to show antisocial behavior into adulthood when compared with other adolescents with CD (Quay, 1987). However, it is not clear whether this poorer outcome was related to the indicators of being undersocialized, to the presence of aggressive behavior, or to the combination of both.

Research, although not directly addressing this question, does suggest that aggressive conduct problems are more stable than nonaggressive conduct problems (Stanger et al., 1997). However, the research on whether aggressive conduct problems predict more problems later in development compared with nonaggressive conduct problems is somewhat mixed. For example, Maughan and colleagues (2000) reported that in a community sample of children ($n = 1,419$) ages 9–13 who were followed through age 16, there was no difference between those with stable high aggressive behavior and those with stable high nonaggressive conduct problems in rate of arrest in adolescence. In contrast, in a sample of boys followed from age 6 to age 15, chronic physical aggression led to more violent delinquency and more serious delinquent acts when controlling for level of nonaggressive conduct problems, whereas nonaggressive conduct problems were only associated with higher levels of theft after controlling for aggressive conduct problems (Nagin & Tremblay, 1999).

Thus there is some evidence to support the clinical importance of physical aggression. That is, physical aggression appears to be relatively stable across the lifespan and is associated with a number of problematic outcomes. Also, when combined with indicators of a lack of empathy and guilt (i.e., undersocialized aggression), it designates a distinct group of children with serious conduct problems who are at risk for worse outcomes. The next important question is whether aggression might also define etiologically distinct subgroups of children with serious conduct problems.

In support of this possibility, research has compared the genetic influences on aggressive and nonaggressive behavior problems and has found that aggressive behavior is more heritable than nonaggressive conduct problems (Tackett, Kreuger, Iacono, & McGue, 2005; Tremblay, 2010). A recent meta-analysis reported that genetic influences account for about 65% of the variance in aggressive behavior, whereas they account for about 48% of the variance in nonaggressive rule-breaking behaviors (Burt, 2009). Of note, these results seem to be consistent across the informants reporting on the aggression, as well as across the genders and ages of the children (Burt, 2009). Further supporting the differences in the genetic influences on the two types of conduct problems, one family study reported specificity in the intergenerational transmission of aggressive and nonaggressive conduct problems. Specifically, aggressive symptoms, but not other forms of conduct problems, were associated with aggression in first-degree biological relatives, whereas nonaggressive conduct problems were associated with rule-breaking symptoms but not aggression in biological relatives (Monuteaux, Fitzmaurice, Blacker, Buka, & Biederman, 2004). However, research has also suggested that there is a substantial degree of shared genetic influences on aggressive and nonaggressive conduct problems, ranging from about 20 to almost 80% of the genetic influences being shared across the two types of behaviors (Bartels et al., 2003; Eley, Lichtenstein, & Stevenson, 1999; Gelhorn et al., 2006), with the shared variance reported to be greater for girls than boys (Eley et al., 1999).

Research has also compared aggressive and nonaggressive conduct problems on their associations with risk factors that could play an important role in their etiology. Negative affectivity, such as high stress reactivity, unpredictable mood changes, neuroticism, and social dominance, are consistently found to be more highly associated with aggression than rule-breaking behavior (Burt & Donnellan, 2008; Burt & Larson, 2007; Tackett, 2010). In contrast, low behavioral control and constraint, or high impulsivity, is more strongly associated with rule-breaking behavior (Burt, 2012; Burt & Donnellan, 2008; Moffitt, 2006; Tackett, 2010). Also, intelligence and executive functioning have been found to be negatively associated with aggression but unrelated to nonaggressive conduct problems (Barker et al., 2007; Hancock, Tapscott, & Hoaken, 2010).

Thus there appear to be several important differences in the correlates to aggressive and nonaggressive forms of conduct problems. These correlates would be consistent with the possibility that children with CD may differ in the causes of their behavior problems depending on whether they show aggression or not. Consistent with this possibility, children with CD that was defined using early definitions of the undersocialized aggressive subtype were more likely to show several neurophysiological correlates to their antisocial behavior, such as low serotonin levels and autonomic irregularities, compared with other children with CD (Lahey, Hart, Pliszka, Applegate, & McBurnett, 1993; Quay, 1993). However, it is again unclear whether these differences were due to the undersocialized or aggressive part of this method for subtyping youth with CD.

Clinical and Etiological Importance of Childhood-Onset versus Adolescent-Onset CD

Despite this evidence supporting both the clinical and etiological utility of using aggression to subtype children with serious conduct problems, a problem with this approach is the fact that the majority of children who show aggression also show other types of behavior problems (Lahey & Loeber, 1994). Thus it is unclear what level of aggression should be required, relative to the level of nonaggressive behavior problems, to designate an "aggressive subtype" of CD (Lahey et al., 1992). As a result, beginning with DSM-IV (American Psychiatric Association, 1994), subtyping approaches in DSM changed from focusing on the type of behavior that was displayed to focusing on the age of onset (i.e., before or after age 10) at which the serious behavior problems began to emerge.

This distinction was based on a rather long history of research on both juvenile delinquency and childhood behavior problems suggesting that the earlier the child behavior problems start, the more likely the child is to have severe impairments that last into adulthood (Moffitt et al., 2008). For example, Farrington, Gallagher, Morley, St. Ledger, and West (1988) reported that boys who were arrested prior to age 12 showed almost twice as many convictions at two later points in time (between the ages of 16 and 18 and between the ages of 22 and 24) compared with boys arrested after 12 years of age. Similarly, Robins (1966) reported that boys referred to a mental health clinic for antisocial behavior prior to age 11 were twice as likely to receive a diagnosis of antisocial personality disorder as adults, as compared with boys who began showing antisocial behavior after age 11. Importantly, these poorer outcomes of early-onset conduct problems are not simply found for antisocial outcomes. In a birth cohort of children in New Zealand followed into adulthood, males who had childhood-onset conduct problems were more than twice as likely to have an anxiety disorder or major depression and more than three times as likely to be drug dependent, to have attempted suicide, and to be homeless by age 32 compared with males whose serious conduct problems began in adolescence (Odgers et al., 2007).

Importantly, the childhood-onset specifier seems to capture youth with CD who are more likely to be aggressive and violent. For example, Tremblay (2010) reviewed several longitudinal studies that investigated trajectories of physical aggression, all of which indicated that serious aggression rarely onsets after early childhood. Furthermore, in a sample of justice-involved adolescents, youth with childhood onset of their antisocial behavior showed higher rates of violent delinquency but not nonviolent delinquency when compared with youth with adolescent onset of their antisocial behavior (Dandreaux & Frick, 2009). Finally, in the New Zealand birth cohort described previously, the rate of violent offending between the ages of 26 and 32 was 32.7% for men who showed a childhood onset to their antisocial behavior and 10.2% for men who showed an adolescent onset to their antisocial behavior (Odgers et al., 2007). In summary, across studies using a variety of methodologies, there appears to be consistent evidence that childhood-onset CD is more likely to involve aggressive behavior than adolescent-onset CD.

In addition to differences in their outcomes and their levels of aggression, there is also extensive research to suggest that the two groups of children with CD formed based on the timing of onset differ on a number of dispositional and contextual risk factors that seem to implicate different etiologies for these two groups (Fairchild, Van Goozen, Calder, & Goodyer, 2013; Frick & Viding, 2009; Moffitt, 2006). To summarize these findings, childhood-onset CD seems to be more strongly related to neuropsychological (e.g., deficits in executive functioning) and cognitive (e.g., low intelligence) deficits. Also, children who show the childhood-onset pattern seem to show more temperamental and personality risk factors, such as impulsivity, attention deficits, and problems in emotional regulation. This group also shows higher rates of family instability and more family conflict, and they have parents who use less effective parenting strategies. When children within the adolescent-onset group differ from control children without conduct problems, it is often in showing higher levels of rebelliousness and being more rejecting of conventional values and status hierarchies (Dandreaux & Frick, 2009; Moffitt, Caspi, Dickson, Silva, & Stanton, 1996).

The different outcomes and risk factors for the two subtypes of antisocial individuals led Moffitt (2006) to propose that children in the childhood-onset group develop their problem behavior through a transactional process involving a difficult and vulnerable child (e.g., impulsive, with verbal deficits) who experiences an inadequate rearing environment (e.g., poor parental supervision, poor quality schools). This dysfunctional transactional process disrupts the child's socialization, leading to enduring vulnerabilities that can negatively affect the child's psychosocial adjustment across the lifespan. In contrast, Moffitt proposed that children in the adolescent-onset pathway show an exaggeration of the normative process of adolescent rebellion. That is, most adolescents show some level of rebelliousness to parents and other authority figures (Brezina & Piquero, 2007). This rebelliousness is part of a process by which the adolescent begins to develop his or her autonomous sense of self and his or her unique identity (Steinberg, 2014). According to Moffitt, the child in the adolescent-onset group engages in antisocial and delinquent behaviors as a misguided attempt to obtain a subjective sense of maturity and adult status in a way that is maladaptive (e.g., breaking societal norms) but encouraged by an antisocial peer group. Given that their behavior is viewed as an exaggeration of a process specific to adolescence, and not due to an enduring vulnerability, their antisocial behavior is less likely to persist beyond adolescence. However, they may still have impairments that persist into adulthood due to the consequences of their adolescent antisocial behavior (e.g., a criminal record, dropping out of school, substance abuse; Odgers et al., 2007).

Thus there is evidence to support the clinical (i.e., more severe, stable, and aggressive behavior) and etiological (i.e., different causal factors) importance of the childhood-versus-adolescent-onset distinction. However, there are also some important limitations to this approach. First, it is not firmly established what should be the exact age at which to differentiate childhood- and adolescent-onset groups and even whether this differentiation should be based on age or on the stage of pubertal development (Frick & Nigg, 2012). This is an important limitation because the use of age of onset over aggression to form subtypes was based at least in part on the rationale that age of onset was easier to assess. Second, there is evidence that this distinction may not be categorical but may best be considered dimensionally (Fairchild et al., 2013; Lahey et al., 2000). That is, a recent review by Fairchild and colleagues (2013) supported the contention that dispositional factors play a greater role in serious conduct problems when the behavior problems start earlier in development. However, their review also suggested that this effect continues into adolescence. Third, there is evidence that there is still substantial variability within the childhood-onset group in terms of both outcome (Fairchild et al., 2013) and etiological factors (Frick, Ray, Thornton, & Kahn, 2014a). This variability in the childhood-onset group has led to attempts to make additional distinctions that could parse this heterogeneity in other clinically and etiologically important ways.

Clinical and Etiological Importance of CU Traits

As noted earlier, DSM-III had a subtype designation for CD called "undersocialized aggressive," but there was a great deal of confusion surrounding the core features of this subtype, which led to its exclusion in the next several versions of the DSM in favor of the focus on age of onset. However, subsequent research has refined the key features of this subtype, particularly by integrating definitions of psychopathic traits in adults with definitions of the affective components of conscience that have been used in developmental research with children (Kochanska, Gross, Lin, & Nichols, 2002; Thompson & Newton, 2010). Explicitly tying the definition to research on psychopathy clarified the key features of the construct, and integrating this with developmental research on conscience development helped to define how these features may be manifested at earlier ages (Frick & Ray, 2015). These indicators formed the criteria for the specifier "with LPE" that was included for the diagnosis of CD in DSM-5 (Kimonis et al., 2015). These criteria explicitly noted that "the indicators of this specifier are those that have often been labeled as callous and unemotional traits in research" (American Psychiatric Association, 2013, p. 471). However, the name was changed to encourage greater use in clinical practice by having a label that accurately conveyed the key parts of the construct but minimized the use of pejorative labels (i.e., *callous*) and did not overstate the potential stability of the symptoms in children (i.e., *traits*; Frick et al., 2014a).

The research on CU traits that resulted in the addition of this specifier in DSM-5 indicated that these traits (1) can be reliably assessed across a wide range of ages from early childhood to young adulthood and (2) differentiate a distinct group of children with severe conduct problems that were not adequately captured by the childhood-onset subtype (Frick & Ray, 2015). That is, Frick and colleagues (2014a) provided a qualitative review of 118 published studies (70 cross-sectional and 48 longitudinal) and reported that in 89% of the studies, CU traits (either alone or with other dimensions of psychopathy) were significantly associated with measures of antisocial and aggressive behavior, with an average correlation of .33. Furthermore, this review reported four studies in which CU traits predicted more problematic outcomes even after controlling for level of aggression and five studies showing that CU traits predicted more severe antisocial outcomes even when controlling for age of onset. Of particular note, in a large high-risk community sample (n = 754), McMahon, Witkiewitz, Kotler, and the Conduct Problems Prevention Research Group (2010) reported that CU traits assessed in the seventh grade significantly predicted adult antisocial outcomes (e.g., adult arrests, adult antisocial personality symptoms) even after controlling for childhood onset of CD.

Research on CU traits has also reported an important link with aggressive behavior. That is, when CU traits are used to divide subgroups of children with serious behavior problems, those high on CU traits appear to be more aggressive. For example, in samples of (1) European American (77%) children in grades 3–7 (n = 1,136) and (2) low-income and largely African American (88%) youth ages 5–18 who were consecutive referrals to a community mental health center (n = 566), elevated CU traits differentiated children with CD who showed higher rates of aggression (Kahn, Frick, Youngstrom, Findling, & Youngstrom, 2012). In a sample of girls ages 6–8 (n = 1,862), those who met criteria for CD and who showed elevated CU traits displayed more bullying and relational aggression (i.e., behavior that harms the relationships of others) both at baseline and at a 6-year follow-up when compared with girls who only met criteria for CD (Pardini, Stepp, Hipwell, Stouthamer-Loeber, & Loeber, 2012). Furthermore, serious juvenile offenders high on CU traits (Kruh, Frick, & Clements, 2005; Lawing, Frick, & Cruise, 2010) and nonreferred children high on both conduct problems and CU traits (Fanti, Frick, & Georgiou, 2009; Frick, Cornell, Barry, Bodin, & Dane, 2003) were more likely to show premeditated and instrumental patterns of aggression when compared with other antisocial youth who showed aggression that was limited to only reactive aggression in response to perceived provocation. Furthermore, in two samples of juvenile offenders, elevated CU traits were associated with violence that resulted in more severe harm to victims (Kruh et al., 2005; Lawing et al., 2010). Thus using CU traits to divide antisocial youth results in groups that often differ in their level, type, and severity of aggression.

There is also substantial evidence to suggest that elevated levels of CU traits designate a group of youth with CD who show different risk factors from other antisocial youth that would seem to implicate distinct causal processes leading to the behavior problems in the two groups. Specifically, Frick and colleagues (2014a) reviewed the available research and concluded that those with elevated CU traits seem to:

- Show conduct problems that are more strongly influenced by genetic factors.
- Be less sensitive to punishment cues, which include responding more poorly to punishment cues after a reward-dominant response set is primed, responding more poorly to gradual punishment schedules, and underestimating the likelihood that they will be punished for misbehavior.
- Endorse more deviant values and goals in social situations, such as viewing aggression as a more acceptable means for obtaining goals, blaming others for their misbehavior, and emphasizing the importance of dominance and revenge in social conflicts.
- Show reduced emotional responsiveness in a number of situations, including showing weaker responses to cues of distress in others, less reactivity to peer provocation, less fear to novel and dangerous situations, and less anxiety over the consequences of their behavior.
- Show conduct problems that are less strongly related to coercive parenting practices but more strongly related to parental warmth.

These findings have led to a number of theories hypothesizing different causal processes underlying the behavior problems in children with and without elevated CU traits. For example, Frick, Ray, Thornton, and Kahn (2014b) have proposed that children with serious conduct problems and elevated CU traits have a temperament (i.e., fearless, insensitive to punishment, low responsiveness to cues of distress in others) that can interfere with the normal development of conscience. For example, Kochanska (1993) proposed that the anxiety and discomforting arousal that follow wrongdoing and punishment are integral in the development of inhibitory control of behavior whereby the child's emotional arousal helps him or her learn to inhibit behavior that hurts others and to inhibit misbehavior, even in the absence of the punishing agent. Thus children who do not show this "transgression-related arousal" may have difficulty internalizing parental norms, especially if parents rely largely on punishment rather than warmth in their discipline (Eisenberg, Eggum, & Edwards, 2010). Blair, Mitchell, and Blair (2005) proposed that a critical process in the development of empathic concern is the ability to encode emotionally valenced stimuli. This ability leads a child to respond to distress cues in others with increased autonomic activity, and this negative emotional response develops before the infant or toddler is cognitively able to take the perspective of others, such as when a young child becomes upset in response to the cries of another child. According to this model, these early negative emotional responses to the distress of others become conditioned to behaviors in the child that lead to distress in others. Through a process of conditioning, the child learns to inhibit such behaviors as a way of avoiding this negative arousal. Fearless children may show problems in the encoding of emotional stimuli and, as a result, may not experience this negative arousal as strongly as other children, leading to problems in the development of empathic concern and perspective taking.

In short, there have been a number of theories about how the unique temperamental features that have been associated with CU traits could explain problems in the development of empathy and guilt, problems that could lead not only to the development of this callous interpersonal style but to the aggressive behavior that often accompanies CU traits. Furthermore, separating out those youth with elevated CU traits helps to clarify how they differ from other children with serious conduct problems. That is, children and adolescents with childhood-onset antisocial behavior with normative levels of CU traits do not typically show problems in empathy and guilt. In fact, they appear to be highly reactive to emotional cues in others, and they are highly distressed by the effects of their behavior on others (Frick & Viding, 2009). Thus the antisocial behavior in this group does not seem to be easily explained by deficits in conscience development. Furthermore, this group that does not show elevated levels of CU traits displays higher levels of emotional reactivity to provocation from others (Frick et al., 2014a). Also, as noted previously, the conduct problems in this group are more strongly associated with hostile/coercive parenting. Based on these findings, it appears that children in this group show a temperament characterized by strong emotional reactivity combined with inadequate socializing experiences that make it difficult for the child to develop the skills needed to adequately regulate his or her emotional reactivity (Frick & Morris, 2004). The resulting problems in emotional regulation can result in the child's committing impulsive and unplanned (i.e., reactive) aggressive and antisocial acts for which he or she may feel remorseful afterward but which he or she may still have difficulty controlling in the future.

Implications

In summary, the available research has supported three possible ways in which aggressive behavior can inform clinical definitions of disorders of conduct in children and adolescents. One is focusing directly on the presence of aggressive behavior within the larger domain of antisocial behavior, and the other two focus on defining subgroups that often show higher rates of aggression (childhood onset) or more severe aggression (with elevated CU traits). Thus all three approaches consider the role of aggression in clinical classifications of children's conduct problems. The lingering question is which of these methods is best (Burt, 2012; Marsee & Frick, 2010).

Available research does not provide a clear answer to this question, and it may depend on the primary goal for making the classification. Because aggression itself is such an important marker of severity, methods that directly focus on the presence of this type of behavior are likely to be most important for determining need for treatment and the level of risk to public safety that the child with serious behavior problems poses. However, it is also important to note that these three methods each seem to account for somewhat unique variance in poor outcomes, suggesting that they each provide important information about prognosis (Burt, 2012; Frick et al., 2014a).

In contrast, the available research suggests that the presence of CU traits may be more important for designating a subgroup of children with serious conduct problems who are highly aggressive but show greater divergence in causal factors that could advance research on the unique etiological pathways to serious conduct problems (Frick et al., 2014a). The theoretical importance of this approach is enhanced by its link to the large body of research on the construct of psychopathy (Blair et al., 2005) and research on the development of conscience (Moul, Killcross, & Dadds, 2012) that can be used to inform theoretical models of aggression. Furthermore, these unique developmental pathways with distinct risk and protective factors could provide important clues to specific targets for intervention that are uniquely tailored to the characteristics of children with and without elevated CU traits (Frick, 2012; Hawes, Price, & Dadds, 2014; Wilkinson, Waller, & Viding, 2016). For example, there is growing evidence that certain forms of positive parenting techniques, such as parental warmth and parental use of positive reinforcement, may be important protective factors for children with elevated CU traits by reducing the level and severity of their conduct problems (Clark & Frick, 2016; Waller et al., 2015). As a result, interventions that focus on increasing these parenting dimensions could prove to be important methods for reducing the level of behavior problems, including aggression, in youth with elevated CU traits (Wilkinson et al., 2016).

Future Directions

Because the various methods differentiating among youth with serious conduct problems all seem to be related to important legal, social, and mental health outcomes, future research should test ways of optimally combining these clinical indicators in ways that are reliable, valid, and useful. For example, the DSM-5 definition has three specifiers for the diagnosis of CD that consider each of these indicators. It includes an onset specifier (childhood vs. adolescent vs. unspecified), the specifier "with LPE" defined by elevated levels for CU traits, and a severity specifier based in part on the amount of harm the child's conduct problems cause to others. Similarly, the Structured Assessment of Violence Risk for Youth (SAVRY; Borum, Bartel, & Forth, 2006) is a clinical method for assessing risk for violence in youth who are in the juvenile justice system. It includes a history of aggression and violence, early initiation of violence, and low empathy and remorse as some of its indicators of risk, and it has shown relatively strong validity for predicting reoffending in adolescents (Borum, Lodewikjs, Bartel, & Forth, 2010; Singh, Grann, & Fazel, 2011).

As noted above, the specifier "CU traits" was added to the DSM-5 classification of CD in part because it designates a group of antisocial youth who are more aggressive and show more premeditated and instrumental aggression and whose aggression results in more severe harm to their victims. However, research has begun to emerge suggesting that there might be some indicators as to which youth with CU traits are most likely to be aggressive. For example, in three samples of detained adolescents, higher intelligence was related to more self-reported aggression and violence in youth high on CU traits, whereas higher levels of intelligence were related to *less* self-reported aggression in those normative on these traits (Baskin-Sommers, Waller, Fish, & Hyde, 2015; Hampton, Drabick, & Steinberg, 2014; Munoz, Frick, Kimonis, & Aucoin, 2008). One possible reason given for this finding is that higher intelligence in adolescents who show a callous disregard for others can result in greater planning for aggression that can be used for gain. Another marker for a higher level of aggression in youth with elevated CU traits is the presence of anxiety (Docherty, Boxer, Huesmann, O'Brien, & Bushman, 2016; Fanti, Demetriou, & Kimonis, 2013; Kimonis, Skeem, Cauffman, & Dmitrieva, 2011). The most common explanation for this finding is that the presence of anxiety is a marker for histories of past trauma and abuse, which lead to problems regulating anger and cognitive biases (e.g., a hostile attributional bias) that promote aggressive responding (Kimonis et al., 2011). However, it is also possible that the higher level of anxiety is simply a marker of the more severe behavioral disturbance in those with CU traits who are also aggressive.

Because the presence of elevated CU traits designates a particularly aggressive group of children and adolescents with behavior problems, advances in the theoretical models for the etiology of CU traits are also likely to lead to advances in knowledge on the causes of aggression. Given the high degree of genetic influence on the conduct problems exhibited by children with elevated CU traits, one particularly promising direction for research is uncovering possible candidate genes that could be involved in conveying this risk. For example, Dadds and colleagues (2014) reported that CU traits were related to greater methylation of the oxytocin receptor gene in a sample of boys ages 4–16. Another promising area of research is studies on early markers of problems in attachment that can predict later CU traits. For example, Bedford, Pickles, Sharp, Wright, and Hill (2015) reported that lower preferential face tracking at 5 weeks of age predicted higher CU traits at age 2½. Such research in young children can also focus on factors that might mitigate the risk for later CU traits. For example, Hyde and colleagues (2016) reported, for an adoption cohort of 561 families, that CU traits at 27 months of age were predicted by biological mothers' antisocial behavior, despite limited or no contact with the biological mother, but that adoptive mothers' use of positive reinforcement as part of their parenting reduced this risk in the child.

This last study has potentially important implications for the prevention of CU traits. Given the link between CU traits and aggression, it is likely that advances in the treatment of children and adolescents with CU traits will lead to advances in the treatment of aggressive behavior as well. Several reviews of the available research on the treatment of CU traits have concluded that youth with CU traits often do not respond as well to many treatments for serious conduct problems and that, when they do respond, they often still end treatment with more severe behavior problems than other children because they enter treatment with a higher level of behavior problems (Frick et al., 2014a; Hawes et al., 2014; Wilkinson et al., 2016). However, all three reviews also concluded that comprehensive treatments that are individually tailored to the specific characteristics of youth with elevated CU traits (e.g., increasing emotional recognition and empathy) or that capitalize on important characteristics of these youth (e.g., motivating the child through self-interest, using positive reinforcement for discipline) can result in reductions in both the child's conduct problems and in the CU traits themselves. Thus, as more treatments are developed and tested based on our expanding knowledge of the causes of CU traits (Kimonis & Armstrong, 2012), it is quite possible that these treatments will also result in reductions in the aggressive behavior displayed by these youth.

Conclusions

In conclusion, aggression has been an integral part of most major methods for classifying disorders of conduct. This focus is supported by research suggesting that aggressive behavior is highly correlated with other types of conduct problems (e.g., rule breaking, oppositional defiance, property destruction). In fact, it is relatively rare for children who show severe patterns of aggressive behavior not to show other types of conduct problems. On the other hand, it is not unusual for children to show nonaggressive conduct problems without any aggressive behavior. Furthermore, aggressive and nonaggressive behavior problems show differences in their onsets (i.e., aggression tends to emerge earlier in development) and their outcomes (i.e., aggression tends to be associated with poorer outcomes).

Based on these differences, there have been a number of different attempts to define subgroups of children with serious conduct problems that reflect these differences. These include defining subtypes of children with serious conduct problems explicitly based on their level of aggression or defining subtypes using other methods (i.e., childhood onset; elevated CU traits) that result in groups that are often more aggressive. Our review revealed that all of these methods have some validity for defining a clinically important subgroup (i.e., one that has more impairment and/or worse outcomes) of children and adolescents with conduct problems. They also each possess some validity for defining etiologically distinct subgroups (i.e., that differ on important causal processes) of youth with conduct problems. However, the research is not clear on which method is *better,* and this may depend on the purpose for making the classification. As a result, many clinical methods for classifying children and adolescents with serious conduct problems, both for use in mental health and juvenile justice settings, attempt to integrate all three methods. This includes the most current definition for CD that is used in DSM-5.

REFERENCES

American Psychiatric Association. (1980). *Diagnostic and statistical manual of mental disorders* (3rd ed.). Washington, DC: Author.

American Psychiatric Association. (1987). *Diagnostic and statistical manual of mental disorders* (3rd ed., rev.). Washington, DC: Author.

American Psychiatric Association. (1994). *Diagnostic and statistical manual of mental disorders* (4th ed.). Washington, DC: Author.

American Psychiatric Association. (2000). *Diagnostic and statistical manual of mental disorders* (4th ed., text rev.). Washington, DC: Author.

American Psychiatric Association. (2013). *Diagnostic and statistical manual of mental disorders* (5th ed.). Arlington, VA: Author.

Barker, E. D., Séguin, J. R., White, H. R., Bates, M. E., Lacourse, É., Carbonneau, R., et al. (2007). Developmental trajectories of male physical violence and theft: Relations to neurocognitive performance. *Archives of General Psychiatry, 64,* 592–599.

Bartels, M., Hudziak, J. J., van den Oord, E. J. C. G., van Beijsterveldt, C. E. M., Rietveld, M. J. H., & Boomsma, D. I. (2003). Co-occurrence of aggressive behavior and rule-breaking behavior at age 12: Multi-rater analyses. *Behavior Genetics, 33,* 607–621.

Baskin-Sommers, A. R., Waller, R., Fish, A. M., & Hyde, L. W. (2015). Callous–unemotional traits trajectories interact with earlier conduct problems and executive control to predict violence and substance use among high-risk male adolescents. *Journal of Abnormal Child Psychology, 43,* 1529–1541.

Bedford, R., Pickles, A., Sharp, H., Wright, N., & Hill, J. (2015). Reduced face preference in infancy: A developmental precursor to callous–unemotional traits? *Biological Psychiatry, 78,* 144–150.

Blair, R. J. R., Mitchell, D., & Blair, K. S. (2005). *The psychopath: Emotion and the brain.* Hoboken, NJ: Wiley-Blackwell.

Borum, R., Bartel, P., & Forth, A. (2006). *Manual for the Structured Assessment for Violence Risk in Youth (SAVRY).* Tampa: Florida Mental Health Institute, University of South Florida.

Borum, R., Lodewikjs, H., Bartel, P., & Forth, A. (2010). Structured Assessment of Violence Risk in Youth (SAVRY). In K. Douglas & R. Otto (Eds.), *Handbook of violence risk assessment* (pp. 63–80). New York: Routledge.

Brezina, T., & Piquero, A. R. (2007). Moral beliefs, isolation from peers, and abstention from peers. *Deviant Behavior, 28,* 433–465.

Broidy, L. M., Nagin, D. S., Tremblay, R. E., Bates, J., Brame, B., Dodge, K. A., et al. (2003). Developmental trajectories of childhood disruptive behaviors and adolescent delinquency: A six-site, cross-national study. *Developmental Psychology, 39,* 222–245.

Burke, J. D., Hipwell, A. E., & Loeber, R. (2010). Dimensions of oppositional defiant disorder as predictors of depression and conduct disorder in girls. *Journal of the American Academy of Child and Adolescent Psychiatry, 49,* 484–492.

Burt, S. A. (2009). Are there meaningful etiological differences within antisocial behavior?: Results of a meta-analysis. *Clinical Psychology Review, 29,* 163–178.

Burt, S. A. (2012). How do we optimally conceptualize the heterogeneity within antisocial behavior?: An argument for aggressive versus non-aggressive behavioral dimensions. *Clinical Psychology Review, 32,* 263–279.

Burt, S. A., & Donnellan, M. B. (2008). Personality correlates of aggressive and non-aggressive antisocial behavior. *Personality and Individual Differences, 44,* 53–63.

Burt, S. A., & Larson, C. L. (2007). Differential affective responses in those with aggressive versus non-aggressive antisocial behaviors. *Personality and Individual Differences, 43,* 1481–1492.

Burt, S. A., Rescorla, L. A., Achenbach, T. M., Ivanova, M. Y., Almqvist, F., Begovac, I., et al. (2015). The association between aggressive and non-aggressive antisocial problems as measured with the Achenbach System of Empirically Based Assessment: A study of 27,861 parent–adolescent dyads from 25 societies. *Personality and Individual Differences, 85,* 86–92.

Clark, J. E., & Frick, P. J. (2016). Positive parenting and callous–unemotional traits: Their association with school behavior problems in young children. *Journal of Clinical Child and Adolescent Psychology.* [Epub ahead of print]

Côté, S. M., Vaillancourt, T., Barker, E. D., Nagin, D., & Tremblay, R. E. (2007). The joint development of physical and indirect aggression: Predictors of continuity and change during childhood. *Development and Psychopathology, 19,* 37–55.

Dadds, M. R., Moul, C., Cauchi, A., Dobson-Stone, C., Hawes, D. J., Brennan, J., et al. (2014). Methylation of the oxytocin receptor gene and oxytocin blood levels in the development of psychopathy. *Development and Psychopathology, 26,* 33–40.

Dandreaux, D. M., & Frick, P. J. (2009). Developmental pathways to conduct problems: A further test of the childhood and adolescent-onset distinction. *Journal of Abnormal Child Psychology, 37,* 375–385.

Docherty, M., Boxer, P., Huesmann, L. R., O'Brien, M., & Bushman, B. J. (2016). Exploring primary and secondary variants of psychopathy in adolescents in detention and in the community. *Journal of Clinical Child and Adolescent Psychology, 45,* 564–578.

Eisenberg, N., Eggum, N. D., & Edwards, A. (2010). Empathy-related responding and moral development. In W. F. Arsenio & E. A. Lemerise (Eds.), *Emotions, aggression, and morality in children: Bridging development and psychopathology* (pp. 115–135). Washington, DC: American Psychological Association.

Eisner, M. P., & Malti, T. (2015). Aggressive and violent behavior. In M. E. Lamb & R. M. Lerner (Eds.), *Handbook of child psychology and developmental science: Vol. 3. Socioemotional processes* (7th ed., pp. 794–841). Hoboken, NJ: Wiley.

Eley, T. C., Lichtenstein, P., & Stevenson, J. (1999). Sex differences in the etiology of aggressive and nonaggressive antisocial behavior: Results from two twin studies. *Child Development, 70,* 155–168.

Fairchild, G., Van Goozen, S. H. M., Calder, A. J., & Goodyer, I. M. (2013). Research review: Evaluating and reformulating the developmental taxonomic theory of antisocial behaviour. *Journal of Child Psychology and Psychiatry, 54,* 924–940.

Fanti, K. A., Demetriou, C. A., & Kimonis, E. R. (2013). Variants of callous–unemotional conduct problems in a community sample of adolescents. *Journal of Youth and Adolescence, 42,* 964–979.

Fanti, K. A., Frick, P. J., & Georgiou, S. (2009). Linking callous–unemotional traits to instrumental and non-instrumental forms of aggression. *Journal of Psychopathology and Behavioral Assessment, 31,* 285–298.

Farrington, D. P., Gallagher, B., Morley, L., St. Ledger, R. J., & West, D. (1988). Are there any successful men from criminogenic backgrounds? *Psychiatry: Journal for the Study of Interpersonal Processes, 51,* 116–130.

Frick, P. J. (2012). Developmental pathways to conduct disorder: Implications for future directions in research, assessment, and treatment. *Journal of Clinical Child and Adolescent Psychology, 41,* 378–389.

Frick, P. J., Cornell, A. H., Barry, C. T., Bodin, S. D., & Dane, H. A. (2003). Callous–unemotional traits and conduct problems in the prediction of conduct problem severity, aggression, and self-report of delinquency. *Journal of Abnormal Child Psychology, 31,* 457–470.

Frick, P. J., Lahey, B. B., Loeber, R., Tannenbaum, L., Van Horn, Y., Christ, M. A. G., et al. (1993). Oppositional defiant disorder and conduct disorder: A meta-analytic review of factor analyses and cross-validation in a clinic sample. *Clinical Psychology Review, 13,* 319–340.

Frick, P. J., & Morris, A. S. (2004). Temperament and developmental pathways to conduct problems. *Journal of Clinical Child and Adolescent Psychology, 33,* 54–68.

Frick, P. J., & Nigg, J. T. (2012). Current issues in the diagnosis of attention-deficit/hyperactivity disorder, oppositional defiant disorder, and conduct disorder. *Annual Review of Clinical Psychology, 8,* 77–107.

Frick, P. J., & Ray, J. V. (2015). Evaluating callous-unemotional traits as a personality construct. *Journal of Personality, 83,* 710–722.

Frick, P. J., Ray, J. V., Thornton, L. C., & Kahn, R. E. (2014a). Can callous–unemotional traits enhance the understanding, diagnosis, and treatment of serious conduct problems in children and adolescents?: A comprehensive review. *Psychological Bulletin, 140,* 1–57.

Frick, P. J., Ray, J. V., Thornton, L. C., & Kahn, R. E. (2014b). A developmental psychopathology approach to understanding callous–unemotional traits in children and adolescents with serious conduct problems. *Journal of Child Psychology and Psychiatry, 55,* 532–548.

Frick, P. J., & Viding, E. M. (2009). Antisocial behavior from a developmental psychopathology perspective. *Development and Psychopathology, 21,* 1111–1131.

Gelhorn, H., Stallings, M., Young, S., Corley, R., Rhee, S. H., Christian, H., et al. (2006). Common and specific genetic influences on aggressive and nonaggressive conduct disorder domains. *Journal of the American Academy of Child and Adolescent Psychiatry, 45,* 570–577.

Hampton, A. S., Drabick, D. A. G., & Steinberg, L. (2014). Does IQ moderate the relation between psychopathy and juvenile offending? *Law and Human Behavior, 38*(1), 23–33.

Hancock, M., Tapscott, J. L., & Hoaken, P. N. S. (2010). Role of executive dysfunction in predicting severity and frequency of violence. *Aggressive Behavior, 36,* 338–349.

Hawes, D. J., Price, M. J., & Dadds, M. R. (2014). Callous–unemotional traits and the treatment of conduct problems in childhood and adolescence: A comprehensive review. *Clinical Child and Family Psychology Review, 17,* 248–267.

Huesmann, L. R., Dubow, E. F., & Boxer, P. (2009). Continuity of aggression from childhood to early adulthood as a predictor of life outcomes: Implications for the adolescent-limited and life-course-persistent models. *Aggressive Behavior, 35,* 136–149.

Hyde, L. W., Waller, R., Trentacosta, C. J., Shaw, D. S., Neidehiser, J. M., Ganiban, J. M., et al. (2016). Heritable and nonheritable pathways to early callous–unemotional behaviors. *American Journal of Psychiatry, 173,* 903–910.

Kahn, R. E., Frick, P. J., Youngstrom, E., Findling, R. L., & Youngstrom, J. K. (2012). The effects of including a callous–unemotional specifier for the diagnosis of conduct disorder. *Journal of Child Psychology and Psychiatry, 53,* 271–282.

Kimonis, E. R., & Armstrong, K. (2012). Adapting parent–child interaction therapy to treat severe conduct problems with callous–unemotional traits: A case study. *Clinical Case Studies, 11,* 234–252.

Kimonis, E. R., Fanti, K. A., Frick, P. J., Moffitt, T. E., Essau, C., Bijjtebier, P., et al. (2015). Using self-reported callous–unemotional traits to cross-nationally assess the DSM-5 "With Limited Prosocial Emotions" specifier. *Journal of Child Psychology and Psychiatry, 56,* 1249–1261.

Kimonis, E. R., Skeem, J. L., Cauffman, E., & Dmitrieva, J. (2011). Are secondary variants of juvenile psychopathy more reactively violent and less psychosocially mature than primary variants? *Law and Human Behavior, 35,* 381–391.

Kochanska, G. (1993). Toward a synthesis of parental socialization and child temperament in early development of conscience. *Child Development, 64,* 325–347.

Kochanska, G., Gross, J. N., Lin, M., & Nichols, K. E. (2002). Guilt in young children: Development, determinants, and relations with a broader system of standards. *Child Development, 73,* 461–482.

Kruh, I. P., Frick, P. J., & Clements, C. B. (2005). Historical and personality correlates to the violence patterns of juveniles tried as adults. *Criminal Justice and Behavior, 32,* 69–96.

Kupfer, D. J., Kuhl, E. A., & Regier, D. A. (2013). DSM-5: The future arrived. *Journal of the American Medical Association, 309,* 1691–1692.

Lahey, B. B., Hart, E. L., Pliszka, S., Applegate, B., & McBurnett, K. (1993). Neurophysiological correlates of conduct disorder: A rationale and a review of research. *Journal of Clinical Child Psychology, 22,* 141–153.

Lahey, B. B., & Loeber, R. (1994). Framework for a developmental model of oppositional defiant disorder and conduct disorder. In D. K. Routh (Ed.), *Disruptive behavior disorders in childhood* (pp. 139–180). New York: Plenum Press.

Lahey, B. B., Loeber, R., Quay, H. C., Frick, P. J., & Grimm, J. (1992). Oppositional defiant disorder and conduct disorders: Issues to be resolved for DSM-IV. *Journal of the American Academy of Child and Adolescent Psychiatry, 31,* 539–546.

Lahey, B. B., Schwab-Stone, M., Goodman, S. H., Waldman, I. D., Canino, G., Rathouz, P. J., et al. (2000). Age and gender differences in oppositional behavior and conduct problems: A cross-sectional household study of middle childhood and adolescence. *Journal of Abnormal Psychology, 109,* 488–503.

Lahey, B. B., van Hulle, C. A., Singh, A. L., Waldman, I. D., & Rathouz, P. J. (2011). Higher order genetic and environmental structure of prevalent forms of child and adolescent psychopathology. *Archives of General Psychiatry, 68,* 181–189.

Lawing, K., Frick, P. J., & Cruise, K. R. (2010). Differences in offending patterns between adolescent sex offenders high or low in callous–unemotional traits. *Psychological Assessment, 22,* 298–305.

Marsee, M. A., & Frick, P. J. (2010). Callous–unemotional traits and aggression in youth. In W. F. Arsenio & E. A. Lemerise (Eds.), *Emotions, aggression, and morality in children: Bridging development and psychopathology* (pp. 137–156). Washington, DC: American Psychological Association.

Maughan, B., Pickles, A., Rowe, R., Costello, E. J., & Angold, A. (2000). Developmental trajectories of aggressive and non-aggressive conduct problems. *Journal of Quantitative Criminology, 16,* 199–221.

McMahon, R. J., Witkiewitz, K., Kotler, J. S., & the Conduct Problems Prevention Research Group. (2010). Predictive validity of callous–unemotional traits measures in early adolescence with respect to multiple antisocial outcomes. *Journal of Abnormal Psychology, 119,* 752–763.

Moffitt, T. E. (2006). Life-course persistent versus adolescence-limited antisocial behavior. In D. Cicchetti & D. J. Cohen (Eds.), *Developmental psychopathology: Vol. 3. Risk, disorder, and adaptation* (2nd ed., pp. 570–598). New York: Wiley.

Moffitt, T. E., Arseneault, L., Jaffee, S. R., Kim-Cohen, J., Koenen, K. C., Odgers, C. L., et al. (2008). Research review: DSM-V conduct disorder: Research needs for an evidence base. *Journal of Child Psychology and Psychiatry, 49,* 3–33.

Moffitt, T. E., Caspi, A., Dickson, N., Silva, P., & Stanton, W. (1996). Childhood-onset versus adolescent-onset antisocial conduct problems in males: Natural history from ages 3 to 18 years. *Development and Psychopathology, 8,* 399–424.

Monuteaux, M. C., Fitzmaurice, G., Blacker, D., Buka, S. L., & Biederman, J. (2004). Specificity in the familial aggregation of overt and covert conduct disorder symptoms in a referred attention-deficit hyperactivity disorder sample. *Psychological Medicine, 34,* 1113–1127.

Moul, C., Killcross, S., & Dadds, M. R. (2012). A model of differential amygdala activation in psychopathy. *Psychological Review, 119,* 789–806.

Munoz, L. C., Frick, P. J., Kimonis, E. R., & Aucoin, K. J. (2008). Verbal ability and delinquency: Testing the moderating role of psychopathic traits. *Journal of Child Psychology and Psychiatry, 49*(4), 414–421.

Nagin, D., & Tremblay, R. E. (1999). Trajectories of boys' physical aggression, opposition, and hyperactivity on the path to physically violent and nonviolent juvenile delinquency. *Child Development, 70,* 1181–1196.

Odgers, C. L., Caspi, A., Broadbent, J. M., Dickson, N., Hancox, R. J., Harrington, H., et al. (2007). Prediction of differential adult health burden by conduct problem subtypes in males. *Archives of General Psychiatry, 64*(4), 476–484.

Pardini, D. A., Frick, P. J., & Moffitt, T. E. (2010). Building an evidence base for DSM-5 conceptualizations of oppositional defiant disorder and conduct disorder: Introduction to the special section. *Journal of Abnormal Psychology, 119,* 683–688.

Pardini, D. A., Stepp, S., Hipwell, A., Stouthamer-Loeber, M., & Loeber, R. (2012). The clinical utility of the proposed DSM-5 callous–unemotional subtype of conduct disorder in young girls. *Journal of the American Academy of Child and Adolescent Psychiatry, 51,* 62–73.

Quay, H. C. (1987). Patterns of delinquent behavior. In H. C. Quay (Ed.), *Handbook of juvenile delinquency* (pp. 118–138). Oxford, UK: Wiley.

Quay, H. C. (1993). The psychobiology of undersocialized aggressive conduct disorder. *Development and Psychopathology, 5,* 165–180.

Robins, L. N. (1966). *Deviant children grown up.* Baltimore: Williams & Wilkins.

Rowe, R., Costello, E. J., Angold, A., Copeland, W. E., & Maughan, B. (2010). Developmental pathways in oppositional defiant disorder and conduct disorder. *Journal of Abnormal Psychology, 119,* 726–738.

Singh, J. P., Grann, M., & Fazel, S. (2011). A comparative study of risk assessment tools: A systematic review and metaregression analysis of 68 studies involving 25,980 participants. *Clinical Psychology Review, 31,* 499–513.

Stanger, C., Achenbach, T. M., & Verhulst, F. C. (1997). Accelerated longitudinal comparisons of aggressive versus delinquent syndromes. *Development and Psychopathology, 9,* 43–58.

Steinberg, L. (2014). *Age of opportunity: Lessons from the new science of adolescence.* Boston: Houghton Mifflin Harcourt.

Stringaris, A., & Goodman, R. (2009). Longitudinal outcome of youth oppositionality: Irritable, headstrong, and hurtful behaviors have distinctive predictions. *Journal of the American Academy of Child and Adolescent Psychiatry, 48,* 404–412.

Tackett, J. L. (2010). Toward an externalizing spectrum in DSM-V: Incorporating developmental concerns. *Child Development Perspectives, 4,* 161–167.

Tackett, J. L., Krueger, R. F., Iacono, W. G., & McGue, M. (2005). Symptom-based subfactors of DSM-defined conduct disorder: Evidence for etiologic distinctions. *Journal of Abnormal Psychology, 114,* 483–487.

Thompson, R. A., & Newton, E. K. (2010). Emotion in early conscience. In W. F. Arsenio & E. A. Lemerise (Eds.), *Emotions, aggression, and morality in children: Bridging development and psychopathology* (pp. 13–31). Washington, DC: American Psychological Association.

Tremblay, R. E. (2003). Why socialization fails: The case of chronic physical aggression. In B. B. Lahey, T. E. Moffitt, & A. Caspi (Eds.), *Causes of conduct disorder and juvenile delinquency* (pp. 182–224). New York: Guilford Press.

Tremblay, R. E. (2010). Developmental origins of disruptive behaviour problems: The original sin hypothesis, epigenetics and their consequences for prevention. *Journal of Child Psychology and Psychiatry, 51,* 341–367.

Waller, R., Gardner, F., Shaw, D. S., Dishion, T. J., Wilson, M. N., & Hyde, L. W. (2015). Callous–unemotional behavior and early-childhood onset of behavior problems: The role of parental harshness and warmth. *Journal of Clinical Child and Adolescent Psychology, 44,* 655–667.

Wilkinson, S., Waller, R., & Viding, E. (2016). Practitioner review: Involving young people with callous–unemotional traits in treatment: Does it work?: A systematic review. *Journal of Child Psychology and Psychiatry, 57,* 552–565.

CHAPTER 3

Developmental Trajectories of Aggression Subtypes

From Early to Late Childhood

JAMIE M. OSTROV, KRISTIN J. PERRY,
and SARAH J. BLAKELY-McCLURE

Brief Introduction

Aggression during childhood has been a topic of study within developmental psychology since the inception of our field. In fact, one of the first issues of the journal *Child Development* included a brief report on egocentric behavior that examined preschool children during free play and included an assessment of aggression (Ezekiel, 1931). This report focused on individual differences in egocentric behavior of preschoolers during free play, and the author attempted to examine changes in egocentric behavior and associations with "aggressive" behavior (e.g., taking toys and "aggression towards other children"; Ezekiel, 1931, p. 75). Ezekiel (1931) reported that over the 3 months of preschool observation, "unaggressive children become more egocentric in their play, changing from the unaggressive to the aggressive" (p. 75). In the same year, at the University of Minnesota, Florence Goodenough (1931) published a report on anger in the young child that would inspire developmental scholars to continue to pursue the study of aggression and associated emotions for decades to come. Furthermore, as a sign of the future research tradition of examining the role of gender in aggression, Hattwick (1937) examined sex differences in behavior of nursery school children attending a public nursery school in Chicago and recorded "aggressive extroverted behavior" (p. 344). Collectively, these historical references suggest that aggression has been a topic of developmental study since the inception of the field and that this has been evidenced by the many hundreds of studies and reviews pertaining to the onset, course, and developmental trajectories associated with aggression in children (e.g., Eisner & Malti, 2015). This chapter adds to this rich tradition by focusing on the various forms and functions of aggressive behavior from early (i.e., 3- to 5-year-olds) to late (i.e., 10-year-olds) childhood. We raise key issues, discuss theoretical and methodological considerations in the developmental study of aggression subtypes during the first decade of life, present major substantive research findings within the literature that support the articulated theory and highlight developmental trajectories, and conclude with implications as well as future directions.

Main Issues

There are several key questions that guide developmental science focused on aggression. These include the delineation of the antecedents (e.g., role of socializing agents), onset, and course (e.g., evidence of continuity) associated with aggression subtypes. More specifically, a goal of contemporary scholars has been to identify specific developmental trajectories associated with individual forms of aggression or the associations between subtypes of aggression. Additionally, scholars have been grappling with associations and predictions of key outcomes, including social-psychological adjustment problems and indices of psychopathology.

The overall definition of aggression is behavior intended to physically or psychologically harm or hurt another person (Eisner & Malti, 2015). Contemporary scholars have recognized the importance of delineating both the different forms or "whats," as well as the different functions or "whys," of aggressive behavior (Little, Jones, Henrich, & Hawley, 2003). We acknowledge that these terms have different historical definitions within the field. For example, within the study of culture and human development, Bornstein (1995) used *form* to imply behavior, activity, or cognition, and *function* was used in reference to the purpose or meaning given to the form (see also Bornstein, 2012). Thus, for example, Bornstein argued that the same form could have different meanings or functions in various contexts. Little and colleagues (2003), as well as Prinstein and Cillessen (2003), have since reintroduced these terms to imply either the way in which the aggressive behavior may manifest (i.e., form) or the reason for the aggressive act (i.e., function), and we therefore use these terms in this chapter. There are numerous forms of aggressive behavior that could be explored herein; however, this material has been presented elsewhere (e.g., Murray-Close, Nelson, Ostrov, Casas, & Crick, 2016). In the present chapter, we generally restrict our scope to two forms (i.e., physical and relational) and two functions (i.e., proactive and reactive) of aggressive behavior that are often studied during childhood (Crick, Ostrov, & Kawabata, 2007).

Physical aggression is defined as the use of physical force or the threat of physical harm to hurt or injure another person; physical aggression includes such behaviors as hitting, kicking, punching, biting, pulling, and taking things away from others (Crick et al., 2006; Eisner & Malti, 2015). *Relational aggression* is defined as the removal or threat of the removal of a relationship with the intent of harming another person in one way or another (Crick & Grotpeter, 1995); relational aggression includes such acts as spreading malicious gossip, rumors, secrets, or lies about a peer, as well as verbal and nonverbal indicators of social exclusion (e.g., "You can't play with us," "You are not my friend anymore," or "You can't come to my birthday party"). Relational aggression is displayed differently across development, with behavior during early childhood typically being more direct, overt, and based on current circumstances (Crick, Ostrov, Appleyard, Jansen, & Casas, 2004). Furthermore, among young children, the identity of the perpetrator is typically known, which is not always the case during later developmental periods (e.g., adolescence) when covert tactics and indirect manifestations of the behavior are common (Crick et al., 2004).

As we have recently stated in a chapter on definitions of aggression (see Ostrov, Blakely-McClure, Perry, & Kamper-DeMarco, 2018; for a historical and comprehensive review, see Murray-Close et al., 2016), there is not consensus within the field (e.g., Archer & Coyne, 2005; Card, Stucky, Sawalani, & Little, 2008; Vaillancourt, 2005), but our interpretation of the current extant literature is that relational aggression is similar to but arguably unique from indirect and social aggression, which are two related and important constructs that appear in the literature. To be fair, depending on the developmental period, the differences may be subtle or perhaps nonexistent (Archer & Coyne, 2005; Card et al., 2008; Coyne, Archer, & Eslea, 2006; Vaillancourt, 2005), but we argue that from a definitional perspective there are unique features that represent potentially important theoretical and applied considerations. Importantly, contemporary researchers qualified the historical definition of the *indirect aggression* construct (e.g., Allport, Burer, & Jandorf, 1941; Buss, 1961; Feshbach, 1969) in meaningful ways. For example, Björkqvist and colleagues argued that indirect aggression is a form of aggression that involves "circumventory behavior" (Lagerspetz, Björkqvist, & Peltonen, 1988, p. 409) and the aggressor "makes it seem as though there has been no intention to hurt at all . . . to remain unidentified" (Björkqvist, Lagerspetz, & Kaukiainen, 1992, p. 118). Theorists who study indirect aggression have also argued that the behaviors require emotional intelligence that would not be present among very young children (Kaukiainen et al., 1999). More recent conceptualizations of indirect aggression acknowledge that the behavior may involve "in rare cases physical" harm via social manipulation (Björkqvist et al., 2001, pp. 112–113), which is not part of the operational definition of the relational aggression construct. In addition, indirect aggression has been conceptualized to include property destruction behaviors (e.g., putting gum on a peer's chair; Goldstein, Tisak, & Boxer, 2002), which would also not apply to the definition of relational aggression. Given the aforementioned definitional considerations, it is not surprising that *indirect aggression,* which is usually displayed anonymously (i.e., the identity of the aggressor is not known to the victim), may be less common in early childhood than in later developmental periods (Vaillancourt, Miller, Fagbemi, Cote, & Tremblay, 2007).

Social aggression is a broader construct and uniquely includes verbal insults and nonverbal aggression such as eye rolling, dirty looks, hair tossing, and glares that are intended to damage the self-esteem and social status of the victim (Galen & Underwood, 1997; Underwood, 2004). Thus a focus on self-esteem and social status, as well as the inclusion of negative facial expressions and verbal insults, make social aggression a construct unique from relational aggression. Relevant findings from indirect and social aggression constructs during early and middle childhood are included in this chapter.

Proactive aggression has been defined as behavior that is purposeful, premeditated, instrumental, or goal oriented (Dodge, 1991). *Reactive aggression* has been defined as behavior that is retaliatory, hostile, or impulsive (Dodge, 1991). Contemporary scholars have been examining the development of both forms (i.e., physical and relational) and functions (i.e., proactive and reactive aggression) by crossing these two dimensions to create four "types" of aggressive behaviors (i.e., proactive physical, proactive relational, reactive physical, reactive relational; Prinstein & Cillessen, 2003). There are interesting developmental trajectories associated with these subtypes of aggression that are reviewed in subsequent sections, but it is important to note that despite high overlap among these constructs (e.g., proactive and reactive relational aggression), there does appear to be utility to examining the unique contribution of these subtypes in longitudinal studies. For example, in our own work with young children (3–5 years old), we have documented that reactive relational aggression predicted increases in peer rejection, whereas proactive relational aggression predicted significant decreases in peer rejection (Ostrov, Murray-Close, Godleski, & Hart, 2013). Collectively, this work suggests the potential for differential developmental trajectories associated with forms and functions of aggression.

Theoretical Considerations

Developmental Psychopathology

As a discipline, developmental psychopathology strives to integrate across frameworks to understand maladaptive behavior and its relation to typical behavior across numerous domains (Cicchetti & Rogosch, 2002). Developmental psychopathology has been defined as "the study of the origins and course of individual patterns of behavioral maladaptation" (Sroufe & Rutter, 1984, p. 18). There is a particular emphasis on elucidating the normative and pathological mechanisms that combine in a dynamic bidirectional fashion to promote maladaptive behavior, as well as on potential moderators that may contribute to different trajectories of maladaptive behavior (Sroufe, 2013; Sroufe & Rutter, 1984). Additionally, in contrast with a medical model of maladaptation, the effect of one factor on behavioral development is considered within the context of all other factors, and thus maladaptation is never the result of a single genetic or environmental trait but is an integrative and cumulative developmental process (Sroufe, 1997). From this perspective, aggression is considered to result from the interaction of normative and maladaptive characteristics at the biological (i.e., genetic, physiological, temperamental), social, and cognitive domains and at multiple levels of analysis (e.g., dyadic and group).

One core concept within the developmental psychopathology framework is the notion of key developmental tasks, which reflect crucial tasks of competence through which adjustment within a developmental period is assessed (for a review, see Masten & Coatsworth, 1998; Sroufe, 2013). From this perspective, increased risk for aggressive behavior may be a result of the child's failure to master key developmental tasks, such as formation of secure attachment in infancy, the development of self-regulation during early childhood, or creating positive competent relationships with peers during middle childhood (Murray-Close et al., 2016; Sroufe, 2013).

A developmental psychopathology perspective would suggest that failure to develop a secure relationship with a primary attachment figure would place children at risk for becoming relationally aggressive. To this end, Michiels, Grietens, Onghena, and Kuppens (2008) proposed a heuristic model whereby the link between nonsupportive or insensitive caregiving and relational aggression in children is mediated by the child's representations of the parent–child relationship (i.e., negative internal working model and lack of secure base). According to this model, a case could be made for links between both avoidant and ambivalent-resistant attachment and relational aggression, but the authors argue that the manifestation of the behavior may change based on the attachment history (e.g., use of the silent treatment for children with avoidant attachment histories and relational aggression directed to close friends for children with ambivalent-resistant histories; Michiels et al., 2008). The link between a history of maltreatment and relational aggression has been documented (Cullerton-Sen et al., 2008; Perry & Price, 2017), and thus, although we are unaware of any current studies, we could also anticipate direct links between Type D, or disorganized, attachment and relational aggression as well. Consistent with this overall approach, a number of scholars have tested links between psychological control, parental support, attachment security, and relational aggression during early (e.g., Hart, Nelson, Robinson, Olsen, & McNeilly-Choque, 1998) and middle (e.g., Park et al., 2005) childhood. There is also evidence for the legacy of these effects well into adolescence (i.e., attachment security may mediate links between parental psychological control and relational aggression within adolescent friendships; Soenens, Vansteenkiste, Goossens, Duriez, & Niemiec, 2008).

Another theoretical approach to the study of aggression is the *social-ecological* approach, wherein behavioral development is theorized to be a product of the bidirectional interaction between individuals and the systems within which they reside (Bronfenbrenner, 1979; Espelage & Swearer, 2010). Within this framework, aggression is maintained through individual factors or youth characteristics (e.g., intelligence, health status, sexual orientation, psychopathology), as well as through cues from the child's peers, teachers, family (e.g., parent–child and sibling relationships), community, media, and culture (Hong & Espelage, 2012).

At an individual level of analysis, temperament, or individual dispositions in social–emotional responding that comprises two central components of reactivity and regulation, may play an important role in the trajectory of a child's aggressive behavior (Lahey & Waldman, 2003). For example, children who have emotion regulation deficits may be at risk for using *reactively* aggressive acts because they may be prone to using aggression when emotionally aroused (Frick & Morris, 2004). Alternatively, children who display callous–unemotional (CU) traits may be probabilistically more likely to engage in *proactive,* instrumental, premeditated, or goal-oriented functions of both physical and relational forms of aggression (e.g., Marsee & Frick, 2007).

In order to address the other levels of analysis and how they interact with the individual level, we consider the seminal theoretical contribution of Robert A. Hinde, who has articulated the importance of the sociocultural structure of the group (Hinde, 1987). Hinde (1987) uses an ethological perspective to argue that multiple levels of analysis should be considered and that the reciprocal dynamic

bidirectional and "dialectical" interactions should be examined among the different levels within the social ecology (p. 21). Moreover, Hinde argues that individual
characteristics (e.g., nervous or endocrine system–mediated processes, gender)
affect behavioral styles, which influence and are influenced by close relationships
with others and, importantly, that the role of these different successive levels of
social complexity obtain their meanings from a given culture. As Hinde states: "Nevertheless group structure, relationships and interactions affect, and are affected by,
the socio-cultural structure" (p. 26).

Social Information-Processing Theory

One social information-processing (SIP) model of children's social adjustment was
developed by Dodge and colleagues (Crick & Dodge, 1994; Dodge, 1986). The SIP
model posits that the child plays an active role in his or her environment, wherein
the child processes cues and makes decisions based on the type of social situation
he or she experiences (Dodge, 1986). The SIP model and associated theoretical
extensions (e.g., Crick & Dodge, 1994; Lemerise & Arsenio, 2000) have been a common organizing framework within the aggression subtypes literature and, as such,
are given an extended review in the present chapter. According to the SIP model,
children have a "database" of past social experiences, including schemas, memories,
and scripts, which guide their behavior and responses in social scenarios (Crick &
Dodge, 1994, p. 76). This database helps guide children's social interactions and
behavior within these interactions through a six-step process: (1) encoding of cues,
(2) interpretation of cues, (3) clarification of goals, (4) response access or construction, (5) response decision, and (6) behavioral enactment (Crick & Dodge, 1994).
One of the most thoroughly researched components of the SIP model is Step 2,
interpretation of cues, for which the majority of the research has focused on hostile attribution biases (HAB), leading researchers to hypothesize that children who
infer hostile intent from an ambiguous provocation are more likely to react with a
display of aggressive behavior (see Orobio de Castro, Veerman, Koops, Bosch, &
Monshouwer, 2002).

Beyond HAB as a risk factor for aggression, Crick, Geiger, and Zimmer-Gembeck (2003) posited a relational vulnerability model, wherein HAB for relational
provocations confers relationally aggressive behavior only for children who are
already vulnerable in their interpersonal relationships (see also Mathieson et al.,
2011). Recent research has supported this hypothesis; for girls in middle childhood,
HAB has been found to be associated only with relational aggression if relational
victimization (i.e., receipt of relational aggression) and emotional distress (i.e.,
emotional sensitivity to relational provocation situations, e.g., being upset when a
peer does not invite one to a party), two relationship vulnerabilities, were elevated
(Mathieson et al., 2011).

There are many similar frameworks to the SIP model of children's adjustment.
For example, Krasnor and Rubin (1981) and Rubin and Krasnor (1986) introduced
an information-processing model of social problem solving. This model articulates
several levels of analysis (e.g., "individual acts" and "social effects") to understand
children's social skills and problem-solving strategies and argues for the importance of examining the child's own affect and relationship quality between children

involved in a social interaction (Rubin, Bream, & Rose-Krasnor, 1991). This model posits, for example, that socially withdrawn children attribute negative events to stable, internal causes and engage in self-blame (Dwyer et al., 2010), which is consistent with the notion of characterological self-blame and Graham and Juvonen's (1998) attribution model of peer victimization.

An additional information-processing script model was also proposed by Huesmann (1988). This model posits that children acquire scripts or cognitive guides for behavior, which are reinforced through observational learning and become more entrenched across development via frequent activation of the scripts (Huesmann, 1988). Moreover, the general aggression model (GAM), as proposed by social psychologists Anderson and Bushman (2002), integrates across several theories, including Huesmann's script theory, and was developed as a parsimonious model to examine multiple motives of aggression. The GAM has been used extensively for understanding the role of exposure to media and subsequent physical and relational aggression in children and adolescents (e.g., Gentile, Coyne, & Walsh, 2010).

Gender-Linked Models

It has been theorized that gender may moderate the SIP patterns that children have, such that gender schemas are relevant to the database and thus are incorporated in every step of the SIP model (see the integrated gender-linked model of aggression subtypes; Ostrov & Godleski, 2010). Gender schemas are influenced by various socialization agents (e.g., family members, peers, media), and these directly and indirectly modify the child's self-construal and gender identity, influencing the child's social knowledge and encoding/interpretation of cues. Beyond socialization, in Step 6 of the SIP model, the child retains information about the utility of the aggressive act, so that gender-consistent acts increase future processing speed and gender-inconsistent acts will be forgotten and avoided and the likelihood of the child using the act in the future is reduced. This history of adaptation (e.g., prior gender and self-relevant experiences) is theorized to directly influence the encoding, storage, and memory retrieval processes (Ostrov & Godleski, 2010). Consistent with this gender-informed SIP model, through socialization and gender schemas, girls may encode, recall, and display more relationally aggressive behaviors, and boys may encode, recall, and display more physically aggressive behaviors (Ostrov, 2008; Ostrov & Godleski, 2010). This integrative SIP model further predicts that due to socialization processes, history of adaptation, and formation of self- and gender-relevant schemas, girls should engage in proportionally more relational aggression than physical aggression, and it further supports the common finding that physical aggression is the modal form of aggression among boys in early and middle childhood. Ettekal and Ladd (2015) found support for the model among girls on a high-relational-aggression and low-physical-aggression trajectory. Specifically, Ettekal and Ladd found that these girls were more likely than girls on other trajectories (e.g., a high co-occurring relational and physical pathway) to more effectively use relational aggression with their peers. Thus, when examining trajectories of aggression, it is still important to consider the potential moderating role of gender.

Gender may also play a role in the relation between aggression and peer victimization. The specificity hypothesis of aggression is consistent with the notion of reciprocity and dynamic bidirectional interactions that Hinde (1987) articulated and proposes that children are victimized based on their own acts of aggression and thus that the type of aggression a child displays should predict reciprocity or the type of victimization they experience (Crick, Casas, & Ku, 1999; Ostrov, 2008). In the specificity model, the relational aggression exhibited by girls will predict future relational victimization, and the physical aggression exhibited by boys will predict future physical victimization (Crick et al., 1999; Ostrov, 2008). There is evidence in support of this theory, as relational aggression uniquely predicts future relational victimization and physical aggression uniquely predicts future physical victimization for children in early childhood (Ostrov, 2008). The converse is also supported: Relational victimization predicts increases only in relational aggression, and physical victimization predicts increases only in physical aggression (Ostrov, 2010). This finding adds support to the specificity hypothesis and underscores the bidirectional nature of the relation between aggression and victimization.

Measures and Methods

Multiple methods can be used to assess aggressive behavior, and thus our focus is on those used in assessments of the developmental trajectories outlined within this chapter. We can assess both physical and relational aggression through parent, teacher, peer, and child reports; structured interviews; and behavioral observations. All of the measures listed below have sound psychometric properties and, as far as we know, are freely available for use by scientists (see the cited references for specific details). Space restrictions preclude a comprehensive review and evaluation of all relevant measures that distinguish between physical and relational aggression (see Crick et al., 2007), so we highlight a few measures and methods in order to demonstrate common approaches to the study of aggression subtypes in childhood.

Teacher, Parent, and Child Reports

A measure that shows considerable promise is the MacArthur Health and Behavior Questionnaire (HBQ), which may be used to study relational and physical aggression among other constructs and has parallel versions for parents and teachers and corresponding self-report versions (Boyce et al., 2002; Essex et al., 2002).

Structured Interviews

The Social Relations Questionnaire (SRQ) is a seven-item structured interview (Lahey et al., 2004) that has been previously used with children and their parents in middle to late childhood to assess the child's relationally aggressive behavior (Tackett & Ostrov, 2010; Tackett, Waldman, & Lahey, 2009). Interviews may present challenges related to the ability of the child to be able to report on his or her own behaviors. Young children may have difficulty providing information about their own behavior, but in our experience developmentally appropriate interview techniques may foster valid reports of aggression among young children.

Peer Reports of Aggression

Peer nomination and peer rating measures are a widely used method to assess peer relations and social behaviors (e.g., Khatri & Kupersmidt, 2003; Prakash & Coplan, 2007). These methods have traditionally been used to assess peer relationships (e.g., likeability, friendship identification; see Rubin, Bukowski, & Bowker, 2015) but also may assess aggression in children. Peer rating systems often have children rate on a scale how aggressive each child is within the classroom or social group. Peer nominations have children list (or point to pictures of their peers) in a limited (up to three) or an unlimited (as many names as they like) manner those children that are aggressive. One typical peer assessment approach is to use the revised class play (Masten, Morison, & Pellegrini, 1985). This instrument was modified by Rubin and colleagues as the "extended class play," which is a psychometrically strong procedure for making distinctions between forms of aggression and social withdrawal, among other peer-relations constructs (see Malti, McDonald, Rubin, Rose-Krasnor, & Booth-LaForce, 2015; Rubin et al., 2015). For example, assessments of relational (e.g., "Someone who spreads rumors so that other people won't like them") and physical aggression (e.g., "Someone who hits, kicks, or punches others") were reliable and associated with theoretically relevant outcomes in a U.S. sample of sixth graders (Bowker & Etkin, 2014).

Structured Observations

Naturalistic observations of aggression can be assessed by the Early Childhood Observation System (ECOS); this observational taxonomy assesses young children's relational and physical aggression (Crick et al., 2006; Ostrov & Keating, 2004). The ECOS uses a focal child sampling with continuous recording approach; each child is observed for 10 minutes per assessment by a trained observer, who is located in an unobtrusive position in the classroom or on the playground. Typically, each child is observed eight times (a total of 80 minutes), and observers record the focal child's engagement in both physical and relational aggression. Responses to aggression are recorded with the ECOS, so it is designed for examining reciprocity, but no known published research has addressed this question. There are additional observational systems that have been used to study relational and physical aggression, including a scan sampling approach (McNeilly-Choque, Hart, Robinson, Nelson, & Olsen, 1996), other direct structured observation approaches (Juliano, Werner, & Cassidy, 2006; McEvoy, Estrem, Rodriguez, & Olson, 2003), as well as semistructured observational paradigms (e.g., Stauffacher & DeHart, 2006) in early childhood. Aggressive behaviors may become more covert with development (Crick et al., 2007), and observations in the school may be challenging to conduct without advanced technology such as remote audiovisual observational systems (e.g., Craig & Pepler, 1997; Pepler & Craig, 1995). In middle childhood, there are also a few observational options for studying both forms of aggression, and these include the use of remote audiovisual assessments of indirect, relational, and physical aggression (Tapper & Boulton, 2000) and systematic lunchroom observations (Putallaz et al., 2007). Additional approaches are available in adolescence that are outside the developmental scope of this chapter (e.g., Underwood, Scott, Galperin, Bjornstad, & Sexton, 2004).

Central Research Findings

Developmental Manifestations

Relational aggression is believed to be manifested differently in the early versus later years of childhood. Rudimentary social exclusion and other relationally aggressive behaviors have been observed in children as young as 30 months of age (Crick et al., 2006). In early childhood studies (i.e., 3–5 years old), relational aggression has been described as being rather direct, with the identity of the perpetrator known to the victim and the content of the aggressive event based on the here and now rather than on a past transgression (Crick et al., 2007). Even when relational aggression is displayed in a more sophisticated or covert way (e.g., spreading a secret), it is done in a relatively overt manner, and all parties are privy to the identity of the aggressor and the content of the act (Ostrov, Woods, Jansen, Casas, & Crick, 2004). In middle childhood, relational aggression becomes a bit more covert and is more likely to be manifested in more sophisticated ways, such as spreading malicious rumors, gossip, and lies about others. The relationship context may also differ from early to middle childhood. That is, relational aggression may be more common among involuntary sibling relationships relative to voluntary friendships in early childhood (Stauffacher & DeHart, 2006).

Physical aggression is also manifested in slightly different ways across early and middle childhood. Comparatively, there are many more studies examining the developmental trajectories of physical aggression relative to relational aggression, and we direct interested readers to prior reviews on physical aggression (see Moffitt, 2007; Tremblay & Nagin, 2005; Vitaro, Boivin, & Tremblay, 2007). One recent and notable study demonstrated that developmental precursors to physical aggression were evident in infancy (i.e., 6 months of age; Hay et al., 2014). Specifically, the authors found that individual differences in early expressions of anger (i.e., temperamental dysregulation) and displays of physical force during infancy were predictive of physically aggressive behavior when the participants were 3 years old (Hay et al., 2014). Importantly, the precursors resembled the later displays of physical aggression. Continuity in behavior was observed for negative emotionality and physical force across the study, and the same social and prenatal risk factors (i.e., male gender, low socioeconomic status, exposure to mother's prenatal smoking, and mother's prenatal mood and antisocial problems) were associated with both precursors to and later manifestations of physical aggression (Hay et al., 2014). A second point to make about the developmental manifestation of physical aggression, and specifically age changes in the morphology of aggression, is that forcibly taking things away from others, or object aggression, is more evident among younger children (Cummings, Iannotti, & Zahn-Waxler, 1989), whereas more sophisticated verbal threats of physical harm rely on the use of expressive language and therefore emerge later (Hartup, 1974). Surprisingly, since Goodenough's (1931) seminal work, the field has not progressed very far, and we still do not have a great understanding of the specific developmental timing associated with different types of physical aggression for typically developing children. That is, it is conceivable that biting peaks at a different age relative to punching and kicking, which presumably require greater motor coordination, but no known work has addressed this topic, and future developmental studies are clearly needed.

Trajectories of Physical Aggression

Generally, children experience an increase in physical aggression from infancy into toddlerhood and early childhood (Naerde, Ogden, Janson, & Zachrisson, 2014) and a decrease in physical aggression beginning around age 5 through middle childhood into preadolescence (Côté, Vaillancourt, LeBlanc, Nagin, & Tremblay, 2006; National Institute of Child Health and Human Development Early Child Care and Research Network (NICHD ECCRN), 2004; Tremblay et al., 2005). With the transition to formal school, and as sanctions increase for displays of physical aggression, the typical developmental trend is a major reduction in hitting, pushing, and engaging in physical fights (NICHD ECCRN, 2004). A small percentage of children do stay elevated relative to their peers (i.e., children classified as life course persistent [LCP]), and they require increased surveillance from mental health professionals (see Moffitt, 1993).

Researchers have identified different trajectories of physical aggression during these periods (Côté et al., 2006; Malti et al., 2015; NICHD ECCRN, 2004; Tremblay et al., 2005). Researchers suggest that there are at least three general physical aggression trajectories and that, although they are slightly different, they are roughly comparable with the three trajectories found in adolescence (e.g., Cleverley, Szatmari, Vaillancourt, Boyle, & Lipman, 2012). The first trajectory is the typical case: Physically aggressive behavior remains infrequent across the different developmental periods (Côté et al., 2006; NICHD ECCRN, 2004; Tremblay et al., 2005). The second trajectory may best be described as involving groups of children who increasingly use physical aggression from infancy into toddlerhood and early childhood, followed by a decrease in aggression as children enter into formal schooling and middle childhood such that by the time children reach preadolescence they almost never use aggression (Côté et al., 2006; NICHD ECCRN, 2004; Tremblay et al., 2005). The majority of children fall into the first two trajectory groupings, such that, even if they exhibit physical aggression early on, this aggression decreases by middle childhood (Côté et al., 2006; NICHD ECCRN, 2004; Tremblay et al., 2005). Lastly, there is a trajectory encompassing a high physically aggressive group which is relatively stable; children in this group demonstrate high levels of physical aggression from infancy into toddlerhood and early childhood and continue to exhibit high levels of physical aggression into middle childhood and preadolescence (Côté et al., 2006; NICHD ECCRN, 2004; Tremblay et al., 2005). It is important to note that even for children in this high physical aggression trajectory, aggression in third grade was not as high as it was at 3 years of age; thus these children experience a decrease in physical aggression but are still consistently higher on physical aggression relative to those on the other trajectories (NICHD ECCRN, 2004). As mentioned above, these children are often described as being on an LCP (Moffitt, 1993) or "early-onset/persistent" pathway (Aguilar, Sroufe, Egeland, & Carlson, 2000).

Despite theory and some findings suggesting particular temperament profiles or neuropsychological functioning deficits (Moffitt, 1993), these findings have not always been replicated in prospective longitudinal research (Aguilar et al., 2000). In fact, a recent meta-analysis revealed that the LCP pathway was predicted by criminal history, aggressive behavior (i.e., both physical and nonphysical forms), and substance use factors, which were all large effects (Assink et al., 2015). Familial and neurocognitive/physiology (i.e., intelligence, verbal ability, resting heart rate) domains accounted for only small effects in the prediction of LCP, and neighborhood factors and physical health factors (e.g., prior head injury) had no effect (Assink et al., 2015). The moderating role of peer rejection and association with delinquent peers in the prediction of LCP status was the strongest during childhood relative to adolescence (Assink et al., 2015).

Trajectories of Relational Aggression

In early childhood, observers have been able to reliably identify relational aggression in children as young as 2½ years old (Crick et al., 2006). Moreover, relational aggression may be more stable across early childhood for girls compared with boys, suggesting that relational aggression may solidify at an earlier age for girls (Crick et al., 2006). As children move from early childhood into middle childhood, they may begin to replace physical aggression with relational aggression because there are fewer social sanctions for relational compared with physical aggression (Murray-Close et al., 2016). In support of this theory, a significant number of children on a decreasing physical aggression trajectory from toddlerhood to middle childhood showed increases in indirect aggression (Côté et al., 2006). This finding was more common for girls compared with boys (Côté et al., 2006). Once children reach middle childhood, developmental trajectories of relational aggression also seem to vary by gender (Murray-Close, Ostrov, & Crick, 2007; Spieker et al., 2012). In one study, from fourth to fifth grade, girls showed an increase over time in the use of relational aggression, whereas boys experienced no change in relational aggression (Murray-Close et al., 2007). Researchers using data (i.e., a composite of mother and teacher reports) from the NICHD Study of Early Child Care and Youth Development found that from ages 8 to 11, gender differences were documented in the unique (i.e., controlling for physical aggression) growth parameters of relational aggression in late middle childhood and specifically revealed that girls had higher intercepts for relational aggression and did not exhibit a declining slope. Boys had lower intercepts and declining slopes from third to sixth grade (Spieker et al., 2012), as predicted by the integrated gender-linked model of aggression subtypes (Ostrov & Godleski, 2010). Moreover, maladaptive outcomes were documented only for girls with higher relational aggression at the intercept or in third grade (Spieker et al., 2012). Researchers using data from the same project found that fifth-grade relational aggression was more strongly predictive of relational aggression for adolescent girls compared with boys, suggesting that relational aggression may be more stable for girls (Blakely-McClure & Ostrov, 2016). Adolescent trajectories of indirect aggression are outside of the scope of the present chapter, but they do suggest three distinct developmental trajectories (i.e., low declining, moderate declining, and high), as well as joint trajectories in which the most common trajectory demonstrated moderate declining levels of both indirect and physical aggression (Cleverley et al., 2012).

Understanding these developmental trajectories is important because physical and relational aggression have also been found to be associated with a host of social-psychological adjustment outcomes across development (see Murray-Close et al., 2016). In sum, the subtypes of aggression described in this chapter have been associated with such externalizing problems as attention-deficit/hyperactivity disorder (ADHD) (Waschbusch, Willoughby, & Pelham, 1998; Zalecki & Hinshaw, 2004), as well as such internalizing problems as depressed affect and anxiety (Murray-Close et al., 2007). Both physical and relational aggression are associated with substance use (e.g., Skara et al., 2008) and personality pathology features (e.g., Tackett, Herzhoff, Reardon, De Clercq, & Sharp, 2014). Relational aggression has also been associated with some adaptive outcomes during middle childhood and early adolescence, which many scholars have termed the "double-edged sword" effect. For example, in one study, on the one hand, relational aggression was associated with such problems as internalizing difficulties, but it was also associated with dynamic increases in friendship intimacy (Murray-Close et al., 2007). Similarly, Banny, Heilbron, Ames, and Prinstein (2011) found that high levels of initial relationally aggressive talk predicted increases in both positive and negative friendship quality 6 months later and argued that relational aggression may be associated with both adaptive and maladaptive outcomes among adolescents with reciprocated friendships. Relatedly, in a sample of fourth graders using the actor–partner interdependence model, boys' best friends' likeability was negatively associated with overt or physical aggression, whereas among girls, best friends' popularity status was positively associated with relational aggression (Peters, Cillessen, Riksen-Walraven, & Haselager, 2010). Interestingly, Malti and colleagues (2015) found that children who were more socially skilled at understanding friendship formation processes (i.e., reciprocity, self-disclosure, and trust) were more likely to be represented in the decreasing trajectory group compared with other aggression groups, which has clear implications for intervention work as children make the transition into early adolescence.

Implications

There are clear intervention implications, depending on the type of aggression that is considered. With that said, it is also highly probable that our lack of attention to other forms of aggression (e.g., verbal aggression; Ostrov & Keating, 2004) and other functions or reasons for engaging in aggression (e.g., avoiding trouble and maintaining relationships within the peer group; Delveaux & Daniels, 2000) limits our understanding of the development of aggression. Collectively, the findings reviewed in this chapter suggest that efforts should continue to develop evidence-based intervention and prevention efforts among young children and school-age children for multiple subtypes of aggression (see Leff, Waasdorp, & Crick, 2010). Admittedly, these efforts may be more challenging for relational aggression, as there appear to be significant social benefits to engaging in relational aggression during middle childhood and adolescence (e.g., Banny et al., 2011; Murray-Close et al., 2007). However, we argue that the costs of the behavior to the aggressor and victim (e.g., Rudolph, Troop-Gordon, Monti, & Miernicki, 2014) justify our intervention efforts.

Future Directions and Conclusions

As reviewed in the preceding sections, there are relatively limited published data on relational aggression trajectories from long-term longitudinal studies in early and middle childhood. In fact, the longest known longitudinal studies have focused on the transition from middle childhood to adolescence (e.g., Spieker et al., 2012) with only a few that address the important transition from preschool to formal school (e.g., Gower, Lingras, Mathieson, Kawabata, & Crick, 2014). Future longitudinal studies are needed to fully examine the onset of relational aggression in the early childhood years and then follow the children as they make the transition to middle childhood and adolescence. It is feasible that relative to physical aggression, the pathways and trajectories that emerge from studies that examine the course of relational aggression from early childhood to adolescence will be different (e.g., Moffitt, 1993).

In conclusion, the study of aggression subtypes during childhood is advancing at a rapid pace. The field has been focusing on the development of physical and relational forms of aggression and proactive and reactive functions of aggression. However, it is clear that longitudinal research, beginning during the infant/toddler years, would allow a stronger perspective on the origins and putative outcomes of various forms and functions of aggressive behavior during the lifespan. Guided by theory and equipped with psychometrically sound methods, we are now well prepared to capitalize on interest in the forms and functions of childhood aggression to enable an improvement in the lives of high-risk children and their families.

ACKNOWLEDGMENTS

Preparation of this chapter was supported by a grant from the National Science Foundation (No. BCS-1450777) to Jamie M. Ostrov. We thank the University at Buffalo Social Development Lab members for comments on a prior draft and give special thanks to Hannah Holmlund for her assistance in the preparation of this chapter. We are also grateful to the directors, teachers, parents, and children who participated in the research described in this chapter.

REFERENCES

Aguilar, B., Sroufe, L. A., Egeland, B., & Carlson, E. (2000). Distinguishing the early-onset/persistent and adolescence-onset antisocial behavior types: From birth to 16 years. *Development and Psychopathology, 12,* 109–132.

Allport, G. W., Bruner, J. S., & Jandorf, E. M. (1941). Personality under social catastrophe: Ninety life-histories of the Nazi revolution. *Character and Personality: A Quarterly for Psychodiagnostic and Allied Studies, 10,* 1–22.

Anderson, C. A., & Bushman, B. J. (2002). Human aggression. *Annual Review of Psychology, 53,* 27–51.

Archer, J., & Coyne, S. M. (2005). An integrated review of indirect, relational, and social aggression. *Personality and Social Psychology Review, 9,* 212–230.

Assink, M., van der Put, C. E., Hoeve, M., de Vries, S. L. A., Stams, G. J. J. M., & Oort, F. J. (2015). Risk factors for persistent delinquent behavior among juveniles: A meta-analytic review. *Clinical Psychology Review, 42,* 47–61.

Banny, A. M., Heilbron, N., Ames, A., & Prinstein, M. J. (2011). Relational benefits of relational aggression: Adaptive and maladaptive associations with adolescent friendship quality. *Developmental Psychology, 47,* 1153–1166.

Björkqvist, K., Lagerspetz, K. M., & Kaukiainen, A. (1992). Do girls manipulate and boys fight?: Developmental trends in regard to direct and indirect aggression. *Aggressive Behavior, 18,* 117–127.

Björkqvist, K., Österman, K., Lagerspetz, K., Landau, S. F., Caprara, G., & Fraczek, A. (2001). Aggression, victimization and sociometric status: Findings from Finland, Israel, Italy and Poland. In J. M. Ramirez & D. S. Richardson (Eds.), *Cross-cultural approaches to research on aggression and reconciliation* (pp. 111–119). Huntington, NY: Nova Science.

Blakely-McClure, S. J., & Ostrov, J. M. (2016). Relational aggression, victimization and self concept: Testing pathways from middle childhood to adolescence. *Journal of Youth and Adolescence, 45,* 376–390.

Bornstein, M. H. (1995). Form and function: Implications for studies of culture and human development. *Culture and Psychology, 1,* 123–137.

Bornstein, M. H. (2012). Cultural approaches to parenting. *Parenting: Science and Practice, 12,* 212–221.

Bowker, J. C., & Etkin, R. G. (2014). Does humor explain why relationally aggressive adolescents are popular? *Journal of Youth and Adolescence, 43,* 1322–1332.

Boyce, W. T., Essex, M. J., Woodward, H. R., Measelle, J. R., Ablow, J. C., Kupfer, D. J., & the MacArthur Assessment Battery Working Group. (2002). The confluence of mental, physical, social, and academic difficulties in middle childhood: I. Exploring the "headwaters" of early life morbidities. *Journal of the American Academy of Child and Adolescent Psychiatry, 41,* 580–587.

Bronfenbrenner, U. (1979). *The ecology of human development: Experiments by nature and design.* Cambridge, MA: Harvard University Press.

Buss, A. H. (1961). *The psychology of aggression.* New York: Wiley.

Card, N. A., Stucky, B. D., Sawalani, G. M., & Little, T. D. (2008). Direct and indirect aggression during childhood and adolescence: A meta-analytic review of gender differences, intercorrelations, and relations to maladjustment. *Child Development, 79,* 1185–1229.

Cicchetti, D., & Rogosch, F. A. (2002). A developmental psychopathology perspective on adolescence. *Journal of Consulting and Clinical Psychology, 70,* 6–20.

Cleverley, K., Szatmari, P., Vaillancourt, T., Boyle, M., & Lipman, E. (2012). Developmental trajectories of physical and indirect aggression from late childhood to adolescence: Sex differences and outcomes in emerging adulthood. *Journal of the American Academy of Child and Adolescent Psychiatry, 51,* 1037–1051.

Côté, S. M., Vaillancourt, T., LeBlanc, J. C., Nagin, D. S., & Tremblay, R. E. (2006). The development of physical aggression from toddlerhood to pre-adolescence: A nationwide longitudinal study of Canadian children. *Journal of Abnormal Child Psychology, 34,* 71–85.

Coyne, S. M., Archer, J., & Eslea, M. (2006). "We're not friends anymore! Unless . . . ": The frequency and harmfulness of indirect, relational, and social aggression. *Aggressive Behavior, 32,* 294–307.

Craig, W., & Pepler, D. J. (1997). Observations of bullying and victimization in the school-yard. *Canadian Journal of School Psychology, 13,* 41–60.

Crick, N. R., Casas, J. F., & Ku, H. (1999). Relational and physical forms of peer victimization in preschool. *Developmental Psychology, 35,* 376–385.

Crick, N. R., & Dodge, K. A. (1994). A review and reformulation of social information processing mechanisms in children's social adjustment. *Psychological Bulletin, 115,* 74–101.

Crick, N. R., Geiger, T. C., & Zimmer-Gembeck, M. J. (2003, April). *Relational vulnerability: A model for understanding girls, aggression, and depressive symptoms.* Paper presented at the biennial meeting of the Society for Research on Child Development, Tampa, FL.

Crick, N. R., & Grotpeter, J. K. (1995). Relational aggression, gender, and social-psychological adjustment. *Child Development, 66,* 710–722.

Crick, N. R., Ostrov, J. M., Appleyard, K., Jansen, E. A., & Casas, J. F. (2004). Relational aggression in early childhood: "You can't come to my birthday party unless. . . ." In M. Putallaz & K. L. Bierman (Eds.), *Aggression, antisocial behavior, and violence among girls: A developmental perspective* (pp. 71–89). New York: Guilford Press.

Crick, N. R., Ostrov, J. M., Burr, J. E., Cullerton-Sen, C., Jansen-Yeh, E., & Ralston, P. (2006). A longitudinal study of relational and physical aggression in preschool. *Journal of Applied Developmental Psychology, 27,* 254–268.

Crick, N. R., Ostrov, J. M., & Kawabata, Y. (2007). Relational aggression and gender: An overview. In D. J. Flannery, A. T. Vazsonyi, & I. D. Waldman (Eds.), *The Cambridge handbook of violent behavior and aggression* (pp. 245–259). New York: Cambridge University Press.

Cullerton-Sen, C., Cassidy, A. R., Murray-Close, D., Cicchetti, D., Crick, N. R., & Rogosch, F. A. (2008). Childhood maltreatment and the development of relational and physical aggression: The importance of a gender-informed approach. *Child Development, 79*(6), 1736–1751.

Cummings, E. M., Iannotti, R. J., & Zahn-Waxler, C. (1989). Aggression between peers in early childhood: Individual continuity and developmental change. *Child Development, 60,* 887–895.

Delveaux, K. D., & Daniels, T. (2000). Children's social cognitions: Physically and relationally aggressive strategies and children's goals in peer conflict situations. *Merrill–Palmer Quarterly, 46,* 672–692.

Dodge, K. A. (1986). A social information processing model of social competence in children. In M. Perlmutter (Ed.), *Minnesota Symposia on Child Psychology: Vol. 18. Cognitive perspectives on children's social and behavioral development* (pp. 77–125). Hillsdale, NJ: Erlbaum.

Dodge, K. A. (1991). The structure and function of reactive and proactive aggression. In D. J. Pepler & K. H. Rubin (Eds.), *The development and treatment of childhood aggression* (pp. 201–218). Hillsdale, NJ: Erlbaum.

Dwyer, K. M., Fredstrom, B. K., Rubin, K. H., Booth-LaForce, C., Rose-Krasnor, L., & Burgess, K. B. (2010). Attachment, social information processing, and friendship quality of early adolescent girls and boys. *Journal of Social and Personal Relationships, 27,* 91–116.

Eisner, M. P., & Malti, T. (2015). Aggressive and violent behavior. In R. M. Lerner (Series Ed.) & M. E. Lamb (Vol. Ed.), *Handbook of child psychology and developmental science: Vol. 3. Socioemotional processes* (7th ed., pp. 795–884). New York: Wiley.

Espelage, D. L., & Swearer, S. M. (2010). A social-ecological model for bullying prevention and intervention: Understanding the impact of adults in the social ecology of youngsters. In D. L. Espelage, S. M. Swearer, & S. R. Jimerson (Eds.), *Handbook of bullying in schools: An international perspective* (pp. 61–72). New York: Routledge/Taylor & Francis Group.

Essex, M. J., Boyce, W. T., Goldstein, L. H., Armstrong, J. M., Kraemer, H. C., Kupfer, D. J., et al. (2002). The confluence of mental, physical, social, and academic difficulties in middle childhood: II. Developing the MacArthur Health and Behavior Questionnaire. *Journal of the American Academy of Child and Adolescent Psychiatry, 41,* 588–603.

Ettekal, I., & Ladd, G. W. (2015). Costs and benefits of children's physical and relational aggression trajectories on peer rejection, acceptance, and friendships: Variations by aggression subtypes, gender, and age. *Developmental Psychology, 51,* 1756–1770.

Ezekiel, L. F. (1931). Changes in egocentricity of nursery school children. *Child Development, 2,* 74–75.

Feshbach, N. D. (1969). Sex differences in children's modes of aggressive responses toward outsiders. *Merrill–Palmer Quarterly, 15,* 249–258.

Frick, P. J., & Morris, A. S. (2004). Temperament and developmental pathways to conduct problems. *Journal of Clinical Child and Adolescent Psychology, 33,* 54–68.

Galen, B. R., & Underwood, M. K. (1997). A developmental investigation of social aggression among children. *Developmental Psychology, 33,* 589–600.

Gentile, D. A., Coyne, S., & Walsh, D. A. (2010). Media violence, physical aggression, and relational aggression in school age children: A short-term longitudinal study. *Aggressive Behavior, 37,* 193–206.

Goldstein, S. E., Tisak, M. S., & Boxer, P. (2002). Preschoolers' normative and prescriptive judgments about relational and overt aggression. *Early Education and Development, 13,* 23–29.

Goodenough, F. L. (1931). *Anger in young children* (Institute of Child Welfare Monograph Series No. 9). Minneapolis: University of Minnesota Press.

Gower, A. L., Lingras, K. A., Mathieson, L. C., Kawabata, Y., & Crick, N. R. (2014). The role of preschool relational and physical aggression in the transition to kindergarten: Links with social-psychological adjustment. *Early Education and Development, 25,* 619–640.

Graham, S., & Juvonen, J. (1998). An attributional approach to peer victimization. In J. Juvonen & S. Graham (Eds.), *Peer harassment in school: The plight of the vulnerable and victimized* (pp. 49–71). New York: Guilford Press.

Hart, C. H., Nelson, D. A., Robinson, C. C., Olsen, S. F., & McNeilly-Choque, M. K. (1998). Overt and relational aggression in Russian nursery-school-age children: Parenting style and marital linkages. *Developmental Psychology, 34,* 687–697.

Hartup, W. W. (1974). Aggression in childhood: Developmental perspectives. *American Psychologist, 29,* 336–341.

Hattwick, L. A. (1937). Sex differences in behavior of nursery school children. *Child Development, 8,* 343–355.

Hay, D. F., Waters, C. S., Perra, O., Swift, N., Kairis, V., Phillips, R., et al. (2014). Precursors to aggression are evident by 6 months of age. *Developmental Science, 17,* 471–480.

Hinde, R. A. (1987). *Individuals, relationships, and culture: Links between ethology and the social sciences.* New York: Cambridge University Press.

Hong, J. S., & Espelage, D. L. (2012). A review of research on bullying and peer victimization in school: An ecological system analysis. *Aggression and Violent Behavior, 17,* 311–322.

Huesmann, L. R. (1988). An information processing model for the development of aggression. *Aggressive Behavior, 14,* 13–24.

Juliano, M., Werner, R. S., & Cassidy, K. W. (2006). Early correlates of preschool aggressive behavior according to type of aggression and measurement. *Journal of Applied Developmental Psychology, 27,* 395–410.

Kaukiainen, A., Björkqvist, K., Lagerspetz, K., Osterman, K., Salmivalli, C., Rothberg, S., et al. (1999). The relationships between social intelligence, empathy, and three types of aggression. *Aggressive Behavior, 25,* 81–89.

Khatri, P., & Kupersmidt, J. (2003). Aggression, peer victimisation, and social relationships among Indian youth. *International Journal of Behavioural Development, 27,* 87–95.

Krasnor, L., & Rubin, K. H. (1981). The assessment of social problem-solving skills in young children. In T. A. Merluzzi, C. R. Glass, & M. Genest (Eds.), *Cognitive assessment* (pp. 452–478). New York: Guilford Press.

Lagerspetz, K. M. J., Björkqvist, K., & Peltonen, T. (1988). Is indirect aggression typical of females?: Gender differences in aggressiveness in 11- to 12-year-old children. *Aggressive Behavior, 14,* 403–414.

Lahey, B. B., Applegate, B., Waldman, I. D., Loft, J. D., Hankin, B. L., & Rick, J. (2004). The structure of child and adolescent psychopathology: Generating new hypotheses. *Journal of Abnormal Psychology, 113,* 358–385.

Lahey, B. B., & Waldman, I. D. (2003). A developmental propensity model of the origins of conduct problems during childhood and adolescence. In B. B. Lahey, T. E. Moffitt, & A. Caspi (Eds.), *Causes of conduct disorder and juvenile delinquency* (pp. 76–117). New York: Guilford Press.

Leff, S. S., Waasdorp, T. E., & Crick, N. R. (2010). A review of existing relational aggression programs: Strengths, limitations, and future directions. *School Psychology Review, 39,* 508–535.

Lemerise, E. A., & Arsenio, W. F. (2000). An integrated model of emotion processes and cognition in social information processing. *Child Development, 71,* 107–118.

Little, T. D., Jones, S. M., Henrich, C. C., & Hawley, P. H. (2003). Disentangling the "whys" from the "whats" of aggressive behaviour. *International Journal of Behavioral Development, 27,* 122–133.

Malti, T., McDonald, K., Rubin, K. H., Rose-Krasnor, L., & Booth-LaForce, C. (2015). Developmental trajectories of peer-reported aggressive behavior: The role of friendship understanding, friendship quality, and friends' aggressive behavior. *Psychology of Violence, 5,* 402–410.

Marsee, M. A., & Frick, P. J. (2007). Exploring the cognitive and emotional correlates to proactive and reactive aggression in a sample of detained girls. *Journal of Abnormal Child Psychology, 35,* 969–981.

Masten, A. S., & Coatsworth, J. D. (1998). The development of competence in favorable and unfavorable environments: Lessons from research on successful children. *American Psychologist, 53,* 205–220.

Masten, A. S., Morison, P., & Pellegrini, D. S. (1985). A revised class play method of peer assessment. *Developmental Psychology, 3,* 523–533.

Mathieson, L. C., Murray-Close, D., Crick, N. R., Woods, K. E., Zimmer-Gembeck, M., Geiger, T. C., et al. (2011). Hostile intent attributions and relational aggression: The moderating roles of emotional sensitivity, gender, and victimization. *Journal of Abnormal Child Psychology, 39,* 977–987.

McEvoy, M. A., Estrem, T. L., Rodriguez, M. C., & Olson, M. L. (2003). Assessing relational and physical aggression among preschool children: Inter-method agreement. *Topics in Early Childhood Special Education, 23,* 53–63.

McNeilly-Choque, M. K., Hart, C. H., Robinson, C. C., Nelson, L., & Olsen, S. F. (1996). Overt and relational aggression on the playground: Correspondence among different informants. *Journal of Research in Childhood Education, 11,* 47–67.

Michiels, D., Grietens, H., Onghena, P., & Kuppens, S. (2008). Parent–child interactions and relational aggression in peer relationships. *Developmental Review, 28,* 522–540.

Moffitt, T. E. (1993). Adolescence-limited and life-course-persistent antisocial behavior: A developmental taxonomy. *Psychological Review, 100,* 674–701.

Moffitt, T. E. (2007). A review of research on the taxonomy of life-course-persistent versus adolescence-limited antisocial behavior. In D. J. Flannery, A. T. Vazsonyi, & I. D. Waldman (Eds.), *The Cambridge handbook of violent behavior and aggression* (pp. 49–76). New York: Cambridge University Press.

Murray-Close, D., Nelson, D. A., Ostrov, J. M., Casas, J. F., & Crick, N. R. (2016). Relational aggression: A developmental psychopathology perspective. In D. Cicchetti (Ed.), *Developmental psychopathology* (3rd ed., pp. 660–722). New York: Wiley.

Murray-Close, D., Ostrov, J. M., & Crick, N. R. (2007). A short-term longitudinal study of growth of relational aggression during middle childhood: Associations with gender, friendship intimacy, and internalizing problems. *Development and Psychopathology, 19,* 187–203.

Naerde, A., Ogden, T., Janson, H., & Zachrisson, H. D. (2014). Normative development of physical aggression from 8 to 26 months. *Developmental Psychology, 50,* 1710–1720.

National Institute of Child Health and Human Development Early Child Care and Research Network. (2004). Trajectories of physical aggression from toddlerhood to middle childhood: III. Person-centered trajectories of physical aggression. *Monographs of the Society for Research in Child Development, 69*(4), 41–49.

Orobio de Castro, B., Veerman, J. W., Koops, W., Bosch, J. D., & Monsouwer, H. J. (2002). Hostile attribution of intent and aggressive behavior: A meta-analysis. *Child Development, 73,* 916–934.

Ostrov, J. M. (2008). Forms of aggression and peer victimization during early childhood: A short-term longitudinal study. *Journal of Abnormal Child Psychology, 36*(3), 311–322.

Ostrov, J. M. (2010). Prospective associations between peer victimization and aggression. *Child Development, 81*(6), 1670–1677.

Ostrov, J. M., Blakely-McClure, S. J., Perry, K. J., & Kamper-DeMarco, K. E. (2018). Definitions: The form and function of relational aggression. In S. Coyne & J. M. Ostrov (Eds.), *Development of relational aggression* (pp. 13–28). New York: Oxford University Press.

Ostrov, J. M., & Godleski, S. A. (2010). Toward an integrated gender-linked model of aggression subtypes in early and middle childhood. *Psychological Review, 117,* 233–242.

Ostrov, J. M., & Keating, C. F. (2004). Gender differences in preschool aggression during free play and structured interactions: An observational study. *Social Development, 13,* 255–277.

Ostrov, J. M., Murray-Close, D., Godleski, S. A., & Hart, E. J. (2013). Prospective associations between forms and functions of aggression and social and affective processes during early childhood. *Journal of Experimental Child Psychology, 116,* 19–36.

Ostrov, J. M., Woods, K. E., Jansen, E. A., Casas, J. F., & Crick, N. R. (2004). An observational study of delivered and received aggression, gender, and social-psychological adjustment in preschool: "This white crayon doesn't work. . . . " *Early Childhood Research Quarterly, 19,* 355–371.

Park, J.-H., Essex, M. J., Zahn-Waxler, C., Armstrong, J. M., Klein, M. H., & Goldsmith, H. H. (2005). Relational and overt aggression in middle childhood: Early child and family risk factors. *Early Education and Development, 16,* 233–256.

Pepler, D. J., & Craig, W. M. (1995). A peek behind the fence: Naturalistic observations of aggressive children with remote audiovisual recording. *Developmental Psychology, 31,* 548–553.

Perry, K. J., & Price, J. M. (2017). The role of placement history and current family environment in children's aggression in foster care. *Journal of Child and Family Studies, 26,* 1135–1150.

Peters, E., Cillessen, A. H. N., Riksen-Walraven, J. M., & Haselager, G. J. T. (2010). Best friends' preference and popularity: Associations with aggression and prosocial behavior. *International Journal of Behavioral Development, 34,* 398–405.

Prakash, K., & Coplan, R. J. (2007). Socio-emotional characteristics and school adjustment of socially withdrawn children in India. *International Journal of Behavioural Development, 31,* 123–132.

Prinstein, M. J., & Cillessen, A. H. N. (2003). Forms and functions of adolescent peer aggression associated with high levels of peer status. *Merrill–Palmer Quarterly, 49,* 310–342.

Putallaz, M., Grimes, C. L., Foster, K. J., Kupersmidt, J. B., Coie, J. D., & Dearing, K. (2007). Overt and relational aggression and victimization: Multiple perspectives within the school setting. *Journal of School Psychology, 45,* 523–547.

Rubin, K. H., Bream, L. A., & Rose-Krasnor, L. (1991). Social problem solving and aggression in childhood. In K. H. Rubin & D. Pepler (Eds.), *The development and treatment of childhood aggression* (pp. 219–248). Hillsdale, NJ: Erlbaum.

Rubin, K., Bukowski, W., & Bowker, J. C. (2015). Children in peer groups. In R. M. Lerner (Series Ed.) & M. H. Bornstein & T. Leventhal (Vol. Eds.), *Handbook of child psychology and developmental science: Vol. 4. Ecological settings and processes* (7th ed., pp. 321–412). New York: Wiley.

Rubin, K. H., & Krasnor, L. R. (1986). Social-cognitive and social behavioral perspectives on problem solving. In M. Perlmutter (Ed.), *Minnesota Symposia on Child Psychology: Vol. 18. Cognitive perspectives on children's social and behavioral development* (pp. 1–68). Hillsdale, NJ: Erlbaum.

Rudolph, K. D., Troop-Gordon, W., Monti, J. D., & Miernicki, M. E. (2014). Moving against and away from the world: The adolescent legacy of peer victimization. *Development and Psychopathology, 26,* 721–734.

Skara, S., Pokhrel, P., Weiner, M. D., Sun, P., Dent, C. W., & Sussman, S. (2008). Physical and relational aggression as predictors of drug use: Gender differences among high school students. *Addictive Behaviors, 33,* 1507–1515.

Soenens, B., Vansteenkiste, M., Goossens, L., Duriez, B., & Niemiec, C. P. (2008). The intervening role of relational aggression between psychological control and friendship quality. *Social Development, 17,* 661–681.

Spieker, S. J., Campbell, S. B., Vandergrift, N., Pierce, K. M., Cauffman, E., Susman, E. J., et al. (2012). Relational aggression in middle childhood: Predictors and adolescent outcomes. *Social Development, 21,* 354–375.

Sroufe, L. A. (1997). Psychopathology as an outcome of development. *Development and Psychopathology, 9,* 251–268.

Sroufe, L. A. (2013). The promise of developmental psychopathology: Past and present. *Development and Psychopathology, 25,* 1215–1224.

Sroufe, L. A., & Rutter, M. (1984). The domain of developmental psychopathology. *Child Development, 55,* 17–29.

Stauffacher, K., & DeHart, G. B. (2006). Crossing social contexts: Relational aggression between siblings and friends during early and middle childhood. *Journal of Applied Developmental Psychology, 27,* 228–240.

Tackett, J. L., Herzhoff, K., Reardon, K. W., De Clercq, B., & Sharp, C. (2014). The externalizing spectrum in youth: Incorporating personality pathology. *Journal of Adolescence, 37,* 659–668.

Tackett, J. L., & Ostrov, J. M. (2010). Measuring relational aggression in middle childhood in a multi-informant multi-method study. *Journal of Psychopathology and Behavioral Assessment, 32,* 490–500.

Tackett, J. L., Waldman, I., & Lahey, B. B. (2009). Etiology and measurement of relational aggression: A multi-informant behavior genetic investigation. *Journal of Abnormal Psychology, 118,* 722–733.

Tapper, K., & Boulton, M. (2000). Social representations of physical, verbal, and indirect aggression in children: Sex and age differences. *Aggressive Behavior, 26,* 442–454.

Tremblay, R. E., & Nagin, D. S. (2005). The developmental origins of physical aggression in humans. In R. E. Tremblay, W. W. Hartup, & J. Archer (Eds.), *Developmental origins of aggression* (pp. 83–106). New York: Guilford Press.

Tremblay, R. E., Nagin, D. S., Séguin, J. R., Zoccolillo, M., Zelazo, P. D., Boivin, M., et al. (2005). Physical aggression during early childhood: Trajectories and predictors. *Canadian Child and Adolescent Psychiatry Review, 14,* 3–9.

Underwood, M. K. (2004). III. Glares of contempt, eye rolls of disgust, and turning away to exclude: Non-verbal forms of social aggression among girls. *Feminism and Psychology, 14,* 371–375.

Underwood, M. K., Scott, B. L., Galperin, M. B., Bjornstad, G. J., & Sexton, A. M. (2004). An observational study of social exclusion under varied conditions: Gender and developmental differences. *Child Development, 75,* 1538–1555.

Vaillancourt, T. (2005). Indirect aggression among humans: Social construct or evolutionary adaptation? In R. E. Tremblay, W. W. Hartup, & J. Archer (Eds.), *Developmental origins of aggression* (pp. 158–177). New York: Guilford Press.

Vaillancourt, T., Miller, J. L., Fagbemi, J., Cote, S., & Tremblay, R. E. (2007). Trajectories and predictors of indirect aggression: Results from a nationally representative longitudinal study of Canadian children aged 2–10. *Aggressive Behavior, 33,* 314–326.

Vitaro, F., Boivin, M., & Tremblay, R. E. (2007). Peers and violence: A two-sided developmental perspective. In D. J. Flannery, A. T. Vazsonyi, & I. D. Waldman (Eds.), *The Cambridge handbook of violent behavior and aggression* (pp. 361–387). New York: Cambridge University Press.

Waschbusch, D. A., Willoughby, M. T., & Pelham, W. J. (1998). Criterion validity and the utility of reactive and proactive aggression: Comparisons to attention deficit hyperactivity disorder, oppositional defiant disorder, conduct disorder, and other measures of functioning. *Journal of Clinical Child Psychology, 27,* 396–405.

Zalecki, C. A., & Hinshaw, S. P. (2004). Overt and relational aggression in girls with attention deficit hyperactivity disorder. *Journal of Clinical Child and Adolescent Psychology, 33,* 125–137.

CHAPTER 4

Behavior Genetics of Aggression

MARA BRENDGEN, FRANK VITARO,
and MICHEL BOIVIN

Brief Introduction

Aggressive behavior during childhood and adolescence is an important risk factor for later serious and persistent adjustment problems in adulthood, including criminal behavior and school dropout, as well as family-related and economic problems (Farrington, 1991). Aggression is also linked to a host of concurrent and future mental and physical health problems for the victims, which can have a negative impact on their socioeconomic well-being in later life (Odgers et al., 2008). Researchers have thus made considerable efforts to uncover what drives individuals to attack and hurt others. Most prominent developmental theories in the 20th century have focused on the role of environmental experiences in explaining interindividual differences in aggressive behavior (e.g., Bandura, 1973; Berkowitz, 1989; Patterson, Reid, & Dishion, 1992). There is increasing evidence, however, that genetic, as well as environmental, factors contribute to shape all aspects of human development—including aggressive behavior (Turkheimer, 2000). Although genetic and environmental influences were initially expected to influence development independently, it is now clear that these forces are likely to interact and to reciprocally influence each other through various mechanisms of gene–environment interplay.

Thus far, the vast majority of studies have examined how genetic factors work together with family-related risk factors or stressful life events (e.g., parental behavior, socioeconomic status, physical or sexual maltreatment) to influence aggressive behavior. However, even young children spend many hours in day care settings or schools, away from their families and in the company of peers. Peers are thus believed to provide another unique context in which children learn social norms and behaviors (Boivin, Vitaro, & Poulin, 2005; Rubin, Bukowski, & Bowker, 2015). In recent years, genetically informed studies have also begun to emerge that investigate the link between the peer environment and aggressive behavior. With a specific focus on the family and the peer environment, this chapter reviews the current state of knowledge from behavior genetic studies on the genetic–environmental etiology of aggressive behavior in children and adolescents.

We first outline two main considerations for understanding the development of aggression: The first refers to the importance of distinguishing different subtypes (i.e., forms and functions) of aggressive behavior; the second refers to the importance of disentangling environmental influences from those that are genetic (i.e., inherent to the individual). The following section describes the various mechanisms of gene–environment interplay as they may relate to the development of aggressive behavior in children and adolescents. Next, we explain the underlying principles of behavior genetic designs. This is followed by an overview of recent behavior genetic findings on the etiology of different forms and functions of aggression, as well as the interplay of genetic factors with the family and the peer environment in this context. Finally, we conclude the chapter by discussing the implications for theory and practice and by outlining future directions in genetically informed research on aggression.

Main Issues

For several decades, the study of aggression has focused on physical aggression. However, individuals can also hurt others through more subtle forms of aggression, for example, through ridicule, social exclusion, or rumor spreading. The victims consider these nonphysical forms of aggression to be as harmful as physical aggression (Crick, Bigbee, & Howes, 1996), with a range of negative effects that include anxiety, depression, and suicide ideation (Owens, Slee, & Shute, 2000). Different labels have been used to describe these forms of aggression, specifically *indirect aggression, relational aggression,* and *social aggression,* but all three terms refer to socially manipulative behavior intended to harm another individual (see Ostrov, Perry, & Blakely-McClure, Chapter 3, this volume). We therefore use the term *social aggression.* Factor analyses show that the distinctiveness of physical and social aggression becomes established early in life and remains stable over the course of middle childhood and into adolescence (Vaillancourt, Brendgen, Boivin, & Tremblay, 2003). However, whereas physical aggression peaks at about 36–48 months and then gradually diminishes over early and middle childhood, social aggression increases from the end of early childhood through middle childhood and early adolescence (Tremblay, 1999). In other words, aggressive behavior may not necessarily decline but may gradually change its form as children grow older. This notion is supported by the considerable correlation between the two forms of aggression (average r = .76; Card, Stucky, Sawalani, & Little, 2008) and by longitudinal research showing that physical aggression predicts an increase in social aggression, but not the other way around (Ojanen & Kiefer, 2013).

In addition to taking different forms, aggressive behavior can also serve different functions (Dodge, 1991). Proactive aggression, which has been described as instrumental, offensive, and "cold-blooded," requires neither provocation nor anger. In contrast, reactive aggression has been described as affective, defensive, and "hot-blooded," involving angry outbursts in response to actual or perceived provocations or threats. At the theoretical level, reactive aggression is related to the frustration–aggression model, which posits that aggression is an angry and hostile response to a perceived threat. In contrast, proactive aggression is consistent with social learning theory, which suggests that aggression serves the purpose of obtaining a desired goal (Card & Little, 2007). At the empirical level, studies show that reactive and proactive aggression are factorially distinct but often co-occur, with correlations reaching $r = .70$ ($\pm$ .15; Vitaro & Brendgen, 2011).

The previously discussed findings show not only that it is often the same children who are physically and socially aggressive toward peers but also that there seems to be a gradual shift from physical to more subtle and often indirect forms of aggression over the course of development. Physical and social aggression might thus share—at least to some extent—common origins that may be rooted either in the child or in his or her environment or both. The possibility of partly common underlying causes should apply even more to proactive and reactive aggression, given their even stronger correlation. By the same token, numerous studies show that—when controlling for their overlap—the different forms and functions of aggression seem to also have partly distinct individual and environmental antecedents and different consequences (Vitaro & Brendgen, 2011). These findings suggest that aggression is not an entirely uniform construct and that distinguishing between different forms or different functions is essential if we are to understand why some children and adolescents aggress against others. When investigating the effects of individual and environmental factors on the etiology of aggression, however, it is difficult to interpret the findings if only one child per family is assessed. For example, the links between a putative environmental variable such as parenting behavior and aggressive behavior in the child may, in fact, be due to the genetic transmission of problem behaviors rather than reflecting a true environmental effect. This confound represents a major challenge for testing causal hypotheses about the developmental origins of aggression. The use of genetically informed designs, which disentangle genetic from environmental influences, allows a better control of this problem (Rutter, Moffitt, & Caspi, 2006).

Theoretical Considerations

In and of itself, even a genetically informed design cannot provide direct and conclusive proof of causation. However, a finding that genetic factors inherent to the child account for the involvement with aggressive friends might indicate that an active selection process, based on heritable personal characteristics, is involved. In this way, genetically informed studies may test theoretical assumptions of child effects on specific (i.e., measured) features of peer relations. Genetically informed designs also permit the assessment of other theoretical models related to the development of aggression. For example, in line with the diathesis–stress model of psychopathology, a genetically informed model can test whether the effect of harsh parental punishment on aggression varies depending on the child's genetic risk for such behavior. Thus, by disentangling genetic from environmental sources of interindividual variation and by examining their different modes of interplay, genetically informed studies can provide useful information for testing causal hypotheses (Rutter et al., 2006). The term *gene–environment interplay* refers to a variety of concepts. However, the two genetic–environmental mechanisms most relevant for understanding the development of aggressive behavior are *gene–environment correlations* and *gene–environment interactions*.

Gene–Environment Correlations

Developmental theorists have suggested for several decades that individuals play a critical role in shaping their environment (Scarr & McCartney, 1983). Many, if not most, of the personal characteristics and behaviors that may influence environmental experiences are partly heritable. As a result, the environment may become influenced, albeit indirectly, by genetic factors. This phenomenon is referred to as a *gene–environment correlation* (*rGE*). Scarr and McCartney (1983) have described three mechanisms whereby genetic factors may influence the environmental experiences of an individual. *Passive* rGE occurs when parents' personal characteristics, which are partly explained by genetic factors, influence the environment they provide for their children. For example, children of parents with a genetic disposition for aggressive behavior may be more likely than others to experience harsh punishment for even minor misdemeanors. The child's genotype, which is inherited from the parents, thus becomes correlated with his or her family environment. This type of rGE is labeled *passive* because the child's environmental experiences are not elicited by the child's own behavior, but rather by parental behavior that is itself genetically influenced and heritable.

In contrast to passive rGE, *selective* rGE and *evocative* rGE involve environmental features that are presumably directly influenced by the child's heritable characteristics. *Selective* (also called *active*) rGE arises when individuals actively select or shape their own environments based on their genetically influenced personal characteristics. Selective rGE would occur, for example, when aggressive adolescents (whose behavior is, in part, genetically influenced) actively select friends with similar behavioral characteristics. Selective rGE may thus be implicated in friendship selection based on personal, heritable characteristics, which could partly account for the similarity between friends. *Evocative* rGE occurs when the child's genetically influenced characteristics lead to specific reactions from the social environment. For example, a genetic disposition for aggression may elicit dislike and rejection from peers, thus generating a correlation between a genetic risk for aggression and the experience of rejection.

Importantly, Scarr and McCartney (1983) suggest that the relative importance of these three forms of rGE may change over development: With increasing autonomy to shape the social world, the role of passive rGE may decline, and selective rGE may increase with age. In contrast, evocative rGE should play a relatively consistent role in shaping environmental experiences.

Gene–Environment Interactions

Gene–environment interactions (G × E) refer to a process whereby (1) the expression of a genetic disposition toward a developmental outcome varies as a function of the environment or (2) the effect of the environment varies depending on an individual's genetic disposition (Shanahan & Hofer, 2005). From a theoretical standpoint, G × E can be expected to be more common than simple additive effects of genetic and environmental factors for basically all aspects of human development, including aggression, because it is consistent with the notion that genes are involved in the adaptation of organisms to environmental conditions (Rutter et al., 2006). Like rGE, G × E may arise through different processes. A *trigger process* occurs when an environmental condition elicits or exacerbates a genetic predisposition for a given outcome or when an environmental condition leads to a given outcome only in individuals with the predisposing genes. When "adverse" environmental conditions and negative outcomes are involved, such as when victimization by peers leads to aggression mainly (or only) in children with a genetic risk for such behavior, the trigger is analogous to a stressor in the *diathesis–stress model*. In contrast, a *suppression process* of G × E may arise when environmental conditions reduce the role of genetic factors in explaining interindividual differences in a behavior or other outcomes. A suppression process of G × E can involve "adverse" environmental conditions, such as exposure to war or famine, which may lead to aggression in a large number of individuals regardless of their genetic dispositions. However, a suppression process can also involve more benign environmental conditions, such as social norms or supportive parenting behaviors, that reduce genetic influence by limiting the expression of individuals' genetic susceptibility for aggression. When a positive environment prevents or reduces the expression of a genetic disposition for problem behavior, researchers sometimes also speak of a *compensation* process of G × E.

Although G × E and rGE have usually been investigated independently, the two processes can and often do co-occur, such that the same environmental factors may simultaneously be involved in both G × E and rGE with respect to a given phenotype (Purcell, 2002). Environmental features that are proximal to the child are most likely to be simultaneously implicated in G × E and rGE (Shanahan & Hofer, 2005). For example, as described in more detail later, behavior genetic studies provide evidence for both G × E and rGE linking aggressive behavior in youth and a problematic relationship with parents. Moreover, similar conjoint effects of gene–environment interplay have been observed that link aggression with environmental experiences outside the family, notably the peer environment.

Measures and Methods

To date, research examining the genetic–environmental etiology of the different forms and functions of aggressive behavior has mostly relied on behavior—also called quantitative–genetic designs. In contrast to molecular genetic studies, in which biological data (e.g., from blood or saliva) are collected to identify particular genes related to a behavior or symptom, behavior genetic studies statistically infer genetic effects without the need for collecting DNA. The relative strength of genetic and environmental effects is instead statistically inferred by examining the phenotypic similarity of family members with varying degrees of genetic relatedness. To this end, behavioral studies can use a variety of research designs, such as the comparison of adopted and biological siblings, or the comparison of identical (monozygotic [MZ]) and fraternal (dizygotic [DZ]) twin pairs growing up together. Biological full siblings share an average of 50% of their genes. Biological half siblings share only one of their two biological parents, and thus share an average of 25% of their genetic material. Adopted siblings and stepsiblings do not share any genetic material. MZ twinning occurs when one egg is fertilized by one sperm and then splits after conception into two genetically identical halves. As such, MZ twins are assumed to share 100% of their genes (barring mutations). DZ twinning occurs when two eggs are fertilized by two separate sperms. DZ twins, like all full siblings, share an average of 50% of their genetic material. One advantage of the twin design over the adoption design is that twins are the same age, which eliminates age difference as a potential source of variability. The assumption underlying all behavior genetic designs is that interindividual differences in a measured outcome (i.e., a phenotype) can be decomposed into three sources of variance: genetic (or heritable) factors, shared (or common) environmental factors, and nonshared (or unique) environmental factors. These three variance components are generally conceived as latent (i.e., unmeasured) variables.

In an adoption design, genetic factors are assumed to be implicated if individuals are "phenotypically" more similar to their biological siblings than to their adopted or stepsiblings. In the classical twin design, genetic influences are indicated when the phenotypic similarity of MZ twin pairs is greater than the phenotypic similarity of DZ twin pairs (Falconer, 1960). Genetic or heritable effects (denoted as h^2) can be approximated as twice the difference between the MZ intrapair correlation and the DZ intrapair correlation, $h^2 = 2(r_{MZ} - r_{DZ})$. For example, if the phenotypic correlation between MZ twins is $r = .60$ and the correlation between DZ twins is $r = .40$, then the genetic effect on this particular phenotype is estimated as $2(.60 - .40) = .40$. In other words, approximately 40% of the interindividual differences in regard to the phenotype under study are due to genetic influences.

Shared environment (denoted as c^2) refers to features of the environment that influence the siblings similarly and, by extension, make them similar to each other. In principle, shared environment may include features both inside (e.g., parental education, family structure) and outside (e.g., neighborhood housing density or crime level) the family. Shared environments may also include peers, such as when siblings share common friends with whom they spend time together. In the classic twin design, shared environment effects can be estimated by subtracting the MZ correlation from twice the DZ correlation, $c^2 = (2r_{DZ}) - r_{MZ}$. Using the twin correlations from our previous example, the shared environment effect would be estimated as $(2 \times .40) - .60 = .20$. In other words, approximately 20% of the interindividual differences in regard to the phenotype under study would be due to shared environmental influences.

Nonshared environment (denoted as e^2) refers to any experiences inside or outside the family—including prenatal experiences—that make siblings dissimilar. For example, although raised in the same family, siblings may be treated differently by their parents, and this, in turn, may lead to differences in their behavior (Conger & Conger, 1994). Moreover, siblings often have different friends or attend different classrooms and are, as a result, exposed to different peer groups (Thorpe & Gardner, 2006). Differential experiences with peers may thus be an important source of nonshared environmental influence during childhood and adolescence. Nonshared environmental effects can be approximated by the extent to which the MZ correlation is less than 1: $e^2 = 1 - r_{MZ}$. Based on the twin correlations from our example, the nonshared environment effect e^2 would be estimated as $1 - .60 = .40$. In other words, approximately 40% of the interindividual differences in regard to the phenotype under study are due to nonshared environmental influences.

Over the past decades, the rapid development of statistical software capabilities has allowed researchers to extend behavior genetic analyses beyond the simple calculation of main effects of genetic and environmental factors. Using structural equation modeling or multilevel regression techniques, the original formulation of variance decomposition proposed by Falconer (1960) has been expanded to incorporate multivariate data (Neale & Cardon, 1992; Ottman, 1994; Purcell & Sham, 2003). This makes it possible, for example, to address questions concerning the underlying causes of comorbidity (i.e., whether the same genetic and environmental factors influence the forms or functions of aggression) or questions concerning developmental (i.e., age-related) changes in the relative influence of genetic and environmental factors on the different types of aggression. Moreover, although genetic and environmental factors are typically conceived as unmeasured variables in behavior genetic studies, specific measured environmental variables can be included to test various theoretical models of gene–environment interplay in the etiology of aggression.

Central Research Findings

Initially, behavior genetic studies mostly focused on estimating and comparing the relative roles of genetic and environmental influences on aggression. More recently, researchers have become increasingly interested in uncovering how genetic liabilities work together with the family or peer environment—either through G × E or rGE—in the development of aggressive behavior. Only a few studies differentiated between different forms or functions of aggression, however. In this section we provide a brief overview of some of the main findings in this context.

Genetic and Environmental Influences on Aggression: Main Effects

Numerous studies have examined the heritability of aggression in humans (for a review, see Tuvblad & Baker, 2011). Although estimates vary depending on the particular measure used and the age range of the sample, the results suggest that around 50% of the variance of aggression is determined by genetic factors. Even stronger average genetic effects were found in a meta-analysis of 103 twin and adoption studies that included only child and adolescent samples, with genetic factors explaining 65% of aggressive behavior in youth (Burt, 2009). The remainder of the variance in physical aggression seems to be influenced mainly by unique or nonshared environmental factors, whereas only a relatively small contribution of environmental sources shared between siblings has been reported in the literature. Findings also suggest that genetic influences on aggressive behavior become increasingly more important, whereas shared environmental effects become less so as children grow into adolescents. As noted by Tuvblad and Baker (2011), however, parents more often serve as reporting sources for aggressive behavior in children than in adolescents. Parental bias may thus lead to overestimation of shared environmental effects and attenuate heritability estimates in childhood. Still, the overall pattern of findings suggests that similarity of aggressive behavior between siblings is mostly due to genetic and not environmental influences. This applies even when comparing different reporting sources, such as mothers and fathers (van den Oord, Verhulst, & Boomsma, 1996), parents, teachers, independent observers, and child self-reports (Arseneault et al., 2003). Existing evidence also suggests that males and females do not differ in terms of the relative magnitude of genetic and environmental effects on aggression.

Although informative, the instruments used to measure aggression vary widely across studies and cover a host of different forms and functions of aggression. As previously mentioned, however, the etiology of the different forms and functions of aggression likely differs to some extent, based both on their theoretical definitions and on empirical evidence from studies using one child per family. The first study to examine the relative contribution of genetic and (shared and nonshared) environmental factors to social aggression compared with physical aggression in childhood used a sample of 6-year-old twin pairs (Brendgen et al., 2005). Strong genetic effects were found for teacher-rated physical aggression, accounting for 63% of the variance, with the remaining variance explained by nonshared environmental influences. In contrast, genetic factors accounted for only 20% of the variance of teacher-rated social aggression, with the remaining variance mostly explained by nonshared environmental influences (60%) but also by shared environmental influences (20%). Further bivariate genetic modeling revealed a strong correlation ($r = .79$) between the genetic factors but a much more modest correlation ($r = .31$) between the nonshared environmental factors contributing to teacher-rated physical and social aggression. A highly similar pattern of results was observed when using peer ratings of social and physical aggression. A similar substantial correlation of genetic factors and a similar weak correlation of environmental factors were also found in a study examining physical aggression versus deceitful behavior (lying, cheating) in 9-year-old children (Barker et al., 2009) and in another study examining physical aggression versus social aggression against the partner in adults (Saudino & Hines, 2007).

Together with the previously mentioned findings of a directional effect from physical aggression to social aggression, the results from these studies may be interpreted in the context of the developmental model of aggressive behavior proposed by Björkqvist, Lagerspetz, and Kaukiainen (1992). Specifically, some children may exhibit genetic liabilities for aggressive behavior in general, which, initially, will be expressed through physical means. Physical aggression is generally not socially accepted, however, and often leads to punishment. At the same time, socializing agents such as peers may foster alternative yet similarly aggressive strategies (i.e., social aggression), either by direct modeling or through reinforcement. As such, many children who initially display physically aggressive behavior may soon learn to use socially more acceptable and less risky aggressive strategies. Whether and when this shift occurs seems to be determined by the extent to which the child is exposed to a social environment that specifically promotes the use of social aggression. The potentially crucial role of the environment in the extent and timing of the development shift in aggressive behavior may also explain findings that social aggression is to a larger extent influenced by environmental factors than physical aggression (Brendgen et al., 2005).

As indicated previously, rates of co-occurrence between the different functions of aggression are even higher than those observed for the different forms. The question arises as to which etiological mechanisms explain the positive correlation between proactive and reactive aggression. A study examining this question was conducted by Tuvblad, Raine, Zheng, and Baker (2009) using a sample of 9- to 14-year-old twins who were assessed twice by their parents over a 2-year period. Using the repeated assessments as indicators of latent variables, the results showed that 80% of the variance of the latent reactive aggression variable and 63% of the variance of the latent proactive aggression variable was explained by genetic factors, with the remainder explained by environmental factors unique to each child for both latent forms of aggression. More importantly, the analyses also revealed that the genetic influences as well as the environmental influences on the latent reactive and proactive aggression variables were the same. These results suggest that proactive and reactive aggression seem to largely share the same etiological origins. Findings from other research indicate, however, that this conclusion may not necessarily provide the whole picture (Paquin, Lacourse, Brendgen, Vitaro, & Dionne, 2014).

Another indication comes from nongenetically informed research showing that reactive and proactive aggression are much less correlated—or even uncorrelated—when controlling for any confound due to the same underlying form (i.e., physical or social; Fite, Stauffacher, Ostrov, & Colder, 2008). To clarify this issue, Brendgen, Vitaro, Boivin, Dionne, and Pérusse (2006) considered not only the overlap between these two functions of aggression but also their overlap with a common underlying form, in this case physical aggression. Similar to the results reported by Tuvblad and colleagues (2009), somewhat stronger genetic effects were found for reactive aggression (accounting for 52% of the variance) than for proactive aggression (accounting for 35% of the variance), with the remaining variance explained by environmental experiences unique to each child. However, proactive and reactive aggression shared 37% of their genetic influences and 18% of their environmental influences. In addition, the inclusion of physical aggression in the model revealed that the genetic factors that were shared by reactive and proactive aggression were those that accounted for a common underlying form (i.e., physical aggression). Apart from the common genetic and environmental effects due to form, reactive and proactive aggression shared no other genetic effects and only few environmental effects. These findings suggest that, once the form of aggression is controlled, both the genetic and the environmental influences on the functions of aggression seem to largely differ. Differential genetic and (largely) differential environmental effects influencing the two functions of aggression are in line with nongenetically informed studies showing that proactive and reactive aggression have different physiological and temperamental correlates and are predicted by different family- and peer-related experiences (for a review, see Vitaro & Brendgen, 2011).

The previously discussed studies provide a first glimpse into the relative roles of genetic and environmental influences on aggressive behavior in children and adolescents. These studies do not inform us, however, about the specific genes and—more important for social scientists—the specific environmental features involved in the development of aggression. Moreover, the sole estimation of main effects presumes that genetic and environmental influences are independent of each other and ignores any possible interplay between genes and the environment.

rGE Linking Child Aggression and the Family Environment

Using the classic twin or the classic adoption design, several researchers have shown that the association between antisocial behavior—including aggression—in offspring and such forms of negative parenting behavior as harsh criticism or punishment can be at least partly explained by common underlying genetic influences (e.g., Button, Lau, Maughan, & Eley, 2008; Jaffee et al., 2004; Narusyte, Andershed, Neiderhiser, & Lichtenstein, 2007). In contrast, more extreme forms of physical child maltreatment are not related to genetically influenced characteristics of the child (Jaffee et al., 2004). The results regarding more "common" forms of negative parenting are typically interpreted as evidence of evocative rGE, that is, as effects of genetically influenced child behavior on the behavior of the parents (Boivin, Pérusse, et al., 2005). Parent-driven effects on parenting, including the effects of the parents' genes indicating passive rGE, are assumed to be included in estimates of the shared environment because these parent-driven effects should affect the two siblings in a similar way (Neiderhiser et al., 2004). However, because genetic and environmental influences can only be estimated for the offspring's behavior in these studies, evocative and passive rGE cannot be clearly distinguished.

The Extended Children of Twins (ECOT) design enables disentangling the contributions of passive rGE and evocative rGE more clearly than the classic twin design or the classic adoption design. This is achieved by combining a sample of children who are twins and their parents (i.e., a child-based design that includes genetic information about the children) with a sample of parents who are twins and their children (i.e., a parent-based design that includes genetic information about the parents; Silberg & Eaves, 2004). In this way, it can be examined whether genetic factors related to the parents' behavior also influence the child or whether genetic factors related to the child's behavior influence the parents (or both). In addition, this type of design can test bidirectional environmental influences between parental and child behavior. Two studies have used the ECOT design to examine the association between negative parenting and antisocial behavior in the offspring. In the first study, it was found that the association between maternal criticism and adolescent externalizing problems was explained by evocative rGE, whereas there was only direct environmental influence of paternal criticism on child externalizing problems (Narusyte et al., 2011). Using a larger sample with more fathers and a wider range of negative parenting (including negativity, conflict, and harsh discipline), Marceau and colleagues (Marceau et al., 2013) extended these conclusions by showing that adolescents' genetically influenced externalizing problems contributed to the evocative rGE underlying both maternal and paternal negativity.

Unfortunately, the antisocial behavior measures in the aforementioned studies included not only aggression but also other externalizing behaviors, such as delinquency and oppositional behavior. This confound was addressed in a more recent study that examined the specific associations of maternal negativity (i.e., harsh punishment and rejection) with aggression and rule breaking, respectively, in a sample of more than 800 families with primary school-age twins (Klahr, Klump, & Burt, 2014). The results revealed that evocative rGE processes are specific to the relation between maternal negativity and child aggression and do not contribute to the association between maternal negativity and the child's nonaggressive rule breaking. In other words, mothers seem to respond with negative behavior to their children's genetically influenced aggressive behavior but not to the children's genetically influenced rule-breaking behavior. However, less than half of the evocative genetic influences on maternal negativity overlapped with genetic influences on child aggression. This suggests that genetically influenced child characteristics other than aggression are also important for evoking negative parenting. There were also substantive shared environmental associations between maternal negativity and child aggression and rule breaking that indicate a potentially causal effect of parenting on these behaviors.

Together, the results from these studies provide strong evidence that children's aggressive behavior, which is partly genetically influenced, may elicit negative behavioral reactions from the parents. In turn, parents' negative behavior may provide an environmental context that further increases the offspring's aggression. It is still unknown, however, whether these processes apply to the same extent to different forms or functions of aggressive behavior.

rGE Linking Child Aggression and the Peer Environment

Genetic factors related to aggression may also influence children's and adolescents' peer-related experiences—most notably, rejection or victimization by peers and affiliation with aggressive friends. Evidence to this effect comes, for instance, from a sample of more than 600 twin pairs followed since birth by our research group (Boivin, Brendgen, Vitaro, Dionne, et al., 2013; Boivin, Brendgen, Vitaro, Forget-Dubois, et al., 2013; Brendgen et al., 2011). Rejection and victimization by peers were assessed longitudinally using peer (i.e., classmates') nominations, as well as teacher and self-reports. By and large, genetic factors accounted for up to 70% of individual differences in peer-related difficulties from kindergarten to grade 4, and more so when stable peer difficulties were considered. Moreover, more than 60% of this influence was explained by genetic factors underlying aggressive behavior. Because individuals are unlikely to deliberately choose to be rejected and victimized, these findings can be interpreted as indicating evocative rGE. Even stronger evidence for evocative rGE comes from an observational study of 5-year old twins, each of whom was paired with an unfamiliar same-sex peer in a peer-play interaction. Results showed that children with a strong genetic disposition for aggressive behavior were more likely to evoke physical or verbal aggression, whereas those with a genetic disposition for prosocial behavior were more often met with friendly behavior from the play partner, thus ruling out passive (parent-influenced) and active (selective) rGE (DiLalla, Bersted, & John, 2015; DiLalla & John, 2014).

It is not known whether rGE processes underlying the link between aggression and peer rejection or victimization exist regardless of the function of the aggressive behavior employed during peer interaction (i.e., proactive or reactive aggression). However, recent findings suggest that the rGE linking aggressive behavior with negative peer treatment applies to *both* physical and social forms of aggression but that it is moderated by the prevailing behavioral norms in the peer group (Brendgen, Girard, Vitaro, Dionne, & Boivin, 2013, 2015). Specifically, children with a strong genetic disposition for either physical or social aggression have been found to be at increased risk of being victimized by their peers only when such behavior is disapproved by the peer group. In contrast, children with a genetic disposition for either physical or relational aggression were *less* likely to be victimized than others in classrooms in which such behavior was highly accepted. These results emphasize that not only heritable characteristics, such as aggression, but also the wider social context play a significant role in how youth are perceived and treated by the larger peer group.

The previously described studies suggest that evocative rGE linking aggressive behavior with negative treatment by parents or peers already occurs at a relatively young age. In contrast, links with deviant peer affiliation—which may to a large extent reflect selective rGE—are observed only in older children and adolescents. To illustrate, in a longitudinal sample of twins, children's own physical aggression was highly heritable, but this genetic liability was unrelated to their friends' physical aggression at ages 6 and 7 (Brendgen, Boivin, Vitaro, Bukowski, et al., 2008; Van Lier et al., 2007). A significant rGE was also absent in the link between children's and their friends' social aggression (Brendgen, Boivin, Vitaro, Bukowski, et al., 2008). However, using the same sample and similar measures, significant genetic influences on friends' aggression were found at ages 10 and 13 (Vitaro et al., 2016). The increasing rGE linking youths' and their friends' aggressive behavior likely reflects selective, not evocative or passive rGE. If passive or evocative rGE processes were involved, evidence of rGE should be found at a younger age. These findings thus accord with the notion that, with age, youth become increasingly autonomous in selecting their friends based on resemblance with their own, partly heritable characteristics.

G × E Linking Child Aggression and the Family Environment

In addition to being influenced by the child's heritable aggressive tendencies (as indicated by rGE), the family environment may also foster aggressive behavior in the child. However, the family environment does not necessarily occur independently of the child's genetic vulnerability for aggression. For instance, using a mixed (i.e., twins, siblings, and nonsiblings) design, Feinberg, Button, Neiderhiser, Reiss, and Hetherington (2007) found that a genetic vulnerability for antisocial behavior (a combination of aggressive and nonaggressive antisocial behaviors) is more readily expressed as actual antisocial behavior when children are exposed to high levels of parental negativity. Other studies indicate that general family dysfunction or parental maltreatment of the child exacerbates the expression of genetic risk associated with antisocial behavior (Button, Scourfield, Martin, Purcell, & McGuffin, 2005; Jaffee et al., 2005). Finally, Cadoret, Yates, Troughton, Woodworth, and Stewart

(1995) used an adoption design in which adopted offspring who were separated at birth from biological parents with documented antisocial personality disorder were followed up as adults. These adoptees were compared with controls whose biological parents showed no psychopathology. Results revealed that only adoptees with biological parents with antisocial personality and an adverse adoptive environment (defined as adoptive parents who had marital problems, were divorced, were separated, or had anxiety conditions, depression, substance abuse and/or dependence, or legal problems) manifested increased conduct problems in adolescence.

Overall, the preceding studies are consistent with a diathesis–stress process of G × E in the interplay between negative family environment and youngsters' genetic liability toward antisocial behavior: At low levels of negative parenting and family dysfunction, the child's genetic liability is not outwardly expressed, or at least less so. However, at high levels of negative parenting and family dysfunction, genetically at-risk children may react with outbursts of anger. A spiraling coercive cycle may result from such encounters that may foster the development of information-processing schemes favorable to aggressive behavior (Patterson et al., 1992). It is important to note, however, that the measures of antisocial behavior in the aforementioned studies included not only aggression but also a host of other, related behaviors (e.g., opposition, difficult temperament, nonviolent delinquency). Moreover, aggression items mostly focused on physical aggression and typically did not include social aggression. Thus it is difficult to judge whether the findings specifically apply to aggressive behavior, let alone whether they vary for different forms or functions of aggression. Indeed, Dodge (1991) proposed, specifically, that reactive aggression should develop in reaction to a harsh, threatening and unpredictable family environment, whereas proactive aggression should thrive in supportive environments that foster the use of aggression as a means to achieve one's goals. Nongenetically informed studies tend to support this theoretical model (Vitaro, Brendgen, & Barker, 2006). The findings of a diathesis–stress process of G × E linking a harsh family environment and child antisocial behavior may thus apply mostly to reactive and physical aggression. Further research is needed to clarify this issue.

G × E Linking Child Aggression and the Peer Environment

More specific evidence of G × E with respect to aggressive behavior comes from studies examining the peer environment. Overall, the findings suggest that negative peer environments tend to promote aggressive behavior, especially in genetically vulnerable youth. For instance, data from a sample of twins assessed in kindergarten revealed that victimized girls showed high levels of generalized aggression mainly if they had a high genetic risk of being aggressive (Brendgen, Boivin, Vitaro, Dionne, et al., 2008). The predictive effect of peer victimization on aggression was much weaker in girls with a very low genetic risk of aggressive behavior. For boys, peer victimization was associated with high levels of aggression independently of their genetic disposition to such behavior. This sex-specific pattern of G × E may be due to the fact that girls perceive aggressive behavior as more unacceptable than boys, even when it is used as a response to an aggressive provocation from peers (Goldstein, Tisak, & Boxer, 2002). When harassed by others, girls may be most likely to behave aggressively if they are genetically disposed to do so. In contrast, because aggressive responses to hostile peer provocations are more acceptable for boys, many victimized boys may retort with aggression regardless of whether or not they have a genetic disposition for such behavior. A follow-up study with the same sample suggests, however, that the presence of positive environmental influences may help alleviate the negative consequences of peer victimization for genetically vulnerable children (Brendgen et al., 2011). Indeed, children with a genetic liability for aggression were less likely to behave aggressively when they had a warm and conflict-free relationship with their teachers. This pattern of G × E is indicative of a compensation process, whereby the presence of a positive environment prevents or reduces the expression of a genetic disposition for aggression. Unfortunately, it is unknown whether these findings apply to both physical and social aggression.

Research also shows that genetic risk for aggression is more readily expressed when youth are exposed to antisocial peers. Most studies in this context have relied on adolescents' reports of their peers' generalized antisocial behavior and have not included measures of aggression per se (Button et al., 2007, 2009; Hicks, South, DiRago, Iacono, & McGue, 2009). Nevertheless, similar findings were observed in studies that specifically focused on aggression and that employed more stringent measures of peers' behavior. The latter findings also suggest that this G × E is not necessarily limited to the adolescent period. This was shown, for instance, in a study of twins in which teacher and peer ratings of aggression were obtained for each twin child and for each twin child's three reciprocal classroom friends in kindergarten (Van Lier et al., 2007). In line with a contextual trigger process of G × E, aggression was most frequently observed in children who were at high genetic risk for such behavior *and* who also affiliated with highly aggressive friends. In contrast, children with very low genetic risk for aggressive behavior showed very low levels of aggression regardless of their friends' behavior. However, a follow-up study conducted with this sample in grade 1 (Brendgen, Boivin, Vitaro, Bukowski, et al., 2008) revealed that this trigger process of G × E holds only for the link between friends' and children's *physical* aggression (i.e., hitting, biting, kicking), not for social aggression. Instead, affiliation with socially aggressive friends seemed to foster relational aggression independently of, and in addition to, the effect of children's genetic disposition for such behavior.

One possible explanation for these distinct genetic–environmental processes may be that social aggression involves rather subtle behaviors that may carry a much lower risk of retribution than physical aggression. Because social aggression is often diffuse and ubiquitous, adults are less likely to intervene against children's use of social aggression compared with physical aggression (Werner, Senich, & Przepyszny, 2006). Social aggression may also offer potential rewards for the perpetrators, as it may promote cohesiveness and closeness among friends who perpetrate these acts against a common "enemy" (Werner & Crick, 2004). Thus children with a genetic disposition for relational aggression may use this behavior toward social gains irrespective of their friends' behavior. Furthermore, the lack of punishment and the potential benefits associated with relational aggression may render children without a genetic disposition susceptible to imitating their friends' behavior. In contrast, physical aggression usually entails negative sanctions from the social environment (Werner et al., 2006). Children who are genetically predisposed to physical aggression may be more impervious to such negative sanctions and thus more vulnerable to the influence of physically aggressive friends than children who lack a genetic predisposition to physical aggression. Interestingly, the environmental effect of friends' social and physical aggression on child aggression was found only for the same type of aggressive behavior in the Brendgen, Boivin, Vitaro, Dionne, and colleagues (2008) study. No crossover links from friends' physical aggression to children's social aggression, or vice versa, were found. These context-specific environmental effects of friends are consistent with findings that social and physical aggression are driven by largely the same underlying genetic dispositions but by mostly different environmental influences (Brendgen et al., 2005).

The larger peer environment beyond the child's immediate friendship group also seems to interact with genetic liabilities to differentially affect the development of physical and social aggression. This was shown in a sample of twins whose physical aggression and relational aggression were measured via peer nominations in the twins' kindergarten classes (Brendgen et al., 2013). Injunctive peer-group norms (i.e., the level of acceptance or rejection of these behaviors in the twins' classrooms) were also assessed. Results showed that peer groups varied considerably in terms of the level of acceptability of both physical and relational aggression. More important, children with a genetic disposition for physical aggression were much more likely to express this trait when their classroom injunctive norms were highly favorable to such behavior than when norms were unfavorable. This "facilitation" effect of favorable peer-group norms and "suppression" effect of unfavorable group norms did not apply to social aggression. Because relational aggression involves circuitous behaviors such as the spreading of malicious rumors about the victim, identifying and punishing the aggressor is often difficult. Children with a genetic disposition for relational aggression may therefore use this behavior regardless of whether peer-group norms are favorable or not. Although replication studies are needed, these results emphasize the potentially diverse transactions at play between genetic factors and the peer environment in the development of different types of aggressive behaviors.

Implications

Behavior genetic studies represent a strong quasi-experimental design for investigating the role of environmental factors and their interplay with genetic dispositions in the development of aggression. Still, behavior genetic studies that specifically focus on aggressive behavior rather than on general antisocial behavior or externalizing problems are surprisingly rare. This is even more the case when it comes to the distinction between different forms or functions of aggressive behavior. Nevertheless, the existing findings indicate that genetic liabilities related to aggression may not only lead to negative social experiences within and outside the family but may also often potentiate the effect of such negative experiences toward a further increase of aggression. The little available evidence further suggests that there are similarities but also important differences in the etiology of the different forms and functions of aggression. Specifically, whereas the different forms of aggression seem, to a large extent, driven by the same underlying genetic influences, environmental influences mostly differ. Moreover, the specific genetic and environmental factors that influence the functions of aggression seem to largely differ, once the form of aggression is controlled. Together, these findings provide compelling support of theoretical models explaining the etiology of physical versus social aggression and of proactive versus reactive aggression, respectively (Björkqvist et al., 1992; Dodge, 1991). They also suggest that preventive intervention programs that use a "one-size-fits-all" approach may not succeed in curbing all types of aggressive behavior.

Because they control for genetic confounds, the findings from behavior genetic studies that include specific measures of the environment can inform the selection of potentially modifiable environmental variables for preventive intervention programs. However, most of the reviewed studies also show that genetic and environmental influences on aggression do not work independently of each other, although these interactive effects may vary according to the form or function of aggression. This is important not only from a theoretical but also from a practical perspective, as it suggests that modification of certain environmental conditions through interventions may work better for some individuals than for others. Eventually, this information might help tailor intervention programs to individual needs, optimizing their efficacy and efficiency.

Future Directions

Behavior genetic studies that statistically infer genetic risk have been and still are instrumental in informing us about the ways genetic factors as a whole may work together with specific, measured features of the environment to shape aggression (Johnson, Penke, & Spinath, 2011). However, these studies rely on a number of assumptions that may not always be tenable (Keller & Coventry, 2005). For example, two important assumptions of the classic twin design are that MZ and DZ twin pairs are influenced to the same extent by their shared environment and that there is no assortative mating by the parents on the trait under study. Violation of one or more of these assumptions may result in either over- or underestimations of the genetic and shared environmental variance components. A related issue refers to the fact that finding evidence of $G \times E$ in the presence of rGE typically requires very large sample sizes (Van Der Sluis, Posthuma, & Dolan, 2012), and many behavior genetic studies have been relatively underpowered. Failure to uncover $G \times E$ in some studies may thus, at least in part, be due to a lack of power rather than true absence of $G \times E$. Sufficiently powered studies are also required to examine potential sex differences in rGE and $G \times E$ linking environmental experiences with aggressive behavior, which have rarely been examined to date. More longitudinal behavior genetic studies are needed to explore developmental changes in the genetic–environmental etiology of aggression. Finally, as already noted, greater specificity in the measurement of aggression is essential, along with a clear distinction between subtypes of aggression, in order to obtain a clear understanding how aggressive behavior develops.

It is also important to note that genetic effect estimates in behavior genetic studies do not reflect the effect of genes per se. Instead, they reflect overall genetic influences that also include any existing nonmeasured rGE and G × E, as described below. Thus findings from behavior genetic studies need to be complemented by molecular genetic studies in order to specify the nature of the genes and biological processes involved in the development of aggressive behavior. To this end, the findings from behavior genetic studies can help inform the selection of environmental variables for testing rGE and G × E in molecular genetic research. Still, the past decades have shown how difficult it is to find specific genes that contribute to phenotypic variance. A recent meta-analysis shows that few genetic markers that have been associated with aggression and violence have withstood replication (Vassos, Collier, & Fazel, 2014). Moreover, multiple genes with very small effects are likely to interact with each other, in addition to interacting with environmental influences, with each resulting effect explaining only a very small portion of the overall variance. Practical limitations usually prohibit detection of such complex interconnections, but failure to account for them necessarily leads to biased or inconclusive study results.

There is increasing evidence, however, that genome function is not so much defined by the individual genotype as by the epigenotype (i.e., the pattern of gene activation). Indeed, the same gene can have very different effects, depending on whether it is "switched" on or off and what other genes are activated. The epigenetic code is laid down during the development of the embryo, but it can be modified by environmental influences (Meaney, 2010). Importantly, these epigenetic changes are not restricted to the prenatal or early childhood period but can also occur later in life (Naumova et al., 2012). Emerging research suggests that environmentally induced epigenetic alterations in genes related to dopamine and serotonin pathways, the hypothalamic–pituitary–adrenal axis, and the immune system may be of specific relevance for the development of aggressive behavior, specifically physical aggression (Waltes, Chiocchetti, & Freitag, 2015). Epigenetic mechanisms may thus play an important role in explaining the G × E that promote aggressive behavior. Integrating measures of epigenetic mechanisms, such as DNA methylation, with twin designs in future studies may offer a promising avenue for examining heritable and environmental influences on aggression (van Dongen et al., 2016).

Conclusions

Behavior genetic research has made important contributions to advancing our understanding of the developmental origins of aggressive behavior. Still, many open questions remain. More studies are needed that integrate a genetically informed design with epigenetic measures and specific environmental measures. As noted by Hatemi, Dawes, Frost-Keller, Settle, and Verhulst (2011, p. 81):

> Only by considering both the environmental and genetic sources of individual differences can we gain a deep understanding of behavior. The more we learn about how genes lead us into environments, affect our interpretations of the exogenous environments we encounter, and how our social environments may change our genetic expression, the more we can contribute to the discipline at large about which environments matter and why.

REFERENCES

Arseneault, L., Moffitt, T. E., Caspi, A., Taylor, A., Rijsdijk, F. V., Jaffee, S. R., et al. (2003). Strong genetic effects on cross-situational antisocial behavior among 5-year-old children according to mothers, teachers, examiner-observers, and twins' self-reports. *Journal of Child Psychology and Psychiatry, 44,* 832–848.

Bandura, A. (1973). *Aggression: A social learning analysis.* Englewood Cliffs, NJ: Prentice-Hall.

Barker, E. D., Larsson, H., Viding, E., Maughan, B., Rijsdijk, F., Fontaine, N., et al. (2009). Common genetic but specific environmental influences for aggressive and deceitful behaviors in preadolescent males. *Journal of Psychopathology and Behavioral Assessment, 31,* 299–308.

Berkowitz, L. (1989). Frustration–aggression hypothesis: Examination and reformulation. *Psychological Bulletin, 106,* 59–73.

Björkqvist, K., Lagerspetz, K. M. J., & Kaukiainen, A. (1992). Do girls manipulate and boys fight?: Developmental trends in regard to direct and indirect aggression. *Aggressive Behavior, 18,* 117–127.

Boivin, M., Brendgen, M., Vitaro, F., Dionne, G., Girard, A., Pérusse, D., et al. (2013). Strong genetic contribution to peer relationship difficulties at school entry: Findings from a longitudinal twin study. *Child Development, 84,* 1098–1114.

Boivin, M., Brendgen, M., Vitaro, F., Forget-Dubois, N., Feng, B., Tremblay, R. E., et al. (2013). Evidence of gene–environment correlation for peer difficulties: Disruptive behaviors predict early peer relation difficulties in school through genetic effects. *Development and Psychopathology, 25,* 79–92.

Boivin, M., Pérusse, D., Dionne, G., Saysset, V., Zoccolillo, M., Tarabulsy, G. M., et al. (2005). The genetic–environmental etiology of parents' perceptions and self-assessed behaviors toward their 5-month-old infants in a large twin and singleton sample. *Journal of Child Psychology and Psychiatry, 46,* 612–630.

Boivin, M., Vitaro, F., & Poulin, F. (2005). Peer relationships and the development of aggressive behavior in early childhood. In R. E. Tremblay, W. W. Hartup, & J. Archer (Eds.), *Developmental origins of aggression* (pp. 376–397). New York: Guilford Press.

Brendgen, M., Boivin, M., Dionne, G., Barker, E. D., Vitaro, F., Girard, A., et al. (2011). Gene–environment processes linking aggression, peer victimization, and the teacher–child relationship. *Child Development, 82,* 2021–2036.

Brendgen, M., Boivin, M., Vitaro, F., Bukowski, W. M., Dionne, G., Tremblay, R. E., et al. (2008). Linkages between children's and their friends' social and physical aggression: Evidence for a gene–environment interaction? *Child Development, 79,* 13–29.

Brendgen, M., Boivin, M., Vitaro, F., Dionne, G., Girard, A., & Pérusse, D. (2008). Gene–environment interactions between peer victimization and child aggression. *Development and Psychopathology, 20,* 455–471.

Brendgen, M., Dionne, G., Girard, A., Boivin, M., Vitaro, F., & Pérusse, D. (2005). Examining genetic and environmental effects on social aggression: A study of 6-year-old twins. *Child Development, 76,* 930–946.

Brendgen, M., Girard, A., Vitaro, F., Dionne, G., & Boivin, M. (2013). Do peer group norms moderate the expression of genetic risk for aggression? *Journal of Criminal Justice, 41,* 324–330.

Brendgen, M., Girard, A., Vitaro, F., Dionne, G., & Boivin, M. (2015). Gene–environment correlation linking aggression and peer victimization: Do classroom behavioral norms matter? *Journal of Abnormal Child Psychology, 43,* 19–31.

Brendgen, M., Vitaro, F., Boivin, M., Dionne, G., & Pérusse, D. (2006). Examining genetic and environmental effects on reactive versus proactive aggression. *Developmental Psychology, 42,* 1299–1312.

Burt, S. A. (2009). Are there meaningful etiological differences within antisocial behavior?: Results of a meta-analysis. *Clinical Psychology Review, 29,* 163–178.

Button, T. M. M., Corley, R. P., Rhee, S. H., Hewitt, J. K., Young, S. E., & Stallings, M. C. (2007). Delinquent peer affiliation and conduct problems: A twin study. *Journal of Abnormal Psychology, 116,* 554–564.

Button, T. M. M., Lau, J. Y. F., Maughan, B., & Eley, T. C. (2008). Parental punitive discipline, negative life events and gene–environment interplay in the development of externalizing behavior. *Psychological Medicine, 38,* 29–39.

Button, T. M. M., Scourfield, J., Martin, N., Purcell, S., & McGuffin, P. (2005). Family dysfunction interacts with genes in the causation of antisocial symptoms. *Behavior Genetics, 35,* 115–120.

Button, T. M. M., Stallings, M. C., Rhee, S. H., Corley, R. P., Boardman, J. D., & Hewitt, J. K. (2009). Perceived peer delinquency and the genetic predisposition for substance dependence vulnerability. *Drug and Alcohol Dependence, 100,* 1–8.

Cadoret, R. J., Yates, W. R., Troughton, E., Woodworth, G., & Stewart, M. A. (1995). Genetic–environmental interaction in the genesis of aggressivity and conduct disorders. *Archives of General Psychiatry, 52,* 916–924.

Card, N. A., & Little, T. D. (2007). Longitudinal modeling of developmental processes. *International Journal of Behavioral Development, 31,* 297–302.

Card, N. A., Stucky, B. D., Sawalani, G. M., & Little, T. D. (2008). Direct and indirect aggression during childhood and adolescence: A meta-analytic review of gender differences, intercorrelations, and relations to maladjustment. *Child Development, 79,* 1185–1229.

Conger, K. J., & Conger, R. D. (1994). Differential parenting and change in sibling differences in delinquency. *Journal of Family Psychology, 8,* 287–302.

Crick, N. R., Bigbee, M. A., & Howes, C. (1996). Gender differences in children's normative beliefs about aggression: How do I hurt thee? Let me count the ways. *Child Development, 67,* 1003–1014.

DiLalla, L. F., Bersted, K., & John, S. G. (2015). Evidence of reactive gene-environment correlation in preschoolers' prosocial play with unfamiliar peers. *Developmental Psychology, 51,* 1464–1475.

DiLalla, L. F., & John, S. G. (2014). Genetic and behavioral influences on received aggression during observed play among unfamiliar preschool-aged peers. *Merrill–Palmer Quarterly, 60,* 168–192.

Dodge, K. A. (1991). The structure and function of reactive and proactive aggression. In D. J. Pepler & K. H. Rubin (Eds.), *The development and treatment of childhood aggression* (pp. 201–218). Hillsdale, NJ: Erlbaum.

Falconer, D. S. (1960). *Introduction to quantitative genetics.* Edinburgh, UK: Oliver & Boyd.

Farrington, D. P. (1991). Childhood aggression and adult violence: Early precursors and later-life outcomes. In D. J. Pepler & K. H. Rubin (Eds.), *The development and treatment of childhood aggression* (pp. 5–29). Hillsdale, NJ: Erlbaum.

Feinberg, M. E., Button, T. M. M., Neiderhiser, J. M., Reiss, D., & Hetherington, E. M. (2007). Parenting and adolescent antisocial behavior and depression: Evidence of genotype × parenting environment interaction. *Archives of General Psychiatry, 64,* 457–465.

Fite, P. J., Stauffacher, K., Ostrov, J. M., & Colder, C. R. (2008). Replication and extension of Little et al.'s (2003) forms and functions of aggression measure. *International Journal of Behavioral Development, 32,* 238–242.

Goldstein, S. E., Tisak, M. S., & Boxer, P. (2002). Preschoolers' normative and prescriptive judgments about relational and overt aggression. *Early Education and Development, 13,* 23–39.

Hatemi, P. K., Dawes, C. T., Frost-Keller, A., Settle, J. E., & Verhulst, B. (2011). Integrating social science and genetics: News from the political front. *Biodemography and Social Biology, 57,* 67–87.

Hicks, B. M., South, S. C., DiRago, A. C., Iacono, W. G., & McGue, M. (2009). Environmental adversity and increasing genetic risk for externalizing disorders. *Archives of General Psychiatry, 66,* 640–648.

Jaffee, S. R., Caspi, A., Moffitt, T. E., Dodge, K. A., Rutter, M., Taylor, A., et al. (2005). Nature × nurture: Genetic vulnerabilities interact with physical maltreatment to promote conduct problems. *Development and Psychopathology, 17,* 67–84.

Jaffee, S. R., Caspi, A., Moffitt, T. E., Polo-Tomas, M., Price, T. S., & Taylor, A. (2004). The limits of child effects: Evidence for genetically mediated child effects on corporal punishment but not on physical maltreatment. *Developmental Psychology, 40,* 1047–1058.

Johnson, W., Penke, L., & Spinath, F. M. (2011). Heritability in the era of molecular genetics: Some thoughts for understanding genetic influences on behavioral traits. *European Journal of Personality, 25,* 254–266.

Keller, M. C., & Coventry, W. L. (2005). Quantifying and addressing parameter indeterminacy in the classical twin design. *Twin Research and Human Genetics, 8,* 201–213.

Klahr, A. M., Klump, K. L., & Burt, S. A. (2014). The etiology of the association between child antisocial behavior and maternal negativity varies across aggressive and non-aggressive rule-breaking forms of antisocial behavior. *Journal of Abnormal Child Psychology, 42,* 1299–1311.

Marceau, K., Horwitz, B. N., Narusyte, J., Ganiban, J. M., Spotts, E. L., Reiss, D., et al. (2013). Gene–environment correlation underlying the association between parental negativity and adolescent externalizing problems. *Child Development, 84,* 2031–2046.

Meaney, M. J. (2010). Epigenetics and the biological definition of gene × environment interactions. *Child Development, 81,* 41–79.

Narusyte, J., Andershed, A.-K., Neiderhiser, J., & Lichtenstein, P. (2007). Aggression as a mediator of genetic contributions to the association between negative parent–child relationships and adolescent antisocial behavior. *European Child and Adolescent Psychiatry, 16,* 128–137.

Narusyte, J., Neiderhiser, J. M., Andershed, A.-K., D'Onofrio, B. M., Reiss, D., Spotts, E., et al. (2011). Parental criticism and externalizing behavior problems in adolescents: The role of environment and genotype–environment correlation. *Journal of Abnormal Psychology, 120,* 365–376.

Naumova, O. Y., Lee, M., Koposov, R., Szyf, M., Dozier, M., & Grigorenko, E. L. (2012). Differential patterns of whole-genome DNA methylation in institutionalized children and children raised by their biological parents. *Development and Psychopathology, 24,* 143–155.

Neale, M. C., & Cardon, L. R. (1992). *Methodology for genetic studies of twins and families.* Dordrecht, The Netherlands: Kluwer Academic.

Neiderhiser, J. M., Reiss, D., Pedersen, N. L., Lichtenstein, P., Spotts, E. L., Hansson, K., et al. (2004). Genetic and environmental influences on mothering of adolescents: A comparison of two samples. *Developmental Psychology, 40,* 335–351.

Odgers, C. L., Moffitt, T. E., Broadbent, J. M., Dickson, N., Hancox, R. J., Harrington, H., et al. (2008). Female and male antisocial trajectories: From childhood origins to adult outcomes. *Development and Psychopathology, 20,* 673–716.

Ojanen, T., & Kiefer, S. (2013). Instrumental and reactive functions and overt and relational forms of aggression: Developmental trajectories and prospective associations during middle school. *International Journal of Behavioral Development, 37,* 514–517.

Ottman, R. (1994). Epidemiologic analysis of gene–environment interaction in twins. *Genetic Epidemiology, 11,* 75–86.

Owens, L., Slee, P., & Shute, R. (2000). "It hurts a hell of a lot . . . ": The effects of indirect aggression on teenage girls. *School Psychology International, 21*, 359–376.

Paquin, S., Lacourse, E., Brendgen, M., Vitaro, F., & Dionne, G. (2014). The genetic–environmental architecture of proactive and reactive aggression throughout childhood. *Monatsschrift für Kriminologie und Strafrechtsreform, 97*, 398–420.

Patterson, G. R., Reid, J. B., & Dishion, T. J. (1992). *A social interactional approach: Vol. 4. Antisocial boys*. Eugene, OR: Castalia.

Purcell, S. (2002). Variance components models for gene–environment interaction in twin analysis. *Twin Research, 5*, 554–571.

Purcell, S., & Sham, P. C. (2003). A model-fitting implementation of the DeFries-Fulker model for selected twin data. *Behavior Genetics, 33*, 271–278.

Rubin, K. H., Bukowski, W. M., & Bowker, J. C. (2015). Children in peer groups. In R. M. Lerner (Ed.), *Handbook of child psychology and developmental science: Vol. 4. Ecological settings and processes* (pp. 175–222). Hoboken, NJ: Wiley.

Rutter, M., Moffitt, T. E., & Caspi, A. (2006). Gene–environment interplay and psychopathology: Multiple varieties but real effects. *Journal of Child Psychology and Psychiatry, 47*, 226–261.

Saudino, K. J., & Hines, D. A. (2007). Etiological similarities between psychological and physical aggression in intimate relationships: A behavioral genetic exploration. *Journal of Family Violence, 22*, 121–129.

Scarr, S., & McCartney, K. (1983). How people make their own environments: A theory of genotype–environment effects. *Child Development, 54*, 424–435.

Shanahan, M., & Hofer, S. (2005). Social context in gene–environment interactions: Retrospect and prospect. *Journal of Gerontology: Series B, 60B*, 65–76.

Silberg, J. L., & Eaves, L. J. (2004). Analysing the contributions of genes and parent–child interaction to childhood behavioral and emotional problems: A model for the children of twins. *Psychological Medicine, 34*, 347–356.

Thorpe, K., & Gardner, K. (2006). Twins and their friendships: Differences between monozygotic, dizygotic same-sex and dizygotic mixed-sex pairs. *Twin Research and Human Genetics, 9*, 155–164.

Tremblay, R. E. (1999). When children's social development fails. In D. P. Keating & C. Hertzman (Eds.), *Developmental health and the wealth of nations: Social, biological, and educational dynamics* (pp. 55–71). New York: Guilford Press.

Turkheimer, E. (2000). Three laws of behavior genetics and what they mean. *Current Directions in Psychological Science, 9*, 160–164.

Tuvblad, C., & Baker, L. A. (2011). Human aggression across the lifespan: Genetic propensities and environmental moderators. *Advances in Genetics, 75*, 171–214.

Tuvblad, C., Raine, A., Zheng, M., & Baker, L. A. (2009). Genetic and environmental stability differs in reactive and proactive aggression. *Aggressive Behavior, 35*, 437–452.

Vaillancourt, T., Brendgen, M., Boivin, M., & Tremblay, R. E. (2003). A longitudinal confirmatory factor analysis of indirect and physical aggression: Evidence of two factors over time? *Child Development, 74*, 1628–1638.

van den Oord, E. J., Verhulst, F. C., & Boomsma, D. I. (1996). A genetic study of maternal and paternal ratings of problem behaviors in 3-year-old twins. *Journal of Abnormal Psychology, 105*, 349–357.

Van Der Sluis, S., Posthuma, D., & Dolan, C. V. (2012). A note on false positives and power in G × E modelling of twin data. *Behavior Genetics, 42*, 170–186.

van Dongen, J., Nivard, M. G., Willemsen, G., Hottenga, J.-J., Helmer, Q., Dolan, C. V., et al. (2016). Genetic and environmental influences interact with age and sex in shaping the human methylome. *Nature Communications, 7*, 1–13.

Van Lier, P., Boivin, M., Dionne, G., Vitaro, F., Brendgen, M., Koot, H., et al. (2007).

Kindergarten children's genetic vulnerabilities interact with friends' aggression to promote children's own aggression. *Journal of the American Academy of Child and Adolescent Psychiatry, 46,* 1080–1087.

Vassos, E., Collier, D. A., & Fazel, S. (2014). Systematic meta-analyses and field synopsis of genetic association studies of violence and aggression. *Molecular Psychiatry, 19,* 471–477.

Vitaro, F., & Brendgen, M. (2011). Subtypes of aggressive behaviors: Etiologies, development and consequences. In T. Bliesener, A. Beelmann, & M. Stemmler (Eds.), *Antisocial behavior and crime: Contributions of theory and evaluation research to prevention and intervention* (pp. 17–38). Goettingen, Germany: Hogrefe.

Vitaro, F., Brendgen, M., & Barker, E. D. (2006). Subtypes of aggressive behaviors: A developmental perspective. *International Journal of Behavioral Development, 30,* 12–19.

Vitaro, F., Brendgen, M., Girard, A., Dionne, G., Tremblay, R. E., & Boivin, M. (2016). Links between friends' physical aggression and adolescents' physical aggression: What happens if gene–environment correlations are controlled? *International Journal of Behavioral Development, 40,* 234–242.

Waltes, R., Chiocchetti, A. G., & Freitag, C. M. (2015). The neurobiological basis of human aggression: A review on genetic and epigenetic mechanisms. *American Journal of Medical Genetics: Part B. Neuropsychiatric Genetics, 171B,* 650–675.

Werner, N. E., & Crick, N. R. (2004). Maladaptive peer relationships and the development of relational and physical aggression during middle childhood. *Social Development, 13,* 495–514.

Werner, N. E., Senich, S., & Przepyszny, K. A. (2006). Mothers' responses to preschoolers' relational and physical aggression. *Journal of Applied Developmental Psychology, 27,* 193–208.

CHAPTER 5

Psychophysiology of Aggression

SUSAN BRANJE and HANS M. KOOT

Brief Introduction

In this chapter we review psychophysiological studies of the development and maintenance of aggression in childhood and adolescence. As aggression is likely to be a function of a complex interplay between individual and social factors, this review is concerned with the role of psychophysiological or neurobiological systems in aggressive behavior of children and adolescents, as well as with the interactions of these systems with social factors. The autonomic nervous system (ANS) and the hypothalamic–pituitary–adrenal (HPA) axis both play important roles in the regulation of stress and decision making, and these stress-regulating mechanisms are thought to be important in understanding individual differences in aggressive behavior (Van Goozen, Fairchild, Snoek, & Harold, 2007). Therefore, we focus on the roles of the ANS and the HPA axis in particular.

Main Issues

Although a large body of literature has addressed psychophysiological correlates of aggressive behavior, the results of these studies are at times quite inconsistent. Contributing to this inconsistency in findings is the heterogeneity in studies in terms of methodological and theoretical issues. We pay attention to a number of these issues, which include the heterogeneity in behavioral constructs and the roles of sex and age.

Different Forms of Antisocial and Aggressive Behavior

Regarding heterogeneity in behavioral constructs, many studies focus on antisocial behavior more generally and do not distinguish aggressive behaviors from other antisocial or externalizing behaviors. Although externalizing behaviors are often significantly and strongly correlated, failing to distinguish them might obscure research findings and interpretations. Different forms of externalizing behavior have a divergent developmental course (Bongers, Koot, van der Ende, & Verhulst, 2004). For example, developmental trajectories of physical violence and theft during adolescence and early adulthood are different and differently related to neurocognitive functioning (Barker et al., 2007). It is thus important to compare the role of psychophysiological processes in externalizing behavior more generally with their role in aggressive behavior more specifically.

Even within the construct of aggression, it is important to distinguish between types of aggressive behaviors, as aggressive acts can differ in their developmental origins, can serve various purposes, and can have diverse consequences (Mullin & Hinshaw, 2007). Different types of aggression, such as reactive and proactive aggression, might have diverging underlying psychophysiological processes. *Reactive aggression* is a defensive response linked to frustration or threat and is exhibited in reaction to provocation. Reactive aggression is impulsive and often accompanied by disinhibition and affective instability and high levels of bodily arousal, but not necessarily by antisocial tendencies. *Proactive aggression,* in contrast, is nonimpulsive, goal directed, and controlled and involves calculated efforts to obtain resources important for the self (Dodge, Harnish, Lochman, Bates, & Pettit, 1997). Proactive aggression often occurs in the context of persistent antisocial behavior. Proactive aggressive individuals are less likely to have unstable affects, and their level of arousal is usually low (Vitiello & Stoff, 1997). Therefore, it is not surprising that the psychophysiological correlates of reactive and proactive aggression differ substantially.

Sex Differences

Research on the associations between aggressive behavior and psychophysiological measures generally tends to focus on boys more than on girls. As recent studies suggest that there are fundamental sex differences in the neural regulation of dominance and aggression (e.g., Terranova et al., 2016), it is important not to generalize findings for boys to girls. Instead, sex differences in the psychophysiological processes underlying aggression need to be taken into account.

Research on the associations between aggressive behavior and psychophysiological measures also tends to focus on aggressive behaviors more typical or salient for boys than for girls (Rappaport & Thomas, 2004). Whereas *physical aggression* is defined as behavior that harms others through damage to their physical well-being, *relational aggression* includes behavior that harms others through damage to relationships or feelings of acceptance, friendship, or group inclusion (Crick & Grotpeter, 1995). When examining gender differences in psychophysiological correlates of aggressive behavior, it is important to consider aggressive behaviors that are more typical for girls as well. Psychophysiological measures might predict different forms of aggression for boys and girls (Powch & Houston, 1996) that are relatively norma-tive and effective in the context of their gender-segregated peer groups (Crick & Grotpeter, 1995).

Age Differences

In addition, it is important to consider age differences in the role of psychophysi-ological processes in aggressive behavior. Although psychophysiological processes are often thought to be an underlying mechanism explaining aggressive behav-ior, these processes might play a more or less important role in aggression at dif-ferent points in childhood and adolescence (Lorber, 2004). Moreover, there are clear developmental changes in psychophysiology (Beauchaine & Webb, 2016). Studies addressing the psychophysiology of aggression should account for the fact that developmental changes in tonic and phasic psychophysiological responding are quite common. These changes occur through various mechanisms, includ-ing increased body and brain size and associated alterations in cardiodynamics, or changes in neural architecture such as maturation of frontal brain structures implicated in self-regulation with effects on autonomic function and other neural systems. These developmental changes have ramifications for measures involving both the ANS and the HPA axis and are important for interpretation of age dif-ferences in associations between aggression and psychophysiological measures. It is therefore essential to address developmental issues in the associations between psychophysiological processes and aggression.

Theoretical Considerations

The ANS and Aggression

The ANS has been thought to play an important role in aggressive behavior. The parasympathetic and sympathetic branches of the ANS are thought to control the "fight-or-flight" stress reaction (Porges, 2007). The sympathetic nervous system (SNS) prepares the body for fight or flight in situations of threat or danger. It is associated with responses such as increased heart rate, blood pressure, cardiac out-put, and skin conductance. The parasympathetic nervous system (PNS) conserves energy and restores the body to a calm state. It is associated with vagally mediated responses, such as decreased heart rate and blood pressure, and increased heart rate variability, or the variation in intervals between heartbeats that varies as a function of respiration. The SNS and PNS in a resting state may reflect individual differences in the capacity to respond adaptively to internal and external demands. Resting activity of the SNS may reflect the individual's preparedness for responding to threat, and resting activity of the PNS may reflect the ability to restore the body's functions after a danger has occurred. SNS-linked cardiac activity has been asso-ciated with approach motivational processes, whereas PNS-linked cardiac activity consistently predicts emotion regulation capabilities (Beauchaine, Gatzke-Kopp, & Mead, 2007). However, in young children, better emotion regulation has also been related to greater sympathetic recovery (Kahle, Miller, Lopez, & Hastings, 2016).

Reactive aggression might be related to autonomic hyperarousal (Scarpa & Raine, 1997). According to frustration–anger models, reactive aggression is associated with heightened emotional and physiological arousal. Such autonomic hyperarousal is thought to reflect an automatic stress response (i.e., a defensive motivational state) and negative emotionality to which children react with aggressive behavior. Aggressive individuals might exhibit exaggerated fight-or-flight responses to provocation (Beauchaine, Katkin, Strassberg, & Snarr, 2001; Rappaport & Thomas, 2004). When aggressive individuals perceive stimuli as threatening, their fight-or-flight systems might be activated, involving parasympathetic withdrawal and relatively dominant sympathetic influence on cardiac activity. These changes result in increases in blood pressure (Gump, Matthews, & Raikkonen, 1999) and heart rate (Beauchaine et al., 2001).

Proactive aggression, in contrast, is thought to be related to autonomic underarousal (Scarpa & Raine, 1997). According to *stimulation-seeking theories,* children might attempt to compensate for physiological underarousal by seeking stimulating and risky situations, such as aggressive acts, to raise their arousal to optimal levels (Raine, Venables, & Mednick, 1997; Zuckerman, 1979). Alternatively, *fearlessness theory* (Raine, 1997, 2002) suggests that underarousal might be an indicator of fearlessness. Fearless children are thought to be more likely to engage in aggression to obtain rewards and status because they are relatively insensitive to the potential negative consequences of aggressive behaviors, such as punishment. A third explanation suggests that individuals with low ANS arousal have difficulty attending and reacting to environmental stimulation and might therefore have a higher chance to develop aggressive behavior (Wilson & Gottman, 1996). These theories suggest that physiologically underaroused children have more difficulty attending to the antecedents or consequences of aggressive behavior because of general low levels of arousal across systems (Van Goozen et al., 2007).

The HPA Axis and Aggression

Whereas the ANS reacts very quickly to threatening events, the HPA axis responds somewhat slower and functions as a "backup" and balancing system (Alink et al., 2006; Sapolsky, Romero, & Munck, 2000). The HPA axis controls a series of neurophysiological processes in response to stressful stimuli (De Kloet, 1991). After exposure to a stressor, stress signals trigger the hypothalamus to secrete corticotropin-releasing hormone, which in turn activates the anterior pituitary to secrete adrenocorticotropic hormone (ACTH) (Vazquez, 1998). ACTH subsequently triggers the release of cortisol by the adrenal glands (Chrousos & Gold, 1992). When cortisol secretion reaches a certain level, it binds to glucocorticoid and mineralocorticoid receptors in the brain, which activate a regulatory feedback mechanism inhibiting the production of the corticotropin-releasing hormone, ACTH, and cortisol, in order to return the system to a prestress or basal state (De Kloet, 1991).

The HPA axis also maintains an underlying diurnal/circadian cortisol rhythm that is independent of stress responses but linked to activity level. At awakening, secretion of cortisol increases, followed by a decrease throughout the day (Edwards, Clow, Evans, & Hucklebridge, 2001), with lowest levels at nighttime, at the start of the sleep cycle. As individual differences exist in the functioning of every step in the circadian rhythm, including the sensitivity to these feedback signals (De Kloet, Joëls, & Holsboer, 2005), links of aggression to both HPA axis reactivity to stress and HPA axis circadian functioning have been examined (Cicchetti & Rogosch, 2001). As with the ANS, aggressive behaviors have been theorized to be associated with both low and high activity of the HPA axis. According to the hypo(re)activity hypothesis of the fearlessness theory (Raine, 1997), a significant negative correlation of cortisol with proactive and reactive aggression will be found. This inverse relation between cortisol (re)activity and aggressive behavior has also been labeled the *blunted stress response* (Van Goozen et al., 2007).

Interaction Effects between Psychophysiological Systems

The combined activity of different psychophysiological systems might predict aggressive behavior better than the activity of either subsystem alone. Activity of both the HPA axis and the SNS generally increases in response to stress. According to the *additive model,* and in line with the low-arousal theory, concurrent low reactivity in both systems is related to elevated levels of (proactive) aggressive behavior (Bauer, Quas, & Boyce, 2002). An alternative hypothesis is, however, that aggressive children are characterized by a mismatch or imbalance in the interplay between different physiological systems involved in the regulation of stress. According to the *interactive model,* asymmetry between the HPA axis and the SNS, with low reactivity in one system together with concurrent high reactivity in the other system, may predict aggressive behavior (Bauer et al., 2002). In this model it is thus suggested that the relation between either of the two systems and disruptive behavior is moderated by the other system.

The balance or interaction between the SNS and PNS within the ANS might also play a role in aggressive behavior. Although, generally, the SNS and PNS display well-coordinated, reciprocal actions, with SNS activity increasing when PSN activity decreases and vice versa, it has been argued that the SNS and PNS can function as two separate dimensions (Berntson, Cacioppo, & Quigley, 1991). These nonreciprocal actions may result in concurrent increases or decreases in both systems and lead to ambiguous effects on physiological arousal (Berntson, Cacioppo, & Quigley, 1993). Indeed, several studies have indicated that concurrent low levels of SNS and PNS are related to juvenile disruptive behavior (Beauchaine et al., 2007; Boyce et al., 2001).

A Biosocial Perspective on Childhood Antisocial Behavior

Psychophysiological factors are thought not only to affect aggressive behavior directly but also to interact with social factors in affecting aggressive behavior (Raine, 2002; Raine, Fung, Portnoy, Choy, & Spring, 2014). According to Raine's (2002) biosocial model, the presence of both biological and social risk factors exponentially increases the extent of antisocial and violent behavior. At the same time, when predicting psychophysiological functioning, social factors moderate the relation between psychophysiological factors and antisocial behavior such that these relations are strongest in those from benign social backgrounds. The latter finding is explained by the "social push" hypothesis, suggesting that when antisocial children lack social factors that "push" or predispose them to antisocial behavior, biological factors are more likely to explain antisocial behavior. Also, the association between life adversities and antisocial behavior might depend on reactivity of the ANS. Children who show blunted physiological responses to stressful life events might be unable to adequately respond to stressful situations (Beauchaine, 2001).

Moreover, the role of social factors in developmental changes in psychophysiology should be considered. Experiences during development might affect psychophysiological functioning and thereby change the role of psychophysiology in aggression. In particular, perinatal and early life adversities might be associated with blunted responses of the ANS, but, in cases of extreme adversities, also with increased ANS reactivity (Obradović, 2013). Because plasticity of the ANS decreases with age, stressful experiences later in life are less likely to affect the reactivity regulation mechanisms of the ANS (Boyce & Ellis, 2005; Gunnar, Wewerka, Frenn, Long, & Griggs, 2009). Prenatal influences, such as fetal exposure to cigarettes or alcohol, or early life stressful experiences are thought to inhibit autonomic functions (Fries, Hesse, Hellhammer, & Hellhammer, 2005), resulting in a low resting heart rate in antisocial individuals. However, it is not clear whether ANS reactivity mediates the relation between early life adversities and antisocial behavior.

The propensity to aggression originating from arousal and heightened or lowered stress reactivity is moderated by cognitive factors. Children displaying antisocial behavior show cognitive deficits in executive functioning and verbal intelligence, which are important for the inhibition of impulses and the finding of alternative forms of social interaction, respectively. Social cognitions are deviant in that aggressive children tend to attribute hostile intent to actions of peers and to expect more instrumental gain from their aggressive actions, are more impaired in moral reasoning, show less sensitivity to others' distress, hold more positive views of aggressive means to obtain goals, tend to blame others for their aggression, and emphasize revenge. Moreover, they have difficulties in reversal learning of tasks involving both rewards and punishments (Kimonis, Frick, & McMahon, 2014).

An important notion is that aggressive behavior has to be unlearned (cf., Tremblay, 2003). Children normally learn to inhibit their natural aggressive impulses in the first 5 years of life (e.g., Alink et al., 2006), mainly based on their interactions with primary caregivers that have an organizing effect on different brain structures, including the HPA axis. Genetic, prenatally acquired, and temperament-based risks that underlie aggression need to be regulated by socialization. Several peculiarities in social cognitions that enhance psychophysiology-dependent aggressive impulses are based on deficits in this learning process, possibly because it contributes to or interacts with deficits in responding to social cues (Blair, 2007).

Measures and Methods

Measures of the ANS

Heart Rate

Heart rate is often used as an indicator of the ANS. Heart rate is controlled by both the parasympathetic and sympathetic branches of the ANS. The heart is subject to influence from the sympathetic and parasympathetic branches of the ANS, and it is subject to neuroendocrine influences as well. Chronotropic (i.e., rate-related) cardiac effects such as heart rate variability are controlled primarily by the PNS, whereas inotropic effects such as contractile force and stroke volume are controlled primarily by the SNS.

Respiratory Sinus Arrhythmia

Respiratory sinus arrhythmia (RSA) is naturally occurring heart rate variability in synchrony with respiration. This is measured by periodic changes in heart rate during a resting state of cardiovascular activity. RSA represents the functionality of vagal tone, which serves as the key component of the PNS. An increase in vagal tone both slows the heart and makes heart rate more variable. During a breathing cycle, the R–R interval, or the time between two of the distinctive, large, upward *R* spikes on an electrocardiogram, is shortened during inhalation, as inhalation temporarily suppresses vagal activity, causing an immediate increase in heart rate. The R–R interval is prolonged during exhalation, which decreases heart rate as it causes vagal activity to resume. Vagal tone (and specifically its influence on heart rate) represents an index for the functional state of the entire PNS.

Resting heart rate and electrodermal activity (EDA) measures reflect the assessment of autonomic activity in the absence of any obvious external stimuli. Heart rate and EDA in response to experimental stimuli are frequently measured in raw form during tasks (task physiology) or expressed as a change from baseline or pre-stimulus levels (physiological reactivity).

Cardiac Pre-Ejection Period

SNS-linked cardiac activity can also be assessed using the pre-ejection period (PEP), an index of the time elapsed between left ventricular depolarization and ejection of blood into the aorta. Shorter intervals represent greater SNS activity.

Salivary Alpha-Amylase

Salivary alpha-amylase is an enzyme produced in the oral mucosa and is an assumptive marker of the adrenergic component of the stress response. Salivary alpha-amylase levels are associated with activity of the sympathetic adrenal medullary system, which is activated by the SNS under stress. Salivary alpha-amylase levels increase under stressful conditions that are also associated with increases in plasma catecholamines, heart rate, systolic blood pressure, PEP, and cardiac output (Skosnik, Chatterton, Swisher, & Park, 2000). However, salivary alpha-amylase can be elevated in response to a stressor independently of serum catecholamines and may reflect a general marker of sympathetic adrenal medullary system activity (van Stegeren, Rohleder, Everaerd, & Wolf, 2006).

Skin Conductance Activity

Skin conductance activity is also referred to as EDA or electrodermal response (EDR). Skin conductance is an indication of psychological or physiological arousal.

Skin resistance varies with the state of sweat glands in the skin. Sweating is controlled by the SNS. If the sympathetic branch of the ANS is highly aroused, sweat gland activity increases, which in turn increases skin conductance. EDA is thus under exclusive control of the SNS (Blascovich & Kelsey, 1990).

Measures of the HPA Axis

Cortisol

Activity of the HPA axis can be estimated using measures of cortisol, which can be assessed in saliva, plasma, or urine. Typically, both basal and stress-induced cortisol levels are used to examine association with aggressive behavior. *Basal* cortisol is often assessed with the cortisol awakening response (CAR). The CAR is superimposed on the circadian rhythm of cortisol secretion, and, in addition to basal activity as reflected by daytime cortisol, it also reflects the reactivity or flexibility of the HPA axis (Fries, Dettenborn, & Kirschbaum, 2009). Basal cortisol is usually assessed with morning cortisol. Cortisol is typically measured in saliva, with samples collected immediately after awakening, then 30 minutes and 60 minutes later (Pruessner et al., 1997). Cortisol *reactivity* is typically assessed as a response to stressful tasks, such as public speaking. Saliva samples are collected at different points during the task to obtain participants' cortisol levels at baseline and at several intervals after the task.

Central Research Findings

ANS (Re)activity

Autonomic Response Measures: Cardiovascular and Electrodermal Activity

Studies of children and adolescents exhibiting antisocial behavior have yielded consistent evidence of lower levels of autonomic activity in comparison with control youth, although associations depend on type of antisocial behavior and psychophysiological measures (Ortiz & Raine, 2004). A relation between resting heart rate and aggressive behavior has been consistently found in several meta-analyses. A meta-analysis of 95 studies (Lorber, 2004) investigated the relations of heart rate with aggression, psychopathy, and conduct problems, thereby distinguishing resting heart rate, test heart rate, and heart rate reactivity. Based on 16 studies, the meta-analysis revealed that lower resting heart rate was weakly related to higher aggression. Age did not significantly moderate this relation. However, whereas higher aggression was reliably associated with heart rate in children and adults, the association was not significant in samples including adolescents. Lower resting heart rate was also negatively related to conduct problems, but not to psychopathy. Heart rate during task activity was not significantly related to aggression, conduct problems, or psychopathy, and this effect was also not moderated by age.

A second meta-analysis, including 46 studies on children and adolescents (Ortiz & Raine, 2004), showed a significant negative relation between resting heart rate and levels of antisocial behavior. This effect was not significantly moderated by gender differences, by use of a psychiatric versus nonpsychiatric control group, by method of assessing heart rate, or by age. Using a sample of 9 studies, antisocial behavior was also found to be negatively associated with heart rate in a stress condition. The meta-analysis did not examine the moderating effect of type of antisocial behavior.

A more recent systematic review and meta-analysis of the relation between resting heart rate and antisocial behavior (Portnoy & Farrington, 2015) included 115 independent effect sizes and yielded a significant negative effect size of $d = -0.20$. Sex and age did not moderate the relation between resting heart rate and antisocial behavior. Antisocial behavior type did not moderate the association. Summary effect sizes were significant for aggression, violence, and behavior problems.

In sum, these meta-analyses demonstrated that the relation between low resting heart rate and antisocial behavior is highly replicable and applies to multiple types of antisocial behavior, including aggression. The relation is also consistently found across children, adolescents, and adults, although some individual studies show exceptions to this pattern. For example, in a recent study among 412 children, lower resting mean heart rate at age 14 months did not predict aggression at age 3 years (Dierckx et al., 2014). The lack of sex differences in the relation between heart rate and antisocial behavior is consistent with the claim that the same risk factors apply to antisocial behavior in both males and females (Moffitt, Caspi, Rutter, & Silva, 2001), despite the fact that females have a higher resting heart rate than males (Voors, Webber, & Berenson, 1982).

Thus studies have consistently shown that children and adolescents who exhibit antisocial behavior, and aggressive behavior more specifically, have lower resting levels of heart rate than control youth (Lorber, 2004; Ortiz & Raine, 2004). The finding of low resting heart rate among children with aggressive behavioral tendencies suggests chronic underarousal in aggressive individuals (Scarpa & Raine, 1997). In response to stressors, children who display aggressive conduct problems tend to have an enhanced heart rate (Lorber, 2004).

Because heart rate is determined by both sympathetic and parasympathetic influences, and because dysregulation in the SNS appears to have different implications for adjustment than dysregulation in the PNS (Beauchaine et al., 2007), several studies have focused on measures more specifically related to SNS or PNS. To study parasympathetic mediation of cardiovascular activity, heart rate reactivity and RSA suppression have been examined most often. Heart rate reactivity, that is, enhanced heart rate variability under circumstances involving stressors or challenges, has been associated with aggressive behavior of children and adolescents (Beauchaine et al., 2001), which suggests weaker vagal–parasympathetic regulation of heart rate activity in exhibiting aggressive conduct problems. Low heart rate variability has also been associated with externalizing problems (Pine, Shaffer, Schonfeld, & Davies, 1997). The meta-analysis by Lorber (2004) found that higher heart rate variability was not significantly associated with higher levels of aggression nor psychopathy, although it was significantly related to higher conduct problems among children and adolescents. Also, aggressive boys have been found to exhibit lower RSA suppression, which is related to attentional and emotional processes, than nonaggressive boys (Calkins & Dedmon, 2000). Similarly, boys who were high on aggression exhibited lower RSA across baselines than boys who were low on aggression. In contrast, no difference in baseline RSA was observed for girls who were high versus low on aggression (Beauchaine, Hong, & Marsh, 2008). In sum, findings with respect to autonomic reactivity to noxious or threatening stimuli have been more mixed, in particular for heart rate reactivity. Lower RSA suppression seems to be more consistently related to more aggressive behavior.

Considering measures of SNS, there is evidence that low skin conductance activity, which is linked to lower behavioral inhibition, accounts for variation in antisocial behavior. In the meta-analysis by Lorber (2004), low resting skin conductance activity was associated with psychopathy and with conduct problems in children, but not with aggressive behavior. Similarly, low task skin conductance activity was associated with psychopathy among adults and with conduct problems in children, but not with aggressive behavior. Higher skin conductance reactivity was positively associated with aggression among adults and negatively associated with psychopathy. Low skin conductance activity has been found to predict the onset of aggression in children and adults. For example, skin conductance activity in 70 typically developing 1-year-old infants at baseline, during an orienting habituation paradigm, and during a fear challenge was significantly and negatively related to mother-reported aggressive behavior at 3 years of age (Baker, Shelton, Baibarazova, Hay, & Van Goozen, 2013). Some studies reported sex differences in associations of skin conductance with aggression. Boys with high levels of aggression did not differ from boys with low levels of aggression in patterns of skin conductance across baselines. In contrast, girls who were aggressive exhibited initially high levels of skin conductance, which then decreased across repeated baseline assessments, whereas girls with low aggression exhibited initially low levels of skin conductance, which then increased across repeated baseline assessments (Beauchaine et al., 2008).

Baseline PEP has been related to reward sensitivity during incentive conditions. Baseline PEP was not significantly related to aggression, but under reward conditions there was significantly less PEP shortening among participants who were high on aggression than among participants who were low on aggression (Beauchaine, 2001). In addition, for male participants only, whereas those who were low on aggression exhibited initial PEP reactivity to incentives, which habituated across trials, those high on aggression exhibited no PEP reactivity to reward (Beauchaine et al., 2008).

In conclusion, studies of parasympathetic and sympathetic activity have generally revealed that aggressive children and adolescents exhibit lower baseline levels of autonomic arousal but higher autonomic reactivity to stressful events. Enhanced heart rate variability under stressful conditions suggests that children and adolescents with aggressive conduct problems have weaker vagal–parasympathetic regulation of heart rate activity (Beauchaine et al., 2001). In addition, lower resting heart rate suggests that these children experience chronic underarousal, and lower skin conductance reflects weak inhibitory capacity, all of which might lower the threshold for impulsive aggressive behavior (Beauchaine et al., 2001). In sum, these findings suggest that aggressive children have difficulties regulating emotions such as anger and tend to react defensively under conditions of threat.

A few studies have examined the role of sensation seeking in the association between parasympathetic and sympathetic activity and aggressive behavior to test whether underarousal leads to more stimulation seeking in order to raise arousal levels (Zuckerman, 1979). A longitudinal study among participants at the ages of 11, 13½, and 16 examined whether fun seeking mediated the relationship between heart rate and antisocial behaviors (Sijtsema et al., 2010). Results showed that heart rate at age 11 was negatively associated with fun seeking at age 13½, and that fun seeking at age 13½ was positively associated with rule breaking at age 16 for both boys and girls. In boys, fun seeking mediated the relation between heart rate and rule breaking but not the relation between heart rate and aggression. Moreover, in girls, heart rate was not significantly associated with aggression at all. Another study examined sensation seeking as a moderator instead of a mediator. A significant relation between low resting heart rate and increased aggression was found, but only for individuals with low levels of sensation seeking (Wilson & Scarpa, 2014). In sum, there seems to be some evidence of relations between heart rate, fun seeking, and conduct problems, but the findings are inconsistent across constructs and gender.

Autonomic Functioning in Proactive and Reactive Aggression

Several researchers have examined whether autonomic functioning is differently related to proactive and reactive aggression. In a meta-analysis including four studies, no significant difference in resting heart rate was found (Portnoy & Farrington, 2015). In a study among 8-year-old children who participated in a task in which they lost a board game and prize to a confederate who cheated, reactive aggression, but not proactive aggression, was significantly and positively related to skin conductance reactivity and negatively to heart rate reactivity (Hubbard et al., 2002). In this study, proactive and reactive aggression were included as predictors simultaneously in the regression to account for the large amount of shared variance between proactive and reactive aggression. Among 42 children ages 6–13 years, resting heart rate was significantly correlated with reactive but not proactive aggression, and no significant correlations were found with skin conductance and heart rate variability (Scarpa, Chiara Haden, & Tanaka 2010). When proactive and reactive aggression were simultaneously included as predictors, reactive aggression was again significantly related to decreased heart rate variability, whereas proactive aggression was significantly related to increased heart rate variability and skin conductance. This pattern of autonomic activity, with parallel effects for parasympathetic and sympathetic activity, is in contrast with predictions made by general arousal theory that heightened sympathetic activity will necessarily be associated with reduced parasympathetic activity.

Additional support for distinct physiological processes underlying different forms of aggression can be found in a growing literature suggesting that callous–unemotional (CU) behaviors and oppositional defiant disorder (ODD) behaviors are associated with distinct psychophysiological profiles (Frick, Ray, Thornton, & Kahn, 2014). Particularly, CU behaviors, including a lack of empathy, lack of guilt, and low emotional responsiveness, tend to be characterized by reduced baseline functioning and blunted physiological responses to stressors. Kavish and colleagues (2017) found that in adolescence lower resting heart rate was related to higher scores on CU and sensation seeking in males, but not in females. Lower baseline RSA, but not heart period, across infancy was found to be associated with both ODD and

CU behaviors in childhood (Wagner et al., 2017). In a different sample, no group differences were observed in children at 6 months of age, but at 15 months of age children with later conduct problems with CU displayed lower levels of heart period and RSA and higher cortisol levels compared with children with conduct problems only and children with no conduct problems (Mills-Koonce et al., 2015). Among male adolescents with disruptive behavior disorder (DBD), adolescents with high CU showed lower resting RSA and less heart rate change from baseline in reaction to sadness than respondents with low CU and controls (De Wied, van Boxtel, Matthys, & Meeus, 2012). Resting heart rate was not different between DBD groups but was significantly lower in adolescents with DBD and with high CU traits compared with controls. Comparably, children with conduct disorder (CD) and high CU traits displayed lower magnitude of heart rate change than both children with CD only and controls (Anastassiou-Hadjicharalambous & Warden, 2008). In sum, the antisocial behavior of children high on CU traits might be due to a combination of underarousal, as indicated by low autonomic activity, and emotional dysregulation, as indicated by their low RSA scores. Children high on CU traits seem to show lower levels of fearfulness and insensitivity to punishment (Fanti, 2016; Frick et al., 2014), and, in line with fearlessness theory, their antisocial and aggressive behavior might result from underarousal.

A study including both physical and relational aggression provided support for the hypothesis that heightened cardiac reactivity to provocation is associated with relational aggression among girls. In contrast, for boys, lower cardiac reactivity was associated with physical aggression. These results suggest that the association between cardiovascular reactivity and aggression differs for males and females and that reactivity following relational provocation may be an especially important predictor of relational aggression among girls (Murray-Close & Crick, 2007).

HPA-Axis Activity

Associations of Aggressive Behavior with Basal Cortisol Levels

Several studies have shown a relation between basal cortisol levels and aggressive behavior. A meta-analysis on the relation between basal cortisol and externalizing behavior showed a significant but small negative relation (Alink et al., 2008). The age of children significantly moderated this relation: Externalizing behavior was associated with higher basal cortisol (hyperactivity) in preschoolers, and with lower basal cortisol (hypoactivity) in elementary school-age children. Among adolescents, cortisol was not significantly related to externalizing behavior. The meta-analysis did not find differences in effects for aggressive behavior compared with other types of externalizing behavior. Similarly, a meta-analysis reported a small to moderate effect across clinical studies in the direction of an inverse relationship between basal cortisol levels and DBD symptoms (Van Goozen et al., 2007). The moderating effect of age on the association between cortisol and aggressive behavior has been attributed to common factors affecting conduct problems and HPA-axis functioning. In early childhood, stress—for example, resulting from harsh and inconsistent parenting—is associated with both conduct problems and heightened cortisol levels. In case of prolonged stress, that is, in case of allostatic load, the HPA axis may downregulate, resulting in lower levels of basal cortisol or hypoactivity (Fries et al., 2005).

Comparable results were reported in a number of recent longitudinal studies. Cortisol levels show modest stability over time, and a study using latent state–trait modeling to distinguish state-like from trait-like sources in basal cortisol levels in youth from the general population revealed that 70% of the variance in cortisol levels could be attributed to state-like sources and 28% to trait-like sources. For boys only, higher levels of externalizing problem behaviors were consistently associated with lower cortisol attributable to trait-like sources across 3 years of behavioral assessment (Shirtcliff, Granger, Booth, & Johnson, 2005). Similarly, a study among 390 adolescents ages 15–17 revealed that adolescents who showed persistent aggressive behavior across the years had decreased cortisol levels at awakening consistently over the years as compared with adolescents with low aggression (Platje et al., 2013). In the same way, low cortisol in preadolescence was associated with more aggressive behavior 5 years later, during middle adolescence. In a sample of adolescent boys, low self-control was identified as the primary personality mediator of the relation between low cortisol and later aggressive behavior (Shoal, Giancola, & Kirillova, 2003). Cortisol was not related to negative emotionality or any of its factors (including trait aggression). Also, young adolescent girls with externalizing behavior problems revealed a significantly higher CAR than girls without behavior problems or girls with comorbid externalizing and internalizing behavior problems. This effect was absent in boys, however (Marsman et al., 2008).

In contrast, several studies showed positive relations between cortisol levels and externalizing behavior in elementary school-age children and adolescents. A study among 1,768 Dutch preadolescents from the general population found small but significant positive correlations between both baseline morning and evening salivary cortisol levels and disruptive behaviors (Sondeijker et al., 2007). Similarly, in a population-based sample of boys who were followed longitudinally from childhood to adolescence, higher cortisol levels at age 13 were found in boys with CD than in boys without CD. In addition, boys with an aggressive form of CD had higher cortisol levels than boys with a covert form of CD (van Bokhoven et al., 2005). Associations between heightened cortisol levels and aggressive behavior have also been reported. For example, in this population-based sample of boys, *reactive* aggression was strongly correlated with heightened cortisol (van Bokhoven et al., 2005). Additionally, a study examining changes in aggressive behavior between the ages of 8 and 10 revealed that boys whose cortisol levels rose most between the ages of 8 and 10 were also those whose aggressive behavior increased most during the same time frame (Azurmendi et al., 2016).

Proactive and Reactive Aggression

A few studies have examined associations between cortisol and aggression separately for proactive and reactive aggression. Among girls admitted for acute psychiatric inpatient treatment, the significant negative correlation between cortisol and aggression seems to be present for both proactive and reactive aggression (Stoppelbein, Greenig, Luebbe, Fite, & Becker, 2014). Tests of indirect effects from cortisol to aggression through subdimensions of psychopathy indicated significant pathways via narcissism to proactive and reactive aggression. Among 245, 15-year-olds from an epidemiological cohort study of children at risk for psychopathology, both reactive and proactive aggression were significantly negatively correlated with plasma cortisol levels in males, but not in females (Poustka et al., 2010). This association between cortisol levels and aggression was found to be mediated by impulsivity rather than by psychopathic traits.

In conclusion, these results suggest that HPA-axis functioning may be differentially relevant in clinical or high-risk samples than at the general population level. Whereas in clinical samples, hypoarousal might be more characteristic of children with high levels of aggression, in population samples, higher aggression might go together with hyperarousal.

Associations of Aggressive Behavior with Cortisol Levels in Reaction to a Stressor

A meta-analysis showed that there was no association between cortisol reactivity and externalizing behaviors, but, again, this meta-analysis did not distinguish between different types of externalizing behaviors (Alink et al., 2008). Reactive aggression significantly predicted total and peak poststress cortisol regardless of stress modality. Proactive aggression was not a predictor of any cortisol index. A comparison of pure reactive, proactive, combined, or nonaggressive children indicated that reactive aggressive children had higher cortisol reactivity than proactive and nonaggressive children. This suggests that an overactive HPA-axis response to stress is associated with reactive aggression, whereas stress-induced HPA-axis variability does not seem to be related to proactive aggression (Lopez-Duran, Hajal, Olson, Felt, & Vazquez, 2009).

Future Directions

The Combined Activity of Different Psychophysiological Systems

The combined activity of different psychophysiological systems might predict aggressive behavior better than the activity of either subsystem alone (Bauer et al., 2002). According to the dual hormone hypothesis, social dominance, including aggressive behavior, is jointly regulated by the hypothalamic–pituitary–gonadal and HPA axes (van Honk, Harmon-Jones, Morgan, & Schutter, 2010). Specifically, testosterone predicts high levels of physical aggression particularly when levels of cortisol are low (Popma et al., 2007). In a nonclinical sample of 259 boys and girls age 17 years, a positive testosterone/cortisol ratio, that is, high testosterone relative to cortisol, was found to be associated with more aggressive behavior. The interaction between testosterone and cortisol was, however, not related to aggressive behavior (Platje et al., 2015). The ratio may reflect an imbalance, leaving the individual more prone to rewarding aspects than to negative implications of aggressive behavior.

Interactions between cortisol and estradiol have also been reported. Among 105 adolescents, those with high estradiol and low cortisol concentrations were found to be at highest risk for externalizing problems, but *only* when personality traits of disagreeableness and emotional instability were high (Tackett et al., 2015).

The asymmetry between salivary cortisol and alpha-amylase reactivity to stress might also be important in understanding aggressive behavior. In a sample of maltreated early adolescents and a control group, interactions between the HPA axis and the SNS were linked with aggressive behavior (Gordis, Granger, Susman, & Trickett, 2006). At lower levels of alpha-amylase reactivity, lower cortisol reactivity corresponded to higher parent-reported adolescent aggression, but at high alpha-amylase reactivity levels, cortisol reactivity was not related to parent-reported adolescent aggression. Thus symmetry in the direction of low activity in both systems was associated with more aggression. Youth with HPA-axis hypoactivity may be less inhibited from engaging in aggressive behavior, but high sympathetic arousal may buffer this effect and protect against development of aggression (Raine, 2005). Youth who have low activity in both systems may be particularly uninhibited and fail to learn from punishment, resulting in higher aggression.

These findings suggest that we need to consider interactions between the HPA axis and the hypothalamic–pituitary–gonadal axis, as well as interactions between the HPA axis and the SNS in understanding aggression. Not all studies find evidence for interaction effects, however. For example, among 48 delinquent male adolescents with and without a DBD and 16 matched normal controls, alpha-amylase and cortisol reactivity, but not heart rate and heart rate variability, were significantly and negatively associated with disruptive behavior, but no significant interactions between these parameters in relation to disruptive behavior were found (de Vries-Bouw et al., 2012). Further research is needed to acquire a better understanding of the ways different psychophysiological systems interact in affecting aggressive behavior.

A Biosocial Perspective on Childhood Antisocial Behavior

Recent studies have examined a wide range of interactions between psychophysiology measures and environmental factors in explaining antisocial behavior and aggression. Several researchers have found that perinatal adversities put youth at a greater risk for antisocial behavior (Beck & Shaw, 2005; Tremblay, 2010). However, not all studies support an interaction between perinatal adversities and psychophysiological functioning in explaining antisocial behavior (e.g., Sijtsema et al., 2015).

Adversities in childhood have also been studied in relation to psychophysiological factors. Marital conflict in childhood affected externalizing problems more strongly among youth with blunted SNS and RSA reactivity (El-Sheikh, Hinnant, & Erath, 2011; Obradović, Bush, & Boyce, 2011). Also, among 334 Hong Kong schoolchildren ages 11–17 years, low resting heart rate interacted with high psychosocial adversity in explaining higher reactive (but not proactive) aggression (Raine et al., 2014). Moreover, adversities during childhood and adolescence were related to antisocial behavior at age 16 only in boys with blunted RSA reactivity and PNS reactivity as shown by PEP reactivity and smaller PEP differences from rest to recovery (Sijtsema et al., 2015). In contrast, for girls with heightened RSA reactivity and larger PEP differences from rest to recovery, childhood adversities were associated with antisocial behavior. Furthermore, negative interaction with parents predicted relative decreases in externalizing behavior for adolescent girls low in resting RSA, whereas the association was nonsignificant for girls with high RSA (van der Graaff et al., 2016). Additionally, among 358 Dutch adolescents, morning cortisol moderated the longitudinal effects of neighborhood density on parent-reported delinquency and aggression and adolescent self-reported delinquency (Yu et al., 2016). More specifically, for adolescents with high levels of cortisol, higher neighborhood density significantly predicted higher levels of parent-reported and adolescent self-reported delinquency and aggression, whereas the association was reversed or nonsignificant for adolescents with low cortisol.

These examples show that there are complex interactions between environmental factors and psychophysiological processes in explaining behavior and that these interactions might differ depending on children's age and gender. More research is needed to acquire a better understanding of the interplay of different factors.

Conclusions

Summarizing the findings presented in this chapter, antisocial behavior in children and adolescents is consistently related to lower levels of autonomic activity and decreased HPA axis activity, although associations tend to vary by type of antisocial behavior and psychophysiological measure (Lorber, 2004; Ortiz & Raine, 2004). The most consistent relations are those between low resting heart rate and cortisol at awakening and antisocial behavior. This relation has been found for various types of antisocial behavior, including aggression, and suggests chronic underarousal in aggressive individuals. Lower RSA suppression also seems to be consistently related to more aggressive behavior. Results for heart rate in reaction to stressors are more inconsistent but suggest enhanced heart rate responses to stressors in children exhibiting aggressive conduct problems specifically (Lorber, 2004). In conclusion, aggressive children and adolescents tend to have lower baseline levels of autonomic arousal yet higher autonomic reactivity to stressful events. Enhanced heart rate variability under stressful conditions might indicate that children and adolescents with aggressive conduct problems have weaker vagal–parasympathetic regulation of heart rate activity (Beauchaine et al., 2001). In addition, lower resting heart rate might indicate that these children experience chronic underarousal, and lower skin conductance might indicate a weaker capacity to inhibit impulses. These processes might lower the threshold for impulsive aggressive behavior (Beauchaine et al., 2001). In sum, these findings suggest that children who display higher levels of aggression have difficulties with regulating emotions such as anger, resulting in enhanced defensive reactivity under conditions of threat.

The association between low heart rate and antisocial behavior can be explained by different theories. First, according to stimulation-seeking theory, low arousal represents an unpleasant physiological state, and antisocial individuals seek stimulation to increase their arousal levels to an optimal or normal level (e.g., Ortiz & Raine 2004; Raine, 2002). The relation between heart rate and antisocial behavior has indeed been found to be mediated by fun seeking (Sijtsema et al., 2010). Second, according to fearlessness theory (Raine, 1997), low levels of arousal during stressful situations are indicative of low levels of fear. This lack of fear is thought to make children less likely to respond to socializing punishments, which may subsequently contribute to poor fear conditioning and poor conscience development.

Third, biosocial theory predicts that psychophysiological factors interact with psychosocial risk factors in predicting antisocial behavior (Raine, 2002). Increasing numbers of researchers have investigated these biosocial interactions, but more research is needed to understand the interplay between biological and social factors.

It is important to note that the functioning of the HPA axis or the ANS might not play a causal role in aggressive behavior, but instead might be a marker for other unmeasured underlying processes that are involved in antisocial behavior, such as genetic factors (see Brendgen, Vitaro, & Boivin, Chapter 4, this volume). Moreover, psychophysiological factors can be both a cause and a consequence of behavior. Most studies on the relation between psychophysiological factors and aggressive behavior are cross-sectional, and we are in need of more longitudinal studies that can inform us about the direction of developmental change between aggressive behavior and psychophysiological processes.

Studies also depicted a differential pattern of psychophysiological activity for reactive versus proactive aggression. These differences are found mainly for psychophysiological reactivity. Reactive aggression seems to be related to decreased heart rate variability and higher cortisol reactivity, whereas proactive aggression appears to be related to increased heart rate variability and lower cortisol reactivity. This suggests that an overactive HPA axis response to stress is associated with reactive aggression, whereas stress-induced HPA axis variability does not seem to be related to proactive aggression (Lopez-Duran et al., 2009). Proactive aggression might occur in situations that require activation of the entire ANS to be prepared to respond to danger but also maintain a calm state in order to intimidate or obtain a goal (Raine, 2002). For situations involving reactive aggression, reduced heart rate variability may reflect heightened negative emotionality. In line with the neurobiological model of reactive aggression (van Goozen et al., 2007), sympathetic underactivity may increase sensitivity to stressors. This apparent discrepancy is in line with the multidimensional nature of autonomic responding, in which the sympathetic and parasympathetic branches of the ANS do not always have to function as coupled dimensions (Berntson et al., 1991). The extent to which high autonomic reactivity is related to aggressive behavior might also be moderated by social context (Ellis & Boyce, 2008). Both supportive, low-stress environments and stressful environments can promote high autonomic reactivity, but only in stressful environments might highly reactive individuals show aggressive behavior. Moreover, the discrepant findings regarding autonomic functioning in reactive aggression and proactive aggression might reflect differences in emotional control or emotion regulation (Beauchaine, 2001). Proactive aggression tends to be associated with higher heart rate variability and enhanced vagal tone, and as such it might be associated with better emotion regulation. Although higher emotional control is generally adaptive, in proactive aggression it might reflect the abilities to show goal-directed aggressive behavior and delay gratification. In contrast, the lower heart rate variability and vagal tone that characterizes reactive aggression might reflect decreased emotion regulation, which might play a role in aggressive outbursts.

In conclusion, research suggests small associations between psychophysiological processes and aggressive behavior, but the patterns of association differ depending on type of aggression. Longitudinal studies are needed in order to delineate the developmental psychophysiological processes that underlie impulsive reactive aggression versus more callous–instrumental forms of proactive aggression.

REFERENCES

Alink, L. R. A., Mesman, J., van Zeijl, J., Stolk, M. N., Juffer, F., Koot, H. M., et al. (2006). The early aggression curve: Development of physical aggression in 10- to 50-month-old children. *Child Development, 77,* 954–966.

Alink, L. R. A., van IJzendoorn, M. H., Bakermans-Kranenburg, M. J., Mesman, J., Juffer, F., & Koot, H. M. (2008). Cortisol and externalizing behavior in children and adolescents: Mixed meta-analytic evidence for the inverse relation of basal cortisol and cortisol reactivity with externalizing behavior. *Developmental Psychobiology, 50,* 427–450.

Anastassiou-Hadjicharalambous, X., & Warden, D. (2008). Physiologically indexed and self-perceived affective empathy in conduct-disordered children high and low on callous–unemotional traits. *Child Psychiatry and Human Development, 39,* 503–517.

Azurmendi, A., Pascual-Sagastizabal, E., Vergara, A. I., Muñoz, J. M., Braza, P., Carreras, R., et al. (2016). Developmental trajectories of aggressive behavior in children from ages 8 to 10: The role of sex and hormones. *American Journal of Human Biology, 28,* 90–97.

Baker, E., Shelton, K. H., Baibarazova, E., Hay, D. F., & Van Goozen, S. H. M. (2013). Low skin conductance activity in infancy predicts aggression in toddlers 2 years later. *Psychological Science, 24,* 1051–1056.

Barker, E. D., Séguin, J. R., White, H. R., Bates, M. E., Lacourse, É., Carbonneau, R., et al. (2007). Developmental trajectories of male physical violence and theft: Relations to neurocognitive performance. *Archives of General Psychiatry, 64,* 592–599.

Bauer, A. M., Quas, J. A., & Boyce, W. T. (2002). Associations between physiological reactivity and children's behavior: Advantages of a multisystem approach. *Journal of Developmental and Behavioral Pediatrics, 23,* 102–113.

Beauchaine, T. P. (2001). Vagal tone, development, and Gray's motivational theory: Toward an integrated model of autonomic nervous system functioning in psychopathology. *Development and Psychopathology, 13,* 183–214.

Beauchaine, T. P., Gatzke-Kopp, L., & Mead, H. K. (2007). Polyvagal theory and developmental psychopathology: Emotion dysregulation and conduct problems from preschool to adolescence. *Biological Psychology, 74,* 174–184.

Beauchaine, T. P., Hong, J., & Marsh, P. (2008). Sex differences in autonomic correlates of conduct problems and aggression. *Journal of the American Academy of Child and Adolescent Psychiatry, 47,* 788–796.

Beauchaine, T. P., Katkin, E. S., Strassberg, Z., & Snarr, J. (2001). Disinhibitory psychopathology in male adolescents: Discriminating conduct disorder from attention-deficit/hyperactivity disorder through concurrent assessment of multiple autonomic states. *Journal of Abnormal Psychology, 110,* 610–624.

Beauchaine, T. P., & Webb, S. J. (2016). Developmental processes. In J. T. Cacioppo, L. G. Tassinary, & G. G. Berntson (Eds.), *Handbook of psychophysiology* (pp. 495–510). Cambridge, UK: Cambridge University Press.

Beck, J. E., & Shaw, D. S. (2005). The influence of perinatal complications and environmental adversity on boys' antisocial behavior. *Journal of Child Psychology and Psychiatry, 46,* 35–46.

Berntson, G. G., Cacioppo, J. T., & Quigley, K. S. (1991). Autonomic determinism: The modes of autonomic control, the doctrine of autonomic space, and the laws of autonomic constraint. *Psychological Review, 98,* 459–487.

Berntson, G. G., Cacioppo, J. T., & Quigley, K. S. (1993). Respiratory sinus arrhythmia:

Autonomic origins, physiological mechanisms, and psychophysiological implications. *Psychophysiology, 30,* 183–196.

Blair, R. J. R. (2007). The amygdala and ventromedial prefrontal cortex in morality and psychopathy. *Trends in Cognitive Sciences, 11,* 387–392.

Blascovich, J., & Kelsey, R. M. (1990). Using electrodermal and measures of arousal in social psychological research. *Review of Personality and Social Psychology, 11,* 45–73.

Bongers, I. L., Koot, H. M., van der Ende, J., & Verhulst, F. C. (2004). Developmental trajectories of externalizing behaviors in childhood and adolescence. *Child Development, 75,* 1523–1537.

Boyce, W. T., & Ellis, B. J. (2005). Biological sensitivity to context: I. An evolutionary-developmental theory of the origins and functions of stress reactivity. *Development and Psychopathology, 17,* 271–301.

Boyce, W. T., Quas, J., Alkon, A., Smider, N. A., Essex, M. J., Kupfer, D. J., et al. (2001). Autonomic reactivity and psychopathology in middle childhood. *British Journal of Psychiatry, 179,* 144–150.

Calkins, S. D., & Dedmon, S. E. (2000). Physiological and behavioral regulation in two-year-old children with aggressive/destructive behavior problems. *Journal of Abnormal Child Psychology, 28,* 103–118.

Chrousos, G. P., & Gold, P. W. (1992). The concepts of stress and stress system disorders: Overview of physical and behavioral homeostasis. *Journal of the American Medical Association, 267,* 1244–1252.

Cicchetti, D., & Rogosch, F. A. (2001). The impact of child maltreatment and psychopathology on neuroendocrine functioning. *Development and Psychopathology, 13,* 783–804.

Crick, N. R., & Grotpeter, J. K. (1995). Relational aggression, gender, and social-psychological adjustment. *Child Development, 66,* 710–722.

De Kloet, E. R. (1991). Brain corticosteroid receptor balance and homeostatic control. *Frontiers in Neuroendocrinology, 12,* 95–164.

De Kloet, E. R., Joëls, M., & Holsboer, F. (2005). Stress and the brain: From adaptation to disease. *Nature Reviews Neuroscience, 6,* 463–475.

de Vries-Bouw, M., Jansen, L., Vermeiren, R., Doreleijers, T., van de Ven, P., & Popma, A. (2012). Concurrent attenuated reactivity of alpha-amylase and cortisol is related to disruptive behavior in male adolescents. *Hormones and Behavior, 62,* 77–85.

De Wied, M., van Boxtel, T., Matthys, W., & Meeus, W. (2012). Verbal, facial and autonomic responses to empathy-eliciting film clips by disruptive male adolescents with high versus low callous–unemotional traits. *Journal of Abnormal Child Psychology, 40,* 211–223.

Dierckx, B., Kok, R., Tulen, J. H. M., Jaddoe, V. W., Hofman, A., Verhulst, F. C., et al. (2014). A prospective study of heart rate and externalising behaviours in young children. *Journal of Child Psychology and Psychiatry, 55,* 402–410.

Dodge, K. A., Harnish, J. D., Lochman, J. E., Bates, J. E., & Pettit, G. S. (1997). Reactive and proactive aggression in school children and psychiatrically impaired chronically assaultive youth. *Journal of Abnormal Psychology, 106,* 37–51.

Edwards, S., Clow, A., Evans, P., & Hucklebridge, F. (2001). Exploration of the awakening cortisol response in relation to diurnal cortisol secretory activity. *Life Sciences, 68,* 2093–2103.

Ellis, B. J., & Boyce, W. T. (2008). Biological sensitivity to context. *Current Directions in Psychological Science, 17,* 183–187.

El-Sheikh, M., Hinnant, J. B., & Erath, S. (2011). Developmental trajectories of delinquency symptoms in childhood: The role of marital conflict and autonomic nervous system activity. *Journal of Abnormal Psychology, 120,* 16–32.

Fanti, K. (2016). Understanding heterogeneity in conduct disorder: A review of psychophysiological studies. *Neuroscience and Biobehavioral Reviews.* [Epub ahead of print]

Frick, P. J., Ray, J. V., Thornton, L. C., & Kahn, R. E. (2014). Annual research review: A developmental psychopathology approach to understanding callous–unemotional traits in children and adolescents with serious conduct problems. *Journal of Child Psychology and Psychiatry and Allied Disciplines, 55,* 532–548.

Fries, E., Dettenborn, L., & Kirschbaum, C. (2009). The cortisol awakening response (CAR): Facts and future directions. *International Journal of Psychophysiology, 72,* 67–73.

Fries, E., Hesse, J., Hellhammer, J., & Hellhammer, D. H. (2005). A new view on hypocortisolism. *Psychoneuroendocrinology, 30,* 1010–1016.

Gordis, E. A., Granger, D. A., Susman, E. J., & Trickett, P. K. (2006). Asymmetry between salivary cortisol and α-amylase reactivity to stress: Relation to aggressive behavior in adolescents. *Psychoneuroendocrinology, 31,* 976–987.

Gump, B. B., Matthews, K. A., & Raikkonen, K. (1999). Modeling relationships among socioeconomic status, cardiovascular reactivity and left ventricular mass in African American and white children. *Health Psychology, 18,* 140–150.

Gunnar, M. R., Wewerka, S., Frenn, K., Long, J. D., & Griggs, C. (2009). Developmental changes in hypothalamus–pituitary–adrenal activity over the transition to adolescence: Normative changes and associations with puberty. *Development and Psychopathology, 21,* 69–85.

Hubbard, J. A., Smithmyer, C. M., Ramsden, S. R., Parker, E. H., Flanagan, K. D., Dearing, K. F., et al. (2002). Observational, physiological, and self-report measures of children's anger: Relations to reactive versus proactive aggression. *Child Development, 73,* 1101–1118.

Kahle, S., Miller, J. G., Lopez, M., & Hastings, P. D. (2016). Sympathetic recovery from anger is associated with emotion regulation. *Journal of Experimental Child Psychology, 142,* 359–371.

Kavish, N., Vaughn, M. G., Cho, E., Barth, A., Boutwell, B., Vaughn, S., et al. (2017). Physiological arousal and juvenile psychopathy: Is low resting heart rate associated with affective dimensions? *Psychiatric Quarterly, 88,* 103–114.

Kimonis, E. R., Frick, P. J., & McMahon, R. J. (2014). Conduct and oppositional defiant disorders. In E. J. Mash & R. A. Barkley (Eds.), *Child psychopathology* (3rd ed., pp. 145–179). New York: Guilford Press.

Lopez-Duran, N. L., Hajal, N. J., Olson, S. L., Felt, B., & Vazquez, D. M. (2009). Hypothalamic pituitary adrenal axis functioning in reactive and proactive aggression in children. *Journal of Abnormal Child Psychology, 37,* 169–182.

Lorber, M. F. (2004). Psychophysiology of aggression, psychopathy, and conduct problems: A meta-analysis. *Psychological Bulletin, 130,* 531–552.

Marsman, R., Swinkels, S. H. N., Rosmalen, J. G. M., Oldehinkel, A. J., Ormel, J., & Buitelaar, J. K. (2008). HPA-axis activity and externalizing behavior problems in early adolescents from the general population: The role of comorbidity and gender (the TRAILS study). *Psychoneuroendocrinology, 33,* 789–798.

Mills-Koonce, W. R., Wagner, N. J., Willoughby, M. T., Stifter, C., Blair, C., Granger, D. A., et al. (2015). Greater fear reactivity and psychophysiological hyperactivity among infants with later conduct problems and callous–unemotional traits. *Journal of Child Psychology and Psychiatry, 56,* 147–154.

Moffitt, T. E., Caspi, A., Rutter, M., & Silva, P. A. (2001). *Sex differences in antisocial behaviour: Conduct disorder, delinquency, and violence in the Dunedin Longitudinal Study.* New York: Cambridge University Press.

Mullin, B. C., & Hinshaw, S. P. (2007). Emotion regulation and externalizing disorders in children and adolescents. In J. J. Gross (Ed.), *Handbook of emotion regulation* (pp. 523–541). New York: Guilford Press.

Murray-Close, D., & Crick, N. R. (2007). Gender differences in the association between cardiovascular reactivity and aggressive conduct. *International Journal of Psychophysiology, 65*, 103–113.

Obradović, J. (2013). How can the study of physiological reactivity contribute to our understanding of adversity and resilience processes in development? *Development and Psychopathology, 24*, 371–387.

Obradović, J., Bush, N. R., & Boyce, W. T. (2011). The interactive effect of marital conflict and stress reactivity on externalizing and internalizing symptoms: The role of laboratory stressors. *Development and Psychopathology, 23*, 101–114.

Ortiz, J., & Raine, A. (2004). Heart rate level and antisocial behavior in children and adolescents: A meta-analysis. *Journal of the American Academy of Child and Adolescent Psychiatry, 43*, 154–162.

Pine, D. S., Shaffer, D., Schonfeld, I. S., & Davies, M. (1997). Minor physical anomalies: Modifiers of environmental risks for psychiatric impairment? *Journal of the American Academy of Child and Adolescent Psychiatry, 36*, 395–403.

Platje, E., Jansen, L. M. C., Raine, A., Branje, T. A. H., Doreleijers, M., de Vries-Bouw, A., et al. (2013). Longitudinal associations in adolescence between cortisol and persistent aggressive or rule-breaking behavior. *Biological Psychology, 93*, 132–137.

Platje, E., Popma, A., Vermeiren, R. R. J. M., Doreleijers, T. A., Meeus, W. H., van Lier, P. A., et al. (2015). Testosterone and cortisol in relation to aggression in a non-clinical sample of boys and girls. *Aggressive Behavior, 41*, 478–487.

Popma, A., Vermeiren, R., Geluk, C. A. M. L., Rinne, T., van den Brink, W., Knol, D. L., et al. (2007). Cortisol moderates the relationship between testosterone and aggression in delinquent male adolescents. *Biological Psychiatry, 61*, 405–411.

Porges, S. W. (2007). The polyvagal perspective. *Biological Psychology, 74*, 116–143.

Portnoy, J., & Farrington, D. P. (2015). Resting heart rate and antisocial behavior: An updated systematic review and meta-analysis. *Aggression and Violent Behavior, 22*, 33–45.

Poustka, L., Maras, A., Hohm, E., Fellinger, J., Holtmann, M., Banaschewski, T., et al. (2010). Negative association between plasma cortisol levels and aggression in a high-risk community sample of adolescents. *Journal of Neural Transmission, 117*, 621–627.

Powch, I. G., & Houston, B. K. (1996). Hostility, anger-in, and cardiovascular reactivity in White women. *Health Psychology, 15*, 200–208.

Pruessner, J. C., Wolf, O. T., Hellhammer, D. H., Buske-Kirschbaum, A., von Auer, K., Jobst, S., et al. (1997). Free cortisol levels after awakening: A reliable biological marker for the assessment of adrenocortical activity. *Life Sciences, 61*, 2539–2549.

Raine, A. (1997). Antisocial behavior and psychophysiology: A biosocial perspective and a prefrontal dysfunction hypothesis. In D. Stoff, J. Breiling, & J. D. Maser (Eds.), *Handbook of antisocial behavior* (pp. 289–304). New York: Wiley.

Raine, A. (2002). Biosocial studies of antisocial and violent behavior in children and adults: A review. *Journal of Abnormal Child Psychology, 30*, 311–326.

Raine, A. (2005). The interaction of biological and social measures in the explanation of antisocial and violent behavior. In D. Stoff & E. Susman (Eds.), *Developmental psychobiology of aggression* (pp. 13–42). New York: Cambridge University Press.

Raine, A., Fung, A. L., Portnoy, J., Choy, O., & Spring, V. L. (2014). Low heart rate as a risk factor for child and adolescent proactive aggressive and impulsive psychopathic behavior. *Aggressive Behavior, 40*, 290–299.

Raine, A., Venables, P. H., & Mednick, S. A. (1997). Low resting heart rate at age 3 years predisposes to aggression at age 11 years: Evidence from the Mauritius Child Health Project. *Journal of the American Academy of Child and Adolescent Psychiatry, 36*, 1457–1464.

Rappaport, N., & Thomas, C. (2004). Recent research findings on aggressive and violent behavior in youth: Implications for clinical assessment and intervention. *Journal of Adolescent Health, 35*, 260–277.

Sapolsky, R. M., Romero, L. M., & Munck, A. U. (2000). How do glucocorticoids influence stress responses?: Integrating permissive, suppressive, stimulatory, and preparative actions. *Endocrine Reviews, 21,* 55–89.

Scarpa, A., Chiara Haden, S., & Tanaka, A. (2010). Being hot-tempered: Autonomic, emotional, and behavioral distinctions between childhood reactive and proactive aggression. *Biological Psychology, 84,* 488–496.

Scarpa, A., & Raine, A. (1997). Psychophysiology of anger and violent behavior. *Psychiatric Clinics of North America, 20,* 375–394.

Shirtcliff, E. A., Granger, D. A., Booth, A., & Johnson, D. (2005). Low salivary cortisol and externalizing behavior problems in youth. *Development and Psychopathology, 17,* 167–184.

Shoal, G. D., Giancola, P. R., & Kirillova, G. P. (2003). Salivary cortisol, personality, and aggressive behavior in adolescent boys: A 5-year longitudinal study. *Journal of the American Academy of Child and Adolescent Psychiatry, 42,* 1101–1107.

Sijtsema, J. J., Van Roon, A. M., Groot, P. F. C., & Riese, H. (2015). Early life adversities and adolescent antisocial behavior: The role of cardiac autonomic nervous system reactivity in the TRAILS study. *Biological Psychology, 110,* 24–33.

Sijtsema, J. J., Veenstra, R., Lindenberg, S., van Roon, A. M., Verhulst, F. C., Ormel, J., et al. (2010). Mediation of sensation seeking and behavioral inhibition on the relationship between heart rate and antisocial behavior: The TRAILS study. *Journal of the American Academy of Child and Adolescent Psychiatry, 49,* 493–502.

Skosnik, P. D., Chatterton, R. T., Swisher, T., & Park, S. (2000). Modulation of attentional inhibition by norephinephrine and cortisol after psychological stress. *International Journal of Psychophysiology, 36,* 59–68.

Sondeijker, F. E. P. L., Ferdinand, R. F., Oldehinkel, A. J., Veenstra, R., Tiemeier, H., Ormel, J., et al. (2007). Disruptive behaviors and HPA-axis activity in young adolescent boys and girls from the general population. *Journal of Psychiatric Research, 41,* 570–578.

Stoppelbein, L., Greenig, L., Luebbe, A., Fite, P., & Becker, S. P. (2014). The role of cortisol and psychopathic traits in aggression among at-risk girls: Tests of mediating hypotheses. *Aggressive Behavior, 40,* 263–272.

Tackett, J. L., Reardon, K. W., Herzhoff, K., Page-Gould, E., Harden, K. P., & Josephs, R. A. (2015). Estradiol and cortisol interactions in youth externalizing psychopathology. *Psychoneuroendocrinology, 55,* 146–153.

Terranova, J. I., Song, Z., Larkin, T. E., II, Hardcastle, N., Norvelle, A., Riaz, A, et al. (2016). Serotonin and arginine–vasopressin mediate sex differences in the regulation of dominance and aggression by the social brain. *Proceedings of the National Academy of Sciences of the USA, 113,* 13233–13238.

Tremblay, R. E. (2003). Why socialization fails: The case of chronic physical aggression. In B. B. Lahey, T. E. Moffitt, & A. Caspi (Eds.), *Causes of conduct disorder and juvenile delinquency* (pp. 182–224). New York: Guilford Press.

Tremblay, R. E. (2010). Developmental origins of disruptive behaviour problems: The "original sin" hypothesis, epigenetics and their consequences for prevention. *Journal of Child Psychology and Psychiatry, 51,* 341–367.

van Bokhoven, I., Van Goozen, S. H. M., van Engeland, H., Schaal, B., Arseneault, L., Séguin, J. R., et al. (2005). Salivary cortisol and aggression in a population-based longitudinal study of adolescent males. *Journal of Neural Transmission, 112,* 1083–1096.

van der Graaff, J., Meeus, W., De Wied, M., Van Boxtel, A., Van Lier, P., & Branje, S. (2016). Respiratory sinus arrhythmia moderates the relation between parent–adolescent relationship quality and adolescents' social adjustment. *Journal of Abnormal Child Psychology, 44,* 269–281.

Van Goozen, S. H. M., Fairchild, G., Snoek, H., & Harold, G. T. (2007). The evidence for a neurobiological model of childhood antisocial behavior. *Psychological Bulletin, 133,* 149–182.

van Honk, J., Harmon-Jones, E., Morgan, B. E., & Schutter, D. J. L. G. (2010). Socially explosive minds: The triple imbalance hypothesis of reactive aggression. *Journal of Personality, 78,* 67–94.

van Stegeren, A., Rohleder, N., Everaerd, W., & Wolf, O. T. (2006). Salivary alpha amylase as marker for adrenergic activity during stress: Effect of betablockade. *Psychoneuroendocrinology, 31,* 137–141.

Vazquez, D. M. (1998). Stress and the developing limbic–hypothalamic–pituitary–adrenal axis. *Psychoneuroendocrinology, 23,* 663–700.

Vitiello, B., & Stoff, D. M. (1997). Subtypes of aggression and their relevance to child psychiatry. *Journal of the American Academy of Child and Adolescent Psychiatry, 36,* 307–315.

Voors, A. W., Webber, L. S., & Berenson, G. S. (1982). Resting heart rate and pressure-rate product of children in a total biracial community. *American Journal of Epidemiology, 16,* 276–286.

Wagner, N., Mills-Koonce, R., Willoughby, M., Propper, C., Rehder, P., & Gueron-Sela, N. (2017). Respiratory sinus arrhythmia and heart period in infancy as correlates of later oppositional defiant and callous–unemotional behaviors. *International Journal of Behavioral Development, 41,* 127–135.

Wilson, B. J., & Gottman, J. M. (1996). Attention: The shuttle between emotion and cognition: Risk, resiliency, and physiological bases. In E. M. Hetherington & E. A. Blechman (Eds.), *Stress, coping and resiliency in children and families* (pp. 189–228). Mahwah, NJ: Erlbaum.

Wilson, L. C., & Scarpa, A. (2014). Aggressive behavior: An alternative model of resting heart rate and sensation seeking. *Aggressive Behavior, 40,* 91–98.

Yu, R., Nieuwenhuis, J., Meeus, W., Hooimeijer, P., Koot, H. M., & Branje, S. J. T. (2016). Biological sensitivity to context: Cortisol awakening response moderates the effects of neighbourhood density on the development of adolescent externalizing problem behaviors. *Biological Psychology, 120,* 96–107.

Zuckerman, M. (1979). *Sensation seeking: Beyond the optimum level of arousal.* Hillsdale, NJ: Erlbaum.

CHAPTER 6

Temperament and Aggression

CHRISTINA C. MOORE, JULIE A. HUBBARD,
and MEGAN K. BOOKHOUT

Brief Introduction

In this chapter, we review theory and research regarding the role of temperament in the development of aggressive behavior in children and adolescents. Recent conceptualizations of temperament define the construct as biologically based individual differences in the domains of motivation, affect, inhibitory control, and attention (Rothbart & Bates, 2006). Temperament is believed to be relatively stable across time and contexts (Rothbart, 2007). Furthermore, theorists recognize the impact of socialization on the stability and change of temperament across development (Rothbart & Derryberry, 1981). Using this framework, we identify temperamental constructs associated with aggressive behavior across development and examine their utility for understanding trajectories of aggression in childhood and adolescence.

Theoretical Considerations

Research on youth temperament and aggression has been conducted in four domains: (1) from the perspective of Rothbart's theory of temperament; (2) within the framework of Gray's psychobiological theory of personality; (3) within the context of investigations of the psychophysiology of aggression; and (4) from the viewpoint of callous–unemotional (CU) traits. The goal of this chapter is to integrate findings from these domains into an understanding of the role of temperament in youth aggression. We begin by describing each domain.

Rothbart explains temperament development through the interaction of biologically driven tendencies and environment (Rothbart, 2007). In this framework, temperament consists of a set of "constitutionally" based individual differences in reactivity and self-regulation. Reactivity refers to the automaticity and strength of typical responses to positive and negative stimuli, and self-regulation refers to the tendency to modulate emotional and behavioral reactivity to positive and negative stimuli (Rothbart & Bates, 2006; Rothbart & Derryberry, 1981). Three temperamental factors are particularly relevant to the study of youth aggression—negative emotionality, effortful control, and sensation seeking. Negative emotionality is conceptualized as the tendency to experience high levels of anger when goals are blocked or excessive fear in the face of novel stimuli. Effortful control refers to efficiency in modulating attention, inhibiting behavioral responses, and activating alternative behavioral responses, particularly in the context of emotion-evoking situations. Finally, sensation seeking is defined as a preference for novel or risky activity (e.g., Rothbart, 1989; Rothbart & Bates, 2006).

Gray (1982, 1987) provides an important neurobiological model of temperament in his reinforcement sensitivity theory. Gray proposes two interdependent systems that serve unique functions, the behavioral inhibition system (BIS) and the behavioral activation system (BAS). The BIS is the aversive punishment system thought to control anxiety and inhibit action to avoid negative consequences; it is mediated by the septohippocampal system (Gray, 1982). The BAS reward system controls positive emotions (Gray, 1990, 1994), as well as anger when rewards are blocked (Harmon-Jones, 2003). This system is less clearly defined in terms of its neural origins, but it may be mediated by dopaminergic pathways. Externalizing behavior is thought to result from a combination of lowered anxiety and concern about negative consequences (decreased BIS) and heightened focus on obtaining rewards due to blunted reward sensitivity (elevated BAS).

Fearlessness and sensation-seeking theories of aggression have emerged from research on the psychophysiology of aggression (Murray-Close, 2013a, 2013b). In fearlessness theory, aggression results from an inability to experience appropriate levels of fear (e.g., Raine, 1996, 2002), which puts youth at increased risk for aggression due to lack of proper socialization via punishment processes (e.g., Fung et al., 2005; Raine, 2002). However, lack of fear has also been operationalized as a preference for new and risky activities (Barry et al., 2000; Levenson, Kiehl, & Fitzpatrick, 1995), which overlaps considerably with a theoretical approach to aggression that emphasizes sensation seeking. In sensation-seeking theory, aggression occurs when individuals experience physiological underarousal and engage in dangerous behaviors to increase arousal to normal thresholds (e.g., Raine, 1996, 2002).

Finally, the study of CU traits has led to important advances in subtyping aggressive youth. CU traits parallel the affective dimension of psychopathy in adults; the construct is defined as deficits in empathy and guilt, failure to put forth effort on important tasks, and shallow emotions (Frick, Ray, Thornton, & Kahn, 2014). Classifying aggressive youth based on whether or not they exhibit CU traits has revealed two subgroups that are distinct in neurocognitive (e.g., Pardini, 2011; Stickle, Kirkpatrick, & Brush, 2009), emotional processing (e.g., Jones, Laurens, Herba, Barker, & Viding, 2009; Willoughby, Waschbush, Moore, & Propper, 2011), and physiological (de Wied, van Boxtel, Matthys, & Meeus, 2012; Fung et al., 2005) correlates. Researchers have attempted to identify the etiological bases of CU traits, and findings have centered around fearlessness and insensitivity to punishment. Thus the study of CU traits has great relevance for our understanding of temperament and aggression.

From these domains of theory and research, two sets of temperamental constructs bearing on the development of youth aggression have emerged. The first set of constructs encompasses negative emotionality and effortful control, whereas the second set incorporates sensation seeking and fearlessness. The goal of this chapter is to organize this work into a cohesive understanding of the role that temperament plays in the trajectories of aggressive youth. First, though, we turn to a brief discussion of the assessment of temperament.

Measures and Methods

In this section, we review the most common means of assessing youth temperament in the aggression literature. Although researchers most often use parent-, teacher-, and self-report questionnaires, we also describe the increasing use of biological measures.

Questionnaires

Rothbart and colleagues have developed a theoretically grounded family of questionnaires to assess temperament based on personality, animal, behavior genetics, and psychophysiological literatures (Rothbart, 1981). Three distinct higher-order factors emerge from these questionnaires in infancy through childhood (Surgency, Negative Affectivity, Effortful Control), with a fourth factor (Affiliativeness) emerging in adolescence (Putnam, Ellis, & Rothbart, 2001). In addition to the higher-order factors of Negative Affectivity and Effortful Control, the subfactor of Sensation Seeking within Surgency is particularly relevant to youth aggression (Putnam et al., 2001).

Subsequently, two questionnaires were developed to tap the constructs of BIS and BAS. The first measure, the Sensitivity to Punishment and Reward Questionnaire, was developed for adults (Torrubia & Tobeña, 1984) and later modified by Colder and O'Connor (2004) for parent report of children and adolescents. The second measure, the BIS–BAS Scale, was developed by Carver and White (1994) and has been modified for use in children (Pagliaccio et al., 2016) and adolescents (Bjørnebekk & Howard, 2012; Gray, Hanna, Gillen, & Rushe, 2016). Factor analyses of these measures differentiate BIS and BAS as separate constructs (e.g., Bjørnebekk & Howard, 2012; Colder & O'Conner, 2004). In addition, BAS further separates into subfactors, with the subfactors most closely linked to youth aggression being Reward Responsiveness and Fun Seeking (Carver & White, 1994; Leone & Russo, 2009; Smillie, Jackson, & Dalgleish, 2006). Reward Responsiveness demonstrates negative relations to aggression because aggressive youth often require higher intensity rewards to reach optimal levels of arousal. In contrast, Fun Seeking, which reflects the desire to seek rewards impulsively, is typically positively related to aggression.

Biological Measures

Questionnaires, however, do not map temperamental traits to specific biological systems and so do not help researchers identify the physiological processes or neurobiological regions associated with the temperamental quality in question. For this reason, in recent years, biological measures have been used to operationalize temperament in relation to youth aggression in theoretically meaningful ways. A thorough discussion of these assessments is beyond the scope of the present chapter. However, the interested reader should refer to an elegant review by Murray-Close (2013a, 2013b) and to Branje and Koot (Chapter 5, this volume). For the purposes of this chapter, we briefly identify common biological measures of temperament and their potential significance to the aggression literature.

Autonomic Psychophysiology

Three autonomic measures have been considered to index temperamental constructs: the sympathetic nervous system (SNS), the pre-ejection period (PEP), and respiratory sinus arrhythmia (RSA). First, lower baseline SNS functioning, particularly low resting heart rate, may mark a tendency toward fearlessness or sensation seeking (see Murray-Close, 2013a, 2013b, for review). In contrast, SNS reactivity may index negative emotionality, especially anger (Hubbard et al., 2002; Rothbart & Bates, 2006).

Second, the PEP, an index of sympathetically controlled cardiac functioning, has been proposed by some theorists as a physiological marker of reward sensitivity (Beauchaine, 2001). Lack of PEP reactivity in response to rewards may reflect underactive BAS functioning, thereby leading externalizing youth toward sensation seeking in order to experience normative levels of reward (Beauchaine, Gatze-Kopp, & Mead, 2007).

Finally, RSA assesses the ebb and flow of heart rate during respiration and is the most common index of vagal tone, the fundamental element of the parasympathetic nervous system. RSA has been positively linked with several facets of effortful control (Chapman, Woltering, Lamm, & Lewis, 2010; Sulik, Eisenberg, Silva, Spinrad, & Kupfer, 2013), including executive functioning (Hansen, Johnsen, & Thayer, 2003; Marcovitch et al., 2010), emotional regulation (Beauchaine, 2001), and behavioral regulation (e.g., Porges, Doussard-Roosevelt, Portales, & Greenspan, 1996). Some theorists have posited that baseline levels of RSA may reflect trait-like emotional reactivity, whereas RSA suppression may signify an individual's ability to regulate emotionality in that moment (Liew et al., 2011).

Neurobiology

Brain imaging studies are a useful source of information about the neural mechanisms underlying temperamental traits. First, the orbitofrontal cortex and medial prefrontal cortex (PFC) are thought to index effortful control (Davidson, 2002; Heatherton, 2011), with positive correlations demonstrated between RSA and medial PFC activity in functional magnetic resonance imaging (fMRI) studies (Beauchaine & Thayer, 2015; Lane et al., 2009). Second, the amygdala is involved in emotional and social processing (Davis & Whalen, 2001) and has been critical in the search for the neurobiological bases of anger reactivity, CU traits, and aggression (Bobes et al., 2013). Finally, both the ventral striatum (Cohn et al., 2015) and the medial PFC (Veroude et al., 2016) are implicated in reward sensitivity.

Central Research Findings

In this section, we review the state of literature on temperament and youth aggression. Results are organized into two sections that parallel the theoretical distinction made above: (1) negative emotionality and effortful control and (2) sensation seeking and fearlessness.

Negative Emotionality and Effortful Control

Negative Emotionality

From infancy, children display individual differences in negative emotional responses to environmental stimuli (Cole, Martin, & Dennis, 2004). Moreover, reactivity to anger appears particularly linked to aggressive behavior. Trait anger and frustration has been linked concurrently with aggression in toddlers (Nærde, Ogden, Janson, & Zachrisson, 2014), children (Park et al., 2005), and adolescents (Ojanen, Findley, & Fuller, 2012). Longitudinally, infant distress in response to frustration predicts aggression 2½ years later (Crockenberg, Leerkes, & Barrig, 2008), and young children who are susceptible to anger are more likely than their agemates to develop externalizing behaviors later in childhood (Arsenio, Cooperman, & Lover, 2000; Lengua & Kovacs, 2005; Rothbart, Ahadi, & Hershey, 1994).

Negative emotionality is particularly relevant for reactive, as opposed to proactive, aggression. Reactive aggression may be best described as angry and dysregulated behavior in response to a perceived provocation, whereas proactive aggression may be described as unemotional behavior purposefully directed toward achieving an instrumental or social goal (Dodge & Coie, 1987). It is no surprise, then, that anger has been uniquely linked to reactive but not proactive aggression (e.g., Bettencourt, Talley, Benjamin, & Valentine, 2006; Xu, Farver, & Zhang, 2009), with investigations conducted as early as the toddler years (Vitaro, Barker, Boivin, Brendgen, & Tremblay, 2006) and using observational or physiological measures of anger (e.g., Hubbard et al., 2002).

The neurobiological roots of the link between anger and reactive aggression may reside in the amygdala (e.g., Blair, Peschardt, Budhani, Mitchell, & Pine, 2006). Individuals with high trait anger display amygdala hyperreactivity in response to displays of angry faces (e.g., Carré, Fisher, Manuck, & Hariri, 2012), and this hyperreactivity extends to neutral faces among chronically aggressive men (Bobes et al., 2013; Pardini & Phillips, 2010), indicating that they may perceive even neutral faces as threatening. Most of these studies have been conducted with adults and need to be replicated with youth. However, both trait anger (Schultz, Izard, & Bear, 2004) and reactive aggression (e.g., Brugman et al., 2015; Hubbard, Dodge, Cillessen, Coie, & Schwartz, 2001) in youth samples have been linked to the tendency to attribute hostile intent to others when ambiguously provoked. When viewed in conjunction with work on amygdala hyperreactivity to threatening faces, these maladaptive neurobiological and social-cognitive processes likely play an important role in triggering reactive aggression among youth (de Castro, Veerman, Koops, Bosch, & Monshouwer, 2002).

Effortful Control

At its most basic, temperament concerns the interplay between emotional reactivity and emotion regulation, a tension at the heart of understanding reactive aggression in youth. As described earlier, the temperamental construct that most closely captures emotion regulation is effortful control, which has been inversely linked to externalizing behavior across numerous studies (Duncombe, Havighurst, Holland, & Frankling, 2013; Eisenberg et al., 1996, 2001; Gilliom, Shaw, Beck, Schonberg, & Lukon, 2002; Rothbart et al., 1994; Valiente et al., 2003), including longitudinal prospective investigations (e.g., Eisenberg et al., 2000; Henry, Caspi, Moffitt, & Silva, 1996). This association may be particularly strong for children who exhibit high levels of negative emotionality (Valiente et al., 2003) or when youth attempt to regulate anger or frustration in particular (e.g., Casey & Schlosser, 1994). Moreover, separate components of effortful control, such as attentional control and inhibitory behavioral control, have demonstrated unique negative associations with externalizing behaviors (Eisenberg et al., 2001, 2005, 2009). Strong inhibitory control, in particular, may buffer youth who tend to experience negative emotions from engaging in externalizing behaviors; in one study of preadolescent boys, a link from increased anger and decreased fearfulness to alcohol use initiation was found only for boys without strong inhibitory control (Pardini, Lochman, & Wells, 2004).

Effortful control is uniquely associated with reactive but not proactive aggression in middle childhood (Rathert, Fite, Gaertner, & Vitulano, 2011) and adolescence (Dane & Marini, 2014). In addition, effortful control moderates the relation between anger and reactive aggression (Xu et al., 2009), such that the relation is significant only at low levels of effortful control. Youth with low resting vagal tone are more likely to engage in reactive aggression (Scarpa, Haden, & Tanaka, 2010; Xu, Raine, Yu, & Krieg, 2014), a finding implicating lower baseline RSA in the regulatory deficits of reactive aggression. In the most current work on the psychophysiology of reactive aggression, researchers examined the interaction of youths' SNS reactivity and RSA in the moment as they were given the opportunity to engage in reactive aggression against a provocative virtual peer; RSA moderated the relation between SNS reactivity and reactive aggression, with children who displayed both elevated SNS reactivity and blunted RSA being particularly likely to respond with reactive aggression when provoked (Moore et al., 2018). Thus deficits in effortful control may play a central role in youths' anger and reactive aggression, and both baseline RSA and RSA reactivity may serve as biomarkers of these deficits.

Sensation Seeking and Fearlessness

Questionnaire measures of sensation seeking are reliably linked to aggression in children (Copeland, Landry, Stanger, & Hudziak, 2004) and adolescents (i.e., Hiramura et al., 2010; Kim et al., 2006; Miller, Zeichner, & Wilson, 2012; Taubitz, Pedersen, & Larson, 2015), as well as to CU traits (Morgan, Bowen, Moore, & Van

Goozen, 2014; Roose, Bijttebier, Van der Oord, Claes, & Lilienfeld, 2013). This finding is consistent with work suggesting that low resting heart rate, considered a physiological indicator of fearlessness and/or sensation seeking, is associated with aggression in youth, with some studies demonstrating unique relations to proactive but not reactive aggression (e.g., Raine, Fung, Portnoy, Choy, & Spring, 2014; Xu et al., 2009, 2014). In a longitudinal study, sensation seeking assessed in early adolescence mediated the relation between low resting heart rate in childhood and aggression in late adolescence among boys (Sijtsema et al., 2010), a finding replicated in a recent concurrent study of adolescent boys (Portnoy et al., 2014). These investigations provide compelling evidence to support sensation-seeking theories of youth aggression, at least among boys.

One mechanism linking sensation seeking and aggression in youth may be empathic responsiveness (Stadler et al., 2007). Aggressive youth display hyporesponsiveness in amygdala activity when viewing fearful faces (Stadler, Poustka, & Sterzer, 2010), a finding especially true for aggressive youth with CU traits (Jones et al., 2009). In a related finding, reduced amygdala activity in response to fearful faces mediated the relation between CU traits and proactive but not reactive aggression (Lozier, Cardinale, Van Meter, & Marsh, 2014). This mechanism may be particularly important for understanding aggressive youths' lack of concern for their victims.

A second mechanism connecting sensation seeking and aggression is blunted reward sensitivity. Youth who do not experience normative levels of positive affect from rewarding experiences may engage in risky activities to increase pleasure. A negative relation emerges between youth aggression and reward responsiveness as assessed through that subfactor of BIS–BAS questionnaires (Taubitz et al., 2015). In addition, physiological and neural evidence of blunted sensitivity or reactivity to rewards is seen in aggressive youth, including blunted PEP reactivity (e.g., Beauchaine et al., 2007; Beauchaine, Hong, & Marsh, 2008) and less ventral striatum activity (Cohn et al., 2015). These findings are paralleled in youth with CU traits, who display medial PFC hypoactivity in anticipation of reward (Veroude et al., 2016).

Low levels of fear and anxiety also characterize both youth with CU traits (Kimonis et al., 2006; Pardini, 2006) and aggressive youth (Barker, Oliver, Viding, Salekin, & Maughan, 2011). Theorists have long postulated that fearlessness is critical to the insensitivity to punishment that aggressive youth display, and this notion is supported in a cross-sectional study demonstrating that insensitivity to punishment mediated the relation between fearlessness and CU traits, which in turn predicted aggressive behavior (Pardini, 2006). In fact, researchers have questioned whether fearlessness and sensation seeking are, in fact, distinct constructs; in a recent study, behavioral sensation seeking was linked to fearlessness assessed neurally via a lessened ability to detect threat in dangerous situations (Mujica-Parodi, Carlson, Cha, & Rubin, 2014). Further support for the close link between the two constructs is found in work suggesting that both sensation seeking (Xu et al., 2009) and fearlessness (Kimonis et al., 2006) are linked to proactive but not reactive aggressive behavior.

The previous section on negative emotionality highlighted links between youth aggression and overreacting with anger in the face of frustration. However, negative emotionality also encompasses particularly fearful responses to novel stimuli, reactions that are quite the opposite of the fearlessness discussed earlier. Two lines of research attempting to reconcile these perspectives suggest that fear may be best conceptualized as a continuous dimension on which both the extremes of fearfulness and fearlessness may result in youth aggression and conduct problems (CP). First, fearfulness is linked to reactive but not proactive aggression, whether fear is operationalized as anxiety (Vitaro, Brendgen, & Tremblay, 2002) or as behavioral inhibition (Miller et al., 2012). Second, youth high on both CP and CU traits are marked by fearlessness, whereas youth high on CP but low on CU traits are characterized by fearfulness. The most methodologically rigorous study to make this second point was conducted by Fanti and colleagues (Fanti, Panayiotou, Lazarou, Michael, & Georgiou, 2016), who compared participants within a community sample on a physiological measure of fear-startle potentiation, as well as questionnaire measures of fearfulness, BIS, and sensitivity to punishment. Groups compared included youth high on both CP and CU traits, youth low on both CP and CU traits, and youth high on one construct but low on the other. Youth high on both CP and CU traits scored the lowest of all four group on all four measures indexing fear, whereas youth high on CP but low on CU traits scored the highest of all four groups on all four fear measures (Fanti et al., 2016).

Implications for Differential
Temperamental Trajectories of Youth Aggression

This literature review suggests that youth aggression may emerge from two distinct temperamental trajectories, with the first characterized by sensation seeking and fearlessness and the second marked by negative emotionality and deficits in effortful control. In this section, these trajectories are explored to understand how temperament may underpin youth aggression.

Trajectory of Sensation Seeking and Fearlessness

The first pathway toward youth aggression has temperamental foundations in fearlessness and sensation seeking. Youth on this trajectory display high levels of CU traits and aggress for proactive reasons of instrumental or social gain. They are distinguished by low resting heart rate (Portnoy et al., 2014; Raine et al., 2014; Sijtsema et al., 2010; Xu et al., 2009, 2014), requiring them to seek out novel and dangerous situations including aggressive actions to increase arousal to optimal levels (Copeland et al., 2004; Hiramura et al., 2010; Kim et al., 2006; Miller et al., 2012; Morgan et al., 2014; Roose et al., 2013; Taubitz et al., 2015; Xu et al., 2009). When they do aggress, they often display a lack of concern for their victims, a tendency perhaps rooted in amygdala hyporesponsiveness to fearful facial expressions (Jones et al., 2009; Lozier et al., 2014; Stadler et al., 2007, 2010; White et al., 2012). At the same time, youth on this trajectory also display fearlessness with regard to their own well-being (Barker et al., 2011; Fanti et al., 2016; Kimonis et al., 2006; Mujica-Parodi et al., 2014). This fearlessness, coupled with blunted reward sensitivity (Beauchaine et al., 2007, 2008; Cohn et al., 2015; Taubitz et al., 2015; Veroude et al., 2016), may lead these youth to be particularly resistant to praise and insensitive to punishment, causing caregivers' traditional socialization approaches to fail (e.g., Barker et al., 2011; Pardini, 2006). In this respect, the temperamental constructs of sensation seeking and fearlessness may be considered at least partially innate, inherited, or hard-wired (Frick & Viding, 2009).

Trajectory of Negative Emotionality and Deficits in Effortful Control

The second pathway toward youth aggression may have its temperamental roots in negative emotionality, including both heightened anger reactivity and fearfulness, as well as deficits in effortful control. Youth on this pathway may tend to anger more easily with less provocation than peers, which can be seen at the neurobiological level in amygdala hyperreactivity to angry faces (Bobes et al., 2013; Carré et al., 2012; Pardini & Phillips, 2010) and at the social-cognitive level in hostile attributional bias (Brugman et al., 2015; de Castro et al., 2002; Hubbard et al., 2001; Schultz et al., 2004). Once angered, they may struggle to regulate angry feelings (Dane & Marini, 2014; Moore et al., 2018; Rathert et al., 2011; Scarpa et al., 2010; Xu et al., 2009, 2014) before resorting to reactive aggression (Bettencourt et al., 2006; Hubbard et al., 2002; Vitaro et al., 2006; Xu et al., 2009). However, once they aggress, these youth may feel remorse, due to low levels of CU traits (Frick, 2012; Frick & Morris, 2004; Frick & White, 2008; Pardini & Frick, 2013). Finally, they may be receptive to praise and amenable to punishment as disciplinary tactics due to normative levels of reward sensitivity and heightened fearfulness and anxiety (Fanti et al., 2016; Miller et al., 2012; Vitaro et al., 2002).

This discussion of the temperamental underpinnings of dysregulated reactive aggression does not imply that these struggles are trait-like or present from birth. Rather, although individual differences in reactivity to emotion-eliciting stimuli may be present from infancy (Arsenio et al., 2000; Lengua & Kovacs, 2005; Rothbart et al., 1994), voluntary control of that reactivity develops later and is less heritable and largely socialized (Beauchaine, 2015). In fact, parental emotion coaching shows positive effects on youth anger regulation and externalizing problems well into adolescence (Shortt, Stoolmiller, Smith-Shine, Mark Eddy, & Sheeber, 2010). Moreover, Beauchaine argues that negative emotionality is not sufficient to lead to conduct-disordered behavior. Instead, he emphasizes that externalizing disorders result from the coupling of this temperamental quality with emotional control deficits conferred through socialization processes that include poor parenting and early life stressors, such as poverty (Hanson, Hair, et al., 2013) and neglect (Hanson, Adluru, et al., 2013). In particular, Beauchaine (2015) argues that emotion dysregulation is learned through repetitive cycles in which aggressive children escape from negative affective exchanges with family members and peers by escalating anger until interactions terminate, resulting in negative reinforcement of the escalation (Patterson, DeBaryshe, & Ramsey, 1989; Snyder, Edwards, McGraw, Kilgore, & Holton, 1994; Snyder & Patterson, 1995; Snyder, Schrepferman, & St. Peter, 1997). Moreover, reactively aggressive children are reinforced not only by escape from others' negative responses but also by escape from their own aversive physiological state (Beauchaine & Zalewski, 2016; Skowron et al., 2011). Thus the temperamental quality of effortful control, in particular, may be heavily affected by socialization processes, a statement in contrast to theoretical conclusions drawn about the etiology of the temperamental traits of sensation seeking and fearlessness.

Distinctiveness of Temperamental Trajectories

Based on this summary, readers may conclude that two distinct trajectories for aggressive youth exist, with one trajectory marked by reactive aggression driven by heightened negative emotionality coupled with deficits in effortful control and the second trajectory characterized by proactive aggression propelled by fearlessness, sensation seeking, and CU traits. However, the correlation between reactive and proactive aggression is consistently high across studies (Card & Little, 2006; Polman, de Castro, Koops, van Boxtel, & Merk, 2007), suggesting that many youth engage in both subtypes of aggressive behavior. To some degree, then, the subtypes of aggression may be more accurately conceptualized as continuous measures of the extent to which youth display each subtype of aggression, rather than as categories into which youth are placed.

However, two recent rigorous investigations suggest that some youth may display reactive aggression only, whereas others display both reactive and proactive aggression. In the first study, self-report data on reactive and proactive aggression from a large sample of adolescents were analyzed using latent class analysis; two latent classes of aggressive adolescents emerged, one that engaged in primarily reactive aggression and a second that displayed both reactive and proactive aggression (Smeets et al., 2016). Similarly, in a recent study of adolescents in community, at-risk residential, and detained samples, cluster analyses of reactive and proactive aggression revealed two aggressive groups, with the first elevated on reactive aggression only and the second elevated on both reactive and proactive aggression. With a few exceptions, these findings were replicated across the three samples, across boys and girls, and across physical and relational aggression (Marsee et al., 2014). These groups differed in severity, with the combined group displaying higher levels of emotion dysregulation, CU traits, and delinquency than the reactive-only group (Marsee et al., 2014). Both studies converged to suggest that few if any youth display proactive aggression only.

Furthermore, when the SNS arousal of youth diagnosed with disruptive behavior disorders was assessed in both a baseline condition and a peer provocation, externalizing youth demonstrated both lower baseline arousal indicative of sensation seeking and fearlessness and greater negative emotional reactivity to the peer provocation than controls (Van Goozen, Matthys, Cohen-Kettenis, Buitelaar, & van Engeland, 2000). These results suggest that aggressive youths' blunted baseline SNS arousal may put them at risk for displaying proactive aggression when faced with the opportunity to aggress for instrumental gain, and their SNS arousal to peer provocation may also increase the chance that they will display reactive aggression. In fact, if aggressive youths' SNS profiles are characterized by both of these patterns, then it follows that many aggressive youth may aggress for both reactive and proactive reasons, albeit in different contexts.

These findings may have important implications for our understanding of multiple temperamental pathways to youth aggression. They suggest a first and less severe pathway characterized primarily by reactive aggression, as well as a second and more severe pathway marked by both types of aggression and CU traits. It may well be that some externalizing youth aggress predominantly when provoked, whereas other disruptive youth aggress both when provoked and to achieve instrumental or social gain (Muñoz, Frick, Kimonis, & Aucoin, 2008). Importantly, the literature reviewed here suggests that the first pathway may be rooted in negative emotionality and deficits in effortful control, whereas the second pathway has a foundation in these temperamental constructs, along with sensation seeking and fearlessness.

A recent fMRI study supports the notion that both youth with and without CU traits evidence anger reactivity when provoked. Compared with a control sample, all adolescents with disruptive behavior disorders displayed reduced amygdala–ventromedial PFC connectivity when provoked, regardless of whether or not they had CU traits, and this reduction predicted their tendency to retaliate during a laboratory task, as well as parent ratings of reactive aggression. These results suggest that all youth with disruptive behavior disorders may be at risk for reactive aggression and propose one neural mechanism of this risk (White et al., 2016).

In many ways, this theory is parallel to Frick's hypothesis of two pathways toward aggressive behavior, with one marked by anger dysregulation and the other by CU traits (Frick, 2012; Frick & Morris, 2004; Frick & White, 2008; Pardini & Frick, 2013). However, the models diverge in that we emphasize that youth on the reactive–proactive pathway also struggle with negative emotionality and emotion dysregulation and, in fact, that their regulatory deficits may be more serious than those of youth who do not evidence CU traits or proactive aggression. Thus we deviate from Frick's thinking by emphasizing that both pathways toward disruptive behavior disorders are characterized by negative emotionality and deficits in effortful control. This point is further emphasized by a recent study suggesting that, among youth with acute CP (criminal or inpatient history), the most aggressive youth displayed both elevated CU traits and elevated anxiety (Euler et al., 2015). Thus it may that the most aggressive youth struggle with negative emotionality and deficits in effortful control with respect not only to anger but also to fear and anxiety. These findings are preliminary, but they suggest that we have much more work to do to fully understand the role of negative emotionality and effortful control in youth aggression across trajectories.

Future Directions

We have outlined two potential trajectories for youth aggression, both characterized by reactive aggression driven by negative emotionality and deficits in effortful control, but only one of which is marked by proactive aggression grounded in CU traits, sensation seeking, and fearlessness. In future studies, researchers should continue to investigate the divergent and convergent temperamental bases for youth aggression across these trajectories. For example, assessing negative emotionality and emotion dysregulation separately for anger versus fear may lead to important advances in our understanding of these trajectories. In addition, as we have seen in a number of recent studies, person-centered approaches to investigating youth aggression and temperament, rather than correlational methods, are likely to continue to advance our knowledge of the various pathways that youth aggression can take.

In addition, further clarity about the etiology of youth aggression may be achieved by mapping behavioral and biological measures of temperament to one another. For example, sensation seeking, but not fearlessness, has been found to mediate the relation between low autonomic arousal and adolescent aggression in two studies (Portnoy et al., 2014; Sijtsema et al., 2010). The continued use of multimethod approaches to assess temperament may help elucidate the mechanisms most relevant for understanding youth aggression.

Finally, associations between temperament and aggression are likely to differ for males and females. As we have seen across many of the studies reviewed, female participants tend to be underrepresented in this work, particularly in samples with severe conduct problems. Furthermore, some investigations of gender as a moderator find that associations between temperament and aggression may not apply to female participants (e.g., Sijtsema et al., 2010), perhaps because females often display lower levels of the temperamental qualities linked to aggressive behavior, suggesting that the temperamental pathways toward aggression may be less applicable to females than males (Else-Quest, Hyde, Goldsmith, & Van Hulle, 2006). As such, the extent to which the work reviewed here can be generalized to females is unclear, and greater attention to this issue is critical.

Conclusions

This review of the current state of research on temperament and youth aggression has revealed important advances but also significant gaps in our understanding of the temperamental underpinnings of trajectories of aggression in children and adolescents. Much work remains as we continue to move forward in our understanding of the multiple pathways toward and subtypes of youth aggression, particularly with respect to temperamental foundations of these trajectories. We feel certain that our field is up to the task and look forward to the exciting advances that are sure to come in the years ahead.

REFERENCES

Arsenio, W. F., Cooperman, S., & Lover, A. (2000). Affective predictors of preschoolers' aggression and peer acceptance: Direct and indirect effects. *Developmental Psychology, 36,* 438–448.

Barker, E. D., Oliver, B. R., Viding, E., Salekin, R. T., & Maughan, B. (2011). The impact of prenatal maternal risk, fearless temperament and early parenting on adolescent callous–unemotional traits: A 14-year longitudinal investigation. *Journal of Child Psychology and Psychiatry, 52,* 878–888.

Barry, C. T., Frick, P. J., DeShazo, T. M., McCoy, M., Ellis, M., & Loney, B. R. (2000). The importance of callous–unemotional traits for extending the concept of psychopathy to children. *Journal of Abnormal Psychology, 109,* 335–340.

Beauchaine, T. P. (2001). Vagal tone, development, and Gray's motivational theory: Toward an integrated model of autonomic nervous system functioning in psychopathology. *Development and Psychopathology, 13,* 183–214.

Beauchaine, T. P. (2015). Future directions in emotion dysregulation and youth psychopathology. *Journal of Clinical Child and Adolescent Psychology, 44,* 875–896.

Beauchaine, T. P., Gatzke-Kopp, L., & Mead, H. K. (2007). Polyvagal theory and developmental psychopathology: Emotion dysregulation and conduct problems from preschool to adolescence. *Biological Psychology, 74,* 174–184.

Beauchaine, T. P., Hong, J., & Marsh, P. (2008). Sex differences in autonomic correlates of conduct problems and aggression. *Journal of the American Academy of Child and Adolescent Psychiatry, 47,* 788–796.

Beauchaine, T. P., & Thayer, J. F. (2015). Heart rate variability as a transdiagnostic biomarker of psychopathology. *International Journal of Psychophysiology, 98,* 338–350.

Beauchaine, T. P., & Zalewski, M. (2016). Physiological and developmental mechanisms of emotional lability in coercive relationships. In T. J. Dishion & J. J. Snyder (Eds.), *Oxford handbook of coercive relationship dynamics* (pp. 39–52). New York: Oxford University Press.

Bettencourt, B. A., Talley, A., Benjamin, A. J., & Valentine, J. (2006). Personality and aggressive behavior under provoking and neutral conditions: A meta-analytic review. *Psychological Bulletin, 132,* 751–777.

Bjørnebekk, G., & Howard, R. (2012). Sub-types of angry aggression in antisocial youth: Relationships with self-reported delinquency and teachers' perceptions of social competence and emotional/behavioural problems. *Personality and Individual Differences, 53,* 312–316.

Blair, R. J. R., Peschardt, K. S., Budhani, S., Mitchell, D. G. V., & Pine, D. S. (2006). The development of psychopathy. *Journal of Child Psychology and Psychiatry, 47,* 262–275.

Bobes, M. A., Ostrosky, F., Diaz, K., Romero, C., Borja, K., Santos, Y., et al. (2013). Linkage of functional and structural anomalies in the left amygdala of reactive-aggressive men. *Social Cognitive and Affective Neuroscience, 8,* 928–936.

Brugman, S., Lobbestael, J., Arntz, A., Cima, M., Schuhmann, T., Dambacher, F., et al. (2015). Identifying cognitive predictors of reactive and proactive aggression. *Aggressive Behavior, 41,* 51–64.

Card, N. A., & Little, T. D. (2006). Proactive and reactive aggression in childhood and adolescence: A meta-analysis of differential relations with psychosocial adjustment. *International Journal of Behavioral Development, 30,* 466–480.

Carré, J. M., Fisher, P. M., Manuck, S. B., & Hariri, A. R. (2012). Interaction between trait anxiety and trait anger predict amygdala reactivity to angry facial expressions in men but not women. *Social Cognitive and Affective Neuroscience, 7,* 213–221.

Carver, C. S., & White, T. L. (1994). Behavioral inhibition, behavioral activation, and affective responses to impending reward and punishment: The BIS/BAS Scales. *Journal of Personality and Social Psychology, 67,* 319–333.

Casey, R. J., & Schlosser, S. (1994). Emotional responses to peer praise in children with and without a diagnosed externalizing disorder. *Merrill–Palmer Quarterly, 40,* 60–81.

Chapman, H. A., Woltering, S., Lamm, C., & Lewis, M. D. (2010). Hearts and minds: Coordination of neurocognitive and cardiovascular regulation in children and adolescents. *Biological Psychology, 84,* 296–303.

Cohn, M. D., Veltman, D. J., Pape, L. E., van Lith, K., Vermeiren, R. R. J. M., van den Brink, W., et al. (2015). Incentive processing in persistent disruptive behavior and psychopathic traits: A functional magnetic resonance imaging study in adolescents. *Biological Psychiatry, 78,* 615–624.

Colder, C. R., & O'Connor, R. M. (2004). Gray's reinforcement sensitivity model and child psychopathology: Laboratory and questionnaire assessment of the BAS and BIS. *Journal of Abnormal Child Psychology, 32,* 435–451.

Cole, P. M., Martin, S. E., & Dennis, T. A. (2004). Emotion regulation as a scientific construct: Methodological challenges and directions for child development research. *Child Development, 75,* 317–333.

Copeland, W., Landry, K., Stanger, C., & Hudziak, J. J. (2004). Multi-informant assessment of temperament in children with externalizing behavior problems. *Journal of Clinical Child and Adolescent Psychology, 33,* 547–556.

Crockenberg, S. C., Leerkes, E. M., & Barrig, P. S. (2008). Predicting aggressive behavior in the third year from infant reactivity and regulation as moderated by maternal behavior. *Development and Psychopathology, 20,* 37–54.

Dane, A. V., & Marini, Z. A. (2014). Overt and relational forms of reactive aggression in adolescents: Relations with temperamental reactivity and self-regulation. *Personality and Individual Differences, 60,* 60–66.

Davidson, R. J. (2002). Anxiety and affective style: Role of prefrontal cortex and amygdala. *Biological Psychiatry, 51,* 68–80.

Davis, M., & Whalen, P. J. (2001). The amygdala: Vigilance and emotion. *Molecular Psychiatry, 6,* 13–34.

de Castro, B. O., Veerman, J. W., Koops, W., Bosch, J. D., & Monshouwer, H. J. (2002). Hostile attribution of intent and aggressive behavior: A meta-analysis. *Child Development, 73,* 916–934.

de Wied, M., van Boxtel, A., Matthys, W., & Meeus, W. (2012). Verbal, facial and autonomic responses to empathy-eliciting film clips by disruptive male adolescents with high versus low callous–unemotional traits. *Journal of Abnormal Child Psychology, 40,* 211–223.

Dodge, K. A., & Coie, J. D. (1987). Social-information-processing factors in reactive and proactive aggression in children's peer groups. *Journal of Personality and Social Psychology, 53,* 1146–1158.

Duncombe, M., Havighurst, S. S., Holland, K. A., & Frankling, E. J. (2013). Relations of emotional competence and effortful control to child disruptive behavior problems. *Early Education and Development, 24,* 599–615.

Eisenberg, N., Cumberland, A., Spinrad, T. L., Fabes, R. A., Shepard, S. A., Reiser, M., et al. (2001). The relations of regulation and emotionality to children's externalizing and internalizing problem behavior. *Child Development, 72,* 1112–1134.

Eisenberg, N., Fabes, R. A., Guthrie, I. K., Murphy, B. C., Maszk, P., Holmgren, R., et al. (1996). The relations of regulation and emotionality to problem behavior in elementary school children. *Development and Psychopathology, 8,* 141–162.

Eisenberg, N., Guthrie, I. K., Fabes, R. A., Shepard, S., Losoya, S., Murphy, B. C., et al. (2000). Prediction of elementary school children's externalizing problem behaviors from attention and behavioral regulation and negative emotionality. *Child Development, 71,* 1367–1382.

Eisenberg, N., Sadovsky, A., Spinrad, T. L., Fabes, R. A., Losoya, S. H., Valiente, C., et al. (2005). The relations of problem behavior status to children's negative emotionality, effortful control, and impulsivity: Concurrent relations and prediction of change. *Developmental Psychology, 41,* 193–211.

Eisenberg, N., Valiente, C., Spinrad, T. L., Cumberland, A., Liew, J., Reiser, M., et al. (2009). Longitudinal relations of children's effortful control, impulsivity, and negative emotionality to their externalizing, internalizing, and co-occurring behavior problems. *Developmental Psychology, 45,* 988–1008.

Else-Quest, N. M., Hyde, J. S., Goldsmith, H. H., & Van Hulle, C. A. (2006). Gender differences in temperament: A meta-analysis. *Psychological Bulletin, 132,* 33–72.

Euler, F., Jenkel, N., Stadler, C., Schmeck, K., Fegert, J. M., Kölch, M., et al. (2015). Variants of girls and boys with conduct disorder: Anxiety symptoms and callous–unemotional traits. *Journal of Abnormal Child Psychology, 43,* 773–785.

Fanti, K. A., Panayiotou, G., Lazarou, C., Michael, R., & Georgiou, G. (2016). The better of two evils?: Evidence that children exhibiting continuous conduct problems high or low on callous–unemotional traits score on opposite directions on physiological and behavioral measures of fear. *Development and Psychopathology, 28,* 185–198.

Frick, P. J. (2012). Developmental pathways to conduct disorder: Implications for future directions in research, assessment, and treatment. *Journal of Clinical Child and Adolescent Psychology, 41,* 378–389.

Frick, P. J., & Morris, A. S. (2004). Temperament and developmental pathways to conduct problems. *Journal of Clinical Child and Adolescent Psychology, 33,* 54–68.

Frick, P. J., Ray, J. V., Thornton, L. C., & Kahn, R. E. (2014). Can callous–unemotional traits enhance the understanding, diagnosis, and treatment of serious conduct problems in children and adolescents?: A comprehensive review. *Psychological Bulletin, 140,* 1–57.

Frick, P. J., & Viding, E. (2009). Antisocial behavior from a developmental psychopathology perspective. *Development and Psychopathology, 21,* 1111–1131.

Frick, P. J., & White, S. F. (2008). Research review: The importance of callous–unemotional traits for developmental models of aggressive and antisocial behavior. *Journal of Child Psychology and Psychiatry, 49,* 359–375.

Fung, M. T., Raine, A., Loeber, R., Lynam, D. R., Steinhauer, S. R., Venables, P. H., et al. (2005). Reduced electrodermal activity in psychopathy-prone adolescents. *Journal of Abnormal Psychology, 114,* 187–196.

Gilliom, M., Shaw, D. S., Beck, J. E., Schonberg, M. A., & Lukon, J. L. (2002). Anger regulation in disadvantaged preschool boys: Strategies, antecedents, and the development of self-control. *Developmental Psychology, 38,* 222–235.

Gray, J. A. (1982). *The neuropsychology of anxiety: An enquiry into the functions of the septohippocampal system.* Oxford, UK: Oxford University Press.

Gray, J. A. (1987). *The psychology of fear and stress.* Cambridge, UK: Cambridge University Press.

Gray, J. A. (1990). Brain systems that mediate both emotion and cognition. *Cognition and Emotion, 4,* 269–288.

Gray, J. A. (1994). Three fundamental emotion systems. In P. Ekman & R. J. Davidson (Eds.), *The nature of emotion* (pp. 243–247). New York: Oxford University Press.

Gray, J. D., Hanna, D., Gillen, A., & Rushe, T. (2016). A closer look at Carver and White's BIS/BAS scales: Factor analysis and age group differences. *Personality and Individual Differences, 95,* 20–24.

Hansen, A. L., Johnsen, B. H., & Thayer, J. F. (2003). Vagal influence on working memory and attention. *International Journal of Psychophysiology, 48,* 263–274.

Hanson, J. L., Adluru, N., Chung, M. K., Alexander, A. L., Davidson, R. J., & Pollak, S. D. (2013). Early neglect is associated with alterations in white matter integrity and cognitive functioning. *Child Development, 84,* 1566–1578.

Hanson, J. L., Hair, N., Shen, D. G., Shi, F., Gilmore, J. H., Wolfe, B. L., et al. (2013). Family poverty affects the rate of human infant brain growth. *PLOS ONE, 8,* e80954.

Harmon-Jones, E. (2003). Anger and the behavioral approach system. *Personality and Individual Differences, 35,* 995–1005.

Heatherton, T. F. (2011). Neuroscience of self and self-regulation. *Annual Review of Psychology, 62,* 363–390.

Henry, B., Caspi, A., Moffitt, T. E., & Silva, P. A. (1996). Temperamental and familial predictors of violent and non-violent criminal convictions: From age 3 to age 18. *Developmental Psychology, 32,* 614–623.

Hiramura, H., Uji, M., Shikai, N., Chen, Z., Matsuoka, N., & Kitamura, T. (2010).

Understanding externalizing behavior from children's personality and parenting characteristics. *Psychiatry Research, 175,* 142–147.

Hubbard, J. A., Dodge, K. A., Cillessen, A. H. N., Coie, J. D., & Schwartz, D. (2001). The dyadic nature of social information processing in boys' reactive and proactive aggression. *Journal of Personality and Social Psychology, 80,* 268–280.

Hubbard, J. A., Smithmyer, C. M., Ramsden, S. R., Parker, E. H., Flanagan, K. D., Dearing, K. F., et al. (2002). Observational, physiological, and self-report measures of children's anger: Relations to reactive versus proactive aggression. *Child Development, 73*(4), 1101–1118.

Jones, A. P., Laurens, K. R., Herba, C. M., Barker, G. J., & Viding, E. (2009). Amygdala hypoactivity to fearful faces in boys with conduct problems and callous–unemotional traits. *American Journal of Psychiatry, 166,* 95–102.

Kim, S. J., Lee, S. J., Yune, S. K., Sung, Y. H., Bae, S. C., Chung, A., et al. (2006). The relationship between the biogenetic temperament and character and psychopathology in adolescents. *Psychopathology, 39,* 80–86.

Kimonis, E. R., Frick, P. J., Boris, N. W., Smyke, A. T., Cornell, A. H., Farrell, J. M., et al. (2006). Callous–unemotional features, behavioral inhibition, and parenting: Independent predictors of aggression in a high-risk preschool sample. *Journal of Child and Family Studies, 15,* 741–752.

Lane, R., McRae, K., Reiman, E., Chen, K., Ahern, G., & Thayer, J. (2009). Neural correlates of heart rate variability during emotion. *NeuroImage, 44,* 213–222.

Lengua, L. J., & Kovacs, E. A. (2005). Bidirectional associations between temperament and parenting and the prediction of adjustment problems in middle childhood. *Journal of Applied Developmental Psychology, 26,* 21–38.

Leone, L., & Russo, P. M. (2009). Components of the behavioral activation system and functional impulsivity: A test of discriminant hypotheses. *Journal of Research in Personality, 43,* 1101–1104.

Levenson, M. R., Kiehl, K. A., & Fitzpatrick, C. M. (1995). Assessing psychopathic attributes in a noninstitutionalized population. *Journal of Personality and Social Psychology, 68,* 151–158.

Liew, J., Eisenberg, N., Spinrad, T. L., Eggum, N. D., Haugen, R. G., Kupfer, A., et al. (2011). Physiological regulation and fearfulness as predictors of young children's empathy-related reactions. *Social Development, 20,* 111–134.

Lozier, L. M., Cardinale, E. M., Van Meter, J. W., & Marsh, A. A. (2014). Mediation of the relationship between callous–unemotional traits and proactive aggression by amygdala response to fear among children with conduct problems. *JAMA Psychiatry, 71,* 627–636.

Marcovitch, S., Leigh, J., Calkins, S. D., Leerks, E. M., O'Brien, M., & Nayena Blankson, A. (2010). Moderate vagal withdrawal in 3.5-year-old children is associated with optimal performance on executive function tasks. *Developmental Psychobiology, 52,* 603–608.

Marsee, M. A., Frick, P. J., Barry, C. T., Kimonis, E. R., Muñoz Centifanti, L. C., & Aucoin, K. J. (2014). Profiles of the forms and functions of self-reported aggression in three adolescent samples. *Development and Psychopathology, 26,* 705–720.

Miller, J. D., Zeichner, A., & Wilson, L. F. (2012). Personality correlates of aggression: Evidence from measures of the five-factor model, UPPS model of impulsivity, and BIS/BAS. *Journal of Interpersonal Violence, 27,* 2903–2919.

Moore, C. C., Hubbard, J. A., Morrow, M. T., Barhight, L. R., Lines, M. M., Rubin, R. M., et al. (2018). *The interaction of sympathetic and parasympathetic psychophysiology on reactive and proactive aggression in real time.* Manuscript under review.

Morgan, J. E., Bowen, K. L., Moore, S. C., & Van Goozen, S. H. M. (2014). The relationship between reward and punishment sensitivity and antisocial behavior in male adolescents. *Personality and Individual Differences, 63,* 122–127.

Mujica-Parodi, L. R., Carlson, J. M., Cha, J., & Rubin, D. (2014). The fine line between "brave" and "reckless": Amygdala reactivity and regulation predict recognition of risk. *NeuroImage, 103*, 1–9.

Muñoz, L. C., Frick, P. J., Kimonis, E. R., & Aucoin, K. J. (2008). Types of aggression, responsiveness to provocation, and callous–unemotional traits in detained adolescents. *Journal of Abnormal Child Psychology, 36*, 15–28.

Murray-Close, D. (2013a). Psychophysiology of adolescent peer relations: I. Theory and research findings. *Journal of Research on Adolescence, 23*, 236–259.

Murray-Close, D. (2013b). Psychophysiology of adolescent peer relations: II. Recent advances and future directions. *Journal of Research on Adolescence, 23*, 260–273.

Nærde, A., Ogden, T., Janson, H., & Zachrisson, H. D. (2014). Normative development of physical aggression from 8 to 26 months. *Developmental Psychology, 50*, 1–11.

Ojanen, T., Findley, D., & Fuller, S. (2012). Physical and relational aggression in early adolescence: Associations with narcissism, temperament, and social goals. *Aggressive Behavior, 38*, 99–107.

Pagliaccio, D., Luking, K. R., Anokhin, A. P., Gotlib, I. H., Hayden, E. P., Olino, T. M., et al. (2016). Revising the BIS/BAS Scale to study development: Measurement invariance and normative effects of age and sex from childhood through adulthood. *Psychological Assessment, 28*, 429–442.

Pardini, D. A. (2006). The callousness pathway to severe violent delinquency. *Aggressive Behavior, 32*, 590–598.

Pardini, D. (2011). Perceptions of social conflicts among incarcerated adolescents with callous–unemotional traits: "You're going to pay. It's going to hurt, but I don't care." *Journal of Child Psychology and Psychiatry, 52*, 248–255.

Pardini, D., & Frick, P. J. (2013). Multiple developmental pathways to conduct disorder: Current conceptualizations and clinical implications. *Journal of the Canadian Academy of Child and Adolescent Psychiatry, 22*, 20–25.

Pardini, D., Lochman, J., & Wells, K. (2004). Negative emotions and alcohol use initiation in high-risk boys: The moderating effect of good inhibitory control. *Journal of Abnormal Child Psychology, 32*, 505–518.

Pardini, D. A., & Phillips, M. (2010). Neural responses to emotional and neutral facial expressions in chronically violent men. *Journal of Psychiatry and Neuroscience, 35*, 390–398.

Park, J. H., Essex, M. J., Zahn-Waxler, C., Armstrong, J. M., Klein, M. H., & Goldsmith, H. H. (2005). Relational and overt aggression in middle childhood: Early child and family risk factors. *Early Education and Development, 16*, 233–258.

Patterson, G. R., DeBaryshe, B. D., & Ramsey, E. (1989). A developmental perspective on antisocial behavior. *American Psychologist, 44*, 329–335.

Polman, H., de Castro, B., Koops, W., van Boxtel, H. W., & Merk, W. W. (2007). A meta-analysis of the distinction between reactive and proactive aggression in children and adolescents. *Journal of Abnormal Child Psychology, 35*, 522–535.

Porges, S. W., Doussard-Roosevelt, J. A., Portales, A. L., & Greenspan, S. I. (1996). Infant regulation of the vagal "brake" predicts child behavior problems: A psychobiological model of social behavior. *Developmental Psychobiology, 29*, 697–712.

Portnoy, J., Raine, A., Chen, F. R., Pardini, D., Loeber, R., & Jennings, J. R. (2014). Heart rate and antisocial behavior: The mediating role of impulsive sensation seeking. *Criminology: An Interdisciplinary Journal, 52*, 292–311.

Putnam, S. P., Ellis, L. K., & Rothbart, M. K. (2001). The structure of temperament from infancy through adolescence. In A. Eliasz & A. Angleitner (Eds.), *Advances in research on temperament* (pp. 165–182). Lengerich, Germany: Pabst.

Raine, A. (1996). Autonomic nervous system factors underlying disinhibited, antisocial, and violent behavior: Biosocial perspectives and treatment implications. In C. F. Ferris & T.

Grisso (Eds.), *Understanding aggressive behavior in children* (pp. 46–59). New York: New York Academy of Sciences.

Raine, A. (2002). Biosocial studies of antisocial and violent behavior in children and adults: A review. *Journal of Abnormal Child Psychology, 30,* 311–326.

Raine, A., Fung, A. L. C., Portnoy, J., Choy, O., & Spring, V. L. (2014). Low heart rate as a risk factor for child and adolescent proactive aggressive and impulsive psychopathic behavior. *Aggressive Behavior, 40,* 290–299.

Rathert, J., Fite, P. J., Gaertner, A. E., & Vitulano, M. (2011). Associations between effortful control, psychological control, and proactive and reactive aggression. *Child Psychiatry and Human Development, 42,* 609–621.

Roose, A., Bijttebier, P., Van der Oord, S., Claes, L., & Lilienfeld, S. O. (2013). Psychopathic traits in youth and associations with temperamental features: Results from a performance-based measure. *Journal of Individual Differences, 34,* 1–7.

Rothbart, M. K. (1981). Measurement of temperament in infancy. *Child Development, 52,* 569–578.

Rothbart, M. K. (1989). Biological processes in temperament. In G. A. Kohnstamm, J. E. Bates, & M. K. Rothbart (Eds.), *Temperament in childhood* (pp. 77–110). New York: Wiley.

Rothbart, M. K. (2007). Temperament, development, and personality. *Current Directions in Psychological Science, 16,* 207–212.

Rothbart, M. K., Ahadi, S. A., & Hershey, K. L. (1994). Temperament and social behavior in childhood. *Merrill–Palmer Quarterly, 40,* 21–39.

Rothbart, M. K., & Bates, J. E. (2006). Temperament. In N. Eisenberg, W. Damon, & R. M. Lerner (Eds.), *Handbook of child psychology: Social, emotional, and personality development* (6th ed., pp. 99–166). Hoboken, NJ: Wiley.

Rothbart, M. K., & Derryberry, D. (1981). Development of individual differences in temperament. In M. E. Lamb & A. L. Brown (Eds.), *Advances in developmental psychology* (Vol. 1, pp. 37–86). Hillsdale, NJ: Erlbaum.

Scarpa, A., Haden, S. C., & Tanaka, A. (2010). Being hot-tempered: Autonomic, emotional, and behavioral distinctions between childhood reactive and proactive aggression. *Biological Psychology, 84,* 488–496.

Schultz, D., Izard, C. E., & Bear, G. (2004). Children's emotion processing: Relations to emotionality and aggression. *Development and Psychopathology, 16,* 371–387.

Shortt, J. W., Stoolmiller, M., Smith-Shine, J., Mark Eddy, J., & Sheeber, L. (2010). Maternal emotion coaching, adolescent anger regulation, and siblings externalizing symptoms. *Journal of Child Psychology and Psychiatry, 51,* 799–808.

Sijtsema, J. J., Veenstra, R., Lindenberg, S., van Roon, A. M., Verhulst, F. C., Ormel, J., et al. (2010). Mediation of sensation seeking and behavioral inhibition on the relationship between heart rate and antisocial behavior: The TRAILS study. *Journal of the American Academy of Child and Adolescent Psychiatry, 49,* 493–502.

Skowron, E. A., Loken, E., Gatzke-Kopp, L., Cipriano-Essel, E., Woehrle, P. L., Van Epps, J. J., et al. (2011). Mapping cardiac physiology and parenting processes in maltreating mother–child dyads. *Journal of Family Psychology, 25,* 663–674.

Smeets, K. C., Oostermeijer, S., Lappenschaar, M., Cohn, M., van der Meer, J. M., Popma, A., et al. (2016). Are proactive and reactive aggression meaningful distinctions in adolescents?: A variable- and person-based approach. *Journal of Abnormal Child Psychology, 45*(1), 1–14.

Smillie, L. D., Jackson, C. J., & Dalgleish, L. I. (2006). Conceptual distinctions among Carver and White's (1994) BAS scales: A reward-reactivity versus trait impulsivity perspective. *Personality and Individual Differences, 40,* 1039–1050.

Snyder, J., Edwards, P., McGraw, K., Kilgore, K., & Holton, A. (1994). Escalation and reinforcement in mother–child conflict: Social processes associated with the development of physical aggression. *Development and Psychopathology, 6,* 305–321.

Snyder, J. J., & Patterson, G. R. (1995). Individual differences in social aggression: A test of a reinforcement model of socialization in the natural environment. *Behavior Therapy, 26,* 371–391.

Snyder, J., Schrepferman, L., & St. Peter, C. (1997). Origins of antisocial behavior: Negative reinforcement and affect dysregulation of behavior as socialization mechanisms in family interaction. *Behavior Modification, 21,* 187–215.

Stadler, C., Poustka, F., & Sterzer, P. (2010). The heterogeneity of disruptive behavior disorders: Implications for neurobiological research and treatment. *Frontiers in Psychiatry, 1,* 21.

Stadler, C., Sterzer, P., Schmeck, K., Krebs, A., Kleinschmidt, A., & Poustka, F. (2007). Reduced anterior cingulate activation in aggressive children and adolescents during affective stimulation: Association with temperament traits. *Journal of Psychiatric Research, 41,* 410–417.

Stickle, T. R., Kirkpatrick, N. M., & Brush, L. N. (2009). Callous–unemotional traits and social information processing: Multiple risk-factor models for understanding aggressive behavior in antisocial youth. *Law and Human Behavior, 33,* 515–529.

Sulik, M. J., Eisenberg, N., Silva, K. M., Spinrad, T. L., & Kupfer, A. (2013). Respiratory sinus arrhythmia, shyness, and effortful control in preschool-age children. *Biological Psychology, 92,* 241–248.

Taubitz, L. E., Pedersen, W. S., & Larson, C. L. (2015). BAS reward responsiveness: A unique predictor of positive psychological functioning. *Personality and Individual Differences, 80,* 107–112.

Torrubia, R., & Tobeña, A. (1984). A scale for the assessment of "susceptibility to punishment" as a measure of anxiety: Preliminary results. *Personality and Individual Differences, 5,* 371–375.

Valiente, C., Eisenberg, N., Smith, C. L., Reiser, M., Fabes, R. A., Losoya, S., et al. (2003). The relations of effortful control and reactive control to children's externalizing problems: A longitudinal assessment. *Journal of Personality, 71,* 1171–1196.

Van Goozen, S. H. M., Matthys, W., Cohen-Kettenis, P. T., Buitelaar, J. K., & Van Engeland, H. (2000). Hypothalamic–pituitary–adrenal axis and autonomic nervous system activity in disruptive children and matched controls. *Journal of the American Academy of Child and Adolescent Psychiatry, 39,* 1438–1445.

Veroude, K., von Rhein, D., Chauvin, R. J. M., van Dongen, E. V., Mennes, M. J. J., Franke, B., et al. (2016). The link between callous–unemotional traits and neural mechanisms of reward processing: An fMRI study. *Psychiatry Research: Neuroimaging, 255,* 75–80.

Vitaro, F., Barker, E. D., Boivin, M., Brendgen, M., & Tremblay, R. E. (2006). Do early difficult temperament and harsh parenting differentially predict reactive and proactive aggression? *Journal of Abnormal Child Psychology, 34,* 681–691.

Vitaro, F., Brendgen, M., & Tremblay, R. E. (2002). Reactively and proactively aggressive children: Antecedent and subsequent characteristics. *Journal of Child Psychology and Psychiatry, 43,* 495–505.

White, M. G., Bogdan, R., Fisher, P. M., Munoz, K. E., Williamson, D. E., & Hariri, A. R. (2012). FKBP5 and emotional neglect interact to predict individual differences in amygdala reactivity. *Genes, Brain, and Behavior, 11,* 869–878.

White, S. F., van Tieghem, M., Brislin, S. J., Sypher, I., Sinclair, S., Pine, D. S., et al. (2016). Neural correlates of the propensity for retaliatory behavior in youths with disruptive behavior disorders. *American Journal of Psychiatry, 173,* 282–290.

Willoughby, M. T., Waschbusch, D. A., Moore, G. A., & Propper, C. B. (2011). Using the ASEBA to screen for callous–unemotional traits in early childhood: Factor structure, temporal stability, and utility. *Journal of Psychopathology and Behavioral Assessment, 33,* 19–30.

Xu, Y., Farver, J. A. M., & Zhang, Z. (2009). Temperament, harsh and indulgent parenting, and Chinese children's proactive and reactive aggression. *Child Development, 80,* 244–258.

Xu, Y., Raine, A., Yu, L., & Krieg, A. (2014). Resting heart rate, vagal tone, and reactive and proactive aggression in Chinese children. *Journal of Abnormal Child Psychology, 42,* 501–514.

CHAPTER 7

Social–Emotional Development and Aggression

TINA MALTI and JU-HYUN SONG

Brief Introduction

Social–emotional development is essential for children's and adolescents' mental health, peer relationships, and learning. This chapter focuses on links between social–emotional development and aggressive behaviors across childhood and adolescence. Social–emotional antecedents and correlates of aggression serve as risk and protective factors in the emergence and development of aggression and can as such provide essential information for the design and planning of intervention strategies. We begin with a description of social–emotional development and the components it entails. Next, we discuss theoretical frameworks that have been introduced to describe social–emotional development and how it relates to aggression. We then describe central findings from empirical research on the associations between core components of social–emotional development and aggression. We conclude the chapter with a discussion of promising areas for future research and practices aimed at improving our understanding of the role of social–emotional development in aggression and promoting social–emotional development to reduce aggression in childhood and adolescence.

Conceptualizations

Social–emotional development includes the process of becoming increasingly able to manage and express various emotions in age- and socially appropriate ways and to effectively engage in social interactions that meet developmental needs (Denham

& Zinsser, 2014). Here we provide a brief description of social–emotional development in childhood and adolescence (for a comprehensive definition of aggression, see Malti & Rubin, Chapter 1, this volume). Key components of social–emotional development include awareness of one's own emotional experiences, emotional responses oriented to others, and capacities to regulate emotional experiences (Malti, Sette, & Dys, 2016). This chapter discusses the three components of social–emotional development—self-conscious emotions (e.g., guilt), other-oriented emotions (e.g., sympathy), and emotion regulation (e.g., regulation of anger)—that are specifically related to the development of aggression from childhood to adolescence. The reason is that well-balanced social–emotional capacities in these domains have been shown to curb aggression and antisocial behaviors (Arsenio, 2014; Colasante, Zuffianò, & Malti, 2015; Malti & Krettenauer, 2013; Olson, Lopez-Duran, Lunkenheimer, Chang, & Sameroff, 2011).

Self-conscious emotions have been defined as emotions triggered by self-reflective processes. Specifically, morally relevant self-conscious emotions are evoked based on one's evaluation of the self in the context of violating a norm (Eisenberg, 2000; Malti, 2016). For example, guilt is a feeling of regret over one's wrongdoing, which thus indicates the activation of internalized moral norms (Malti, Gummerum, Keller, & Buchmann, 2009).

Other-oriented emotions are described as affective responses that stem from the understanding and evaluation of another's emotional state or behavior in relation to social or moral norms (Eisenberg, Spinrad, & Morris, 2014; Malti, Sette, & Dys, 2016). A widely studied other-oriented emotion is sympathy, which involves feelings of concern for others as well as cognitive understanding of others' perspective, which thus can be differentiated from early-emerging empathy (i.e., experience of the same or similar emotion as the distressed other without distance between the self and the other; Davidov, Zahn-Waxler, Roth-Hanania, & Knafo, 2013; Eisenberg et al., 2014). Another other-oriented emotional response that is closely connected to aggression is anger. Anger is broadly defined as a negative affective reaction to the perception of a personal threat or provocation (Lazarus, 1991).

Emotion regulation is defined as the capacity to manage the experience and expression of affective states (Eisenberg, Spinrad, & Eggum, 2010). As a component of self-regulation, it is biologically based, yet also shaped by contextual influences and maturational processes (Eisenberg et al., 2010; Posner & Rothbart, 2000).

Theoretical Considerations

Over the past decades, several models and frameworks have been developed to conceptualize the theoretical foundations for social–emotional development in childhood and adolescence. Although it is beyond the scope of this chapter to provide a comprehensive review of the various theoretical accounts, we highlight some central assumptions and approaches that have relevance for aggression. Social–emotional skills typically entail abilities to form, maintain, and support social relationships, as well as emotional capacities such as emotion expression and management, empathy, and emotion regulation in ways that are developmentally appropriate (Denham, 2006; Saarni, 1999). Social–emotional development is therefore linked to child well-being, academic learning, and quality of relationships with peers. On the other hand, a lack of core social and emotional skills can contribute to the development of aggressive antisocial behaviors. Central to engaging in competent social behavior is balancing self-oriented needs and desires with other-oriented responsibilities in an age-appropriate manner; this involves understanding of one's own internal affective states, understanding and appreciating the emotional experiences of others, and coordinating and integrating one's own and others' perspectives (Rose-Krasnor, 1997).

Developmental scientists have emphasized the transactional nature of social–emotional capacities from early on (Rose-Krasnor, 1997). Thus age-appropriate levels of social–emotional functioning emerge through interactions between the child and his or her social partners (Rose-Krasnor & Denham, 2009). As such, there is natural fluctuation in every individual's skill level, depending on the partner and his or her characteristics, as well as the quality of the interaction between the two (see Vygotsky, 1978).

Our own theoretical framework for social–emotional development has focused on conceptualizing three core components and their development in social interactions: an understanding of emotions in the self and other, the age-appropriate expression of emotions, and the ability to regulate emotional arousal (Malti, Sette, & Dys, 2016). The framework includes the taxonomy of social–emotional development, in which the structure and function of social–emotional development is described along two core organizational principles. First, the principle of self- and other-orientation is an organizational principle used to understand whether the component of emotional responding is (more) focused on the self (e.g., self-conscious emotional responses), the other (e.g., other-oriented emotions such as sympathy), or both in a way that is adequate for their age and development (Malti, Sette, & Dys, 2016; see Malti & Noam, 2016). The second core organizational principle refers to overregulation and underregulation. This principle helps identify the extent to which the individual is able to regulate and balance his or her own and others' emotions in a manner that is adequate for their development (Eisenberg, 2000).

This framework links the core components of social–emotional development to aggression and antisocial behavior, as well as to kindness and prosocial behavior. Specifically, the integration of others' and oneself's perspectives that transcends one's own standpoint may ultimately lead to other-oriented sympathy and impede aggression (Malti & Dys, 2017; Malti & Ongley, 2014). The model also acknowledges that there is a basic human need to demonstrate emotional control and flexibility by regulating one's own emotions. This regulatory capacity affects our behavioral responses to varying situational demands. Both processes—the integration of perspectives and regulation of emotions—underlie growth, decline, and transformation in our social behavior. Experiencing self- and other-oriented emotions is thus likely to become increasingly intertwined across development as emotion understanding, expression, and regulation become increasingly coordinated (Thompson, 2011). As a consequence, the role of self- and other-oriented emotions in aggressive behavior outcomes may become increasingly complex.

In the following sections, we briefly discuss selected, central components of the development of self-conscious emotions, other-oriented emotions, and emotion regulation, and theoretically expected links with aggressive behaviors (Eisenberg, 2000; Malti & Ongley, 2014). We focus on social–emotional responding in the contexts of social conflict due to their multifaceted nature; these situations help us understand how children negotiate and integrate considerations such as "not harming others" versus "being fair." The development of self-conscious and other-oriented emotional responses and emotion regulation capacities has been shown to impede antisocial, selfishly motivated behaviors (Arsenio, 2014; Malti & Krettenauer, 2013).

Development of Self-Conscious Emotional Responses and Aggression

Developmentally, self-conscious emotions strongly increase from early to middle childhood. The prototypical self-conscious emotion is guilt. Although children show early forms of guilt-induced behaviors such as gaze aversion or bodily tension around age 4 (Kochanska, Barry, Aksan, & Boldt, 2008), they attribute negative feelings to themselves as transgressors around age 8 (for a review, see Arsenio, 2014). Yet interindividual differences in the anticipation of guilt remain well into adolescence and beyond. A combination of multiple factors contributes to interindividual differences in guilt, most likely due to temperamental differences and cognitive restraints in early childhood, but more possibly due to motivational variation, desires, and self-interests in later childhood and beyond (for a review, see Malti, 2016).

Experiencing guilt has been identified as a crucial factor for the prevention of aggressive behaviors (for a review, see Arsenio, 2014; Kochanska, Barry, Jimenez, Hollatz, & Woodard, 2009; for a meta-analysis, see Malti & Krettenauer, 2013). The reason is that guilt serves as an important emotional marker that highlights the negative consequences of aggressive behaviors for the perpetrator due to its aversive emotional nature. Thus experiencing feelings of guilt is expected to potentially reduce the recurrence of aggression, whereas the lack thereof underlies maladaptive aggressive behaviors (Arsenio, Gold, & Adams, 2006; Eisner & Malti, 2015).

Development of Other-Oriented Emotional Responses and Aggression

The most widely investigated other-oriented emotional responses are empathy and sympathy (Eisenberg, 2000). Empathy stems from the comprehension of another's emotional state and resembles the other person's feelings. Unlike empathy, sympathy (i.e., concern for others) does not necessarily involve feeling the same emotion that the other person is experiencing. Sympathy is considered to provide immediate feedback for discouraging aggressive acts by orienting the perpetrator to the pain suffered by the victim (Arsenio, 2014). Some studies suggest that there is little change in sympathy across early childhood (e.g., Vaish, Carpenter, & Tomasello, 2009), whereas others show an increase in concern for others from early childhood to early adolescence (Eisenberg et al., 2014; Malti, Eisenberg, Kim, & Buchmann, 2013). Empirical research has confirmed a theoretically expected negative link between empathy or sympathy and aggression, albeit frequently in the small to medium effect-size range (Jolliffe & Farrington, 2006; van Noorden, Haselager, Cillessen, & Bukowski, 2015). Nevertheless, these findings collectively point to the importance of connecting to the feelings of others' pain in preventing aggression and antisocial behaviors.

Anger, on the other hand, involves an intense affective reaction to threat and provocations from others (real or perceived) and a fight-or-flight response. Developmental research has shown evidence to support a normative decrease in negative emotionality from preschool years to early adolescence (e.g., Murphy, Eisenberg, Fabes, Shepard, & Guthrie, 1999). Despite this normative decline, proneness to experience anger is expected to be strongly associated with aggression across the development because anger and arousal are often expressed through aggression (Berkowitz, 1989). Empirical findings indeed suggest that anger is related to higher aggression toward others (Arsenio, Cooperman, & Lover, 2000) and particularly related to higher reactive and overt forms of aggression (Hubbard, McAuliffe, Morrow, & Romano, 2010).

Development of Emotion Regulation and Aggression

Emotion regulation is one of the most widely studied social–emotional factors in relation to aggression, especially considering the influence of developing self-regulation capacities on the normative decline in aggression during preschool years (Alink et al., 2006; Eisenberg et al., 2010; Eisner & Malti, 2015). As a subcomponent of top-down self-regulation, emotion regulation shows gradual mean-level increase up to early adulthood but moderate rank-order stability in early childhood that increases with age (for a review, see Bridgett, Burt, Edwards, & Deater-Deckard, 2015).

The inability to modulate negative emotional responses is critical to the development of aggression, especially for children prone to experience negative affect, such as anger (Olson et al., 2011). Also, poor positive emotion regulation has been related to happy victimization (i.e., attributing positive emotions to the wrongdoer in a hypothetical transgression story; Arsenio et al., 2006), which is related to aggression across childhood and adolescence (Malti & Krettenauer, 2013). Importantly, emotion regulation is not independent of self-conscious emotions and other-oriented emotional responses but, rather, critical for buffering detrimental effects of the absence of one another against the development of aggression (Malti, Sette, & Dys, 2016). What is less understood is whether and how various regulatory capacities underlie children's self-conscious and other-oriented emotions. For instance, it remains unclear which components of emotion regulation (e.g., ability to control impulses and manage emotions, behavioral expression of emotions) are central to promoting the emergence of self-conscious and other-oriented emotions.

Social–Emotional Development and Aggression Subtypes

One issue that rises from the literature on social–emotional development and aggression is the specificity of their associations between the subtypes of aggression. The ways in which social–emotional factors are involved in aggressive behaviors may depend on the function or motivation behind aggression (Hubbard et al., 2010). Some scholars also argue that it is the function that aggression serves that matters in how maladaptive or adaptive aggression can be for one's social and emotional well-being (Hawley & Vaughn, 2003; Vitaro, Brendgen, & Barker, 2006). Based on its function, aggression can be broadly categorized into proactive and reactive subtypes. Both subtypes involve intention to harm others, but proactive aggression is "cold blooded" and involves stimulus-seeking behaviors that are goal oriented, whereas reactive aggression is "hot-headed," defensive harming of others in reaction to perceived provocation or threats (Arsenio, Adams, & Gold, 2009; see also Malti & Rubin, Chapter 1, this volume). This categorization of behaviors is useful for understanding the developmental mechanisms underlying the complex associations between social–emotional development and aggression. Indeed, studies that have distinguished subtypes of aggression have identified their differential links to social–emotional development.

In the following section, we review the empirical literature on associations between social–emotional development and overt aggression. We also describe some of the unique associations between proactive and reactive types of aggression with social–emotional development.

Central Research Findings

In this section, we take a comprehensive, but not exhaustive, approach to reviewing the literature on social–emotional development and children's and adolescents' aggression and related externalizing behaviors. Because the literature linking various components of social–emotional development to aggression is extensive and reviewed more generally elsewhere (e.g., Eisner & Malti, 2015; Malti, Colasante, & Jambon, Chapter 11, this volume), this section primarily reviews the recent literature with a focus on the three core components of social–emotional development (i.e., self-conscious emotion, other-oriented emotion, emotion regulation) that have been theorized to be linked closely to aggression and its development from childhood to adolescence.

One issue with the individual differences in the development of aggression is whether and how they are related to social–emotional development across different developmental periods. Few studies have directly examined codeveloping trajectories of aggression and social–emotional skills (Zuffianò, Colasante, Buchmann, & Malti, 2017), but developmental (dis)continuities in the associations between social–emotional development and aggression can be inferred from longitudinal studies and cross-sectional studies targeting different age groups. Research examining the moderating effect of age can also shed lights on how social–emotional development influences the progression of aggression in a developmentally sensitive manner. For example, if the association between social–emotional development and aggression becomes weaker with age, this suggests that the association may be largely explained by intrapersonal, developmental changes in social–emotional development; children acquire social–emotional capacities as they mature, capacities that may become less responsible for the changes in aggressive tendencies once they reach a certain level of threshold. If the association continues to remain strong with age, this may imply that the interindividual differences in social–emotional development are relatively stable across development (i.e., dispositional, trait-like) and that these individual differences may be largely accountable for the development of aggression. To address this issue, we discuss developmental continuities and discontinuities in the relations between aggression and the three chosen aspects of social–emotional development.

Self-Conscious Emotion and Aggression across Development

As a self-conscious emotion, guilt has been inversely related to aggression in both childhood and adolescence (for a review, see Malti & Krettenauer, 2013). In early childhood, children's development of conscience (i.e., a broader construct encompassing guilt) at 52 months negatively predicted disruptive behaviors at 67 months (Kochanska et al., 2008). Also, boys between ages 7 and 13 with clinical levels of aggression reported less guilt in response to aggression vignettes compared with nonaggressive boys (Orobio de Castro, Merk, Koops, Veerman, & Bosch, 2005). Moreover, guilt moderated the link between anger and aggression in children who were 4, 8, and 12 years of age, such that high anger was related to high aggression only for children with low guilt (Colasante et al., 2015).

As such, across normative and clinical levels of aggression, the inverse relation between guilt and aggression seems to be stable across childhood and adolescence without being moderated by age, which suggests that interindividual differences—rather than intrapersonal change—in dispositional guilt may be playing an important role (Malti & Krettenauer, 2013). For example, a study on dispositional guilt found that it was negatively related to aggression and positively related to cognitive reappraisal of the self's role in responding to hypothetical anger-inducing situations (e.g., "It was partly my fault"; "Maybe I should have been more careful") in both children and adults (Tangney, Wagner, Hill-Barlow, Marschall, & Gramzow, 1996). This suggests that guilt may suppress aggressive behaviors directly through an online negative emotional feedback mechanism, and indirectly through individual differences in the social-cognitive process that allows reevaluation of the situation. Guilt, however, should be distinguished from shame; shame is another self-conscious emotion but one that focuses on the negative aspects of the *self* for a wrongdoing rather than focusing on the *behavior,* as with guilt (Tracy & Robins, 2006). Whereas guilt proneness is known to be a protective factor for anger and violence (for a review, see Tangney, Stuewig, & Mashek, 2007), shame proneness is considered a maladaptive emotion (Barret, Zahn-Waxler, & Cole, 1993; Luby et al., 2009) that is positively associated with aggression across the lifespan (Bennett, Sullivan, & Lewis, 2005; Tangney et al., 1996). Thus it would be important to distinguish guilt from shame in understanding the role of self-conscious emotions in developing aggression.

Some studies have suggested evidence for the specificity of the link between guilt and aggression subtypes. Compared with reactive aggression, proactive aggression has been more strongly associated with deficiencies in feeling guilt. In a sample of adolescents, proactive aggression was related to higher expectation for happiness after engaging in aggressive behaviors (Arsenio et al., 2009). Similarly, incarcerated adolescent boys who engaged in high levels of proactive aggression were more likely to expect to feel positive emotion following aggression than did more reactively aggressive boys (Smithmyer, Hubbard, & Simons, 2000). Deficiencies in guilt response may be due to low levels of autonomic and affective arousal in children and adolescents with high proactive aggressive tendencies (Arsenio et al., 2009). More studies need to examine whether these biologically based deficiencies in self-conscious emotions can be compensated for by cognitive or behavioral interventions.

Other-Oriented Emotion and Aggression across Development

As an other-oriented moral emotion, sympathy buffers the risk for developing aggression. Despite the developmental changes in sympathy, many studies have replicated the negative association between sympathy and aggression in different age groups (e.g., Schultz, Izard, & Bear, 2004; Strayer & Roberts, 2004), suggesting the continuity of the inverse link across childhood and adolescence (for a review, see van Noorden et al., 2015). Others found that the negative relation between sympathy and aggression becomes stronger later in development. For example, a review on the association between sympathy and aggression reported that the negative link was more consistently found in adolescents than in children (e.g., Lovett & Sheffield, 2007). One interpretation for the age difference deals with methodology because the measures used for younger children often do not distinguish empathy (or emotional contagion) from sympathy. Alternatively, younger children may indeed experience more emotional contagion than other-oriented sympathy in empathy-inducing situations because of their rudimentary emotion regulation skills. For example, a previous study on early aggression and sympathy found that toddlers who were rated as aggressive showed other-oriented behaviors more quickly in the empathy-eliciting situations (e.g., another child crying). Possibly, this occurred because aggressive children were less aroused by others' distress, which allowed them to orient to others rather than to struggle with their own distress (Gill & Calkins, 2003). However, this is likely to be true only in the early years, when children do not have effective emotion regulation skills and thus easily overwhelmed by empathy-eliciting situations.

Another possible explanation for the stronger link between sympathy and aggression in later childhood is that there may be an actual decline in sympathy from earlier levels or a delay in the development of sympathy over a period of time among aggressive children. To test this hypothesis, a longitudinal study examined the development of concern for others in children with normative, subclinical, or clinical levels of externalizing problems (Hastings, Zahn-Waxler, Robinson, Usher, & Bridges, 2000). This study found no group differences in concern for others at 4–5 years of age, but children with clinical levels of problems showed a significant decrease in their concern for others, as well as lower levels of concern relative to the other groups at 6–7 years. Longitudinally, however, they found that concern for others at an earlier time point (i.e., 4–5 years of age) predicted decreases in the severity of externalizing problems at later time points, up to 9–10 years of age. Therefore, deficiencies in sympathy as a correlate of aggression may not be readily detectable until after the preschool years, but fostering sympathy early on might still be important for reducing aggression over time.

Although sympathy is expected to provide immediate feedback for discouraging aggressive acts by orienting the perpetrator to the pain suffered by the victim (Arsenio, 2014), this curbing mechanism of sympathy on aggression may not be strong for children with high proactive aggression. For proactively aggressive children, viewing distress in the victim may be rewarding as a sign of goal achievement, which brings positive emotions (Orobio de Castro et al., 2005). Thus these children may understand the victim's pain and distress but not necessarily feel concern (i.e., sympathy) for the victim. Supporting this idea, proactive aggression was negatively related to sympathy while controlling for reactive aggression in children ages 5, 7, and 10 (Peplak & Malti, 2016). Similarly, proactively aggressive adolescents focused less on the negative emotional consequences in others than on the instrumental gains of aggression (Arsenio et al., 2009).

Another other-oriented emotion that is closely associated with aggression is anger. Normative developmental trajectories of aggression and anger show decline from the peak around early preschool age and into middle childhood (Alink et al., 2006; Murphy et al., 1999), facilitated by advancing self-regulatory competencies (Olson et al., 2011). But children who remained anger prone and poorly regulated at age 5 showed more externalizing problems at home until age 6 and at school until age 8 (Rydell, Berlin, & Bohlin, 2003). Similarly, children who were highly aggressive displayed a greater number of angry nonverbal cues and more physiological arousal during a frustrating task at age 8 (Hubbard et al., 2002). Anger proneness was also related to, and predictive of, externalizing problems in middle childhood and early adolescence (Eisenberg et al., 2009).

When other self-conscious and other-oriented emotions were considered simultaneously, anger proneness was robustly related to aggression in both children and adolescents if not buffered by high guilt and sympathetic tendencies (Colasante et al., 2015). Not only dispositional anger, but also daily spikes in anger, were positively associated with aggression in 4- and 8-year-olds, supporting the notion that fluctuation in anger is an important antecedent of aggressive behaviors (Colasante, Zuffianò, & Malti, 2016; Egger & Angold, 2006; Hubbard et al., 2010). Consistent with these findings, many researchers consider aggression as mainly driven by dysregulated angry feelings (Lochman, Barry, Powell, & Young, 2010). Moreover, aggressive children may experience more anger and hostility over time due to peer conflict and rejection (Rubin, Bukowski, & Laursen, 2009), creating a bidirectional feedback loop between anger and aggression.

Anger is particularly relevant to reactive rather than proactive aggression, given that reactive aggression is motivated by reaction to perceived threats whereas proactive aggression is goal and reward-oriented. Previous evidence suggests that reactive aggression may be partly based on temperamental characteristics, such as low threshold to aversive stimuli and tendency to react emotionally (Vitaro, Brendgen, & Tremblay, 2002). In fact, reactive aggression was related to high levels of skin conductance—which indicates emotional arousal—and angry nonverbal reactions to stressors during a frustrating task in early-school-age children (Hubbard et al., 2002).

Emotion Regulation and Aggression across Development

Developmental researchers have argued that the decline in aggression after age 3 might be due to growing skills of self-regulation that can replace physical aggression with alternative strategies to manage frustration during conflicts (Côté, Tremblay,

Nagin, Zoccolillo, & Vitaro, 2002). Early strategies for regulating arousal develop into a diverse repertoire of coping skills for inhibiting behaviors and expressing context-appropriate emotions, which leads to a decline in disruptive behaviors, including aggression, over time (Calkins & Degnan, 2006). The mean-level change pattern of emotion regulation shows a gradual increase over time up to early adulthood, but there is a moderately high level of rank-order stability (see Bridgett et al., 2015, for a review). Therefore, one can expect the continuity in the link between emotion regulation and aggression independent from intrapersonal developmental change in regulatory capacities. Anger reactivity or dysregulated emotion may not in itself be sufficient for the expression of aggressive behavior, but the combination of high anger reactivity and poor regulatory competencies can be, and this is considered an early risk factor for childhood aggression (Degnan, Calkins, Keane, & Hill-Soderlund, 2008). Thus emotion regulation is closely related to developmental trajectories of aggression and cannot be separate from an understanding of the link between anger and aggression.

Numerous studies indeed support the developmental continuity in the inverse link between emotion regulation and aggression, suggesting that poor regulation of negative emotion is a risk factor for aggression consistently across development. Toddlers with high levels of externalizing problems showed more emotional venting and temper tantrums and fewer regulatory behaviors than other children during observed emotion regulation tasks (Calkins & Dedmon, 2000). In trajectory analyses, emotion regulation at age 2 negatively predicted membership in chronic-clinical levels of externalizing problems from age 2 to 4 in girls (Hill, Degnan, Calkins, & Keane, 2006). Also, extremely low or high emotion expressiveness and physiological dysregulation were associated with higher externalizing symptoms in preschoolers (Cole, Zahn-Waxler, Fox, Usher, & Welsh, 1996). Similarly, high levels of unregulated expression of anger during free play in the preschool years predicted aggressive behaviors 2–4 years later (Eisenberg et al., 1999). In a sample of adolescents, emotion dysregulation was found to be a mediator between stressful life events such as peer victimization and later aggressive behaviors (Herts, McLaughlin, & Hatzenbuehler, 2012; McLaughlin, Hatzenbuehler, Mennin, & Nolen-Hoeksema, 2011).

Dysregulated negative emotion, as well as anger proneness, is more closely related to reactive aggression than to proactive aggression, both conceptually and empirically. Reactive aggression, by definition, is driven by difficulties in regulating aggressive impulses provoked by others. Reactively aggressive children are characterized by high sympathetic arousal, impulsivity, and anger reactivity (Raine et al., 2006). Reactive aggression has also been associated with hostile attribution bias in ambiguous situations (see Orobio de Castro, Veerman, Koops, Bosch, & Monshouwer, 2002, for a review), which is closely related to poor regulation of anger; dysregulated emotional responses to stressors can lead to social information-processing deficits in decoding social cues (Crick & Dodge, 1996; Dodge et al., 2003). As a consequence, children with poor regulation and hostile attribution bias can show reactive aggression because they view their own aggression as provoked and legitimate, although they are aware of moral rules as valid and personally binding (Arsenio, 2014). Also, children who were reactively aggressive between ages 10 and

12 were rated by their caregivers as having been more reactive to social or nonsocial disturbances and more inattentive and impulsive by age 6, suggesting that they were deficient in emotion regulation and attention control from early on (Vitaro et al., 2002).

Summary

Main research findings reviewed in this section support the idea that different aspects of social—emotional development show different patterns of continuities in their relations to the development of aggression. Our review suggests that guilt and regulation of anger are consistently related to lower aggression across development, suggesting the importance of their dispositional interindividual differences, whereas sympathy seems to be more strongly related to lower aggression after a certain developmental period, which emphasizes the role of developmental maturation of the ability. More studies are needed to explore other aspects of social—emotional development in relation to aggression while considering the developmental continuity and discontinuity to understand the mechanism underlying the influence of social—emotional development on aggression.

Although many studies have examined various facets of social—emotional development, the three core facets have been mostly examined as independent factors contributing to the development of aggression rather than in relation to one another. Only a few studies have considered the interactions among multiple social—emotional components in predicting aggression. For example, moral emotions moderated the link between anger and aggression in children who were 4, 8, and 12 years of age, such that high anger was related to high aggression only for children with low guilt or low sympathy (Colasante et al., 2015). Also, guilt predicted prosocial behavior for children who showed low sympathy between ages 4 and 12, suggesting compensatory roles of different emotions for social—behavioral outcomes (Ongley & Malti, 2014). These findings provide various avenues for aggression interventions that are based in social—emotional developmental theory and research.

Implications and Conclusions

Social—emotional development is essential for an understanding of the emergence, stability, and change in aggression across childhood and adolescence. Thus well-regulated self-conscious emotions and other-oriented responsibilities can often prevent and reduce aggression in children and adolescents, whereas their absence or imbalance likely contributes to maintenance or increases in aggressive behaviors over time. Empirical work supports the long-standing argument that age-appropriate social—emotional capacities curb aggressive behaviors in children and adolescents. This chapter provided a select review of theoretical approaches and research on the relation between social—emotional capacities and aggression with a focus on developmental continuity and change, as well as specificity pertaining to the subtypes of aggression.

Self-conscious emotions, such as guilt, and other-oriented emotions, such as sympathy, as well as age-appropriate levels of emotion regulation, have been shown to relate to lower levels of aggression across childhood and adolescence. Some components of social–emotional development, such as sympathy, appear more strongly related to lower aggression in later childhood or adolescence, suggesting some developmental changes in its role as a buffer. For other components, such as guilt and negative emotion regulation, interindividual differences seem to be important even from early childhood, as their associations with aggression tend to stay stable across development, supporting its developmental continuity. Research has also shown some specificity in the links between social–emotional development and aggression subtypes. For instance, deficiencies in guilt and sympathy are particularly more relevant to proactive aggression, whereas dysregulated negative emotion (e.g., anger) is a key characteristic and motivator of reactive aggression. Based on the theoretical and empirical evidence, intervention efforts for reducing childhood and adolescence aggression are expected to target the core aspects of social–emotional development in a developmentally sensitive manner.

A promising future direction for research includes the investigation of various social emotions and their joint role in the emergence and development of aggression. For instance, one area that needs further investigation is the distinctive roles of moral and amoral anger. Moral anger is a specific case of anger, which can be experienced when individuals perceive disrespect or injustice that harms cooperation within a group (Kurzban, DeScioli, & O'Brien, 2007). Moral anger can motivate moralistic aggression, which can take many forms, including punishment (if imposed by specified agencies) or revenge/reactive aggression (if delivered by individuals), aiming to restore balance in the group (Miller, 2001). Given the distinct triggers of moral anger and its motivations for aggression, social and psychological consequences of moral anger may be different from that of amoral anger and aggression. Also, distinguishing guilt from shame and sympathy from empathy would be critical in understanding the clear mechanisms for how self-conscious and other-oriented emotions intervene in the development of aggression. Failing to distinguish these constructs may lead to ambiguous and unclear results, as they are differentially associated with aggression (e.g., Tangney et al., 2007).

Another direction for future research is to examine dynamics within the core social–emotional factors in relation to aggression. Understanding the bidirectional associations among these factors across development, as well as their interaction effects on aggression, will contribute to discovering multiple avenues for developmentally sensitive interventions for aggression (e.g., Colasante et al., 2015).

Finally, future research would benefit from considering social–emotional development as a mediator of biological factors contributing to aggression and its trajectories. Besides physiological correlates of aggression, such as low heart rate (Portnoy & Farrington, 2015; see Colasante & Malti, 2017), burgeoning fields of genetic research have been focusing on identifying pathways from genetic risks to aggressive behaviors (Hyde, 2015). Family characteristics or demographic factors have been studied as potential moderators of genetic influences (Moffitt, Caspi, &

Rutter, 2005), but psychological mechanisms underlying the interactions between genes and social factors are largely unknown. Investigating the mediating roles of social–emotional development would not only contribute to theorizing on the mechanisms underlying the gene–aggression relation but also inform practitioners what to target among intrachild-level developmental factors for children who have a high genetic risk for developing aggression.

The current state of knowledge on normative social–emotional development, as well as links to aggressive behaviors in children and adolescents, calls for a systematic translation to practice. In line with this argument, researchers have emphasized that it is time to apply the extensive knowledge on children's and adolescents' normative social–emotional development to refine existing practices, as well as generate new developmentally tailored strategies aimed at reducing aggression. For example, a practitioner's understanding of normative development of sympathy can help determine if, and by how much, a child (or a classroom) is developmentally normative, delayed, or advanced in sympathy (Malti, Chaparro, Zuffianò, & Colasante, 2016). Consistent with this effort, many existing evidence-based programs that aim to promote social–emotional development in school settings include some degree of between-grade differentiation in their curricula (Durlak, Weissberg, Dymnicki, Taylor, & Schellinger, 2011). However, most programs do not adjust their curricula for possible developmental differences in social–emotional responding *within* grades. This is surprising because there is much variability between children of the same chronological age. Therefore, future work may focus on the systematic translation of knowledge on normative levels of social–emotional development into intervention strategies for reducing aggression.

Other, related open questions concern the issue of how many (and which) dimensions of social–emotional responding should be targeted in intervention approaches, as well as generating responses to the questions *when, to whom,* and *how.* In a recent review, we found that evidence-based programs targeting several components of social–emotional development simultaneously were more effective in mitigating conduct problems and promoting academic functioning (Malti, Chaparro, et al., 2016). This finding suggests that it may be beneficial to target various components of social–emotional responding, as they may work in consort to reduce aggression and improve children's and adolescents' positive outcomes. Similarly, intervention timing and duration need to be explored further. For instance, there is some evidence to suggest that social–emotional interventions that commence earlier in development (e.g., during preschool and kindergarten) are more effective in promoting social–emotional development (Malti, Chaparro, et al., 2016). What remains to be seen is whether and how developmentally tailored interventions in other important periods of social–emotional development (e.g., puberty) compare with early childhood interventions to reduce aggression and related externalizing behaviors in terms of effectiveness. In sum, future work is needed to promote the translation of social–emotional development research into practice, to enhance practitioners' understanding of normative development, and to integrate social–emotional knowledge and assessment tools into clinical decision making and use of intervention strategies aimed at treating aggression, both between and within age groups.

ACKNOWLEDGMENTS

This research was supported by the Social Sciences and Research Council of Canada (SSHRC) and a Canadian Institutes of Health Research (CIHR) Foundation Scheme grant awarded to Tina Malti (Grant Number: FDN-148389).

REFERENCES

Alink, L. A., Mesman, J., van Zeijl, J., Stolk, M. N., Juffer, F., Koot, H. M., et al. (2006). The early childhood aggression curve: Development of physical aggression in 10- to 50-month-old children. *Child Development, 77*(4), 954–966.

Arsenio, W. (2014). Moral emotion attributions and aggression. In M. Killen & J. Smetana (Eds.), *Handbook of moral development* (2nd ed., pp. 235–255). New York: Psychology Press.

Arsenio, W. F., Adams, E., & Gold, J. (2009). Social information processing, moral reasoning, and emotion attributions: Relations with adolescents' reactive and proactive aggression. *Child Development, 80*(6), 1739–1755.

Arsenio, W. F., Cooperman, S., & Lover, A. (2000). Affective predictors of preschoolers' aggression and peer acceptance: Direct and indirect effects. *Developmental Psychology, 36*(4), 438–448.

Arsenio, W., Gold, J., & Adams, E. (2006). Children's conceptions and displays of moral emotions. In M. Killen & J. Smetana (Eds.), *Handbook of moral development* (pp. 581–610). Mahwah, NJ: Erlbaum.

Barret, K. C., Zahn-Waxler, C., & Cole, P. M. (1993). Avoiders vs. amenders: Implications for the investigation of guilt and shame during toddlerhood? *Cognition and Emotion, 7*(6), 481–505.

Bennett, D., Sullivan, M., & Lewis, M. (2005). Young children's adjustment as a function of maltreatment, shame, and anger. *Child Maltreatment, 10*(4), 311–323.

Berkowitz, L. (1989). Frustration–aggression hypothesis: Examination and reformulation. *Psychological Bulletin, 106*, 59–73.

Bridgett, D. J., Burt, N. M., Edwards, E. S., & Deater-Deckard, K. (2015). Intergenerational transmission of self-regulation: A multidisciplinary review and integrative conceptual framework. *Psychological Bulletin, 141*(3), 602–654.

Calkins, S. D., & Dedmon, S. E. (2000). Physiological and behavioral regulation in two-year-old children with aggressive/destructive behavior problems. *Journal of Abnormal Child Psychology, 28*(2), 103–118.

Calkins, S. D., & Degnan, K. A. (2006). Temperament in early development. In M. Hersen & J. C. Thomas (Eds.), *Comprehensive handbook of personality and psychopathology* (pp. 64–84). Hoboken, NJ: Wiley.

Colasante, T., & Malti, T. (2017). Resting heart rate, guilt, and sympathy: A developmental psychophysiological study of physical aggression. *Psychophysiology, 54*(11), 1770–1781.

Colasante, T., Zuffianò, A., & Malti, T. (2015). Do moral emotions buffer the anger–aggression link in children and adolescents? *Journal of Applied Developmental Psychology, 41*, 1–7.

Colasante, T., Zuffianò, A., & Malti, T. (2016). Daily deviations in anger, guilt, and sympathy: A developmental diary study of aggression. *Journal of Abnormal Child Psychology, 44*(8), 1515–1526.

Cole, P. M., Zahn-Waxler, C., Fox, N. A., Usher, B. A., & Welsh, J. D. (1996). Individual differences in emotion regulation and behavior problems in preschool children. *Journal of Abnormal Psychology, 105*(4), 518–529.

Côté, S., Tremblay, R. E., Nagin, D., Zoccolillo, M., & Vitaro, F. (2002). The development of impulsivity, fearfulness, and helpfulness during childhood: Patterns of consistency and change in the trajectories of boys and girls. *Journal of Child Psychology and Psychiatry, 43*(5), 609–618.

Crick, N., & Dodge, K. (1996). Social information-processing mechanisms in reactive and proactive aggression. *Child Development, 67*(3), 993–1002.

Davidov, M., Zahn-Waxler, C., Roth-Hanania, R., & Knafo, A. (2013). Concern for others in the first year of life: Theory, evidence, and avenues for research. *Child Development Perspective, 7*(2), 126–131.

Degnan, K. A., Calkins, S. D., Keane, S. P., & Hill-Soderlund, A. L. (2008). Profiles of disruptive behavior across early childhood: Contributions of frustration reactivity, physiological regulation, and maternal behavior. *Child Development, 79*(5), 1357–1376.

Denham, S. A. (2006). Social–emotional competence as support for school readiness: What is it and how do we assess it? *Early Education and Development, 17,* 57–89.

Denham, S. A., & Zinsser, K. M. (2014). Social and emotional learning during early childhood. In T. P. Gullotta & M. Bloom (Eds.), *Encyclopedia of primary prevention and health promotion* (2nd ed., pp 926–935). New York: Springer.

Dodge, K. A., Lansford, J. E., Burks, V. S., Bates, J. E., Pettit, G. S., Fontaine, R., et al. (2003). Peer rejection and social information-processing factors in the development of aggressive behavior problems in children. *Child Development, 74*(2), 374–393.

Durlak, J., Weissberg, R., Dymnicki, A., Taylor, R., & Schellinger, K. (2011). The impact of enhancing students' social and emotional learning: A meta-analysis of school-based universal interventions. *Child Development, 82,* 405–432.

Egger, H. L., & Angold, A. (2006). Common emotional and behavioral disorders in preschool children: Presentation, nosology, and epidemiology. *Journal of Child Psychology and Psychiatry, 47*(3), 313–337.

Eisenberg, N. (2000). Empathy and sympathy. In M. Lewis & J. M. Haviland-Jones (Eds.), *Handbook of emotions* (2nd ed., pp. 677–691). New York: Guilford Press.

Eisenberg, N., Fabes, R. A., Murphy, B. C., Shepard, S., Guthrie, I. K., Mazsk, P., et al. (1999). Prediction of elementary school children's socially appropriate and problem behavior from anger reactions at age 4–6 years. *Journal of Applied Developmental Psychology, 20,* 119–142.

Eisenberg, N., Spinrad, T. L., & Eggum, N. D. (2010). Emotion-related self-regulation and its relation to children's maladjustment. *Annual Review of Clinical Psychology, 6,* 495–525.

Eisenberg, N., Spinrad, T. L., & Morris, A. (2014). Empathy-related responding in children. In M. Killen & J. Smetana (Eds.), *Handbook of moral development* (2nd ed., pp. 184–207). New York: Psychology Press.

Eisenberg, N., Valiente, C., Spinrad, T. L., Liew, J., Zhou, Q., Lasoya, S. H., et al. (2009). Longitudinal relations of children's effortful control, impulsivity, and negative emotionality to their externalizing, internalizing, and co-occurring behavior problems. *Developmental Psychology, 45*(4), 988–1008.

Eisner, M. P., & Malti, T. (2015). Aggressive and violent behavior. In M. E. Lamb (Ed.), *Handbook of child psychology and developmental science: Vol. 3. Socioemotional processes* (7th ed., pp. 794–841). Hoboken, NJ: Wiley.

Gill, K. L., & Calkins, S. D. (2003). Do aggressive/destructive toddlers lack concern for others?: Behavioral and physiological indicators of empathic responding in 2-year-old children. *Development and Psychopathology, 15,* 55–71.

Hastings, P. D., Zahn-Waxler, C., Robinson, J., Usher, B., & Bridges, D. (2000). The development of concern for others in children with behavior problems. *Developmental Psychology, 36*(5), 531–546.

Hawley, P. H., & Vaughn, B. E. (2003). Aggression and adaptation: The bright side to bad behavior: Introduction to special volume. *Merrill–Palmer Quarterly, 49*(3), 239–244.

Herts, K. L., McLaughlin, K. A., & Hatzenbuehler, M. L. (2012). Emotion dysregulation as a mechanism linking stress exposure to adolescent aggressive behavior. *Journal of Abnormal Child Psychology, 40*(7), 1111–1122.

Hill, A. L., Degnan, K. A., Calkins, S. D., & Keane, S. P. (2006). Profiles of externalizing behavior problems for boys and girls across preschool: The roles of emotion regulation and inattention. *Developmental Psychology, 42*(5), 913–928.

Hubbard, J. A., McAuliffe, M. D., Morrow, M. T., & Romano, L. J. (2010). Reactive and proactive aggression in childhood and adolescence: Precursors, outcomes, processes, experiences, and measurement. *Journal of Personality, 78,* 95–118.

Hubbard, J. A., Smithmyer, C. M., Ramsden, S. R., Parker, E. H., Flanagan, K. D., Dearing, K. F., et al. (2002). Observational, physiological, and self–report measures of children's anger: Relations to reactive versus proactive aggression. *Child Development, 73*(4), 1101–1118.

Hyde, L. W. (2015). Developmental psychopathology in an era of molecular genetics and neuroimaging: A developmental neurogenetics approach. *Developmental Psychopathology, 27*(2), 587–613.

Jolliffe, D., & Farrington, D. P. (2006). Examining the relationship between low empathy and bullying. *Aggressive Behavior, 32*(6), 540–550.

Kochanska, G., Barry, R. A., Aksan, N., & Boldt, L. J. (2008). A developmental model of maternal and child contributions to disruptive conduct: The first six years. *Journal of Child Psychology and Psychiatry, 49*(11), 1220–1227.

Kochanska, G., Barry, R. A., Jimenez, N. B., Hollatz, A. L., & Woodard, J. (2009). Guilt and effortful control: Two mechanisms that prevent disruptive developmental trajectories. *Journal of Personality and Social Psychology, 97*(2), 322–333.

Kurzban, R., DeScioli, P., & O'Brien, E. (2007). Audience effects on moralistic punishment. *Evolution and Human Behavior, 28,* 75–84.

Lazarus, R. S. (1991). Progress on a cognitive–motivational–relational theory of emotion. *American Psychologist, 46*(8), 819–834.

Lochman, J. E., Barry, T., Powell, N., & Young, L. (2010) Anger and aggression. In D. Nangle, D. Hansen, C. Erdley, & P. Norton (Eds.), *Practitioner's guide to empirically based measures of social skills* (pp. 155–166). New York: Springer.

Lovett, B. J., & Sheffield, R. A. (2007). Affective empathy deficits in aggressive children and adolescents: A critical review. *Clinical Psychology Review, 27,* 1–13.

Luby, J., Belden, A., Sullivan, J., Hayen, R., McCadney, A., & Spitznagel, E. (2009). Shame and guilt in preschool depression: Evidence for elevations in self-conscious emotions in depression as early as age 3. *Journal of Child Psychology and Psychiatry, 50*(9), 1156–1166.

Malti, T. (2016). Toward an integrated clinical-developmental model of guilt. *Developmental Review, 39,* 16–36.

Malti, T., Chaparro, M. P., Zuffianò, A., & Colasante, T. (2016). School-based interventions to promote empathy-related responding in children and adolescents: A developmental analysis. *Journal of Clinical Child and Adolescent Psychology, 45*(6), 718–731.

Malti, T., & Dys, S. P. (2017). From being nice to being kind: Development of prosocial behaviors. *Current Opinion in Psychology, 5*(20), 45–49.

Malti, T., Eisenberg, N., Kim, H., & Buchmann, M. (2013). Developmental trajectories of sympathy, moral emotion attributions, and moral reasoning: The role of parental support. *Social Development, 22*(4), 773–793.

Malti, T., Gummerum, M., Keller, M., & Buchmann, M. (2009). Children's moral motivation, sympathy, and prosocial behavior. *Child Development, 80*(2), 442–460.

Malti, T., & Krettenauer, T. (2013). The relation of moral emotion attributions to prosocial and antisocial behavior: A meta-analysis. *Child Development, 84*(2), 397–412.

Malti, T., & Noam, G. G. (2016). Social–emotional development: From theory to practice. *European Journal of Developmental Psychology, 13*(6), 652–665.

Malti, T., & Ongley, S. F. (2014). The development of moral emotions and moral reasoning. In M. Killen & J. Smetana (Eds.), *Handbook of moral development* (2nd ed., pp. 163–183). New York: Psychology Press.

Malti, T., Sette, S., & Dys, S. P. (2016). Social–emotional responding: A perspective from developmental psychology. Retrieved from *http://onlinelibrary.wiley.com/doi/10.1002/9781118900772.etrds0415/abstract.*

McLaughlin, K. A., Hatzenbuehler, M. L., Mennin, D. S., & Nolen-Hoeksema, S. (2011). Emotion dysregulation and adolescent psychopathology: A prospective study. *Behaviour Research and Therapy, 49*(9), 544–554.

Miller, D. T. (2001). Disrespect and the experience of injustice. *Annual Review of Psychology, 52*, 527–553.

Moffitt, T. E., Caspi, A., & Rutter, M. (2005). Strategy for investigating interactions between measured genes and measured environments. *Archives of General Psychiatry, 62*(5), 473–481.

Murphy, B. C., Eisenberg, N., Fabes, R. A., Shepard, S., & Guthrie, I. K. (1999). Consistency and change in children's emotionality and regulation: A longitudinal study. *Merrill-Palmer Quarterly, 45*(3), 413–444.

Olson, S. L., Lopez-Duran, N., Lunkenheimer, E. S., Chang, H., & Sameroff, A. J. (2011). Individual differences in the development of early peer aggression: Integrating contributions of self-regulation, theory of mind, and parenting. *Development and Psychopathology, 23*, 253–266.

Ongley, S. F., & Malti, T. (2014). The role of moral emotions in the development of children's sharing behavior. *Developmental Psychology, 50*(4), 1148–1159.

Orobio de Castro, B., Merk, W., Koops, W., Veerman, J. W., & Bosch, J. D. (2005). Emotions in social information processing and their relations with reactive and proactive aggression in referred aggressive boys. *Journal of Clinical Child and Adolescent Psychology, 34*, 105–116.

Orobio de Castro, B., Veerman, J. W., Koops, W., Bosch, J. D., & Monshouwer, H. J. (2002). Hostile attribution of intent and aggressive behavior: A meta-analysis. *Child Development, 73*(3), 916–934.

Peplak, J., & Malti, T. (2016) "That really hurt, Charlie!": Investigating the role of sympathy and moral respect in children's aggressive behavior. *Journal of Genetic Psychology, 178*(2), 89–101.

Portnoy, J., & Farrington, D. P. (2015) Resting heart rate and antisocial behaviour: An updated systematic review and meta-analysis. *Aggression and Violent Behavior, 22*, 33–45.

Posner, M., & Rothbart, M. (2000). Developing mechanisms of self-regulation. *Development and Psychopathology, 12*(3), 427–441.

Raine, A., Dodge, K., Loeber, R., Gatzke-Kopp, L., Lynam, D., Reynolds, C., et al. (2006). The reactive–proactive aggression questionnaire: Differential correlates of reactive and proactive aggression in adolescent boys. *Aggressive Behavior, 32*(2), 159–171.

Rose-Krasnor, L. (1997). The nature of social competence: A theoretical review. *Social Development, 6*, 111–135.

Rose-Krasnor, L., & Denham, S. (2009). Social–emotional competence in early childhood. In K. H. Rubin, W. M. Bukowski, & B. Laursen (Eds.), *Handbook of peer interactions, relationships, and groups* (pp. 162–179). New York: Guilford Press.

Rubin, K. H., Bukowski, W. M., & Laursen, B. (Eds.). (2009). *Handbook of peer interactions, relationships, and groups.* New York: Guilford Press.

Rydell, A., Berlin, L., & Bohlin, G. (2003). Emotionality, emotion regulation, and adaptation among 5- to 8-year-old children. *Emotion, 3,* 30–47.

Saarni, C. (1999). *The development of emotional competence.* New York: Guilford Press.

Schultz, D., Izard, C. E., & Bear, G. (2004). Children's emotion processing: Relations to emotionality and aggression. *Development and Psychopathology, 16*(2), 371–387.

Smithmyer, C. M., Hubbard, J. A., & Simons, R. F. (2000). Proactive and reactive aggression in delinquent adolescents: Relations to aggression outcome expectancies. *Journal of Clinical Child Psychology, 29,* 86–93.

Strayer, J., & Roberts, W. (2004). Empathy and observed anger and aggression in five-year-olds. *Social Development, 13,* 1–13.

Tangney, J. P., Stuewig, J., & Mashek, D. J. (2007). Moral emotions and moral behavior. *Annual Review of Psychology, 58,* 345–372.

Tangney, J. P., Wagner, P. E., Hill-Barlow, D., Marschall, D. E., & Gramzow, R. (1996). Relation of shame and guilt to constructive versus destructive responses to anger across the lifespan. *Journal of Personality and Social Psychology, 70*(4), 797–809.

Thompson, R. A. (2011). Emotion and emotion regulation: Two sides of the developing coin. *Emotion Review, 3,* 53–61.

Tracy, J., & Robins, R. (2006). Appraisal antecedents of shame and guilt: Support for a theoretical model. *Personality and Social Psychology Bulletin, 32*(1), 1339–1351.

Vaish, A., Carpenter, M., & Tomasello, M. (2009). Sympathy through affective perspective taking and its relation to prosocial behavior in toddlers. *Developmental Psychology, 45*(2), 534–543.

van Noorden, T. H. J., Haselager, G. J. T., Cillessen, A. H. N., & Bukowski, W. M. (2015). Empathy and involvement in bullying in children and adolescents: A systematic review. *Journal of Youth and Adolescence, 44*(3), 637–657.

Vitaro, F., Brendgen, M., & Barker, E. (2006). Subtypes of aggressive behaviors: A developmental perspective. *International Journal of Behavioral Development, 30,* 12–19.

Vitaro, F., Brendgen, M., & Tremblay, R. E. (2002). Reactively and proactively aggressive children: Antecedent and subsequent characteristics. *Journal of Child Psychology and Psychiatry, 43*(4), 495–505.

Vygotsky, L. S. (1978). *Mind in society: The development of higher psychological processes.* Cambridge, MA: Harvard University Press.

Zuffianò, A., Colasante, T., Buchmann, M., & Malti, T. (2017). The codevelopment of sympathy and overt aggression from middle childhood to early adolescence. *Developmental Psychology.* [Epub ahead of print]

CHAPTER 8

Social-Cognitive Development and Aggression

JENNIFER E. LANSFORD

Brief Introduction

This chapter focuses on the role of social-cognitive factors in aggression at different stages of development across childhood and adolescence. The chapter begins by outlining two main issues: how social-cognitive development unfolds over time and how social-cognitive biases develop. I then summarize the main theories that have been proposed to account for how social cognition is related to aggressive behavior. Next, I describe measures and methods that have been used to study social cognition in relation to aggression before describing central research findings from empirical studies. I then turn to implications of the findings in terms of interventions targeting social cognition as a way to reduce aggression and policies that have been shaped by knowledge of how exposure to aggressive media shapes children's social cognition and aggression. Finally, the chapter ends with a consideration of directions for future theory and research.

Main Issues

In understanding social-cognitive development and aggression, the main issues are twofold. The first set of issues involves development as a chronological sequence from infancy to adulthood, with the development of social-cognitive abilities a normative progression that either inhibits or enables aggressive behavior at different life stages. The second set of issues involves the development of biases in social cognition that can serve as risk factors for aggressive behavior.

With respect to normative development, newborns are not thought to be able to behave aggressively in the way that aggression is usually defined, which involves the intention to cause harm (DeWall, Anderson, & Bushman, 2012). Because, developmentally, newborns are not yet capable of behaving intentionally, any harm they might cause (e.g., biting while nursing, pulling a parent's hair) would not be described as aggressive by traditional standards. Indeed, parents who inappropriately attribute intentionality to their infants are at greater risk of abusing them than are parents who recognize that infants do not yet have the cognitive capacity to cause harm intentionally (Rodriguez, 2010).

Aggressive behavior characterized by the intention to cause harm emerges in the toddler years, when rates of aggressive behavior are higher than at any other point in the lifespan (Anderson & Huesmann, 2003). Children at this stage of development do not yet have the verbal capacity to express their desires or reason with others in complex ways, so they may resort to physical force to take toys they want or to express their displeasure. Physical aggression generally decreases after age 3 (Tremblay, 2000). With improvements in perspective taking and theory of mind that come during the preschool years (approximately 3–4 years), children become better able to understand that other people have thoughts and desires that are not the same as their own (Wellman, 2014), which leads to increases in empathy and a decrease in physically aggressive behavior. Physical aggression continues to decrease into middle childhood and adolescence, so that by the time adolescents reach high school, physical aggression is no longer developmentally normative as it was during early childhood. In contrast, verbal aggression increases after age 3 (Tremblay, 2000) and takes on a more hostile tone around age 7 years, with name calling and ridiculing (Coie & Dodge, 1998). Some of the same social-cognitive abilities that lead to a decrease in physical aggression may lead to an increase in relational aggression. That is, by better understanding the nature of social relationships, children become able to manipulate those relationships by exclusion, by spreading malicious rumors, or by other social means to inflict harm to relationships (Crick & Grotpeter, 1995).

With respect to the second set of issues, biases in social-cognitive development that can lead to aggression, several risk factors are important. Exposure to violence in the neighborhood, the home, or the peer group is an important risk factor for social-cognitive biases, as well as aggressive behavior (e.g., Dodge, Bates, & Pettit, 1990; Schwartz & Proctor, 2000). This exposure can be direct, in the case of witnessing crime in the neighborhood, being abused by parents, or being victimized by peers, or the exposure can come through media, such as playing violent video games or watching violent television programs (Anderson & Bushman, 2001). These risk factors alter the development of social cognition in ways that increase the likelihood that individuals will behave aggressively and expose children to opportunities to learn aggression by observing others behaving aggressively and to opportunities in which children themselves can try aggression. For example, if children are abused by their parents, children learn to expect others to act with hostile intent and that using aggression is accepted in interpersonal interactions (Dodge et al., 1990). With repeated exposure, aggression becomes easily accessible to children as a behavioral response in social situations, which increases children's propensity to aggress in the future. Understanding how early relationships set the stage for later behaviors both within that relationship and in other relationships is consistent with attachment theory (e.g., Bretherton & Munholland, 1999) and coercion theory (e.g., Snyder, Reid, & Patterson, 2003), which also describe how patterns of interaction learned in families generalize to other relationships.

It is important to consider two overarching aspects of social cognition: latent mental structures and online processing (Crick & Dodge, 1994). Latent mental structures include general knowledge and cognitive schemas that individuals bring to particular situations; these latent structures reduce individuals' online workload by providing shortcuts that reduce complexity when individuals encounter new situations. Individuals' biologically based capacities for memory, processing speed, attention, and emotionality, in conjunction with an existing database of knowledge drawn from prior experiences, affect what individuals perceive and process in new situations (Lemerise & Arsenio, 2000).

Cognitive schemas and scripts are mental representations that develop over time through repeated experiences with particular social situations that help people process future situations more efficiently. Schemas involve general categories; scripts involve a more specific set of automatic actions. Rather than approaching each new social situation as a novelty, individuals bring to a new social situation schemas and scripts that they have developed through previous social situations, generally making new situations less cognitively taxing. Normative beliefs about aggression have been described as an example of a script particularly relevant for understanding aggression (Huesmann & Guerra, 1997). That is, if a girl believes it is acceptable to hit another child to obtain a desired outcome or to retaliate for a perceived wrong, then she will be more likely to behave aggressively than if she does not hold the normative belief about the acceptability of aggression. Normative beliefs can be either situation specific (e.g., "If others hit you first, it is OK to hit them back") or general (e.g., "It is OK to hit others").

As individuals encounter social situations that require them to encode, interpret, evaluate, and act on social cues, they may engage in either controlled or automatic processing (Schneider & Chein, 2003). If an individual stops to consider different options and carefully evaluates the situation, he or she is engaging in controlled processing, whereas if the individual responds quickly without consciously processing of the situation, he or she is engaging in automatic processing. As children develop, their responding becomes more automatic because they have an increasing knowledge base of similar situations to which they have responded in the past, allowing them to respond more quickly to new situations. For aggressive children, aggressive scripts contribute to more automatic aggressive responding in new social situations.

Theoretical Considerations

Several theories describe social cognitive pathways to aggression. Guerra (2010) characterized such theories as encompassing social knowledge stored in memory, as well as specific information-processing skills that address the questions of (1)

What happened and what does this mean? (2) What do I want? (3) What are my options? and (4) What should I do? Answering these questions ultimately leads to a decision that does or does not result in aggression.

Social information-processing (SIP) theory is typically characterized as having six steps (i.e., encoding, making attributions, clarifying goals, generating responses, evaluating responses, and enacting responses) through which individuals progress as they respond to social stimuli (Crick & Dodge, 1994). First, *encoding* is the process by which individuals take in information about the situation. Individuals who behave aggressively are hypervigilant to hostile cues, inattentive to relevant nonhostile cues, or both (Dodge et al., 1990). Second, *making attributions* involves drawing conclusions about why individuals in a social situation behaved as they did. Individuals who behave aggressively are more likely to make hostile attributions for others' actions (e.g., to believe that others intended to be mean or cause something bad to happen), whereas individuals who do not behave aggressively are more likely to make benign or neutral attributions (e.g., to believe that others caused harm by accident; Dodge, Price, Bachorowski, & Newman, 1990; Orobio de Castro, Veerman, Koops, Bosch, & Monshouwer, 2002). Third, *clarifying and selecting goals* involves determining what one's desired outcome is. Individuals who behave aggressively are more likely to have goals that involve retaliation, demonstrating dominance, or obtaining some instrumental end rather than a social goal that involves maintaining harmony with others (Crick & Dodge, 1994). Fourth, *generating responses* involves coming up with possible ways to respond to a given social situation. Compared with individuals who do not behave aggressively, individuals who behave aggressively generate fewer possible responses overall and generate a larger proportion of aggressive responses (Asarnow & Callan, 1985). Fifth, *evaluating responses* is the process by which individuals weigh the costs and benefits of behaving in particular ways. Individuals who behave aggressively are likely to deem aggressive responses to be easier to enact; more likely to be effective; more likely to be approved by others; and more likely to lead to desired instrumental, interpersonal, and intrapersonal outcomes than are individuals who do not behave aggressively (Crick & Ladd, 1990; Dodge & Crick, 1990). Sixth, *enacting a response* is the behavior that ultimately results from the social-cognitive steps leading up to it. Individuals who are skilled in behaving aggressively but lack skills in enacting nonaggressive responses are more likely to act aggressively (Dodge, McClaskey, & Feldman, 1985).

Although individuals often have or lack biases across these different steps, it is possible for individuals to have biases in some but not other SIP steps (Lansford et al., 2006). For example, if individuals have deficits in the early steps of encoding and making attributions but do not have deficits in the later steps of generating and evaluating responses, they may not behave aggressively because adaptive later processing steps are able to compensate for biased early ones. Psychometric analyses support the discriminative validity of the distinct steps in the multistep SIP model (Dodge, Laird, Lochman, Zelli, & Conduct Problems Prevention Research Group, 2002); although individuals who have biases in one processing step are at increased risk for biases in others, each step also contributes unique value to understanding links between social cognition and aggression.

Lemerise and Arsenio (2000) present a theoretical model that integrates emotion with the SIP model described by Crick and Dodge (1994). In this integrative model, Lemerise and Arsenio explain how emotions can serve motivational, communicative, and regulatory functions in social encounters that are distinguishable from cognition, which involves attention, learning, memory, and logic. Emotions help individuals narrow behavioral choices to ones that lead to positive "gut feelings"; cognitive processes are more efficient when they only need to attend to this smaller pool of choices (Damasio, 1994). For each of the six SIP steps, emotion can affect social-cognitive processes and, ultimately, aggressive behavior. At the steps of encoding and making attributions about others' intentions, specific emotions, as well as overall mood and level of arousal, can influence what individuals notice in a given situation. Individuals are more likely to recall information that is congruent with their current mood, so if they enter a situation feeling angry and emotionally aroused, they will be more likely to encode environmental cues and make attributions that are consistent with feelings of anger than if they enter a situation feeling happy and content. To encode and interpret social cues in an unbiased way, individuals must take into account their own emotion cues, as well as others' emotion cues. For example, taking into account whether a peer is angry will help a child make an accurate attribution regarding the peer's intent in an ambiguous situation (Lemerise & Arsenio, 2000). Children who behave aggressively are less skilled at reading their own and others' emotional cues and have less empathy (Lemerise & Arsenio, 2000). At the goal clarification step, emotions can lead an individual to focus on a particular goal (Lemerise & Arsenio, 2000). For example, children who are feeling angry are more likely to focus on instrumental goals (e.g., getting a toy, by force if necessary), whereas children who are feeling happy more likely to focus on goals that will maintain their positive mood. Peers' affective cues can also influence children's goals, with peers' positive affect promoting affiliative goals and peers' negative affect discouraging affiliative goals (Sroufe, Schork, Motti, Lawroski, & LaFreniere, 1984). Children may choose goals that lead to avoidance if they are overwhelmed by their own or others' emotions. Goals will also be influenced by emotional ties between individuals involved in the interaction (e.g., relational goals would be facilitated if the individuals in the encounter are friends, whereas revenge goals would be more likely if the individuals in the encounter are enemies; Bowker, Rubin, Rose-Krasnor, & Booth-LaForce, 2007; Burgess, Wojslawowicz, Rubin, Rose-Krasnor, & Booth-LaForce, 2006).

At the response generation and evaluation steps, experiencing particular emotions may make it more likely that individuals will access and positively evaluate some responses rather than others. In addition, if children are experiencing strong emotions, they may be too overwhelmed to generate a large number of possible responses and carefully evaluate them from different perspectives (Lemerise & Arsenio, 2000). By contrast, children who are skilled at regulating emotions even in provocative situations may be better able to generate a variety of possible responses and evaluate them from multiple perspectives, ultimately leading to a more competent response (Saarni, 1999). An important aspect of Crick and Dodge's (1994) model involves children's evaluations of the emotional outcomes associated with different possible responses. In addition, children may be more willing to consider others' reactions to a given response if they have a close emotional connection and are motivated for others to like them (Burgess et al., 2006; Lemerise & Arsenio, 2000).

At the enactment step, if children are calm they may be better able to use their knowledge of acceptable behaviors to control their own behavior, but if children are emotionally aroused, it may be more difficult for children to put their knowledge of acceptable behavior into practice (Underwood, 1997). Furthermore, children who are good at reading emotional cues may be able to use these cues to assess whether their behavioral response has been effective and to make adjustments to future actions accordingly (Lemerise & Arsenio, 2000). Across all steps, the intensity of emotions and individuals' skill at regulating emotions are important potential moderators of the cognitive processes (Eisenberg & Fabes, 1992; Eisenberg, Fabes, Nyman, Bernzweig, & Pinuelas, 1994; Saarni, 1999).

The general aggression model (GAM; Anderson & Bushman, 2002), like SIP theory, outlines a set of cognitive mechanisms that lead to aggressive behavior. The GAM proposes that knowledge structures developed during the course of experiences in different situations affect individuals' perceptions, interpretations, decisions, and behavior in new situations. A particular situation may activate a knowledge structure that triggers affective and behavioral scripts that in turn make it more likely that an individual will behave aggressively (e.g., if anger and retaliation scripts are activated). The GAM has been applied to understanding how exposure to violent media can lead to aggression by altering cognition, affect, and arousal. Namely, individuals learn ways to aggress, come to hold attitudes and beliefs that are more accepting of aggression, are primed to perceive and expect aggression, are desensitized to aggression, and have higher levels of physiological arousal when they are exposed repeatedly to violent media (Anderson & Bushman, 2001). The association between exposure to violent media and aggressive behavior is nearly as strong as the link between smoking and lung cancer and is stronger than many other widely accepted links (e.g., condom use and reduced risk of HIV/AIDS; Bushman & Anderson, 2001). Although aggressive children are more likely to select violent media, violent media contribute above and beyond selection effects to the development of aggressive behavior through processes specified in the GAM (Bushman & Anderson, 2001).

Huesmann's (1988, 1998) theory of social cognition emphasizes three main components: cognitive schemas that serve as models of the world, cognitive scripts that guide social behavior, and normative beliefs about the appropriateness of aggression. Individuals who behave aggressively have cognitive schemas that portray the world as a hostile place, cognitive scripts stored in memory that emphasize aggressive responses, and normative beliefs that characterize aggression as acceptable. Children develop these schemas, scripts, and normative beliefs through social learning, such as observing role models behaving aggressively (Bandura, 1973, 1986).

If children repeatedly witness aggression, they habituate to it, making it a less aversive experience and making it more likely that children will retrieve aggressive scripts when it is time for them to act (Huesmann, 1998). According to Huesmann's (1988) model, children's evaluations of scripts they could enact is dependent upon three factors. First, children predict the consequences of using the script, such as whether it will lead to desired short- and long-term outcomes; focusing only on short-term outcomes is more likely to lead to aggressive behavior than is thinking about long-term consequences. Second, children evaluate their ability to carry out the script; children may behave aggressively if they have low self-efficacy for nonaggressive scripts. Third, children are more likely to internalize and act on scripts that they believe are consistent with internalized social norms.

Huesmann's (1988) model then describes four reasons that children may behave aggressively despite negative consequences. First, children may not evaluate the consequences of aggression accurately, either because they misjudge the social situation or focus only on short-term outcomes, such as obtaining an instrumental goal. Second, children may not hold any alternate scripts and so resort to aggression because it is easier to enact than more mentally and socially complex prosocial behaviors. Third, children may alter their cognitive schema to justify aggression, such as by adopting an "eye for an eye" mentality. Fourth, children may select into environments in which aggression is accepted, such as by choosing aggressive peers with whom to affiliate.

The mechanisms proposed in these theoretical models account for links between social cognition and aggression during adulthood as well as childhood. In addition, these models have sometimes been tailored to apply to particular situations. For example, to explain parents' potential for physical child abuse, Milner (1993, 2003) proposed a four-step model of parents' SIP that shares many features with the Crick and Dodge (1994) model of children's SIP. The four steps in Milner's model involve perceiving social behavior, interpreting and evaluating social behavior, integrating information and selecting a response, and finally implementing the response. Likewise, to explain why parents aggress toward their children, Azar (1986) proposed a multifactorial model that includes both intrapersonal and contextual risk factors. Making negative attributions and holding developmentally inappropriate expectations about children's behaviors constitute primary intrapersonal risk factors in the model (Azar, 1986).

Traditional theoretical formulations have focused on social cognition in relation to physical aggression, but a different set of social-cognitive processes may be related to the development of indirect, social, or relational aggression. For example, relationally aggressive children have been found to make more hostile attributions and feel more distressed in relational provocation situations than nonaggressive children (Crick, 1995).

Measures and Methods

Measures of social cognition often include hypothetical vignettes presented either in videos, on storyboards, or orally (e.g., Dodge et al., 2002). Generally, the vignette depicts a provocation (e.g., milk being spilled on a child) or social exclusion (e.g., a child being ignored upon trying to enter a peer group) that has ambiguous intent. After viewing or listening to the vignette, the child is asked a series of questions to assess social-cognitive processing of the vignette. For example, the child would be asked to recount what happened (to assess encoding of the presented information), why the negative event happened (to assess hostile attribution biases), what his or her goal would be in that situation, what he or she would do in that situation (to assess response generation), and whether he or she believes a series of different aggressive and nonaggressive responses would be effective and viewed favorably (to assess response evaluation).

Several questionnaire measures have been used to assess other aspects of social cognition. For example, cognitive schemas have been measured by the Young Schema Questionnaire, which has items capturing a number of maladaptive schemas such as emotional deprivation, abandonment, mistrust/abuse, and failure (Young, 1994). The Normative Beliefs about Aggression scale asks individuals to rate whether physical and verbal aggression is acceptable in general and in a range of specific situations (Huesmann & Guerra, 1997).

In addition, a number of open-ended tasks have been used to tap into social-cognitive processes. For example, sentence completion tasks in which individuals are provided with a sentence stem and asked to complete the sentence (e.g., "When I am the last one to sit down at a lunch table with other kids, they usually _____") are sometimes used to assess cognitive schemas about particular situations or individuals (Burks, Laird, Dodge, Pettit, & Bates, 1999). Word association tasks in which individuals are provided with a word such as *school, best friend,* or *parents* and asked to say the first thing that comes to mind in connection with that word have been coded for aggressive and nonaggressive associations (Bushman, 1998). Sometimes measures of psychophysiology such as blood pressure, heart rate reactivity, and skin conductance are administered in conjunction with vignette- or task-based measures to be able to assess physiological arousal in potentially provocative situations (e.g., Crozier et al., 2008).

Central Research Findings

A wide range of risk factors, including childhood adversities such as exposure to community violence, interparental conflict, poverty, harsh and inconsistent parenting, and affiliation with deviant peers, to name a few, predict the development of aggression (e.g., Dishion, Spracklen, Andrews, & Patterson, 1996; Gershoff & Grogan-Kaylor, 2016; Guerra, Huesmann, & Spindler, 2003). However, these risk factors do not just have direct effects on the development of aggression; rather, they operate indirectly by increasing social-cognitive biases and deficits that then lead to aggressive behavior. It is social-cognitive functioning that predicts whether an individual will behave aggressively in the moment.

A large body of research demonstrates that particular patterns of social cognition are related to the development of aggressive behavior, but the ways in which social cognition and aggressive behavior are related may change somewhat over the course of development. For example, children's self-efficacy beliefs related to aggression become more strongly related to aggressive behavior in adolescence than they were during early childhood (Davis-Kean et al., 2008). Other studies also have found that beliefs become better predictors of future behavior after approximately age 8 (Huesmann & Guerra, 1997; Parsons & Ruble, 1977; Spencer & Bornholt, 2003). For example, although exposure to community violence predicted aggressive behavior for 5- to 8- and 9- to 12-year-olds, this association was mediated by social cognition only for the 9- to 12-year-olds (Guerra et al., 2003). A developmental shift occurs in the relation between beliefs and behaviors such that early in elementary school, children's aggressive behaviors predict their beliefs about the appropriateness of aggression, whereas in later elementary school, children's beliefs about the appropriateness of aggression predict their aggressive behaviors (Huesmann & Guerra, 1997). These changes over time may be related to cognitive developments that occur during the age "5- to 7-year shift" (Sameroff & Haith, 1986; White, 1965).

Social cognition and aggression continue to develop through adolescence and into adulthood, and links between social cognition and aggression may continue to change over time. For example, response evaluation and decision steps of the SIP model are more strongly related to aggression during adolescence than childhood (Fontaine, Yang, Dodge, Pettit, & Bates, 2009). Adults' SIP in relation to peers mediated the links between harsh parenting and peer rejection during childhood and aggression toward peers in adulthood (Pettit, Lansford, Malone, Dodge, & Bates, 2010). Empirical research also has examined different aspects of parents' social-cognitive biases. For example, parents who have an external locus of control and believe that their child is responsible for parent–child interactions are more likely to abuse their child and respond with a harsh and angry disciplinary style (Rodriguez, 2010). The most frequently studied aspect of parents' social cognition in relation to aggression toward children is mothers' hostile attributions (e.g., Mac-Brayer, Milich, & Hundley, 2003; Nix et al., 1999).

Researchers have investigated both how social-cognitive biases develop and how such biases come to shape aggressive behavior. One of the key factors of understanding social-cognitive development in relation to aggression is that the development of social-cognitive biases in response to environmental stressors often provides a mediating link between these environmental stressors and aggressive behavior. Parents' physical abuse and peers' rejection are two environmental stressors that have been particularly well studied both in relation to social-cognitive biases and children's aggressive behavior. Indeed, harsh parenting in the first 5 years of life predicts social-cognitive biases and deficits into adulthood (Pettit et al., 2010). When children are physically abused by parents, it can be adaptive in the short term for abused children to become hypervigilant to environmental cues signaling threat (Dodge et al., 1990). However, when abused children generalize this hypervigilance to the peer group, they are likely to perceive threat where none exists and to respond in ways that are maladaptive in the long term in the peer group.

If children are rejected by their peers, this may contribute to deficits in social information processing, both because of the negative experience of rejection and because rejection deprives children of opportunities to interact with peers in ways that would promote socially competent processing of social information (Dodge et al., 2003). That is, children who are rejected by peers have fewer social interactions in which they can learn to attend to relevant cues and to respond prosocially and have more interactions that would foster their belief that peers' intentions are hostile (Trachtenberg & Viken, 1994). Errors in encoding relevant social cues, making hostile attributions in ambiguous or benign situations, and generating fewer and more hostile possible responses in hypothetical social situations have all been associated with peer rejection (e.g., Dodge et al., 2003; Waldman, 1996).

Many mechanisms that have been proposed for the development of aggressive behavior hinge on social-cognitive processes. Deviancy training is the process by which peers reinforce one another's antisocial beliefs and behaviors in a cycle that leads to the dispersion and escalation of antisocial behavior (Dishion et al., 1996). For example, if an adolescent's peers laugh in response to a story about the adolescent's misbehavior or join in with stories about their own misbehaviors, problem behavior is positively reinforced within the group. In such a peer group, norms about the desirability of antisocial behavior are perpetuated, and the members come to define themselves in terms of their deviancy. When social institutions such as schools and the juvenile justice system also categorize individuals into "deviant" groups (e.g., by placing them in alternative schools or the juvenile justice system), this can further solidify adolescents' identity in reference to their problem behaviors and lead to self-fulfilling prophecies (Johnson, Simons, & Conger, 2004).

Different cognitive schemas have been found to be associated with different aspects of SIP, and SIP, in turn, has been found to mediate the relation between cognitive schemas and aggressive behavior. For example, in a longitudinal study of adolescents, cognitive schemas involving justification of violence, mistrust, and narcissism longitudinally predicted SIP, and SIP predicted reactive aggression. In particular, justification of violence predicted aggressive response access, narcissism predicted anger and aggressive response access, and mistrust predicted more hostile attributions and less anger (Calvete & Orue, 2012).

Differences in social-cognitive processes may also predict aggressive behaviors with different functions (Dodge & Coie, 1987). Reactive aggression, which is characterized as an angry, retaliatory response to provocation, has been found experimentally to be predicted when inappropriate hostile attributions are made in the face of ambiguous or benign social stimuli (Dodge & Coie, 1987). Proactive aggression, in contrast, is characterized as an instrumental behavior that seeks to obtain some desired outcome and is associated with evaluating aggression positively (Smithmyer, Hubbard, & Simons, 2000) and holding instrumental (e.g., obtaining a toy) rather than relational (e.g., becoming friends) goals in social interactions (Crick & Dodge, 1996).

Empirical studies of links between social cognition and aggression, gender, culture, and individual differences have received attention both in terms of whether these factors contribute to mean differences in social cognition, aggression, or both and in terms of whether these factors moderate associations between social cognition and aggression.

Gender

Although mean-level differences between males and females in aggressive behavior are well documented for direct aggression, particularly physical aggression (Archer, 2004), findings regarding mean differences in indirect aggression are more mixed, with meta-analyses generally suggesting no consistent gender differences (Card, Stucky, Sawalani, & Little, 2008). Mean-level differences between males' and females' social-cognitive biases have been reported in some situations. For example, males may be more likely than females to misinterpret peers' intentions in conflictual situations because such situations may be more likely to trigger scripts and schemas that males develop in competitive contexts with peers (especially those involving physical confrontations; Ruble, Martin, & Berenbaum, 2006). Likewise, females may be more likely than males to misinterpret romantic partners' intentions because of insecurity about relationships and jealousy that have developed in emotionally intense friendships (Connolly, Craig, Goldberg, & Pepler, 2004). In addition, males are more likely than females to fantasize about violence and to believe that aggression is acceptable in certain situations (Guerra et al., 2003). Regardless of gender differences or similarities in mean levels of aggressive behavior or social-cognitive biases, though, links between social-cognitive variables and aggressive behavior are generally consistent for males and females (e.g., Guerra et al., 2003). However, in some studies, the link between beliefs about the acceptability of aggression and aggressive behavior has been found to be stronger for boys than girls (Huesmann & Guerra, 1997), perhaps because the measures focused on direct aggression, which is more commonly used by boys than girls. Nevertheless, for both males and females, more social-cognitive biases are related to more aggressive behavior.

Culture

At the community level, children who live in dangerous neighborhoods or societies that value and endorse violence are more likely to behave aggressively (Skinner et al., 2014). According to the cultural spillover theory of violence, if people live in a society that condones violence for legitimate purposes, such as in childrearing or in punishing criminals, violence in one domain tends to generalize, or spill over, into other domains, so that people are more likely to use aggression either for socially legitimate or criminal purposes (Baron & Straus, 1989). For example, cultures of violence have been found to be characterized by co-occurring war, homicide, assault, combative sports, and severe punishment of criminals (Ember & Ember, 1994). Corporal punishment of children has been found to be part of a broader culture of violence (Ember & Ember, 2005). Individuals living within cultures of violence may adopt norms regarding the acceptability of aggression and may model aggression they witness, following social learning mechanisms. Cognitions that normalize violence may mediate the association between exposure to violence and aggressive behavior (Ng-Mak, Salzinger, Feldman, & Stueve, 2002).

Nisbett and Cohen (1996) have described a "culture of honor" akin to a culture of violence. When an experimental confederate provoked male college students, males from the southern United States were more than twice as likely to experience anger, almost twice as likely to generate an aggressive response to a provocative hypothetical vignette, and more likely to attribute hostile intent to a provocateur than were males from the northern United States. Males in the southern United States, compared with males in the northern United States, were more likely to interpret interpersonal slights as threats to their honor and to react aggressively when so provoked. According to Nisbett and Cohen, these regional differences can be attributed to a "culture of honor" in the southern United States that emphasizes respect and heightened motivation to maintain one's honor. Thus community-level norms and values become internalized in a way that can increase risk for aggressive behavior, which is consistent with higher levels of violence in the southern than northern United States.

Despite cultural differences in some groups being more attuned to perceived slights than others, processes linking social-cognitive biases and aggression show cultural similarities. In a study of children in nine countries (China, Colombia, Italy, Jordan, Kenya, Philippines, Sweden, Thailand, and the United States), country differences in children's hostile attributions accounted for a significant portion of country differences in aggressive behavior problems (Dodge et al., 2015). Children were presented with 10 hypothetical vignettes depicting an ambiguous situation and asked to attribute the likely intent of the provocateur (coded as benign or hostile) and to predict how they would respond in that situation (coded as nonaggression or reactive aggression). Mothers and children independently rated the child's aggressive behavior. In every cultural group, in those situations in which a child attributed hostile intent to a peer, that child was more likely to report that he or she would respond with reactive aggression than in situations when that same child attributed benign intent. Across children, hostile attributional bias scores predicted higher mother- and child-rated aggressive behavior problems, even controlling for prior aggression. Cultural-group differences in the tendency for children to attribute hostile intent statistically accounted for a significant portion of group differences in aggressive behavior problems, suggesting a psychological mechanism for group differences in aggressive behavior.

Individual Differences

Several types of individual differences might affect the relation between social cognition and aggression. For example, impulsivity has been found to moderate the association between adolescents' positive endorsement of aggressive responses in vignettes depicting hypothetical, ambiguous social situations and subsequent aggressive behavior in such a way that the association is not significant for adolescents low in impulsivity but is significant for adolescents who are moderately or highly impulsive (Fite, Goodnight, Bates, Dodge, & Pettit, 2008). Impulsive individuals may immediately act on responses they initially evaluate as positive, whereas nonimpulsive individuals may pause to reflect more on long-term consequences and integrate other information before acting on responses they initially perceive as being positive (Fite et al., 2008).

Individual differences in emotional responsivity and emotion regulation may also moderate the link between social cognition and aggression. For example, children who are emotionally labile and have difficulty regulating their emotions may have a harder time suppressing aggressive responses in the face of provocation, and the link between social-cognitive biases and aggressive behavior may be more pronounced than in children who are better at controlling their emotions (Eisenberg et al., 1994). High emotionality is not related to more behavior problems unless it is coupled with poor regulation skills (Eisenberg et al., 1996; Rubin, Coplan, Fox, & Calkins, 1995). Individuals with callous–unemotional traits, characterized by lack of empathy and use of others for personal gain, are at higher risk for aggressive behavior (Frick & White, 2008), likely in part because their social-cognitive processes are less likely to evaluate responses with respect to their impact on others. In addition, individuals who are moderately aggressive may be more susceptible to deviant peer influences that would lead to greater aggression, whereas nonaggressive individuals may have enough protective factors or disinclination to aggress to avoid such peer influences, and highly aggressive individuals may already be far enough along on an aggressive path that additional peer influence has relatively little sway (Dodge, Dishion, & Lansford, 2006).

Implications

Clearly, to prevent aggressive behavior, the best option would be to prevent children's exposure to community violence, harsh parenting, peer rejection, and other environmental risks that directly predict aggression. However, when primary prevention is not possible, social cognition provides an intermediate intervention point. In longitudinal studies of social cognition and aggression, aggression has been found to be more stable over time than is social cognition (Lansford, Malone, Dodge, Pettit, & Bates, 2010). Without intervention, aggression has been estimated to be as stable over time as intelligence. In a review of 16 early longitudinal studies, the stability correlation for aggression was .69 over a 5-year period and .60 over a 10-year period (Olweus, 1979). Likewise, in a 22-year longitudinal study, the most aggressive 8-year-olds in the sample continued to be the most aggressive 30-year-olds, with a stability of .50 for boys and .35 for girls over this 22-year period (Huesmann, Eron, Lefkowitz, & Walder, 1984). Because social cognition is less stable than aggression (especially during the early school years) and because of the well-documented links between social cognition and aggression, social cognition provides an important intervention target.

Classroom interventions such as the Promoting Alternative Thinking Strategies (PATHS) curriculum and the Second Step program target social-cognitive and social–emotional skills as mechanisms through which to decrease aggression and promote prosocial behavior. In rigorous evaluations, PATHS has been demonstrated to be effective as a universal prevention program that decreases aggression by promoting self-control, emotional understanding, positive self-esteem, relationships, and interpersonal problem-solving skills (e.g., Greenberg, Kusche, Cook, & Quamma, 1995). PATHS is a social–emotional learning curriculum delivered in elementary school classrooms. Compared with control groups who have not participated in PATHS, children randomized to classrooms delivering the PATHS program have been found to be better at recognizing others' feelings, resolving peer conflicts, and demonstrating social competence and to have fewer externalizing and internalizing behavior problems (Greenberg et al., 1995).

Like PATHS, Second Step is delivered as a classroom-based program in elementary or middle schools. Children complete activities designed to help them recognize and manage emotions, communicate clearly, make responsible decisions, and solve problems effectively. In randomized controlled trials, compared with children in control schools that did not participate in Second Step, children in intervention schools have been shown to have better social–emotional competence (Low, Cook, Smolkowski, & Buntain-Ricklefs, 2015) and to engage in less physical aggression (Espelage, Low, Polanin, & Brown, 2013).

A program specifically targeting relationally aggressive girls is the Preventing Relational Aggression in Schools Everyday (PRAISE) Program, which involves 20 sessions that are co-led by classroom teachers and therapists (Leff et al., 2010). The intervention has been found to be effective for girls but not boys in improving SIP and anger management techniques, as well as lowering levels of relational aggression.

In addition to contributing to interventions designed to reduce social-cognitive biases and aggressive behaviors, theory and research on social-cognitive development and aggression have been used to inform policies such as restrictions on sales of violent video games to minors and requiring warning labels on packaging to notify parents of violent content; for example, such laws were passed by the California State Legislature in 2005 (AB 1179; *http://leginfo.legislature.ca.gov/faces/billNavClient.xhtml?bill_id=200520060AB1179*). The video game industry, under the auspices of the Entertainment Merchants Association, challenged the law in *Brown v. Entertainment Merchants Association,* a case that ultimately went to the Supreme Court. In an amicus brief in support of the California law, resolutions by the American Psychological Association and American Academy of Pediatrics were cited regarding the strength of research evidence supporting links between exposure to violent media and aggressive behavior (see Sacks, Bushman, & Anderson, 2011). Ultimately, the Supreme Court ruled the California law a violation of First Amendment rights to free speech, but the case remains an example of how high-quality research should be used to attempt to drive evidence-based policies.

Future Directions

One direction for future research is to understand whether and how social-cognitive processes may account for intergenerational continuity in aggressive behavior. Parents' social-cognitive biases have been found to predict the use of corporal punishment (Lansford et al., 2014), and parents' use of corporal punishment predicts children's future social-cognitive biases (Weiss, Dodge, Bates, & Pettit, 1992) and children's aggressive behavior (Gershoff & Grogan-Kaylor, 2016). Future research could elucidate this full developmental cascade model. An additional direction for future research is to advance understanding of resilience from a social-cognitive standpoint. For example, although exposure to environmental risks such as neighborhood violence, child abuse, and peer rejection is associated with social-cognitive biases and aggressive behaviors on average, not all individuals exposed to these environmental risks develop social-cognitive biases or aggressive behavior (Masten, 2014). A better understanding of protective factors involved in resilience has the potential to contribute to future interventions.

Burgeoning research in neuroscience has begun to elucidate neural mechanisms underlying both social cognition and aggressive behavior. For example, neuroimaging studies have shown that the medial frontal cortex, which includes brain regions responsible for monitoring outcomes that are associated with rewards and punishments and are also involved in making inferences about others' thoughts, is important to social-cognitive processes (Amodio & Frith, 2006). Advances in neuroscience also have facilitated understanding of how infants' and young children's brains develop in ways that promote social cognition (Grossmann, 2015). Neuroscience remains an area ripe for further research on links between social-cognitive development and aggression.

Although theory and research on links between social-cognitive development and aggression are well established, theory and research on links between social-cognitive development and prosocial behaviors are less well characterized. An important future direction will be expanding social-cognitive theories to encompass aspects of knowledge structures and processing that not only do not promote aggression but that also promote prosocial behavior. Likewise, empirical research could move toward understanding unique social-cognitive mechanisms that might be involved in prosocial development.

Conclusion

Theoretical models of how social-cognitive development is related to aggressive behavior are well specified, both in terms of development at different points in the lifespan and in terms of how specific biases in cognitive schemas, scripts, and SIP are expected to relate to aggressive behavior. The tenets of the major social-cognitive theories have received considerable empirical support from studies employing a range of methods, including responses to hypothetical, provocative vignettes and task-based measures. Consistent with hypotheses generated from the theories, rigorous interventions that have attempted to reduce aggressive behavior by altering social cognition have shown promise with children and adolescents.

REFERENCES

Amodio, D. M., & Frith, C. D. (2006). Meeting of minds: The medial frontal cortex and social cognition. *Nature Reviews Neuroscience, 7,* 268–277.

Anderson, C. A., & Bushman, B. J. (2001). Effects of violent video games on aggressive behavior, aggressive cognition, aggressive affect, physiological arousal, and prosocial behavior: A meta-analytic review of the scientific literature. *Psychological Science, 12,* 353–359.

Anderson, C. A., & Bushman, B. J. (2002). Human aggression. *Annual Review of Psychology, 53,* 27–51.

Anderson, C. A., & Huesmann, L. R. (2003). Human aggression: A social-cognitive view. In M. A. Hogg & J. Cooper (Eds.), *SAGE handbook of social psychology* (pp. 296–323). Thousand Oaks, CA: SAGE.

Archer, J. (2004). Sex differences in aggression in real-world settings: A meta-analytic review. *Review of General Psychology, 8,* 291–322.

Asarnow, J. R., & Callan, J. W. (1985). Boys with peer adjustment problems: Social cognitive processes. *Journal of Consulting and Clinical Psychology, 53,* 80–87.

Azar, S. T. (1986). A framework for understanding child maltreatment: An integration of cognitive behavioral and developmental perspectives. *Canadian Journal of Behavioural Science, 18,* 340–355.

Bandura, A. (1973). *Aggression: A social learning analysis.* New York: Holt.

Bandura, A. (1986). *Social foundations of thought and action: A social-cognitive theory.* Englewood Cliffs, NJ: Prentice Hall.

Baron, L., & Straus, M. A. (1989). *Four theories of rape in American society: A state-level analysis.* New Haven, CT: Yale University Press.

Bowker, J. C., Rubin, K. H., Rose-Krasnor, L., & Booth-LaForce, C. L. (2007). Good friendships, bad friends: Friendship factors as moderators of the relation between aggression and social information processing. *European Journal of Developmental Psychology, 4,* 415–434.

Bretherton, I., & Munholland, K. A. (1999). Internal working models in attachment relationships: A construct revisited. In J. Cassidy & P. R. Shaver (Eds.), *Handbook of attachment: Theory, research, and clinical applications* (pp. 89–111). New York: Guilford Press.

Burgess, K. B., Wojslawowicz, J. C., Rubin, K. H., Rose-Krasnor, L., & Booth-LaForce, C. (2006). Social information processing and coping styles of shy/withdrawn and aggressive children: Does friendship matter? *Child Development, 77,* 371–383.

Burks, V. S., Laird, R. D., Dodge, K. A., Pettit, G. S., & Bates, J. E. (1999). Knowledge structures, social information processing, and children's aggressive behavior. *Social Development, 8,* 220–235.

Bushman, B. J. (1998). Priming effects of media violence on the accessibility of aggressive constructs in memory. *Personality and Social Psychology Bulletin, 24,* 537–545.

Bushman, B. J., & Anderson, C. A. (2001). Media violence and the American public: Scientific facts versus media misinformation. *American Psychologist, 56,* 477–489.

Calvete, E., & Orue, I. (2012). Social information processing as a mediator between cognitive schemas and aggressive behavior in adolescents. *Journal of Abnormal Child Psychology, 40,* 105–117.

Card, N. A., Stucky, B. D., Sawalani, G. M., & Little, T. D. (2008). Direct and indirect aggression during childhood and adolescence: A meta-analytic review of gender differences, intercorrelations, and relations to maladjustment. *Child Development, 79,* 1185–1229.

Coie, J. D., & Dodge, K. A. (1998). Aggression and antisocial behavior. In W. Damon & N. Eisenberg (Eds.), *Handbook of child psychology: Vol. 3. Social, emotional, and personality development* (pp. 779–862). New York: Wiley.

Connolly, J., Craig, W., Goldberg, A., & Pepler, D. (2004). Mixed-gender groups, dating, and romantic relationships in early adolescence. *Journal of Research on Adolescence, 14,* 185–207.

Crick, N. R. (1995). Relational aggression: The role of intent attributions, feelings of distress, and provocation type. *Development and Psychopathology, 7,* 313–322.

Crick, N. R., & Dodge, K. A. (1994). A review and reformulation of social information-processing mechanisms in children's social adjustment. *Psychological Bulletin, 115,* 74–101.

Crick, N. R., & Dodge, K. A. (1996). Social information-processing mechanisms in reactive and proactive aggression. *Child Development, 67,* 993–1002.

Crick, N. R., & Grotpeter, J. K. (1995). Relational aggression, gender, and social-psychological adjustment. *Child Development, 66,* 710–722.

Crick, N. R., & Ladd, G. W. (1990). Children's perceptions of the outcomes of aggressive strategies: Do the ends justify being mean? *Developmental Psychology, 26,* 612–620.

Crozier, J. C., Dodge, K. A., Fontaine, R. G., Lansford, J. E., Bates, J. E., Pettit, G. S., et al. (2008). Social information processing and cardiac predictors of adolescent antisocial behavior. *Journal of Abnormal Psychology, 117,* 253–267.

Damasio, A. R. (1994). *Descartes' error: Emotion, reason, and the human brain.* New York: Avon Books.

Davis-Kean, P. E., Huesmann, L. R., Jager, J., Collins, W. A., Bates, J. E., & Lansford, J. E.

(2008). Changes in the relation of self-efficacy beliefs and behaviors across development. *Child Development, 79,* 1257–1269.

DeWall, C. N., Anderson, C. A., & Bushman, B. J. (2012). Aggression. In H. Tennen, J. Suls, & I. B. Weiner (Eds.), *Handbook of psychology* (2nd ed., Vol. 5, pp. 449–466). Hoboken, NJ: Wiley.

Dishion, T. J., Spracklen, K. M., Andrews, D. W., & Patterson, G. R. (1996). Deviancy training in male adolescent friendships. *Behavior Therapy, 27,* 373–390.

Dodge, K. A., Bates, J. E., & Pettit, G. S. (1990). Mechanisms in the cycle of violence. *Science, 250,* 1678–1683.

Dodge, K. A., & Coie, J. D. (1987). Social-information-processing factors in reactive and proactive aggression in children's peer groups. *Journal of Personality and Social Psychology, 53,* 1146–1158.

Dodge, K. A., & Crick, N. R. (1990). Social information-processing bases of aggressive behavior in children. *Personality and Social Psychology Bulletin, 16,* 8–22.

Dodge, K. A., Dishion, T. J., & Lansford, J. E. (2006). Deviant peer influences in intervention and public policy for youth. *Social Policy Report, 20,* 1–19.

Dodge, K. A., Laird, R., Lochman, J., Zelli, A., & Conduct Problems Prevention Research Group. (2002). Multidimensional latent-construct analysis of children's social information processing patterns: Correlations with aggressive behavior problems. *Psychological Assessment, 14,* 60–73.

Dodge, K. A., Lansford, J. E., Burks, V. S., Bates, J. E., Pettit, G. S., Fontaine, R., et al. (2003). Peer rejection and social information-processing factors in the development of aggressive behavior problems in children. *Child Development, 74,* 374–393.

Dodge, K. A., Malone, P. S., Lansford, J. E., Sorbring, E., Skinner, A. T., Tapanya, S., et al. (2015). Hostile attributional bias and aggressive behavior in global context. *Proceedings of the National Academy of Sciences of the USA, 112,* 9310–9315.

Dodge, K. A., McClaskey, C. L., & Feldman, E. (1985). A situational approach to the assessment of social competence in children. *Journal of Consulting and Clinical Psychology, 53,* 334–353.

Dodge, K. A., Price, J. M., Bachorowski, J., & Newman, J. P. (1990). Hostile attributional biases in severely aggressive adolescents. *Journal of Abnormal Psychology, 99,* 385–392.

Eisenberg, N., & Fabes, R. A. (1992). Emotion regulation and the development of social competence. In M. S. Clark (Ed.), *Review of personality and social psychology: Vol. 14. Emotion and social behavior* (pp. 119–150). Newbury Park, CA: SAGE.

Eisenberg, N., Fabes, R. A., Guthrie, I. K., Murphy, B. C., Maszk, P., Holmgren, R., et al. (1996). The relations of regulation and emotionality to problem behavior in elementary school children. *Development and Psychopathology, 8,* 141–162.

Eisenberg, N., Fabes, R. A., Nyman, M., Bernzweig, J., & Pinuelas, A. (1994). The relations of emotionality and regulation to children's anger-related reactions. *Child Development, 65,* 109–128.

Ember, C. R., & Ember, M. (1994). War, socialization, and interpersonal violence: A cross-cultural study. *Journal of Conflict Resolution, 38,* 620–646.

Ember, C. R., & Ember, M. (2005). Explaining corporal punishment of children: A cross-cultural study. *American Anthropologist, 107,* 609–619.

Espelage, D. L., Low, S., Polanin, J. R., & Brown, E. C. (2013). The impact of a middle school program to reduce aggression, victimization, and sexual violence. *Journal of Adolescent Health, 53,* 180–186.

Fite, J. E., Goodnight, J. A., Bates, J. E., Dodge, K. A., & Pettit, G. S. (2008). Adolescent aggression and social cognition in the context of personality: Impulsivity as a moderator of predictions from social information processing. *Aggressive Behavior, 34,* 511–520.

Fontaine, R. G., Yang, C. M., Dodge, K. A., Pettit, G. S., & Bates, J. E. (2009). Development of response evaluation and decision (RED) and antisocial behavior in childhood and adolescence. *Developmental Psychology, 45,* 447–459.

Frick, P. J., & White, S. F. (2008). The importance of callous–unemotional traits for the development of aggressive and antisocial behavior. *Journal of Child Psychology and Psychiatry, 49,* 359–375.

Gershoff, E. T., & Grogan-Kaylor, A. (2016). Spanking and child outcomes: Old controversies and new meta-analyses. *Journal of Family Psychology, 30,* 453–469.

Greenberg, M. T., Kusche, C. A., Cook, E. T., & Quamma, J. P. (1995). Promoting emotional competence in school-aged children: The effects of the PATHS curriculum. *Development and Psychopathology, 7,* 117–136.

Grossmann, T. (2015). The development of social brain functions in infancy. *Psychological Bulletin, 141,* 1266–1287.

Guerra, N. (2010). *Cognitive-behavioral foundations of aggression and violence.* White paper, University of California, Riverside, CA. Retrieved from *http://stopyouthviolence.ucr.edu/website_pages/Social%20Cognition%20White%20Paper.pdf.*

Guerra, N. G., Huesmann, L. R., & Spindler, A. (2003). Community violence exposure, social cognition, and aggression among urban elementary school children. *Child Development, 74,* 1561–1576.

Huesmann, L. R. (1988). An information processing model for the development of aggression. *Aggressive Behavior, 14,* 13–24.

Huesmann, L. R. (1998). The role of social information processing and cognitive schema in the acquisition and maintenance of habitual aggressive behavior. In R. E. Geen & E. Donnerstein (Eds.), *Human aggression: Theories, research, and implications for policy* (pp. 73–109). New York: Academic Press.

Huesmann, L. R., Eron, L. D., Lefkowitz, M. M., & Walder, L. O. (1984). Stability of aggression over time and generations. *Developmental Psychology, 20,* 1120–1134.

Huesmann, L. R., & Guerra, N. G. (1997). Children's normative beliefs about aggression and aggressive behavior. *Journal of Personality and Social Psychology, 72,* 408–419.

Johnson, L. M., Simons, L., & Conger, R. D. (2004). Criminal justice system involvement and continuity of youth crime: A longitudinal analysis. *Youth and Society, 36,* 3–29.

Lansford, J. E., Malone, P. S., Dodge, K. A., Crozier, J. C., Pettit, G. S., & Bates, J. E. (2006). A 12-year prospective study of patterns of social information processing problems and externalizing behaviors. *Journal of Abnormal Child Psychology, 34,* 715–724.

Lansford, J. E., Malone, P. S., Dodge, K. A., Pettit, G. S., & Bates, J. E. (2010). Developmental cascades of peer rejection, social information processing biases, and aggression during middle childhood. *Development and Psychopathology, 22,* 593–602.

Lansford, J. E., Woodlief, D., Malone, P. S., Oburu, P., Pastorelli, C., Skinner, A. T., et al. (2014). A longitudinal examination of mothers' and fathers' social information processing biases and harsh discipline in nine countries. *Development and Psychopathology, 26,* 561–573.

Leff, S. S., Waasdorp, T. E., Paskewich, B., Gullan, R. L., Jawad, A., MacEvoy, J. P., et al. (2010). The Preventing Relational Aggression in Schools Everyday (PRAISE) program: A preliminary evaluation of acceptability and impact. *School Psychology Review, 39,* 569–587.

Lemerise, E., & Arsenio, W. (2000). An integrated model of emotion processes and cognition in social information processing. *Child Development, 71,* 107–118.

Low, S., Cook, C. R., Smolkowski, K., & Buntain-Ricklefs, J. (2015). Promoting social–emotional competence: An evaluation of the elementary version of *Second Step. Journal of School Psychology, 53,* 463–477.

MacBrayer, E. K., Milich, R., & Hundley, M. (2003). Attributional biases in aggressive children and their mothers. *Journal of Abnormal Psychology, 112,* 698–708.

Masten, A. S. (2014). *Ordinary magic: Resilience in development.* New York: Guilford Press.

Milner, J. S. (1993). Social information processing and physical child abuse. *Clinical Psychology Review, 13,* 275–294.

Milner, J. S. (2003). Social information processing in high-risk and physically abusive parents. *Child Abuse and Neglect, 27,* 7–20.

Ng-Mak, D. S., Salzinger, S., Feldman, R., & Stueve, A. (2002). Normalization of violence among inner-city youth: A formulation for research. *American Journal of Orthopsychiatry, 72,* 92–101.

Nisbett, R. E., & Cohen, D. (1996). *Culture of honor: The psychology of violence in the South.* Boulder, CO: Westview Press.

Nix, R. L., Pinderhughes, E. E., Dodge, K. A., Bates, J. E., Pettit, G. S., & McFadyen-Ketchum, S. (1999). The relation between mothers' hostile attribution tendencies and children's externalizing behavior problems: The mediating role of mothers' harsh discipline practices. *Child Development, 70,* 896–909.

Olweus, D. (1979). Stability of aggressive reaction patterns in males: A review. *Psychological Bulletin, 85,* 852–875.

Orobio de Castro, B., Veerman, J. W., Koops, W., Bosch, J. D., & Monshouwer, H. J. (2002). Hostile attribution of intent and aggressive behavior: A meta-analysis. *Child Development, 73,* 916–934.

Parsons, J. E., & Ruble, D. N. (1977). The development of achievement-related expectancies. *Child Development, 48,* 1075–1079.

Pettit, G. S., Lansford, J. E., Malone, P. S., Dodge, K. A., & Bates, J. E. (2010). Domain specificity in relationship history, social-information processing, and violent behavior in early adulthood. *Journal of Personality and Social Psychology, 98,* 190–200.

Rodriguez, C. M. (2010). Parent–child aggression: Association with child abuse potential and parenting styles. *Violence and Victims, 25,* 728–741.

Rubin, K. H., Coplan, R. J., Fox, N. A., & Calkins, S. D. (1995). Emotionality, emotion regulation, and preschoolers' social adaptation. *Development and Psychopathology, 7,* 49–62.

Ruble, D. N., Martin, C., & Berenbaum, S. (2006). Gender development. In W. Damon & R. M. Lerner (Series Eds.) & N. Eisenberg (Vol. Ed.), *Handbook of child psychology: Vol. 3. Personality and social development* (6th ed., pp. 858–932). New York: Wiley.

Saarni, C. (1999). *The development of emotional competence.* New York: Guilford Press.

Sacks, D. P., Bushman, B. J., & Anderson, C. A. (2011). Do violent video games harm children?: Comparing the scientific amicus curiae experts in Brown v. Entertainment Merchants Association. *Northwestern University Law Review, 106,* 1–12.

Sameroff, A. J., & Haith, M. M. (1986). *The five- to seven-year shift.* Chicago: University of Chicago Press.

Schneider, W., & Chein, J. M. (2003). Controlled and automatic processing: Behavior, theory, and biological mechanisms. *Cognitive Science, 27,* 525–559.

Schwartz, D., & Proctor, L. J. (2000). Community violence exposure and children's social adjustment in the school peer group: The mediating roles of emotion regulation and social cognition. *Journal of Consulting and Clinical Psychology, 68,* 670–683.

Skinner, A. T., Bacchini, D., Lansford, J. E., Godwin, J., Sorbring, E., Tapanya, S., et al. (2014). Neighborhood danger, parental monitoring, harsh parenting, and child aggression in nine countries. *Societies, 4,* 45–67.

Smithmyer, C. M., Hubbard, J. A., & Simons, R. F. (2000). Proactive and reactive aggression in delinquent adolescents: Relations to aggression outcome expectancies. *Journal of Clinical Child Psychology, 29,* 86–93.

Snyder, J. J., Reid, J. B., & Patterson, G. R. (2003). A social learning model of child and adolescent antisocial behavior. In B. B. Lahey, T. E. Moffitt, & A. Caspi (Eds.), *The causes of conduct disorder and juvenile delinquency* (pp. 27–48). New York: Guilford Press.

Spencer, F. H., & Bornholt, L. (2003). A model of children's cognitive functioning and cognitive self concepts. *Australian Journal of Learning Disabilities, 8,* 4–8.

Sroufe, L. A., Schork, E., Motti, F., Lawroski, N., & LaFreniere, P. (1984). The role of affect in social competence. In C. E. Izard, J. Kagan, & R. B. Zajonc (Eds.), *Emotions, cognition, and behavior* (pp. 289–319). New York: Cambridge University Press.

Trachtenberg, S., & Viken, R. J. (1994). Aggressive boys in the classroom: Biased attributions or shared perceptions? *Child Development, 65,* 829–835.

Tremblay, R. E. (2000). The development of aggressive behavior during childhood: What have we learned in the past century? *International Journal of Behavioral Development, 24,* 129–141.

Underwood, M. K. (1997). Peer social status and children's understanding of the expression and control of positive and negative emotions. *Merrill–Palmer Quarterly, 43,* 610–634.

Waldman, I. D. (1996). Aggressive boys' hostile perceptual and response biases: The role of attention and impulsivity. *Child Development, 67,* 1015–1033.

Weiss, B., Dodge, K. A., Bates, J. E., & Pettit, G. S. (1992). Some consequences of early harsh discipline: Child aggression and a maladaptive social-information-processing style. *Child Development, 63,* 1321–1335.

Wellman, H. M. (2014). *Making minds: How theory of mind develops.* New York: Oxford University Press.

White, S. H. (1965). Evidence for a hierarchical arrangement of learning processes. In L. P. Lipsitt & C. C. Spiker (Eds.), *Advances in child development and behavior* (pp. 187–220). New York: Academic Press.

Young, J. E. (1994). *Cognitive therapy for personality disorders: A schema-focused approach* (2nd ed.). Sarasota, FL: Professional Resource Press.

PART II

AGGRESSION IN CONTEXT

CHAPTER 9

Parenting, Parent–Child Relationships, and the Development of Aggression during Childhood and Adolescence

K. LEE RABY and GLENN I. ROISMAN

Brief Introduction

The scientific study of parental contributions to aggression during childhood and adolescence transcends several academic disciplines. In developmental psychology, several theoretical accounts emphasize that one of the central tasks of parenting is to help children effectively manage the desire to harm others (for a historical overview, see Maccoby, 2007). In addition, research in the area of clinical psychology has consistently identified various forms of poor parenting as risk factors for later aggression and other forms of delinquency (e.g., Pinquart, 2017). These findings have inspired intervention efforts that target parenting behaviors as a means of reducing the prevalence of aggression and antisocial behavior during childhood and adolescence (e.g., Kaminski, Valle, Filene, & Boyle, 2008). Each of these academic disciplines has a distinct body of research devoted to understanding how experiences with parents shape the development of aggression, resulting in an expansive literature on this broad topic. Nonetheless, the theoretical and practical importance of the topic continues to attract scholarly attention.

The purpose of this chapter is to survey the scientific literature pertinent to the significance of experiences with parents for the development of aggression during childhood and adolescence. In the first section, we describe the overarching issues that distinguish the major theoretical accounts regarding parental contributions to the development of aggression. In the second section, we review the specific theoretical perspectives that have arguably been most valuable in stimulating research in this area. In the third section, we summarize the relevant research findings. Wherever possible, we highlight findings from meta-analyses or large-sample investigations, as such studies provide the most precise estimates of the associations of interest. We also give special attention to findings from genetically informed and experimental designs, as these approaches afford more rigorous tests of parents' potential environmentally mediated causal effects on children's aggressive behaviors. In the fourth section, we describe the implications of these findings for our basic understanding of the developmental origins of aggression, as well as for prevention and intervention programs aimed at reducing the prevalence of these harmful behaviors. In the final section, we describe promising areas of research that address newer theoretical ideas or incorporate methodological advances.

This chapter focuses exclusively on theory and research regarding the implications of parental behaviors, parent–child interactions, and parent–child relationships for the development of aggression among children. We do not review the literature regarding the potential consequences of parental characteristics (e.g., teenage parenthood or psychopathology) or family structure (e.g., single parenthood or divorce). That said, it is widely assumed that parent–child interactions represent one of the pathways by which these factors influence children's development (Belsky, 1984). Moreover, although this chapter only addresses children's experiences with parents, this is not meant to suggest that experiences with parents are solely responsible for, or even are the largest contributors to, the development of aggression. There is a general consensus among aggression scholars that there are multiple developmental pathways to aggression and that these pathways are shaped by the interplay between experiences with parents, child characteristics, family-level processes, experiences in other interpersonal contexts, and broader contextual forces (Dishion & Patterson, 2016; Moffitt, 1993). This view is consistent with the broader developmental-systems perspective, which emphasizes that both competent and problematic forms of developmental adaptation emerge from and are maintained by the continuous transactions across multiple levels of analysis (e.g., Cicchetti & Tucker, 1994; Sameroff, 2010). That said, parental contributions have a somewhat privileged status within theory and research regarding the development of aggression. This likely is based partly on the assumption that experiences with parents have a substantial influence on children's developmental adaptation and partly on the view that parent–child interactions represent a node in the complex network of factors contributing to aggression that may be especially amenable to clinical intervention.

Main Issues

The various theoretical perspectives concerning the contributions of parenting to the development of aggression differ with respect to three overarching issues. The first concerns the specific features of experiences with parents that are believed to be influential in the development of aggression. Theoretical accounts have emphasized different *content* of the parent–child experiences, resulting in a fairly large number of almost certainly correlated constructs. The features of the parent–child experiences can also be characterized at different *levels of analysis*. Hinde (1987) described several "levels of social complexity," including the actions of an individual person in a social situation, the interactions between two or more individuals, and the resulting relationship between the individuals (i.e., the pattern of interactions across time and corresponding interpersonal expectations). Consistent with this framework, theories of the developmental origins of aggression differ in their emphasis on parents' behavior toward a child (e.g., parents' discipline practices), the back-and-forth exchanges between parents and children (e.g., coercive cycles), and the child's internalization of the relationship (e.g., attachment security). The distinction between individual and dyadic levels of analysis (which includes interaction and relationship levels of analysis) reflects a difference in children's developmental outcomes being viewed either as a consequence of parents' socialization efforts or as a process of individual adaptation that emerges out of parent–child relationships (Maccoby, 2007; Sroufe, 1990).

The second overarching issue involves the specific period of development in which parent–child experiences occur. Theories differ in their emphases on whether experiences with parents during infancy and early childhood, middle childhood, or adolescence are most significant in the development of aggression. This issue of developmental timing is intertwined with the issue of which features of parent–child experiences are relevant for later aggression. The reason is that the tasks of parenting change as children develop and encounter novel challenges during each phase of life (e.g., Sroufe, Egeland, Carlson, & Collins, 2005). For this reason, theories that focus on the emergence of aggression during the first few years of life tend to emphasize different features of experiences with parents than theories that focus on the relevance of parents for aggression during middle childhood or adolescence.

The third issue involves the specific mechanisms that are theorized to account for the influence of parent–child experiences on aggressive behavior. This issue involves three specific questions: What are the specific characteristics that are shaped by interactions with parents? How are these characteristics carried forward across time? And, finally, how do these characteristics influence children's aggressive behavior at later ages and in novel interpersonal contexts? In addressing these questions, theoretical perspectives have tended to emphasize children's behavioral patterns in interpersonal situations and children's social cognitions. As we discuss in the later section "Future Directions," one of the more recent developments has been the focus on specifying how alterations to the structure and functioning of neurobiological systems mediate the associations between parent–child experiences and the development of aggression.

Theoretical Considerations

In this section, we summarize key theoretical ideas about the role of parent–child experiences in the development of aggression during childhood and adolescence. We have organized the ideas of three major theoretical perspectives: theories regarding parent–child attachment, theories regarding social learning processes, and theories regarding parental control. These theoretical perspectives have had substantial heuristic value for this topic, in part because they describe the specific aspects of the parent–child experiences that are thought to be relevant for the development of aggression and provide guidance regarding the potential mechanisms of influence.

Attachment Theory

For the last half century, attachment theory has served as one of the dominant theoretical accounts regarding the consequences of early caregiving experiences for subsequent social–emotional adaptation. One of the fundamental tenets of attachment theory is that human infants share a universal propensity to elicit or actively seek physical proximity with their caregivers during times of distress. Bowlby (1982) proposed that the tendency to form these attachment relationships was the product of evolutionary pressures given that these relationships help promote the survival of young infants. Infants are also expected to vary in the degree to which they achieve a sense of security in their attachment relationships, with these individual differences being a function of the degree to which caregivers sensitively respond to infants' cues and behaviors (Ainsworth, Blehar, Waters, & Wall, 1978). Moreover, the security of infants' attachment relationships is believed to provide the foundation for a set of mental representations regarding close relationships that are carried forward across development and assist in organizing individuals' thoughts, feelings, and behavior in later interpersonal situations. For example, Sroufe and colleagues (Sroufe, Carlson, Levy, & Egeland, 1999) have argued that children with insecure attachment representations have less positive expectations of others, have less competent social skills, experience more difficulties building the emotional connections necessary for empathically responding to others, and are less effective at regulating feelings of anger. As a result, children who experienced insensitive caregiving and/or who formed insecure attachment relationships during the first few years of life are expected to experience more conflict and to behave more aggressively within their family and peer relationships during early childhood.

Some attachment scholars have further hypothesized that early caregiving experiences and attachment patterns continue to shape aggressive outcomes during later developmental periods. Specifically, children may elicit or actively seek interpersonal experiences later in life that are consistent with the attachment-related representations that they formed during infancy, and attachment representations established early in life may persistently bias children's interpretations of later interpersonal events (Bowlby, 1988; Sroufe et al., 1999). According to this perspective, early experiences with caregivers exert an enduring influence on individuals' aggressive behavior that persists into adulthood (Sroufe, Egeland, & Kreutzer, 1990).

Social Learning Perspectives

The social learning perspective includes multiple theoretical ideas regarding the contributions of parent–child experiences to the development of aggression. There are two commonalities of these theories. The first is the assumption that aggressive behavior emerges and is maintained across childhood and adolescence because of general learning processes, including reinforcement and imitation. The second is the emphasis on negative parental behaviors—such as hostility, rejection, and conflict—during the developmental periods of early and middle childhood.

A highly influential idea within the social learning perspective is that children learn by imitating the behavior of others (i.e., observational learning; Bandura,

1973). One implication of this idea is that parents who interact with their children in a harsh, punitive, and forceful manner may be modeling aggressive behaviors and implicitly communicating that these types of behaviors are normative and acceptable. Moreover, if parents achieve their immediate goals through these behaviors (e.g., increasing child compliance through harsh discipline), children may learn that these behaviors are an effective strategy for responding to interpersonal problems. Ultimately, these beliefs are expected to lead to aggressive behavior in children.

Patterson's (1982) coercion theory builds on the observational learning ideas by proposing that aggression emerges from the bidirectional interactions between parents and children. According to this theory, aggression is not simply the result of children passively observing their parents' caustic behaviors and then imitating them in novel situations. Instead, aggression is thought to result from a cycle of coercive parent–child exchanges. For example, a child may angrily resist the parent's attempts to set a behavioral limit on his or her behavior. If the parent responds with harsh discipline, this may exacerbate the child's aggressive behavior. This escalating pattern likely will culminate in either the parent giving up, which inadvertently reinforces the child's oppositional and aggressive behavior, or the parent winning the argument, which reinforces the parent for intensifying the hostile interaction. When repeated over time, these coercive parent–child interactions are believed to canalize a pattern of aggressive behavior that the child eventually carries into situations outside the family context (Patterson, DeBaryshe, & Ramsey, 1989).

The social information-processing model proposes that harsh parent–child interactions not only promote children's aggressive behavior but also lead to biases in how children cognitively process information from social situations (Crick & Dodge, 1994; Dodge, 1986). In particular, earlier experiences with their parents are thought to guide how children encode and interpret information about interpersonal events, which, in turn, influence children's behavioral responses. Children with histories of harsh parental care may be more likely to incorrectly attribute hostile intentions in ambiguous situations. These children's hostile attribution biases have been suggested as a cognitive mechanism underlying associations between harsh and hostile parent–child interactions and the development of aggressive behavior across childhood and adolescence.

Theories of Parental Control

Similar to social learning, there are several interrelated theoretical ideas regarding the significance of parental control for the development of aggression. Many of these ideas have their conceptual origins in Baumrind's (1966) typology of parental control. Within this perspective, authoritarian parenting was defined as having high and uncompromising expectations for the child's behavior, as well as a willingness to use punitive force to achieve child compliance. Permissive parenting, on the other hand, was characterized by a general acceptance of the child's behavior and few demands on the child. The third type of parental control was viewed as an optimal blend of the authoritarian and permissive parenting styles. Specifically, authoritative parenting was defined as establishing developmentally appropriate standards for the child's behavior, directing the child's behavior by explaining the rationale for the rules, and using inductive discipline techniques to enforce rules.

The authoritative parental style was assumed to lead to more competent forms of developmental adjustment, including fewer aggressive behaviors, by promoting the child's cooperation with and eventual internalization of the behavioral standards (Baumrind, 1966).

Maccoby and Martin (1983) reconceptualized Baumrind's (1966) parenting type classifications as quadrants in a two-dimensional space. The first dimension reflected the degree of parental responsiveness and support versus parental rejection and hostility. The second dimension captured the degree to which the parent attempted to control the child's behavior by establishing and enforcing limits versus being indulgent of their children. Within this two-dimensional framework, authoritative parenting was viewed as the combination of high support and high control, authoritarian parenting as the combination of low support and high control, and permissive parenting as high support but low control. In addition, this framework also identified a fourth parenting style, referred to as neglectful parenting, which represented the combination of low support and low control.

A second extension of Baumrind's early ideas involved Barber's (1996) distinction between behavioral and psychological control. Whereas behavioral control reflects parents' attempts to guide their children's behaviors by setting rules, monitoring their children, and enforcing rules with consistent discipline, psychological control involves parental actions that undermine the child's autonomy and manipulate the child's cognitions or emotions. Examples of psychological control include diminishing or ridiculing the child's opinions or beliefs or attempting to control the child by using guilt or withdrawing affection. Although the use of behavioral control strategies are expected to be inversely associated with aggression, psychological control is hypothesized to predict higher levels of aggression.

Central Research Findings

Attachment Theory

Attachment researchers have studied the consequences of children's early caregiving experiences for later aggression outcomes in a number of ways. Historically, one of the most common research strategies has been to investigate the degree to which observations of the security of children's early attachment relationships are associated with the emergence of aggressive behaviors during childhood. Some the most influential early findings on this topic were based on the Minnesota Longitudinal Study of Risk and Adaptation, a prospective study of, originally, 267 participants born into poverty. Erickson, Sroufe, and Egeland (1985) provided initial evidence that preschool-age children with histories of insecure infant–caregiver attachments—especially insecure–avoidant attachments—exhibited more teacher-reported physical and verbal aggression than children with early histories of secure attachments. Similarly, Troy and Sroufe (1987) reported that children who had formed avoidant attachments to their parents as infants were more likely to be physically or verbally aggressive toward a playmate during observed one-on-one peer interactions. Taken together, these findings suggested that forming an insecure–avoidant attachment during infancy confers a risk for later aggressive behavior, presumably because of feelings of anger stemming from early experiences of rejection by their caregivers.

These early studies were followed by a large corpus of research regarding the role of early parent–child relationships in later aggressive behaviors. A recent meta-analysis of this area of research, which included data from nearly 60 reports comprising approximately 6,000 individuals, indicated that forming an insecure attachment during infancy is associated with increased risk for externalizing behaviors (Fearon, Bakermans-Kranenburg, van IJzendoorn, Lapsley, & Roisman, 2010). However, insecure–avoidant attachments were not uniquely associated with later externalizing behaviors within this large dataset, as the effects for each of the subtypes of attachment insecurity did not differ from one another. The combined effect size of early attachment insecurity for later externalizing problems was d = .31, which is small according to Cohen's (1992) criteria. However, the effect size did not diminish as the temporal lag between the measurements of early attachment and aggressive behavior problems increased. In other words, the consequences of early attachment insecurity for later aggressive behaviors appeared to persist from early childhood through adolescence.

A second research strategy inspired by attachment theory has involved investigating the predictive effects of children's experiences of sensitive versus insensitive caregiving during the first few years of life for later behavior problems. For example, in a relatively large sample of over 1,000 rural families, observations of sensitive care during the first 3 years of life were consistently associated with fewer parent-reported externalizing behavior problems between the ages of 3 and 7 years (r's between –.23 and –.33; Sulik et al., 2015). These results are generally consistent with findings from the large sample Study of Early Child Care and Youth Development, a separate longitudinal study of over 1,000 families. Specifically, Roisman and Fraley (2012b) reported that early experiences of sensitive caregiving consistently predicted fewer teacher-reported externalizing behavior problems during early childhood through midadolescence, and the overall magnitude of the associations at each age were relatively stable (r's were around –.25). This suggests that the predictive effects of early sensitive caregiving for teacher-reported externalizing behavior problems did not diminish with time. These enduring associations with teacher-reported externalizing behavior problems were not accounted for by indices of early contextual risk (e.g., family income, maternal depression, single parent) or sensitive caregiving during later development periods. Importantly, although the associations between early sensitivity and *mother*-reported externalizing behavior problems were statistically significant at each age, the predictive effects systematically decreased with time (i.e., the correlation diminished from –.23 during early childhood to –.14 during adolescence).

Because many of the studies regarding the potential consequences of early sensitive caregiving for the development of aggression involved biologically related parent–child pairs, they could not rule out the possibility that the associations were due to genetic factors shared between parents and children. Potential genetic confounding represents a serious threat to causal inferences in this area, as variation in both parenting and children's aggressive behaviors are heritable (Burt, 2009; Klahr

& Burt, 2014; see Brendgen, Vitaro, & Boivin, Chapter 4, this volume). Indeed, findings from genetically informed studies suggest that the associations between early experiences of sensitive caregiving and child aggression–related behavior problems are partially accounted for by shared genetic variation. For example, among a sample of approximately 150 children adopted within the first 6 months of life, observations of sensitive caregiving were not significantly associated with teacher-reported aggressive behaviors during middle childhood or adolescence (van der Voort, Linting, Bakermans-Kranenburg, & van IJzendoorn, 2013). In addition, an analysis of data from more than 400 twins indicated that the negative association between early supportive parenting and externalizing behavior problems during kindergarten were largely accounted for by shared genetic factors (Roisman & Fraley, 2012a). In fact, only a quarter of the overall correlation of $r = -.11$ was estimated to be due to the shared environment in this sample.

Randomized controlled trials represent another strategy for evaluating whether early sensitive caregiving experiences have environmentally mediated effects on the development of aggression in children. Because families are randomly assigned to receive either a control intervention or an intervention that aims to improve parents' sensitive caregiving, any subsequent group differences in the functioning of the children are presumed to reflect a causal effect of the intervention-induced changes in parenting on children's behaviors. There is a robust body of evidence indicating that sensitivity-focused interventions are effective at improving the security of children's attachments to their caregivers (Bakermans-Kranenburg, van IJzendoorn, & Juffer, 2003). In addition, evidence is emerging that these interventions may also lead to reductions in children's behavior problems. For example, preschool-age children whose caregivers received a sensitivity-focused intervention have been reported to exhibit less anger during interactions with their caregivers (Lind, Bernard, Ross, & Dozier, 2014) and have fewer parent-reported externalizing behavior problems (Velderman et al., 2006) than children whose parents did not receive the intervention.

A fifth strategy for evaluating the significance of early attachment experiences for aggression involves examining the development of children who have been adopted internationally. Many of these children spent a portion of their preadoptive lives in a group-based or institutional caregiving setting. These environments are generally characterized by high child-to-caregiver ratios, frequent caregiver turnover, and a lack of care that is responsive to the child's individual needs (van IJzendoorn et al., 2011). Because these children are typically adopted into highly enriching family environments, this represents a natural experiment that disentangles early and later experiences (Rutter, 2007). Consistent with the idea that disturbances in early infant–caregiver relationships have a unique influence on later development, children who have been adopted internationally are at greater risk for externalizing behavior problems after being adopted, especially if they experienced more severe preadoptive deprivation (Juffer & van IJzendoorn, 2005). The Bucharest Early Intervention Project provided even more direct evidence for the causal contributions of early social deprivation experiences. Children living in an institutional environment who were randomly assigned to receive foster care exhibited fewer externalizing behavior problems at age 12 years than their peers who had been assigned to remain in institutional care (Humphreys et al., 2015).

Social Learning Perspectives

One of the more controversial questions that stems from the social learning perspective on parental contributions to children's aggression is whether the use of corporal punishment has iatrogenic effects. This question has inspired scores of studies on the consequences of spanking. A meta-analysis of the research findings on this topic from the last 50 years indicated that the use of physical punishment has a small but positive association with aggressive behavior ($d = .33$; Gershoff & Grogan-Kaylor, 2016). A common critique of this literature is that this association may not reflect social causation but rather may be due to parents' relying on physical discipline because their children are highly aggressive (i.e., child evocative effects). However, studies involving twin and adoption studies indicate that the associations between physical punishment and children's externalizing behavior problems are partially but not entirely due to children's genetic characteristics (for a review, see Jaffee, Strait, & Odgers, 2012). Emerging experimental evidence also suggests that decreases in the use of parental physical punishment may lead to fewer behavioral problems in children (e.g., Gershoff, Lee, & Durrant, 2017). However, because these interventions tend to target multiple parenting behaviors, it is not clear that the reduced use of harsh discipline is solely responsible for the corresponding reductions in children's aggressive behaviors.

Experiencing physical abuse, a more extreme form of harsh parenting that has the potential to result in physical injury to a child, is also assumed to promote the development of aggressive behavior in children. A highly influential narrative review concluded that there is strong evidence from retrospective and prospective longitudinal studies that childhood physical abuse is associated with increased risk for aggression, crime, and violence (Gilbert et al., 2009). In addition, there is a small but statistically significant meta-analytic association between prospective measures of childhood physical abuse and aggression-related outcomes ($r = .11$; Braga, Goncalves, Basto-Pereira, & Maia, 2017). Findings from a large twin sample indicated that the associations between maternal reported child physical abuse and children's aggression and antisocial behavior at age 5 years were largely independent of children's genetic characteristics (Jaffee et al., 2004). In contrast, twin studies that have focused on aggression-related outcomes at later ages have produced mixed results regarding the degree to which associations with childhood maltreatment were due to genetic confounding (e.g., Forsman & Langstrom, 2012; Schulz-Heik et al., 2010). These inconsistencies may be attributable to use of retrospective, self-report measures of maltreatment, which tend to show larger genetic contributions than prospective, independent assessments of childhood maltreatment.

Consistent with the principles of coercion theory, in-depth microanalyses of parent–child exchanges and longitudinal analyses indicate that parent–child interactions characterized by escalating dyadic conflict and reciprocal hostility are associated with the development of noncompliant and aggressive behavior in children (for a review, see Dishion & Patterson, 2016). Meta-analyses also indicate that negative parenting behaviors such as parental harshness, hostility, and rejection are robustly associated with relational and physical aggression during childhood and adolescence (Kawabata, Alink, Tseng, van IJzendoorn, & Crick, 2011; Pinquart, 2017). That said, the associations appear to be small to moderate in overall size (i.e., equivalent to correlations between .11 and .20). Dozens of parenting-focused interventions indicate that coercive parent–child dynamics have a causal role in the development of aggression. Specifically, parent training programs that encourage using noncoercive discipline strategies, such as time-outs, and promoting more positive parent–child interactions are an effective means of modifying children's externalizing behaviors (Kaminski et al., 2008).

The social information-processing model of aggression involves two central hypotheses: (1) Harsh parent–child experiences result in a tendency for children to attribute hostile intentions to other individuals; and (2) this hostile attribution bias leads to aggressive behavior. Results from the Child Development Project, a multisite longitudinal study of more than 500 children, indicated that experiencing harsh discipline or physical abuse does in fact predict a greater hostile attribution bias, and this attributional bias was associated with teacher reports of aggressive behavior (Dodge, Bates, & Pettit, 1990). These early findings have been supported by subsequent research with independent samples. For example, separate meta-analyses have concluded that this bias in children's processing of social information is predicted by harsh parenting experiences and positively associated with aggressive behavior (Luke & Banerjee, 2013; Orobio de Castro, Veerman, Koops, Bosch, & Monshouwer, 2002). However, the size of these associations appears to be conditional on the stimuli used to assess children's hostile attribution biases.

Parental Control

Early research from Baumrind and others consistently demonstrated that the authoritative style of parenting was associated with fewer behavior problems (e.g., Baumrind, 1966; Maccoby & Martin, 1983). In contrast, indulgent parenting and/or inconsistent discipline—characteristics of the neglectful and permissive parenting styles—appeared to provide insufficient limits on children's aggressive impulses. Strict and rigid parental control—which is characteristic of authoritarian parenting—have been associated with high levels of aggressive, delinquent, and antisocial behavior. Quantitative reviews of this literature have supported the idea that both the lack of behavioral control and the authoritative use of control are associated with the development of aggressive behavior (Pinquart, 2017). However, as with the other forms of parenting, these associations appear to be small to moderate in overall magnitude.

Parents' use of psychological control has also been implicated as a predictor of problematic adjustment during childhood and adolescence, including children's aggression-related outcomes (e.g., Barber, 1996). A meta-analysis of over 150 studies indicated that psychological control has a small to moderate association with aggression ($r = .21$; Pinquart, 2017). Nelson and Crick (2002) proposed that parental psychological control may also be associated with children's use of relational aggression, which involves damaging others' feelings of inclusion in a group or specific friendships via social exclusion or gossiping. Indeed, there is a positive but weak meta-analytic association between parental psychological control and relational aggression during childhood and adolescence ($r = .05$; Kawabata et al. 2011).

The associations between aspects of parental control and children's aggression-related behavior problems commonly are assumed to reflect the causal effects of parenting on the adjustment of children and adolescents. However, the recent debate regarding parental monitoring and adolescents' behavior problems highlights the child's active role in these processes. Specifically, Kerr and Stattin (2000) demonstrated that parents' knowledge of adolescents' whereabouts, friends, and activities is not simply the product of parents' monitoring efforts but rather is largely due to adolescents' willingness to disclose this information to their parents. Moreover, adolescents' disclosures—but not parents' monitoring attempts—are consistently associated with fewer problem behaviors, as well as declines in behavior problems across time (for a review, see Keijser, 2016). These findings have challenged researchers to reinterpret the associations between parental knowledge and adolescents' behavior outcomes as potentially reflecting an adolescent-driven process, though of course adolescent disclosures may have their own origins in the quality of the earlier caregiving environment.

The question concerning the direction of effect in correlational findings applies beyond parental monitoring. For example, individual differences in adolescents' adjustment have been reported to lead to changes in authoritative and neglectful parenting styles rather than vice versa (Kerr, Stattin, & Özdemir, 2012). Moreover, behavioral genetics studies have demonstrated that parent-report, child-report, and observational assessments of parental control are associated with the child's genetic characteristics (Klahr & Burt, 2014), which further suggest evocative effects on parents' attempts to direct the child's behavior. Thus there is a critical need for further research that critically evaluates the possibility of reciprocal effects between parents' attempts to exercise authority and adolescents' aggression behaviors.

Implications

Overall, a substantial body of research indicates that experiences with parents—including insensitive caregiving and insecure attachments early in development, harsh and coercive parent–child interactions during childhood, and a lack of appropriate parental guidance and control during adolescence—are associated with the emergence and maintenance of aggression during childhood and adolescence. These correlational findings, though, appear partially accounted for by aggressive children evoking these responses from parents and genetic factors shared between parents and children. That said, studies that have used research designs that control for these types of processes—including genetically informed studies, natural experiments, and interventions with random assignment to treatment—support the theoretical ideas purporting a causal influence of insensitive and coercive parenting on the development of aggression during childhood and adolescence. Taken together, these findings are also consistent with the more general idea from developmental psychopathology that behavioral and psychological disturbances, including manifestations of aggression, are not simply inherent characteristics of the individual but rather are the products of a series of adaptations to individuals' local environments (Cicchetti, 1993; Sroufe, 1997).

The findings from this body of research also have implications for the prevention or treatment of aggression among children and adolescents. In fact, much of the research in this area has been motivated by the desire to identify environmental risk factors that could be modified to reduce the prevalence of aggression and other harmful behaviors. Efforts are already under way—and have been for some time—to translate these research findings into interventions that effectively prevent or help reduce aggression during childhood and adolescence by altering various aspects of parent–child interactions (e.g., Kaminski et al., 2008; Lind et al., 2014). These programs represent valuable, empirically supported tools for clinicians and mental health providers who work with children at high risk for aggressive outcomes.

Future Directions

Although there has been substantial progress in our understanding of parental contributions to aggression in recent decades, there are several outstanding questions. The first is whether childhood experiences with parents have long-term consequences for aggression that extend beyond childhood and adolescence and into the years of adulthood. Individuals who display elevated aggressive behavior early in development are thought to be especially likely to be engaged in a pattern of increasingly destructive behavior that persists across the life course (Moffitt, 1993; Patterson et al., 1989). Although it was originally assumed that antisocial behavior that initially appears during adolescence may be limited to that developmental period (e.g., Moffitt, 1993), longitudinal studies have revealed that individuals who display adolescent-onset behavior problems are at greater risk for continuing to display externalizing behavior problems during early adulthood compared with individuals with histories of no behavior problems during childhood or adolescence (for a review, see Fairchild, Van Goozen, Calder, & Goodyer, 2013). Thus, given the stability of aggressive behavior across development, it is possible that parental experiences that lead to aggressive behavior during childhood or adolescence may also increase risk for various forms of aggression during adulthood. Indeed, prospective, longitudinal studies indicate that individuals who were maltreated during childhood are more likely to experience violence in their romantic relationships (Widom, Czaja, & Dutton, 2014), maltreat their own children (Thornberry & Henry, 2013), and engage in criminal behavior during late adolescence and early adulthood (Gilbert et al., 2009). However, there are fewer prospective, longitudinal investigations of the potential long-term consequences of more normative variations in parent–child experiences for aggression-related outcomes during adulthood.

A related but still distinct question is whether the effects of parent–child relationship experiences for children's aggressive behaviors diminish in their overall magnitude or are relatively stable across development. For example, some scholars have argued that childhood experiences with parents have a concurrent causal effect on children's functioning but that these effects fade with time (Clarke & Clarke, 2000; Kagan, 1980). Fraley, Roisman, and Haltigan (2013) referred to this as a *revisionist* model of development, as it implies that consequences of early experiences with parents are eventually "overwritten" by subsequent experiences. In contrast, others have argued that parent–child relationship experiences leave an indelible imprint on children's functioning that endures across development (e.g., Sroufe et al., 1990). This *enduring effects* model of development (Fraley et al., 2013) proposes that negative childhood experiences with parents not only initiate a pattern of aggressive behavior during childhood but also continuously influence individuals' propensity to behave in an aggressive manner across the life course.

Conclusively answering this question requires shifting from focusing on the association between parent–child experiences and children's aggressive behavior during only one developmental period to focusing on the overall patterns of associations with aggressive behavior at multiple ages. Recently, Fraley and colleagues (2013) recommended a set of analytic techniques that can be leveraged for distinguishing between the revisionist and the enduring effects models of development. These analytic procedures have been used to demonstrate that early experiences of insensitive caregiving during the first few years of life appear to have enduring associations with individuals' externalizing behavior problems through adolescence (Roisman & Fraley, 2012b). A potentially fruitful future direction would be applying these analytic tools to evaluate whether there are enduring consequences of other parent–child experiences.

A third question is *through what mechanisms* various parent–child experiences contribute to children's aggressive outcomes during these different developmental periods. Although children's behavioral and cognitive processes have traditionally been emphasized, there is growing interest in the specific alterations to the structure and functioning of children's neurobiological systems that mediate parental effects on the development of aggression (e.g., Van Goozen, Fairchild, Snoek, & Harold, 2007). Indeed, developmental neuroscience research is beginning to provide evidence of the specific neurobiological systems that are tuned by experiences with parents, including the hypothalamus–pituitary–adrenal axis and central nervous system processes (Belsky & de Haan, 2011; Gunnar & Quevedo, 2007). In addition, there is accumulating evidence that aggressive behavior during childhood is associated with disturbances in similar systems (Alegria, Radua, & Rubia, 2016; Alink et al., 2008). Although these findings are promising, the thoughtful integration of information across multiple levels of analysis likely will be needed to fully understand the mechanisms responsible for mediating the consequences of parent–child relationship experiences for children's aggressive behavior.

A fourth question is why children differ in their responses to parent–child experiences. One intriguing idea is that children's genetically based characteristics dampen or amplify the effects of their experiences with parents on aggressive behavior. For example, both diathesis–stress and differential-susceptibility models suggest that some children are more strongly affected by negative parenting experiences than others (Belsky & Pluess, 2009). In a landmark study, Caspi and colleagues (2002) indicated that the consequences of childhood maltreatment for later antisocial and violent behavior varied as a function of individuals' genetic makeup. Specifically, the harmful effects of maltreatment were greater among males carrying the low-activity variant of the gene that encodes for the monoamine oxidase-A enzyme, which is involved in the metabolism of neurotransmitters. This initial finding sparked an ever-expanding body of research into the possibility that associations between parenting experiences and children's behavior problems may be moderated by genetic variants related to the functioning of dopaminergic or serotonin neurotransmitter systems. Although the original Caspi and colleagues finding has been replicated in several independent samples (Byrd & Manuck, 2014),

many other similar candidate gene-by-environment (G × E) results have proven difficult to replicate. One reason for this is that the effect sizes of individual genetic
variants appear to be exceedingly small, thereby requiring large sample sizes to reliably detect such G × E interactions. A potentially fruitful strategy is to use information from meta-analyses to create polygenetic risk scores (Chabris, Lee, Cesarini,
Benjamin, & Laibson, 2015). Because these scores aggregate the individual contributions of a number of genetic variants, they may represent a more statistically
powerful, and therefore reliable, approach to testing whether children's genetic
characteristics moderate parental contributions to aggression.

A fifth question is how the various parent–child relationship experiences work
together across childhood and adolescence to influence the development of aggression. As we have highlighted throughout the chapter, different theoretical perspectives emphasize different features of experiences with parents during different
developmental periods. Many of the empirical studies in this area were intended
to test ideas from only one theoretical perspective. This has resulted in a somewhat
fragmented understanding of the cumulative contributions of the role of parents to
the emergence, maintenance, or desistance in aggression across the first two decades
of life. Integrating the various theoretical ideas will require careful consideration
of the distinctions and relations between the levels of social organization described
by Hinde (1987), including the behavior of the parent, the reciprocal interactions
between parents and children, and the resulting parent–child relationship.

A noteworthy example of this is Kochanska and colleagues' (e.g., Kochanska,
Barry, Stellern, & O'Bleness, 2009) efforts to integrate ideas regarding the significance of early attachment relationships and parents' use of control. These scholars
have proposed that the early attachment relationship establishes the emotional context for parents' later attempts to set limits and exercise control over the children's
behaviors. Consistent with this idea, parents' use of physical control while establishing limits appears to lead to children's oppositional behavior during interactions
with parents and to eventual disruptive behavior problems only for children with
histories of insecure infant–caregiver attachments. These findings illustrate how
integrating various theoretical perspectives and considering how several aspects
of the parent–child relationship may illuminate a more complete understanding
of how experiences with parents shape children's trajectories of social–emotional
development.

Finally, as researchers investigate the answers to these and other questions, it
is critical to continue to leverage research designs that afford stronger tests of the
potential effects of experiences with parents for the development of aggression.
Because each of the various research designs has unique strengths and weaknesses,
converging evidence from multiple types of studies allow for the most compelling
conclusions. Multiwave longitudinal designs can help clarify the degree to which
the associations between parent–child relationship experiences and children's
aggressive outcomes may be due to social causation or evocative processes. In
addition, recent research in this and other domains has highlighted the inferen-
tial errors attached to the use of between-person data to reach conclusions about
within-person processes (e.g., Keijser, 2016). There also are a range of genetically
informed designs that allow for testing whether the associations are consistent with
genetically or environmentally mediated effects (Jaffee et al., 2012; Rutter, 2007).

Intervention studies offer powerful tests of the causal effects of parenting by randomly assigning parents to receive an intervention that aims to change parents' behaviors and evaluating whether enrollment in the intervention leads to reductions in children's aggressive behaviors. In addition to their value for theory testing, randomized controlled trials offer the added benefit of developing empirically evaluated programs that can be implemented in an effort to reduce the prevalence of aggressive behavior. Intervention studies can also be used to test whether there are reciprocal effects of experiences with parents and children's aggressive behavior by targeting children's aggressive behaviors and evaluating whether this results in changes to parent–child interactions and relationships.

Conclusions

The scientific study of parental contributions to aggression represents a relatively mature area of scholarship. A large body of research involving a diverse set of research designs has lent support for the theoretical accounts regarding the consequences of parent–child relationships for children's developmental trajectories of aggression. These findings have also supported the creation and evaluation of interventions that help prevent or treat childhood aggression by modifying parent–child interactions. A pressing challenge for this area of research is to continue shifting from addressing whether experiences with parenting matter for the development of aggression to specifying more precisely the magnitude of such associations and clarifying the developmental processes underlying *why* such associations obtain and *for whom*. Ultimately, these research investments will help extend our understanding of the interpersonal origins of aggression and may provide avenues for more effectively intervening with high-risk children and their families.

REFERENCES

Ainsworth, M. D. S., Blehar, M., Waters, E., & Wall, S. (1978). *Patterns of attachment: A psychological study of the Strange Situation*. Hillsdale, NJ: Erlbaum.

Alegria, A. A., Radua, J., & Rubia, K. (2016). Meta-analysis of fMRI studies of disruptive behavior disorders. *American Journal of Psychiatry, 173,* 1119–1130.

Alink, L. R. A., van IJzendoorn, M. H., Bakermans-Kranenburg, M. J., Mesman, J., Juffer, F., & Koot, H. M. (2008). Cortisol and externalizing behavior in children and adolescents: Mixed meta-analytic evidence for the inverse relation of basal cortisol and cortisol reactivity with externalizing behavior. *Developmental Psychobiology, 50,* 427–450.

Bakermans-Kranenburg, M. J., van IJzendoorn, M. H., & Juffer, F. (2003). Less is more: Meta-analyses of sensitivity and attachment interventions in early childhood. *Psychological Bulletin, 129,* 195–215.

Bandura, A. (1973). *Aggression: A social learning analysis*. Englewood Cliffs, NJ: Prentice-Hall.

Barber, B. K. (1996). Parental psychological control: Revisiting a neglected construct. *Child Development, 67,* 3296–3319.

Baumrind, D. (1966). Effects of authoritative control on child behavior. *Child Development, 37,* 887–907.

Belsky, J. (1984). The determinants of parenting: A process model. *Child Development, 55,* 83–96.

Belsky, J., & de Haan, M. (2011). Annual research review: Parenting and children's brain development: The end of the beginning. *Journal of Child Psychology and Psychiatry, 52,* 409–428.

Belsky, J., & Pluess, M. (2009). Beyond diathesis–stress: Differential susceptibility to environmental influence. *Psychological Bulletin, 135,* 885–908.

Bowlby, J. (1982). *Attachment and loss: Vol. 1. Attachment.* New York: Basic Books. (Original work published 1969)

Bowlby, J. (1988). Developmental psychiatry comes of age. *American Journal of Psychiatry, 145,* 1–10.

Braga, T., Goncalves, L. C., Basto-Pereira, M., & Maia, A. (2017). Unraveling the link between maltreatment and juvenile antisocial behavior: A meta-analysis of prospective longitudinal studies. *Aggression and Violent Behavior, 33,* 37–50.

Burt, S. A. (2009). Are there meaningful etiological differences within antisocial behavior?: Results of a meta-analysis. *Clinical Psychology Review, 29,* 163–178.

Byrd, A. L., & Manuck, S. B. (2014). MAOA, childhood maltreatment, and antisocial behavior: Meta-analysis of a gene–environment interaction. *Biological Psychiatry, 75,* 9–17.

Caspi, A., McClay, J., Moffitt, T. E., Mill, J., Martin, J., Craig, I. W., et al. (2002). Role of genotype in the cycle of violence in maltreated children. *Science, 297,* 851–854.

Chabris, C. F., Lee, J. J., Cesarini, D., Benjamin, D. J., & Laibson, D. I. (2015). The fourth law of behavior genetics. *Current Directions in Psychological Science, 24,* 304–312.

Cicchetti, D. (1993). Developmental psychopathology: Reactions, reflections, projections. *Developmental Review, 13,* 471–502.

Cicchetti, D., & Tucker, D. (1994). Development and self-regulatory structures of the mind. *Development and Psychopathology, 6,* 533–549.

Clarke, A. M., & Clarke, A. D. B. (2000). *Early experience and the life path.* London: Jessica Kingsley.

Cohen, J. (1992). A power primer. *Psychological Bulletin, 112,* 155–159.

Crick, N. R., & Dodge, K. A. (1994). A review and reformulation of social information-processing mechanisms in children's social adjustment. *Psychological Bulletin, 115,* 74–101.

Dishion, T. J., & Patterson, G. R. (2016). The development and ecology of antisocial behavior: Linking etiology, prevention, and treatment. In D. Cicchetti (Ed.), *Developmental psychopathology: Vol. 3. Maladaptation and psychopathology* (3rd ed., pp. 647–678). Hoboken, NJ: Wiley.

Dodge, K. A. (1986). A social information processing model of social competence in children. In M. Perlmutter (Ed.), *The Minnesota Symposium on Child Psychology: Vol. 18. Cognitive perspectives on children's social and behavioral development* (pp. 77–125). Hillsdale, NJ: Erlbaum.

Dodge, K. A., Bates, J. E., & Pettit, G. S. (1990). Mechanisms in the cycle of violence. *Science, 250,* 1678–1683.

Erickson, M. F., Sroufe, L. A., & Egeland, B. (1985). The relationship between quality of attachment and behavior problems in preschool in a high-risk sample. In I. Bretherton & E. Waters (Eds.), Growing points of attachment theory and research. *Monographs of the Society for Research in Child Development, 50,* 147–166.

Fairchild, G., Van Goozen, S. H. M., Calder, A. J., & Goodyer, I. M. (2013). Research review: Evaluating and reformulating the developmental taxonomic theory of antisocial behaviour. *Journal of Child Psychology and Psychiatry, and Allied Disciplines, 54,* 924–940.

Fearon, R. P., Bakermans-Kranenburg, M. J., van IJzendoorn, M. H., Lapsley, A. M., & Roisman, G. I. (2010). The significance of insecure attachment and disorganization in the development of children's externalizing behavior: A meta-analytic study. *Child Development, 81,* 435–456.

Forsman, M., & Langstrom, N. (2012). Child maltreatment and adult violent offending: Population-based twin study addressing the "cycle of violence" hypothesis. *Psychological Medicine, 42,* 1977–1983.

Fraley, R. C., Roisman, G. I., & Haltigan, J. D. (2013). The legacy of early experiences in development: Formalizing alternative models of how early experiences are carried forward over time. *Developmental Psychology, 49,* 109–125.

Gershoff, E. T., & Grogan-Kaylor, A. (2016). Spanking and child outcomes: Old controversies and new meta-analyses. *Journal of Family Psychology, 30,* 453–469.

Gershoff, E. T., Lee, S. J., & Durrant, J. E. (2017). Promising intervention strategies to reduce parents' use of physical punishment. *Child Abuse and Neglect, 71,* 9–23.

Gilbert, R., Widom, C., Browne, K., Fergusson, D., Webb, E., & Janson, S. (2009). Burden and consequences of child maltreatment in high-income countries. *Lancet, 373,* 68–81.

Gunnar, M., & Quevedo, K. (2007). The neurobiology of stress and development. *Annual Review of Psychology, 58,* 145–173.

Hinde, R. A. (1987). *Individuals, relationships, and culture: Links between ethology and the social sciences.* Cambridge, UK: Cambridge University Press.

Humphreys, K. L., Gleason, M. M., Drury, S. S., Miron, D., Nelson, C. A., Fox, N. A., et al. (2015). Effects of institutional rearing and foster care on psychopathology at age 12 years in Romania: Follow-up of an open, randomised controlled trial. *Lancet Psychiatry, 2,* 625–634.

Jaffee, S. R., Caspi, A., Moffitt, T. E., Polo-Tomas, M., Price, T. S., & Taylor, A. (2004). The limits of child effects: Evidence for genetically mediated child effects on corporal punishment but not on physical maltreatment. *Developmental Psychology, 40,* 1047–1058.

Jaffee, S. R., Strait, L. B., & Odgers, C. L. (2012). From correlates to causes: Can quasi-experimental studies and statistical innovations bring us closer to identifying the causes of antisocial behavior? *Psychological Bulletin, 138,* 272–295.

Juffer, F., & van IJzendoorn, M. H. (2005). Behavior problems and mental health referrals of international adoptees: A meta-analysis. *Journal of the American Medical Association, 293,* 2501–2515.

Kagan, J. (1980). Four questions in psychological development. *International Journal of Behavioral Development, 3,* 231–241.

Kaminski, J., Valle, L., Filene, J., & Boyle, C. (2008). A meta-analytic review of components associated with parent training program effectiveness. *Journal of Abnormal Child Psychology, 36,* 567–589.

Kawabata, Y., Alink, L. R., Tseng, W. L., van IJzendoorn, M. H., & Crick, N. R. (2011). Maternal and paternal parenting styles associated with relational aggression in children and adolescents: A conceptual analysis and meta-analytic review. *Developmental Review, 31,* 240–278.

Keijser, L. (2016). Parental monitoring and adolescent problem behaviors: How much do we really know? *International Journal of Behavioral Development, 40,* 271–281.

Kerr, M., & Stattin, H. (2000). What parents know, how they know it, and several forms of adolescent adjustment: Further support for a reinterpretation of monitoring. *Developmental Psychology, 36,* 366–380.

Kerr, M., Stattin, H., & Özdemir, M. (2012). Perceived parenting style and adolescent adjustment: Revisiting directions of effects and the role of parental knowledge. *Developmental Psychology, 48,* 1540–1553.

Klahr, A. M., & Burt, S. A. (2014). Elucidating the etiology of individual differences in parenting: A meta-analysis of behavioral genetic research. *Psychological Bulletin, 140,* 544–586.

Kochanska, G., Barry, R. A., Stellern, S. A., & O'Bleness, J. J. (2009). Early attachment organization moderates the parent–child mutually coercive pathway to children's antisocial
conduct. *Child Development, 80,* 1288–1300.

Lind, T., Bernard, K., Ross, E., & Dozier, M. (2014). Intervention effects on negative affect
of CPS-referred children: Results of a randomized clinical trial. *Child Abuse and Neglect,
38,* 1459–1467.

Luke, N., & Banerjee, R. (2013). Differentiated associations between childhood maltreatment experiences and social understanding: A meta-analysis and systematic review.
Developmental Review, 33, 1–28.

Maccoby, E. E. (2007). Historical overview of socialization research and theory. In J. E. Grusec & P. D. Hastings (Eds.), *Handbook of socialization: Theory and research* (pp. 13–41).
New York: Guilford Press.

Maccoby, E. E., & Martin, J. A. (1983). Socialization in the context of the family: Parent–
child interaction. In P. H. Mussen (Series Ed.) & E. M. Hetherington (Vol. Ed.), *Handbook of child psychology: Vol. 4. Socialization, personality, and social development* (4th ed.,
pp. 1–101). New York: Wiley.

Moffitt, T. E. (1993). Adolescence-limited and life-course-persistent antisocial behavior: A
developmental taxonomy. *Psychological Review, 100,* 674–701.

Nelson, D. A., & Crick, N. R. (2002). Parental psychological control: Implications for child-
hood physical and relational aggression. In B. K. Barber (Ed.), *Intrusive parenting:
How psychological control affects children and adolescents* (pp. 161–189). Washington, DC:
American Psychological Association.

Orobio de Castro, B., Veerman, J. W., Koops, W., Bosch, J. D., & Monshouwer, H. J. (2002).
Hostile attribution of intent and aggressive behavior: A meta-analysis. *Child Development, 73,* 916–934.

Patterson, G. R. (1982). *Coercive family process.* Eugene, OR: Castalia.

Patterson, G. R., DeBaryshe, B. D., & Ramsey, E. (1989). A developmental perspective on
antisocial behavior. *American Psychologist, 44,* 329–335.

Pinquart, M. (2017). Associations of parenting dimensions and styles with externalizing
problems of children and adolescents: An updated meta-analysis. *Developmental Psychology, 53,* 873–932.

Roisman, G. I., & Fraley, R. C. (2012a). A behavior–genetic study of the legacy of early caregiving experiences: Academic skills, social competence, and externalizing behavior in
kindergarten. *Child Development, 83,* 728–742.

Roisman, G. I., & Fraley, R. C. (2012b). The legacy of early interpersonal experience. In J.
B. Benson (Ed.), *Advances in child development and behavior* (Vol. 42, pp. 79–112). Burlington, VT: Academic Press.

Rutter, M. (2007). Proceeding from observed correlation to causal inference: The use of
natural experiments. *Perspectives on Psychological Science, 2,* 377–395.

Sameroff, A. (2010). A unified theory of development: A dialectic integration of nature and
nurture. *Child Development, 81,* 6–22.

Schulz-Heik, R. J., Rhee, S. H., Silvern, L. E., Haberstick, B. C., Hopfer, C., Lessem, J. M.,
et al. (2010). The association between conduct problems and maltreatment: Testing
genetic and environmental mediation. *Behavior Genetics, 40,* 338–348.

Sroufe, L. A. (1990). An organizational perspective on the self. In D. Cicchetti & M. Beeghly
(Eds.), *The self in transition: Infancy to childhood* (pp. 281–307). Chicago: University of
Chicago Press.

Sroufe, L. A. (1997). Psychopathology as an outcome of development. *Development and Psychopathology, 9,* 251–268.

Sroufe, L. A., Carlson, E. A., Levy, A. K., & Egeland, B. (1999). Implications of attachment
theory for developmental psychopathology. *Development and Psychopathology, 11,* 1–13.

Sroufe, L. A., Egeland, B., Carlson, E., & Collins, W. A. (2005). Placing early attachment experiences in developmental context: The Minnesota Longitudinal Study. In K. E. Grossmann, K. Grossmann, & E. Waters (Eds.), *Attachment from infancy to adulthood: The major longitudinal studies* (pp. 48–70). New York: Guilford Press.

Sroufe, L. A., Egeland, B., & Kreutzer, T. (1990). The fate of early experience following developmental change: Longitudinal approaches to individual adaptation in childhood. *Child Development, 61,* 1363–1373.

Sulik, M. J., Blair, C. B., Mills-Koonce, R., Berry, D. J., Greenberg, M., & the Family Life Project Investigators. (2015). Early parenting and the development of externalizing behavior problems: Longitudinal mediation through children's executive function. *Child Development, 86,* 1588–1603.

Thornberry, T. P., & Henry, K. L. (2013). Intergenerational continuity in maltreatment. *Journal of Abnormal Child Psychology, 41,* 555–569.

Troy, M., & Sroufe, L. A. (1987). Victimization among preschoolers: Role of attachment relationship history. *Journal of American Academy of Child and Adolescent Psychiatry, 26,* 166–172.

van der Voort, A., Linting, M., Bakermans-Kranenburg, M. J., & van IJzendoorn, M. H. (2013). Delinquent and aggressive behaviors in early-adopted adolescents: Longitudinal predictions from child temperament and maternal sensitivity. *Children and Youth Services Review, 35,* 439–446.

Van Goozen, S. H. M., Fairchild, G., Snoek, H., & Harold, G. T. (2007). The evidence for a neurobiological model of childhood antisocial behavior. *Psychological Bulletin, 133,* 149–182.

van IJzendoorn, M. H., Palacios, J., Sonuga-Barke, E. J. S., Gunnar, M. R., Vorria, P., McCall, R. B., et al. (2011). Children in institutional care: Delayed development and resilience. In R. B. McCall, M. H. van IJzendoorn, F. Juffer, C. J. Groark, & V. K. Groza (Eds.), Children without permanent parents: Research, practice, and policy. *Monographs of the Society for Research on Child Development, 76,* 8–30.

Velderman, M. K., Bakermans-Kranenburg, M. J., Juffer, F., van IJzendoorn, M. H., Mangelsdorf, S. C., & Zevalking, J. (2006). Preventing preschool externalizing behavior problems through video-feedback intervention in infancy. *Infant Mental Health Journal, 27,* 466–493.

Widom, C. S., Czaja, S., & Dutton, M. A. (2014). Child abuse and neglect and intimate partner violence victimization and perpetration: A prospective investigation. *Child Abuse and Neglect, 38,* 650–663.

CHAPTER 10

Aggression and Functioning
with Peers

WILLIAM M. BUKOWSKI and FRANK VITARO

Brief Introduction

It would not be unreasonable to expect the association between aggression and peer relations to be relatively simple. Aggression is typically seen as a negative form of behavior. It is, by definition, a form of behavior intended to cause harm. It is known to disrupt human functioning. Moreover, aggressive individuals are at risk for maladaptive outcomes. In contrast, peer relations are seen as having either very positive or very negative features. Relations with peers promote well-being, and they form important functions that add to healthy development (Rubin, Bukowski, & Bowker, 2015). Interactions and relationships with peers can also have negative effects (Vitaro, Boivin, & Bukowski, 2009). Experiences with peers such as exclusion, victimization, and friendlessness are known to have negative effects on well-being (Bukowski, Castellanos, Vitaro, & Brendgen, 2015). What's so difficult about expecting aggression to be negatively associated with the positive forms of peer relations and to be positively associated with the negative forms?

The problem with this view is its naive simplicity. Aggression and peer relations are complex phenomena. Both are composed of multiple processes and features that are manifested in diverse ways and serve a broad set of purposes. The attributes and mechanisms of aggression and peer relations are too complex and multifaceted to be conceived of according to a binary positive–negative scheme. Instead, they intersect in many ways that vary across individuals, age, and contexts. Our goal in this chapter is to discuss what we know about peer relations and aggression. Our discussion is based on an understanding of the basic types of experiences that children have with their peers and on a view of the basic processes that underlie these experiences. We take a process-oriented approach in which we show how aggression is implicated in what goes on between peers and how these experiences affect subsequent well-being and functioning.

As a means of helping our readers, we can state at the outset the conclusions we reach. We conclude that (1) aggression plays a complicated role in children's experiences with peers; (2) it can promote and deter attraction; (3) it can facilitate formation of friendship and can function to disrupt friendship; (4) it can be a form of incompetence and of competence; (5) it can promote status within the group and it can be the consequence of status; and (6) its effects vary across forms of aggression and as a function of participants' personal characteristics, notably age, sex, and behavior profile, and as a function of contextual/cultural factors. None of our conclusions can be seen as simple.

Before we begin, a final word of introduction is needed. For most children, the peer group is probably the context in which aggression is produced, experienced, and observed most frequently. Some children, of course, see and experience aggression in their families, either as part of the interaction between their parents or as the experiences they have with parents and siblings (see Raby & Roisman, Chapter 9, this volume). For most children, however, the peer group is the primary context for aggressive behavior. For this reason, it is a fundamental context for the emergence and control of aggression.

We start our discussion with a description of the features and processes of the peer system. We then turn our attention to a discussion of the measures used to study aggression among peers. Next, we provide a summary of what we believe we currently know about peer relations and aggression. Finally, we provide some forward-thinking ideas in a conclusion section about what is needed in contemporary research on aggression.

Main Issues

What and Where Are Peer Relations?

To understand how aggression intersects with peer relations, one needs to have a view of what the term *peer relations* means. The term *peer relations* refers to the broad set of features and experiences that are relevant to what goes on between children and their agemates. The features and experiences implicated in peer relations are vast and diverse. They differ from each other in many ways, including their personal orientation, their structural properties, and their location at different levels of social complexity. *Personal orientation* refers to the degree to which they involve movement toward others, movement against others, or movement away from others (Bukowski, Laursen, & Rubin, 2018). Movement toward others is seen in forms of sociability, liking, attraction, altruism, inclusion, and cohesion. Movement against others is seen in forms of harm, conflict, victimization, exclusion, and aggression. Movement away from others is seen in forms of withdrawal or avoidance, which minimize interactions with others.

The *structural properties* of the features of peer relations refer to the positive and negative links a child has with peers. An interest in structural features was initially seen in Moreno's landmark publication *Who Shall Survive?* (1934). These features refer to the attractions and repulsions that occur between peers. They can be conceptualized as features of an individual, such as the degree to which a child is accepted (i.e., seen as a friend) or rejected (i.e., seen as an undesirable child) by peers, or as feature of groups, such as the number of links that exist between group members and the degree to which there are imbalances between members in the degree to which they are connected to others (Rubin et al., 2015).

Social complexity refers to the multiple level of experiences in which peer relations occur. Peer researchers have typically organized different forms of experiences with peers according to a three-level model. These levels are the individual, the dyad, and the group (Rubin et al., 2015). This three-level scheme is largely taken from the six-level model described by Hinde and Stevenson-Hinde (1987). The six levels in their model included (1) underlying *biological and psychological processes*; (2) characteristics of the *individual*; (3) *interpersonal interactions*; (4) forms, features, and qualitative aspects of *relationships*; (5) the social *group*(s) within which individuals and their interpersonal relationships are clustered; and (6) society/culture. At the level of the *individual* are the goals, tendencies, characteristics, and developmental histories that children bring to their experiences with peers. The level of the dyad includes *interactions* and *relationships*. Interactions refer to what children do with each other when they are together in person or connected via media and communication devices. Relationships are made up of the internalized representations and expectations that members of the dyad have of each other and of their interactions. Relationships are presumed to derive both from within individual features (e.g., temperament) and from the quality of experienced interpersonal interactions with specific others. Security and intimacy are important features of relationships (Furman & Buhrmester, 1985; Wood, Bukowski, & Santo, 2017), but so are conflict and jealousy. Finally, the levels of the individual and the dyad are situated within *groups*. Groups are networks of individuals and relationships with more or less clearly defined boundaries (see Sijtsema & Ojanen, Chapter 12, this volume). Some groups, such as school classrooms, have clear boundaries; the boundaries of other groups, such as a clique, are fuzzy. The structure within a group comes from the affective and interactive links between their members and by the types of behaviors, attitudes, and goals that are common to them. Groups differ from each other in their norms and shared conventions. These features of a group affect what is expected of group members, and they influence the type and range of relationships and interactions that are likely or permissible within the group. Groups have properties and processes that affect the degree to which members of the group can influence each other.

In Hinde and Stevenson-Hinde's (1987) model, the level of society/culture is treated as an overriding structure that ascribes meaning to constructs and experiences found at the other levels (Rubin, Oh, Menzer, & Ellison, 2011). Consistent with Geertz's (1973) meaning-based approach to anthropology, the cultural context is seen as a "significative" system that assigns value to individual-, dyadic-, or group-level variables. For example, the degree to which aggression is tolerated in a peer group may vary as a function of the degree of individualism within the current cultural context.

Like any other categorical model, this three-level scheme has its limitations. The most critical is the lack of clarity as to where some constructs are situated. For example, knowing that a child is aggressive in a particular group may reveal something about the child's behavioral tendencies and also something about the group's capacity to elicit aggressive behavior.

One form of overlap between the three levels serves as a strength of the model rather than as a limitation. This critical overlap is their interrelatedness in the dynamic processes that take place within peer interactions and relationships at the levels of the group and dyad. Consider, for example, the behaviors that are characteristic of a friendship between two peers. What these friends do with each other (i.e., how they interact with each other) will depend on what each of the two individual children brings to the friendship. Consider also that a child's experiences of interacting with a particular friend can lead to changes in how the child behaves. Similar points can be made about the level of the group. The behavior of individual children can change as they conform to group norms or as they internalize the forms of behavior that are characteristic of the group.

Two points are implicit to this description of a multilevel approach. The first is that the basic processes of peer experiences typically involve measures from different levels of complexity. The second is that aspects of aggression can exist at all of these levels and that individual differences can exist at each of these levels. Some children are more aggressive than others, and some children are more tolerant or accepting of aggression than are others. Dyads differ in their level of aggression and in the degree to which aggression is seen as a normal way of behaving. Differences exist also between the level of aggression seen in the behaviors of some groups (i.e., descriptive norms) and in how much aggression is seen as normative (i.e., injunctive norms).

What Are the Basic Processes of the Peer System?

At the risk of minimizing the vast number of processes that occur within the peer system, one can argue that the peer system involves five basic interrelated processes. They can be conceived of as attraction, status hierarchies, influence, co-construction, and internalization. These processes are themselves made up of more specific constructs and mechanisms.

Attraction refers to the differences in children's preferences for associating with some peers more than others. It can be understood from two different perspectives. One perspective emphasizes the importance of the features of attractive peers. The premise of a features approach is that children with particular characteristics will be more or less attractive to their peers. The features that promote attraction are believed to be those that (1) make a person interesting and engaging, (2) conform to normative expectations, and (3) facilitate another's person's functioning (see Rubin et al., 2015). The emphasis on the features model has been seen since the earliest days on peer research (see Monroe, 1898).

Another perspective on attraction concerns the importance of similarity (Laursen, 2017). The hypothesis that similarity underlies attraction as a formal model in psychological research is at least 50 years old (Hinde, 1966). The argument can be stated simply: Beginning in the preschool years, children appear to be attracted to, and to become friends with, peers whose behavioral tendencies are similar to their own (Rubin, Lynch, Coplan, Rose-Krasnor, & Booth, 1994). Similarity between friends has been shown on several dimensions of behavior, including prosocial and antisocial behaviors (Haselager, Hartup, van Lieshout, & Riksen-Walraven, 1998) shyness and internalized distress (Rubin, Wojslawowicz, Burgess, Rose-Krasnor, & Booth-LaForce, 2006), and academic achievement and motivation (Liu & Chen, 2003). The extent of similarity appears to vary across friendships. Hamm (2000), for example, showed that similarity among friends on a particular dimension varied across children largely according to the importance the child ascribed to it. For example, similarity to one's friend on academic performance was highest among children who saw academic performance as important. The similarity model is relational in the sense that the importance of any particular feature will vary as a function of the degree to which it is a feature of other members of the group.

Attraction can be further dissected into the processes of acceptance and rejection, or liking and disliking. This distinction recognizes that these two forms of affect are not polar opposites. That is, the absence of acceptance (i.e. not being attracted to someone) does not imply the presence of rejection or repulsion, just as the absence of disliking does not imply the presence of liking. The point of this distinction is that attraction is made up of two intertwined systems, one having to do with positive affect that brings peers together and one that has to do with negative affect that keeps them apart.

Status hierarchies refer to the differential levels of power and influence that exist within a group (Bukowski & Sippola, 2001; Sijtsema & Ojanen, Chapter 12, this volume). Two forces account for the presence of status hierarchies in groups. First, in order to evolve in adaptive ways, groups need leaders who use power to make decisions and to establish norms and expectations. As a consequence, in most groups a power hierarchy will emerge so that the group can maintain its membership and respond to internal and external demands. Second, typically within groups there are differences between individual members in the need for dominance and control. As a function of these differences, some individuals will have more influence than others. In peer groups, status is typically manifested as popularity.

Peer influence refers to the processes by which peers affect each other's behavior. One of the oldest hypotheses about peer relations is that children shape other's behaviors via the mechanisms of reinforcement and imitation. Laboratory-based analogue studies have provided compelling evidence that children imitate their peers and that children's behavior can be shaped by reinforcements received from peers (see Hartup, 1964). Findings from studies of the effects of imitation indicated that children use each other as sources of information about the forms of behavior that are most appropriate for functioning with peers. More recently, these processes were conceived of as forms of coordinated exchange-based action that creates exclusive interdependencies between peers that lead to increased levels of interpersonal similarity (Laursen, 2017). In turn, this similarity increases the interconnection between peers and promotes further similarity.

Whereas attraction has to do with an affective process and peer influence is typically studied with behavioral indicators, *co-construction* is a cognitive process that is promoted by peer interaction. Both Piaget and Vygotsky have credited peer interaction with a role in the development of children's conceptions of social life. Piaget (1932) emphasized the role of peer discourse, conflict resolution, and negotiation as the interactional contexts in which social constructs were developed. Piaget believed that in their interactions with peers, children could examine conflicting ideas, understand different points of view, and reconcile the differences between them. Vygotsky (Tudge, 1992; Vygotsky, 1978) also emphasized the importance of peer interaction, especially as it would promote the internalization of social concepts, norms, and values.

The fifth and final process we describe is similar to the process of co-construction in the sense that it involves internalization (i.e., a process of self-perception based on others' views of oneself). Theory from Vygotsky and from a set of sociologists known collectively as the symbolic interactionists (e.g., Mead, 1934) and the views of the American psychiatrist Harry Stack Sullivan support the claim that people define themselves according to how they believe they are perceived by others. According to the symbolic interactionists, children's internalizations of how they are perceived and treated by others not only form the basis of the self-concept but also of how they perceive and treat others. Mead (1934) claimed that exchanges among peers that involve power, cooperation, competition, conflict, and/or friendly discussion provide a basic platform for developing a sense of one's basic characteristics and of how one can and should treat other people.

Measures: What Types of Aggression Are Studied in Peer Research?

Before turning our attention to the question of how aggression is implicated in the processes we have just described, it is important for us to identify the kinds of aggression that are studied in peer research and how these forms of aggression are assessed (see Ostrov, Perry, & Blakely-McClure, Chapter 3, this volume). Procedures to measure aggression in childhood and early adolescence have typically relied on peer assessment procedures to provide efficient, reliable, and valid indices of multiple forms of aggression (see Bukowski, Cillessen, & Velasquez, 2012). Peer assessment procedures use a questionnaire-based format in which the participants indicate which of their peers participating in the study fit particular items that describe forms of behavior. Persons are given scores according to how often they are chosen for each item. Typically, items used in peer assessments to measure aggression emphasize either different forms or different "functions" of aggression. The two forms of aggression that have received the most attention are physical aggression and relational aggression (Ostrov et al., Chapter 3, this volume). Whereas physical aggression is carried out directly via actions such as hitting or pushing, relational aggression is carried out indirectly via efforts to disrupt a person's interactions with others or to negatively affect their reputations. The two functions that have been studied the most are proactive and reactive aggression. Proactive aggression occurs without provocation, whereas reactive aggression follows provocation. Example items (taken from Bukowski, Schwartzman, Santo, Bagwell, & Adam, 2009) are: "Someone who gets into physical fights" for physical aggression; "Someone who tells lies about others" for relational aggression; "Someone who can get into fights even if no one has bothered him/her" for proactive aggression, and "Someone who can get into fights but only when someone has bothered him/her first" for reactive aggression. These types of aggression have received the lion's share of attention in peer research.

In the next sections we turn our attention to the ways that aggression is implicated in the basic processes of peer interactions and relationships.

Attraction: Aggression, Rejection, and Acceptance

The role of aggression in the processes of attraction can be assessed according to the constructs of rejection and acceptance. It can also be seen from the perspective of popularity. The most attention has been paid to, and the clearest findings can be seen in, research on rejection. We start with a thorough discussion of rejection and aggression and then turn our attention to acceptance.

From Aggression to Peer Rejection

There is ample evidence showing that aggression predicts attraction and social preference at the peer-group level, although it is not the only predictor (Bierman, Kalvin, & Heinrichs, 2015). However, aggression specifically predicts the negative side of peer preference, that is, rejection/disliking, but not the positive side, that is, acceptance/liking (see Crick, Murray-Close, Marks, & Mohajeri-Nelson, 2009). Exceptions may nevertheless exist depending on the subtypes of aggressive behaviors under study. For example, Tseng, Banny, Kawabata, Crick, and Gau (2013) found that relational aggression during the elementary school years predicts both peer rejection and social acceptance, whereas physical aggression predicts only peer rejection. Participants' sex may also play a moderating role in this context, as the links between relational aggression and peer rejection are generally stronger in girls than in boys (Zimmer-Gembeck, Geiger, & Crick, 2005). Furthermore, the link between aggression and rejection may vary depending on children's age and the functions of aggression. Dodge, Coie, Pettit, and Price (1990) addressed this issue by looking at the association between aggression and rejection in play groups involving first- and third-grade boys. They also looked at different forms of aggressive behavior, including reactive aggression and instrumental aggression (a type of proactive aggression used to control resources), bullying (a type of proactive aggression used to dominate others), and rough play. Both reactive aggression and instrumental aggression, but not rough play, were associated with peer rejection at the end of the play sessions at both ages. Bullying was also related to peer rejection, but only among third graders, suggesting a heightened risk for proactively aggressive children to be rejected by middle childhood compared with early childhood. Combining these results with other findings showing that reactive aggression is repeatedly associated with heightened risk for peer rejection during the preschool years and during adolescence (Ostrov, Murray-Close, Godleski, & Hart, 2013; Prinstein & Cillessen, 2003), it is possible to conclude with some confidence that the relation between reactive aggression and rejection is stable across different developmental periods. In contrast, the pattern of associations between proactive aggression and peer rejection seems to vary with age in an apparent curvilinear mode. Hence, although proactive aggression has been linked to an increased risk for peer rejection during middle childhood (Dodge et al., 1990), it has been linked to a lowered risk for peer rejection during the preschool years (Ostrov et al., 2013) and during adolescence (Boivin, Hymel, & Hodges, 2001), although this might vary depending on the specific type of proactive aggression involved (i.e., instrumental vs. bullying; Prinstein & Cillessen, 2003). Finally, the association between aggression and rejection may vary depending on local norms. Indeed, the correlations between peer rejection and aggression are attenuated in classrooms in which the prevalence of aggression is high (Barth, Dunlap, Dane, Lochman, & Wells, 2004; Boivin, Dodge, & Coie, 1995; Stormshak et al., 1999). The above studies addressed the question of whether different types of aggressive behaviors determine peer rejection for different age groups and in different social ecologies. They did not address the question of whether peer rejection predicts an increase in different types of aggression with children and adolescents exposed to different contexts.

From Peer Rejection to Aggression

There is substantial evidence from correlational studies indicating that peer rejection predicts later aggressive behaviors, as well as other forms of maladjustment, even after controlling for baseline levels of aggressive behavior (see reviews by Bierman, 2004; Prinstein & Giletta, 2016). In addition, the longitudinal associations between peer rejection and aggression have been shown to be bidirectional (Lansford, Malone, Dodge, Pettit, & Bates, 2010; van Lier & Koot, 2010), possibly leading to an increasing spiraling association over time (but see Ladd, 2006, for an exception). This bidirectional association between peer rejection and aggression, and other externalizing problems, may begin early in childhood and persist over a number of years (Sturaro, van Lier, Cuijpers, & Koot, 2011). However, the precise role of peer rejection as an additive risk factor, a mediator, or a moderator remains unsettled. The view of peer rejection as an additive risk factor (i.e., as a main effect) proposes that peer rejection uniquely and independently contributes to the development of aggressive behaviors, above and beyond preexisting personal characteristics and other environmental stressors. There is evidence to support this view. To illustrate, peer rejection in elementary school has been found to predict later teacher-rated aggression above and beyond previous aggressive behaviors, concurrent peer victimization, and involvement in mutual friendships (Ladd & Troop-Gordon, 2003). Peer rejection during late childhood has also been found to predict the persistence of aggressive behavior into early adulthood (Rabiner, Coie, Miller-Johnson, Boykin, & Lochman, 2005). However, there is evidence that this "effect" of peer rejection affects reactive more than proactive aggression, at least in the short term (Dodge et al., 2003).

Another view posits that peer rejection is part of a developmental chain and mediates the association between children's behavior problems and later adjustment problems, with or without a residual additive effect of its own. For example, peer rejection has been found to partially mediate the link between personal characteristics such as disruptiveness or a difficult temperament and the growth of conduct problems over the following years (Buil, van Lier, Brendgen, Koot, & Vitaro, 2017), although only for boys in some studies (Snyder, Prichard, Schrepferman, Patrick, & Stoolmiller, 2004).

A third view posits that the association between peer rejection and aggression or other adjustment problems may be moderated by children's characteristics or contextual factors. This form of interaction is, in fact, a conditional variant of the main effect model; it simply posits that the contribution of peer rejection to the outcome is significant but conditional on participants' characteristics or contextual factors. To illustrate, Dodge and his colleagues (2003) found that persistent peer rejection beginning in kindergarten predicted growth in aggression, but only for children who were initially high on aggression, particularly reactive aggression. In another study, the link between one form of peer rejection, that is, peer victimization, and aggression was modulated by children's genetic risk for aggression, albeit only in girls. For boys, peer victimization was related to aggression regardless of the child's genetic risk for such behavior (Brendgen et al., 2008).

There is also a second form of the interaction view, as peer rejection might moderate the association between personal or socioenvironmental factors and aggression. From this perspective, peer rejection is the implicit moderator and personal or socioenvironmental characteristics are the main predictor. For example, the predictive association between aggression and later violence was found to be exacerbated for individuals who were rejected by their peers (DeRosier, Kupersmidt, & Patterson, 1994). Peer rejection has also been found to heighten the level of antisocial behavior resulting from a process known as deviancy training that often takes place among aggressive children or adolescents (Snyder, 2010). Importantly, it appears that it is peer rejection, and not peer acceptance, that is the active moderating force with respect to the link between aggression and later adjustment problems (Prinstein & La Greca, 2004).

Explanatory Mechanisms

Three mechanisms may account for the putative main or moderating "effect" of peer rejection on aggression. These mechanisms are not mutually exclusive, and they may differ as a function of the form of peer rejection (i.e., overt vs. covert) and the type of aggressive behavior under scrutiny. First, peer rejection (especially of the covert type, in which aggressive children are avoided by mainstream peers) reduces opportunities for rejected children to learn and to practice developmentally appropriate problem-solving skills (Coie, 1990). Missed learning opportunities explain why aggressive children who are rejected do not tend to decrease their aggressive behaviors with age as other children do (Broidy et al., 2003). Second, peer rejection (especially of the overt type, which involves open confrontation) can alter children's social information-processing abilities. Specifically, overt peer rejection could increase children's hypervigilance to hostile cues and their tendency to react aggressively in conflictual or threatening situations (Dodge et al., 2003; Lansford et al., 2010). Finally, peer rejection may encourage affiliation with other aggressive children who are also isolated from the peer group, further increasing their insulation from nonaggressive peers and their exposure to influence processes typical of aggressive dyads and cliques (Fabes, Hanish, & Martin, 2003).

Peer rejection, peer victimization, popularity, participation in a friendship, affiliation with aggressive friends, and friendship quality are theoretically and empirically distinct (Bukowski & Hoza, 1989). For example, many rejected children have at least one reciprocated friend and are not victimized (Gest, Graham-Bermann, & Hartup, 2001), whereas some aggressive adolescents are perceived as popular although they are disliked by the majority of their classmates (Bukowski, 2011; Prinstein & Cillessen, 2003). In turn, some aggressive children enjoy high-quality friendships, although friendships among aggressive friends are generally low in quality (Grotpeter & Crick, 1996). Yet peer rejection, peer victimization, popularity, participation in a friendship, affiliation with aggressive friends, and friendship quality may not operate independently. They may influence each other over time according to a cascade model, as suggested decades ago (e.g., Dishion, Patterson, Stoolmiller, & Skinner, 1991; Patterson, DeBaryshe, & Ramsey, 1989), or they may conspire together in a coactive or synergetic mode, possibly starting at an early age, as they tend to co-occur already in kindergarten (Snyder et al., 2008). A cascade model implies that different peer experiences operate in a sequential or a transactional mode, partially or totally mediating the link between early risk factors and later aggression. In contrast, a coaction model implies that different peer experiences work additively and independently (i.e., in parallel) in predicting children's or adolescents' aggressive behaviors, above and beyond early and concurrent risk factors. Finally, a synergetic model implies that different peer experiences interact with each other, potentiating their respective effects. A cascade model and a coactive model are in line, respectively, with a mediational or a main effect view of peer rejection and friendships, whereas a synergetic model is in line with an interactive view.

Two studies, to our knowledge, examined whether peer rejection and friends' aggressiveness operate according to a cascade or a coactive model in predicting the evolution of aggressive/disruptive behaviors from childhood to adolescence. In the first study, Laird, Jordan, Dodge, Pettit, and Bates (2001) did not find support for a cascade model, as adolescent-reported antisocial peer involvement played no role with respect to the relation between childhood peer rejection and adolescent behavior problems. In contrast, Vitaro, Pedersen and Brendgen (2007) found support for a cascade model. More specifically, peer rejection and friends' self-reports of aggressive/disruptive behavior during childhood mediated, in sequence, albeit partially, the link between early disruptiveness and interpersonal violence during adolescence. Other studies examined different peer experiences concurrently at one time point only, mainly during childhood (Powers, Bierman, & Conduct Problems Prevention Research Group, 2013; Snyder et al., 2008; Werner & Crick, 2004). These studies found support for a parallel-coactive model, in which peer rejection and friends' aggressiveness independently and simultaneously predict changes in aggressive/disruptive behavior.

Although the focus of most studies was on the interplay between peer rejection and affiliation with aggressive friends, some examined the interplay between other types of peer difficulties, such as peer victimization, friendlessness (i.e., having no friends), and friendship quality. These studies are reviewed next, after a quick overview of how these peer difficulties are linked to each other over time. Ladd and Troop-Gordon (2003) found that rejection was predictive of later victimization and that victimization reciprocally influenced later peer rejection throughout elementary school. According to these authors, peer rejection also predicted friendlessness, but friendlessness did not contribute to the development of other forms of peer adversities. These results partly concord with a study by Salmivalli and Isaacs (2005) showing that peer rejection unilaterally predicted friendlessness; however, in contrast to Ladd and Troop-Gordon, Salmivalli and Isaacs did not find reciprocal links between peer rejection and peer victimization, only unilateral links from peer rejection to peer victimization.

Ladd and Troop-Gordon (2003) further found that peer rejection and peer victimization independently contributed to children's externalizing problems. However, these results were partly contradicted by Bierman and colleagues (2015) who reported that peer rejection, but not peer victimization, contributed to young adolescents' delinquent behaviors, as well as school difficulties, whereas peer victimization uniquely predicted adolescent depressed mood and social problems. These two groups of authors were nevertheless in accord regarding the specific contribution of friendlessness. Similarly to others (van Lier & Koot, 2010; Vitaro et al., 1997), they found no contribution of friendship participation when the outcome referred to externalizing problems. This statement, however, may need to be qualified by personal or contextual factors given that for rejected children, having mutual friends was found to be related to an increase in their aggressive behaviors, probably because their friends are aggressive and their friendships are of low quality (Kupersmidt, Burchinal, & Patterson, 1995; Lansford, Yu, Pettit, Bates, & Dodge, 2014). However, as already mentioned, aggressive children sometimes enjoy positive friendships. In this case, it is worth noting that a high-quality friendship can mitigate the usual spiral found between aggression and social-cognitive bias or lead to a decrease in aggression opposite to, and independent from, friends' aggression (Bowker, Rubin, Rose-Krasner, & Booth-Laforce, 2007; Salvas et al., 2011).

Some final comments are in order. First, most of the above studies used longitudinal designs spanning sometimes several years, although the number of studies covering more than one developmental period remains scarce. Second, all the above studies controlled for baseline behavior problems and some, in addition, controlled for concurrent behavior problems and autoregressive paths through the use of a cross-lagged design. Third, all the above studies reported a link between baseline behavior problems, especially aggression, and peer experiences, and many reported a residual link between baseline or concurrent behavior problems and their outcomes. Yet none of the above studies examined the conjoint role of two or more types of peer experiences longitudinally while simultaneously distinguishing between forms and functions of aggression. The only researchers who simultaneously examined the contribution of popularity (social reputation) and peer rejection (social preference) found that both types of peer status measures independently contributed to an increase in different types of aggressive behavior during adolescence (i.e., overt, relational, and reputational), although the increase for overt aggression was limited to girls (Prinstein & Cillessen, 2003). These researchers, like others, however, did not take into account the overlap between different types of aggressive behavior. Moreover, few of the above studies examined the possible moderating role of important personal factors. As noted throughout this chapter, the nature, consequences, and interplay of different peer experiences can vary as a function of children's age and sex. However, whether participants' developmental profiles also play a role with respect to the strength and the timing of the association between different peer experiences and changes in aggression remains unknown. Resolving this issue may help reconcile the complex and sometimes contradictory pattern of results in reference to the interplay between different peer experiences. Simply said, it is possible that peer rejection and selection of aggressive friends or friend-lessness operate concurrently, starting in early childhood for early starters who are prone to behavior problems. For late starters, however, a sequential mediational model is more plausible; in this case, early peer rejection, which does not necessarily derive from aggression, may leave rejected children isolated from the normative peer group and slowly drive them toward other rejected youth, some of whom are aggressive (see Chen, Drabick, & Burgers, 2015, for a similar model). Early starters are defined as children, mostly boys, who engage in antisocial behavior, mostly of the aggressive type, early in life, whereas late starters are defined as children who engage in antisocial behavior, mostly of the nonaggressive type, by early adolescence (Moffitt, 1993; Patterson et al., 1989).

Moderators should also include important contextual factors, such as social norms toward aggression, which may vary among classrooms, sexes, and developmental periods, thereby possibly affecting the interplay between different types of peer experiences and aggressive behavior. Two types of social norms have been identified: descriptive and injunctive. *Descriptive* norms correspond to the degree to which aggressive behavior is displayed by members of a particular group, whereas *injunctive* norms reflect the degree of acceptability of aggression within the group. Yet few studies have examined how social norms affect the impact of peer experiences, such as peer rejection and affiliation with aggressive peers, on children's aggression. For example, some researchers found that the social preference of aggressive children varied depending on social norms (Stormshak et al., 1999): Among boys, aggression was positively, not negatively, associated with social preference in the most aggressive classrooms.

Descriptive norms may also determine the number of aggressive friends a child can nominate. This may simply be a function of the greater density of aggressive children in aggressive classrooms. Hence, children in aggressive classrooms are likely to have more aggressive friends than similar children in nonaggressive classrooms because aggressive children are less disliked in these classrooms. Hence, social norms may indirectly affect children's aggression through their impact on peer acceptance or rejection and the availability of aggressive friends. As shown by Powers and colleagues (2013) and others (Boivin et al., 1995; Stormshak et al., 1999), social norms can also affect levels of children's aggression, possibly because deviancy training at the group level is more prevalent or because genetic dispositions toward aggression can be more easily expressed without risk for sanctions (Vitaro et al., 2015; see Brendgen, Vitaro, & Boivin, Chapter 4, this volume). Finally, social norms can exacerbate the impact of peer rejection or affiliation with deviant friends, although no study to our knowledge reported evidence in this regard. In all cases, social norms may be an important contextual factor to consider, in addition to personal characteristics, when examining the interplay between peer rejection and children's or adolescents' aggressive behaviors.

Acceptance and Aggression

In contrast to research on aggression and rejection, research on the association between aggression and acceptance has been less frequent, less thorough, and less conclusive. The available evidence indicates that, at best, the association between aggression and acceptance is weak (Rubin et al., 2015). Evidence from studies done in a prior era of peer research indicated that, although children who are rejected by peers typically showed higher levels of aggression, children who are accepted by peers do not, on average, differ from others on aggression (Rubin, Bukowski, & Parker, 2006). When accepted children do engage in aggressive behavior, it tends to resemble assertiveness rather than disruptiveness or harmful forms of action that are likely to impede the goals of their peers (Newcomb, Bukowski & Pattee, 1993).

There may be four explanations for this weak association between aggression and acceptance. One is consistent with a features model. It recognizes that aggression is correlated with features that may be seen as positive and that promote attraction. In spite of the trouble they cause, some aggressive children can be exciting and amusing and can have a positive place in the peer-group hierarchy. These correlated features may function to minimize the negative consequences of aggression on liking, leading to weak associations between these measures.

A second explanation takes a dyadic perspective and uses a similarity model (Bukowski, Sippola, & Newcomb, 2000). It recognizes that liking occurs at the level of the person and that children may be drawn to peers to whom they are similar. According to this view, aggressive children will be attracted to other aggressive children, whereas nonaggressive children will not be. Assuming there are more nonaggressive children than aggressive children, these similarity-based attraction patterns would lead to a mild negative association between aggression and attraction. Evidence on the effects of this similarity-based explanation can be found in Bukowski and colleagues (2000).

A third explanation emphasizes developmental variations. Moffitt (1993) has proposed that in early adolescence aggression is seen more favorably than in childhood. Instead of being viewed as a form of harmful disruptiveness, it is perceived as a form of adult-like power and assertiveness. Accordingly, aggression becomes normative, rather than non-normative. As a consequence, it functions as a source of attraction instead of as a form of repulsion.

A fourth explanation also emphasizes the concept of normativeness. As already discussed, individuals and groups have norms, or standards, regarding the "acceptability" of particular acts. Insofar as the degree to which a child is accepted by peers derives from whether the child engages in normative behaviors, and if norms vary across groups and individuals, then the association between acceptance and a form of behavior will vary as a function of group norms. Behaviors that are universally valued will, for the most part, show a positive correlation with peer acceptance; when the normativeness of a behavior varies across groups, its association with acceptance will also vary. As a result, the overall association between acceptance and aggression may be weak.

Peer Influence

The current literature on peer influence and aggression is robust. Many effects have been widely replicated, and researchers have used sophisticated and powerful designs to examine the degree of influence between friends. The typical model used to assess peer influence is relatively simple, but it involves an important difference from most studies of children's behavior. It typically consists of a two-wave longitudinal cross-lagged panel design. It differs from other uses of this design in its use of a friendship dyad, rather than an individual child, as the unit of analysis. With this approach, at each of the two times, there is a measure of the variable of interest for each of the two friends in the dyad. The degree of peer influence is shown by the extent to which each friend's score at Time 1 predicts the other friend's score at Time 2. Although the dyad is the unit of analysis in this model, one can assess whether one friend has more influence than the other friend. There is extensive evidence that peers in a dyad become more similar to each other as a function of the continuity of their friendship. The evidence, recently reviewed by Laursen (2017), shows that this process can affect the level of a child's aggressive behavior and that the higher-status member of a dyad has a stronger effect on the partner than does the lower-status member (another example of the intricate and interdependent nature of different aspects of peer relationships). There is also evidence that when the dyad initially presents an unreciprocated level of liking (i.e., one child has chosen a peer as a friend, but the peer had not chosen him or her), the child who was not chosen at first shows a higher level of change (Bukowski & Adams, 2005).

As mentioned earlier, the effects of peer influence on aggressive behavior have been attributed to mechanisms of reinforcement and imitation that fit within the rubric known as *deviancy training* (Dishion, McCord, & Poulin, 1999). This term refers to the processes of praise, encouragement, imitation, and expectancy by which children increase the level of *aggression* or *antisocial behavior* in their peers. Essentially, deviancy training occurs when children model and reward aggressive behaviors in each other; the process by which these exchanges take place is thought to increase individual tendencies in aggressiveness and to strengthen ties to aggressive and substance-abusing friends and delinquent peer groups. In this regard, deviancy training "hits" at all levels of the social complexity. However, coercion processes and victimization among aggressive dyads or aggressive clique members may also be at work (Vitaro et al., 2011).

Aggression and Status (Popularity)

A third basic process of the peer system is the emergence of status hierarchies. There is no shortage of evidence that aggression appears to promote a child's status in the peer group (Hawley, Little, & Pasupathi, 2002; Lease, Kennedy, & Axelrod, 2002). Typically, studies of the association between aggression and popularity are framed according to fundamental aspects of group process, such as dominance, resource control, and use of retaliatory gestures between group members (Hawley, 2003). Children who show an above-average level of aggression and who use aggression for instrumental reasons are perceived to be more popular in their groups than are children who are low in aggression or whose aggression is especially high (Hawley, 2003; Prinstein & Cillessen, 2003).

Although the association between aggression and popularity may be seen even during early childhood (Vaughn, Vollenweider, Bost, Azria-Evans, & Snider, 2003), this association becomes stronger during early adolescence (Cillessen & Mayeux, 2004; Prinstein & Cillessen, 2003). It is important to recognize that although aggression is positively associated with popularity during early adolescence (Cillessen & Mayeux, 2004;), it is not related to acceptance (Buskirk et al., 2004). Moderately aggressive children are given status and power within the peer group, but they do not receive affection from peers. This pattern raises the question: In what ways are aggressive children competent and in what ways are they incompetent (Bukowski, 2003)?

The observation that aggression and status are interrelated confirms ideas about group functioning and about how groups reward persons who facilitate a group's functioning (Bukowski & Sippola, 2001). In contrast to the level of dyad, where the primary rewards may be affection and security, the primary rewards available at the level of the group are power, attention, and status. These rewards appear to be provided to group leaders even though their behavior may, at times, include a larger coercive or aggressive component than is seen among other children. This tendency to ascribe power and status to moderately aggressive individuals may be more pronounced in adolescence, when aggression is seen as a more normative entity than among children (Moffitt, 1993). As a result, status, leadership, and aggression may often go together, especially for young adolescents (Prinstein & Cillessen, 2003).

Aggression and Co-construction

Of all the basic processes of peer interactions, the one that has received the least attention is co-construction. How children's interactions with their peers influence their thoughts about aggression is an understudied phenomenon. It is known that children vary in their tolerance of aggression and that these differences are associated with experiences with peers (Ellis, Chung-Hall, & Dumas, 2013). Nevertheless, the degree to which this association is due to co-construction is not clear.

Aggression and Internalization

The association between aggression and internalization is also understudied. Although one can reasonably hypothesize that acting in aggressive ways and being seen as aggressive will promote a view of oneself as an aggressive individual, evidence of this association is weak (Rubin et al., 2015). This lack of evidence that aggressive children will see themselves in this way likely occur for two reasons. First, there is evidence that aggressive children are more likely than other boys and girls to have an inflated sense of self and that this form of self-distortion will support the continuity of aggressive behavior (Bukowski, Schwartzman, Santo, Bagwell, & Adams, 2009). These distortions are known to be more strongly related to reactive aggression than to proactive aggression and more strongly related to relational aggression than to physical aggression. Second, if it is the case that aggressive children can achieve a place of status in the peer group, then when aggressive children think about themselves, they may be inclined to emphasize their presumably more positive features than their level of aggression behavior.

Future Directions

In this final section, we present a blueprint for where research on peer relations and aggression may go in the next wave of studies. We propose nine new directions: (1) sticking close to the definition of aggression; (2) distinguishing between subtypes of aggressive behavior; (3) understanding the mechanisms of reward within the peer system; (4) examining different types of peer experiences specifically and repeatedly; (5) examining links between peer experiences and behaviors other than aggressiveness (e.g., prosociality, well-being, and internalizing problems); (6) assessing mediators and moderators of the links either from personal characteristics to peer experiences or from peer experiences to personal development; (7) considering genetic factors; (8) conducting experimental prevention studies; and (9) examining contextual variations.

Sticking Close to the Definition

Nearly every definition of aggression includes harm as a central component. Harm is invoked as a defining feature of aggression in the definitions that are found in scholarly articles about aggression (Cohen, Hsueh, Russell, & Ray, 2006; Coie & Dodge, 2006; Loeber & Hay, 1997). The specific role that harm is given in these definitions is that of an effect. The definitions state explicitly that harm is the immediate result or effect of an aggressive behavior. A presumed repercussion of the definitional necessity of harm is that an act cannot be designated as aggressive unless it is shown to be harmful. Moreover, the meaning or interpretation of findings related to aggression needs to recognize how it is that an aggressive act or an aggressive person has been harmful and what the meaning of this harm is for other social processes, such as being liked or being seen as popular by one's peers.

Currently, the emphasis on harm in research on aggression is largely implicit. Although harm is recognized as a critical feature of aggression, the explicit emphasis on it in the measurement of aggression or in efforts to understand findings related to aggression has been exceedingly rare. Instead, items used to measure aggression emphasize either different forms of aggression (i.e., relational or physical) or different "functions" (i.e., proactive or reactive). The absence of a concern with harm in the measure of aggression is potentially problematic in two ways. The first is that measures of aggression, such as those that are derived from peer assessment techniques, may have a limited validity because they do not index a fundamental component of aggression. If we do not know that a behavior leads to harm, then how do we know whether it is a form of aggression?

The second problem may be more limiting. The interpretation and understanding of variations in findings observed with different measures of aggression is the ultimate goal of research on aggression. If the findings observed with measures of aggression cannot be understood through an explicit consideration of harmful effects, then the full meaning of these findings cannot be known. For these reasons, it would appear that harm as an effect of aggression needs to be assessed as part of the study of aggression and peer relations. This premise serves as the justification of the proposed studies.

Distinguishing between Subtypes of Aggressive Behavior

Once the above issue is resolved, it is necessary to integrate it in the distinction of different subtypes of aggressive behaviors based on their forms and/or their functions, as their links to different peer experiences may be specific. This echoes a call made some 30 years ago by Coie, Dodge, and Kupersmidt (1990). Yet most researchers keep using broadband measures of aggression or, worse, measures that encompass both aggressive and nonaggressive behaviors. It is also imperative to measure different types of aggressive behavior concurrently and repeatedly to control for their overlap and monitor their evolution carefully.

Understanding the Mechanisms of Reward within the Peer System

A long-standing and fundamental point of theory on peer research is that experiences with peers can be conceived of as rewards (Hartup, 1983). These experiences can be affective, as in the experience of being accepted by peers, or they can derive from the power and status that is ascribed to popular children. Although these experiences are recognized as rewards, they are rarely studied as such. That is, they have not been studied according to their capacity to maintain or increase the frequency of the behaviors to which they are associated. This sort of assessment can be applied easily to the understanding of the stability of aggression. If experiences such as acceptance and being treated as having high status among peers are forms of reward, then these experiences will function to maintain or even promote the level of child's aggression, possibly by inflating aggressive children's positive self-views or by supporting the value of aggression as an acceptable means to achieve personal goals. Studies of these effects would not be difficult. They can be done easily with the existing datasets of many labs that study peer relations.

Examining Different Types of Peer Experiences Specifically and Repeatedly

If we want to determine the specific contribution of each type of peer experience and examine their dynamic interplay, it is imperative to measure them distinctively and to measure them across different developmental periods in the same study. It is also imperative that we use specific measures to index specific aspects of peer experiences (e.g., peer rejection, peer acceptance, popularity); at this moment, it seems that peer rejection, but not peer acceptance, contributes to children's and adolescents' aggression.

Examining Links between Peer Experiences and Behaviors Other Than Aggressiveness

Although friendship participation for rejected children had no main effect in some studies and a negative effect in others in reference to externalizing problems, it nonetheless predicted decreased internalizing problems (i.e., feelings of loneliness and depressed mood) in a number of other studies (Laursen, Bukowski, Aunola, & Nurmi, 2007; Pedersen, Vitaro, Barker, & Borge, 2007), unless the friends were also aggressive (Brendgen, Vitaro, & Bukowski, 2000). This may be the case because participation in a friendship provides emotional and instrumental supports that may compensate for negative peer experiences, or it may buffer the risk of further rejection or victimization, provided the friendship is of high quality (Bagwell, Newcomb, & Bukowski, 1998; Hodges, Boivin, Vitaro, & Bukowski, 1999). Depending on the research question, it could be useful and informative to include other behavioral outcomes besides aggression when studying the interplay of different types of peer experiences.

Assessing Mediators and Moderators

If we want to clarify the processes through which peer experiences influence personal development and help resolve inconsistencies between studies, as suggested in the last section, future studies need to include theoretically relevant mediators and moderators. Mediators that might help explain the link between peer experiences and personal development can refer to intra- or interpersonal processes such as those described in this chapter. They can also refer to biological mechanisms and epigenetic processes triggered by peer experiences (see, e.g., Vaillancourt, Hymel, & McDougall, 2013, in reference to peer victimization). Factors that could moderate the link between peer experiences and personal development, notably aggression, can be many, but they should include participants' genetic risks or developmental profiles with respect to aggression. Indeed, there is evidence from behavior, and molecular, genetic studies that peer rejection and friends' aggression can moderate the expression of genetic dispositions toward aggression or, inversely, can be moderated by one's genetic makeup (see Brendgen et al., Chapter 4, this volume).

Considering Genetic Factors

Behavior genetic (mostly twin) studies have found that between 40 and 60% of individual differences in aggressive behavior in childhood and adolescence is accounted for by genetic factors, whereas shared and nonshared environmental factors (such as peer rejection, friendship participation, or friends' aggression) explain the remaining variation (Burt, 2009). Genetic sources of variance have been found for all types of aggressive behavior, although they tend to be stronger for physical and proactive aggression than for social and reactive aggression (see Brendgen et al., Chapter 4, this volume). Behavior genetic studies have also shown that both peer rejection and affiliation with aggressive friends can be influenced by individuals' heritable characteristics, indicating a gene–environment correlation (see Brendgen, Ouellet-Morin, & Boivin, 2018). Future studies need to account for these genetic effects if they want to provide a clearer picture of the impact of peer rejection or friends' aggression on aggressive behavior in children and adolescents.

Conducting Experimental Prevention Studies

Although they are an improvement over nongenetically controlled studies, genetically controlled studies remain correlational in nature. Therefore, if we want to claim causality, it is necessary to resort to experimental manipulations. There have been a number of studies that managed to do so despite the delicate nature of the peer experiences involved. These studies need to be acknowledged and continued if we want to convince ourselves and others of the central role played by peer experiences in regard to aggression and other important developmental outcomes for children and adolescents. In terms of peer rejection, a study by Reijntjes, Kamphuis, Prinzie, and Telch (2010) serves as an example. These authors randomly assigned 11-year-old children to conditions in which they received either negative or positive feedback from peers after completing personal profiles that would be evaluated online by peers. After the experimental manipulation, participants were given an opportunity to aggress against the same peers who evaluated them. As expected, aggression was higher in the negative feedback condition, but this effect was moderated by individual characteristics: Children high on alienation reacted more aggressively than children low on alienation.

In terms of exposure to aggressive peers, an interesting example comes from a study by Cohen and Prinstein (2006), who led adolescents participating in a computerized chatroom activity to believe that they were interacting with other students who perceived aggressive behaviors in positive ways. Peers' social status was also experimentally manipulated; participants were randomly assigned to conditions in which peers' status was either high or low. Overall, peer influence on aggressive/risk behaviors was strongest in the high-peer-status condition. This effect was, in turn, moderated by participants' characteristics. Adolescents low on social anxiety conformed only to high-status peers, whereas socially anxious adolescents were equally influenced by low- and high-status peers. There is also evidence from intervention studies that directly manipulated exposure to aggressive peers. For instance, Dishion and colleagues reported that an intervention delivered to delinquent/aggressive youth as a group inadvertently resulted in an increase in teacher-reported delinquency (i.e., rule breaking) in comparison with a randomly assigned control condition (Poulin, Dishion, & Burraston, 2001). Detailed observations revealed that deviancy training during the group sessions partly explained the increase in delinquency (Patterson, Dishion, & Yoerger, 2000). As important are experimental studies showing that exposure to normative peers or improvement in friendship quality among aggressive friends can result in a reduction in aggression and other undesirable outcomes, through processes that remain to be clarified. Although promising and innovative, the number of studies that used prosocial peers or targeted friendship quality as a means to improve aggressive children's behaviors are still too rare on which to base firm conclusions about their effectiveness (see, e.g., Feldman & Caplinger, 1983; Salvas, Vitaro, Brendgen, & Cantin, 2016). This is a promising line of research in need of new experimental manipulations in the form of prevention/intervention programs.

Examining Contextual Variations

At the outset of this chapter, we noted that peer relations need to be understood at different levels of social complexity. We also noted that different contexts have different norms and that these norms and expectations will influence the level of tolerance for aggressive behavior. With respect to sociocultural contextual factors, it is likely that basic features such as individualism, collectivism, and the acceptance of power differentials will affect the level of aggressive behavior. One can hypothesize that in contexts that favor individualism, there may be a heightened tolerance or acceptance of aggression as a form of culturally sanctioned behavior. In contrast, the tolerance of aggression may be weakened by the presence of collectivism as a cultural value. One can also hypothesize that the association between aggression and status may be stronger in contexts that accept the existence of power differentials.

Conclusions

The goal of this chapter was to provide a view of the intersection between aggression and peer relations. We have shown that the associations between them are complex and that they are implicated in many processes that occur at different levels of analysis. We have shown also that in spite of the vast literature on this topic, there are great gaps in what we know. Peer researchers have at their disposal a broad and rich set of measures, methods, ideas, and processes that can be used profitably to understand how peer experiences and aggression fit together to affect each other and to affect development.

REFERENCES

Bagwell, C. L., Newcomb, A. F., & Bukowski, W. M. (1998). Preadolescent friendship and peer rejection as predictors of adult adjustment. *Child Development, 69,* 140–153.

Barth, J. M., Dunlap, S. I., Dane, H., Lochman, J. E., & Wells, K. C. (2004). Classroom environment influences on aggression, peer relations, and academic focus. *Journal of School Psychology, 42*(2), 115–133.

Bierman, K. L. (2004). *Peer rejection: Developmental processes and intervention strategies.* New York: Guilford Press.

Bierman, K. L., Kalvin, C. B., & Heinrichs, B. S. (2015). Early childhood precursors and adolescent sequelae of grade school peer rejection and victimization. *Journal of Clinical Child and Adolescent Psychology, 44*(3), 367–379.

Boivin, M., Dodge, K. A., & Coie, J. D. (1995). Individual–group behavioral similarity and peer status in experimental play groups: The social misfit revisited. *Journal of Personality and Social Psychology, 69*(2), 269–279.

Boivin, M., Hymel, S., & Hodges, E. (2001). Toward a process view of peer rejection and harassment. In J. Juvonen & S. Graham (Eds.), *Peer harassment in school: The plight of the vulnerable and victimized children* (pp. 265–289). New York: Guilford Press.

Bowker, J. C., Rubin, K. H., Rose-Krasnor, L., & Booth-LaForce, C. (2007). Good friendships, bad friends: Friendship factors as moderators of the relation between aggression and social information processing. *European Journal of Developmental Psychology, 4*(4), 415–434.

Brendgen, M., Boivin, M., Vitaro, F., Girard, A., Dionne, G., & Pérusse, D. (2008). Gene–environment interaction between peer victimization and child aggression. *Development and Psychopathology, 20*(2), 455–471.

Brendgen, M., Ouellet-Morin, I., & Boivin, M. (2018). Peer relations and psychosocial development: Perspectives from genetic approaches. In W. M. Bukowski, B. Laursen, & K.

H. Rubin (Eds.), *Handbook of peer interactions, relationships, and groups* (2nd ed., pp. 123–140). New York: Guilford Press.

Brendgen, M., Vitaro, F., & Bukowski, W. M. (2000). Deviant friends and early adolescents' emotional and behavioral adjustment. *Journal of Research on Adolescence, 10*(2), 173–189.

Broidy, L. M., Nagin, D. S., Tremblay, R. E., Bates, J. E., Brame, B., Dodge, K. A., et al. (2003). Developmental trajectories of childhood disruptive behaviors and adolescent delinquency: A six-site, cross-national study. *Developmental Psychology, 39*(2), 222–245.

Buil, M., van Lier, P. A. C., Brendgen, M., Koot, H. M., & Vitaro, F. (2017). Developmental pathways linking childhood temperament with antisocial behavior and substance use in adolescence: Explanatory mechanisms in the peer environment. *Journal of Personality and Social Psychology, 112*(6), 948–966.

Bukowski, W. M. (2003). What does it mean to say that aggressive children are competent or incompetent? *Merrill–Palmer Quarterly, 49*, 390–400.

Bukowski, W. M. (2011). Popularity as a social concept: Meanings and significance. In A. H. C. Cillessen, D. Schwartz, & L. Mayeux (Eds.), *Popularity in the peer system* (pp. 3–24). New York: Guilford Press.

Bukowski, W. M., & Adams, R. (2005). Peer relations and psychopathology: Markers, mechanisms, mediators, moderators, and meanings. *Journal Clinical Child and Adolescent Psychology, 34*, 3–10.

Bukowski, W. M., Castellanos, S., Vitaro, F., & Brendgen, M. (2015). Socialization and experiences with peers. In J. E. Grusec & P. D. Hastings (Eds.), *Handbook of socialization: Theory and research* (2nd ed., pp. 228–250). New York: Guilford Press.

Bukowski, W. M., Cillessen, A. H. N., & Velasquez, A. M. (2012). The use of peer ratings in developmental research. In B. Laursen, T. Little, & N. Card (Eds.), *Handbook of developmental research methods* (pp. 211–228). New York: Guilford Press.

Bukowski, W. M., & Hoza, B. (1989). Popularity and friendship: Issues in theory, measurement, and outcome. In T. Berndt & G. Ladd (Eds.), *Peer relationships in child development* (pp. 15–45). New York: Wiley.

Bukowski, W. M., Laursen, B., & Rubin, K. H. (2018). Peer relations: Past, present, and promise. In W. M. Bukowski, B. Laursen, & K. H. Rubin (Eds.), *Handbook of peer interactions, relationships, and groups* (2nd ed., pp. 3–20). New York: Guilford Press.

Bukowski, W. M., Schwartzman, A. E., Santo, J. B., Bagwell, C., & Adams, R. (2009). Reactivity and distortions in the self: Narcissism, types of aggression, and the functioning of the HPA axis during early adolescence. *Development and Psychopathology, 21*, 1249–1262.

Bukowski, W. M., & Sippola, L. K. (2001). Groups, individuals, and victimization: A view of the peer system. In J. Juvonen & S. Graham (Eds.), *Peer harassment in school* (pp. 355–377). New York: Guilford Press.

Bukowski, W. M., Sippola, L., & Newcomb, A. F. (2000). Variations in patterns of attraction to same- and other-sex peers during early adolescence. *Developmental Psychology, 36*, 147–154.

Burt, S. A. (2009). Are there meaningful etiological differences within antisocial behavior?: Results of a meta-analysis. *Clinical Psychology Review, 29*(2), 163–178.

Buskirk, A. A., Rubin, K. H., Burgess, K., Booth-LaForce, C. L., & Rose-Krasnor, L. (2004, March). *Loved, hated . . . but never ignored: Evidence for two types of popularity.* Paper presented at The Many Faces of Popularity symposium at the biennial meeting of the Society for Research in Adolescence, Baltimore.

Chen, D. N., Drabick, D. A. G., & Burgers, D. E. (2015). A developmental perspective on peer rejection, deviant peer affiliation, and conduct problems among youth. *Child Psychiatry and Human Development, 46*(6), 823–838.

Cillessen, A. H. N., & Mayeux, L. (2004). From censure to reinforcement: Developmental changes in the association between aggression and social status. *Child Development, 75*, 147–163.

Cohen, G. L., & Prinstein, M. J. (2006). Peer contagion of aggression and health risk behavior among adolescent males: An experimental investigation of effects on public conduct and private attitudes. *Child Development, 77*(4), 967–983.

Cohen, R., Hsueh, Y., Russell, K. M., & Ray, G. E. (2006). Beyond the individual: A consideration of context for the development of aggression. *Aggression and Violent Behavior 11,* 341–351.

Coie, J. D. (1990). Toward a theory of peer rejection. In S. R. Asher & J. D. Coie (Eds.), *Peer rejection in childhood* (pp. 365–402). New York: Cambridge University Press.

Coie, J., & Dodge, K. (2006). Aggression and antisocial behavior. In W. Damon (Series Ed.) & N. Eisenberg (Vol. Ed.), *The handbook of child psychology* (pp. 779–862). New York: Wiley.

Coie, J. D., Dodge, K. A., & Kupersmidt, J. B. (1990). Peer group behavior and social status. In S. R. Asher & J. D. Coie (Eds.), *Peer rejection in childhood* (pp. 17–59). Cambridge, UK: Cambridge University Press.

Crick, N. R., Murray-Close, D., Marks, P. E. L., & Mohajeri-Nelson, N. (2009). Aggression and peer relationship in school-age children: Relational and physical aggression in group and dyadic contexts. In K. H. Rubin, W. M. Bukowski, & B. Laursen (Eds.), *Handbook of peer interactions, relationships and groups* (pp. 287–302). New York: Guilford Press.

DeRosier, M. E., Kupersmidt, J. B., & Patterson, C. J. (1994). Children's academic and behavioral adjustment as a function of the chronicity and proximity of peer rejection. *Child Development, 65,* 1799–1813.

Dishion, T. J., McCord, J., & Poulin, F. (1999). When interventions harm: Peer groups and problem behavior. *American Psychologist, 54*(9), 755.

Dishion, T. J., Patterson, G. R., Stoolmiller, M., & Skinner, M. L. (1991). Family, school, and behavioral antecedents to early adolescent involvement with antisocial peers. *Developmental Psychology, 27*(1), 172–180.

Dodge, K. A., Coie, J. D., Pettit, G. S., & Price, J. M. (1990). Peer status and aggression in boys' groups: Developmental and contextual analyses. *Child Development, 61,* 1289–1309.

Dodge, K. A., Lansford, J. E., Burks, V. S., Bates, J. E., Pettit, G. S., Fontaine, R., et al. (2003). Peer rejection and social information-processing factors in the development of aggressive behavior problems in children. *Child Development, 74*(2), 374–393.

Ellis, W. E., Chung-Hall, J., & Dumas, T. M. (2013). The role of peer group aggression in predicting adolescent dating violence and relationship quality. *Journal of Youth and Adolescence, 42,* 1–13.

Fabes, R. A., Hanish, L. D., & Martin, C. L. (2003). Children at play: The role of peers in understanding the effects of child care. *Child Development, 74*(4), 1039–1043.

Feldman, R. A., & Caplinger, T. E. (1983). The St. Louis experiment: Treatment of antisocial youths in prosocial peer groups. In J. R. Kluegel (Ed.), *Evaluating juvenile justice* (pp. 121–148). Beverly Hills, CA: SAGE.

Furman, W., & Buhrmester, D. (1985). Children's perceptions of the personal relationships in their social networks. *Developmental Psychology, 21*(6), 1016–1024.

Geertz, C. (1973). *The interpretation of cultures: Selected essays.* New York: Basic Books.

Gest, S. D., Graham-Bermann, S. A., & Hartup, W. W. (2001). Peer experience: Common and unique features of number of friendships, social network centrality, and sociometric status. *Social Development, 10*(1), 23–40.

Grotpeter, J. K., & Crick, N. R. (1996). Relational aggression, overt aggression, and friendship. *Child Development, 67*(5), 2328–2338.

Hartup, W. W. (1964). Friendship status and the effectiveness of peers as reinforcing agents. *Journal of Experimental Child Psychology, 1*(2), 154–162.

Hartup, W. W. (1983). Peer relations. In P. H. Mussen (Series Ed.) & E. M. Hetherington (Vol. Ed.), *Handbook of child psychology: Vol. 4. Socialization, personality, and social development* (pp. 103–196). New York: Wiley.

Haselager, G. J. T., Hartup, W. W., van Lieshout, C. F. M., & Riksen-Walraven, J. M. A.

(1998). Similarities between friends and nonfriends in middle childhood. *Child Development, 69*(4), 1198–1208.

Hamm, J. V. (2000). Do birds of a feather flock together?: The variable bases for African American, Asian American, and European American adolescents' selection of similar friends. *Developmental Psychology, 36*(2), 209–219.

Hawley, P. H. (2003). Strategies of control, aggression, and morality, in preschoolers: An evolutionary perspective. *Journal of Experimental Child Psychology, 85,* 213–235.

Hawley, P. H., Little, T. D., & Pasupathi, M. (2002). Winning friends and influencing peers: Trategies of peer influence in late childhood. *International Journal of Behavioral Development, 26*(5), 466–474.

Hinde, R. A. (1966). *Animal behavior: A synthesis of ethology and comparative psychology.* New York: McGraw-Hill

Hinde, R. A., & Stevenson-Hinde, J. (1987). Interpersonal relationships and child development. *Developmental Review, 7*(1), 1–21.

Hodges, E. V. E., Boivin, M., Vitaro, F., & Bukowski, W. M. (1999). The power of friendship: Protecting against an escalating cycle of peer victimization. *Developmental Psychology, 35*(1), 94–101.

Kupersmidt, J. B., Burchinal, M., & Patterson, C. J. (1995). Developmental patterns of childhood peer relations as predictors of externalizing behavior problems. *Development and Psychopathology, 7,* 825–843.

Ladd, G. W. (2006). Peer rejection, aggressive or withdrawn behavior, and psychological maladjustment from ages 5 to 12: An examination of four predictive models. *Child Development, 77*(4), 822–846.

Ladd, G. W., & Troop-Gordon, W. (2003). The role of chronic peer difficulties in the development of children's psychological adjustment problems. *Child Development, 74,* 1344–1367.

Laird, R. D., Jordan, K. Y., Dodge, K. A., Pettit, G. S., & Bates, J. E. (2001). Peer rejection in childhood, involvement with antisocial peers in early adolescence, and the development of externalizing behavior problems. *Development and Psychopathology, 13*(2), 337–354.

Lansford, J. E., Malone, P. S., Dodge, K. A., Pettit, G. S., & Bates, J. E. (2010). Developmental cascades of peer rejection, social information-processing biases, and aggression during middle childhood. *Development and Psychopathology, 22*(3), 593–602.

Lansford, J. E., Yu, T. Y., Pettit, G. S., Bates, J. E., & Dodge, K. A. (2014). Pathways of peer relationships from childhood to young adulthood. *Journal of Applied Developmental Psychology, 35*(2), 111–117.

Laursen, B. (2017). Making and keeping friends: The importance of being similar. *Child Development Perspectives, 11*(4), 282–289.

Laursen, B., Bukowski, W. M., Aunola, K., & Nurmi, J.-E. (2007). Friendship moderates prospective associations between social isolation and adjustment problems in young children. *Child Development, 78,* 1395–1404.

Lease, A. M., Kennedy, C. A., & Axelrod, J. L. (2002). Children's social constructions of popularity. *Social Development, 11,* 87–109.

Liu, M., & Chen, X. (2003). Friendship networks and social, school and psychological adjustment in Chinese junior high school students. *Psychology in the Schools, 40*(1), 5–17.

Loeber, R., & Hay, D. (1997). Key issues in the development of aggression and violence from childhood to early adulthood. *Annual Review of Psychology, 48,* 371–410.

Moffitt, T. E. (1993). Adolescence-limited and life-course-persistent antisocial behavior: A developmental taxonomy. *Psychological Review, 100*(4), 674–701.

Mead, G. H. (1934). *Mind, self, and society.* Chicago: University of Chicago Press.

Monroe, W. S. (1898). Discussion and reports. Social consciousness in children. *Psychological Review, 5*(1), 68.

Moreno, J. L. (1934). *Who shall survive?: A new approach to the problem of human interrelations* (Nervous and Mental Disease Monograph Series, No. 58). Washington, DC: Nervous and Mental Disease.

Newcomb, A. F., Bukowski, W. M., & Pattee, L. (1993). Children's peer relations: A meta-analytic review of popular, rejected, neglected, controversial, and average sociometric status. *Psychological Bulletin, 113,* 99–128.

Ostrov, J. M., Murray-Close, D., Godleski, S. A., & Hart, E. J. (2013). Prospective associations between forms and functions of aggression and social and affective processes during early childhood. *Journal of Experimental Child Psychology, 116*(1), 19–36.

Patterson, G. R., DeBaryshe, B. D., & Ramsey, E. (1989). A developmental perspective on antisocial behavior. *American Psychologist, 44*(2), 329–335.

Patterson, G. R., Dishion, T. J., & Yoerger, K. (2000). Adolescent growth in new forms of problem behavior: Macro-and micro-peer dynamics. *Prevention Science, 1*(1), 3–13.

Pedersen, S., Vitaro, F., Barker, E. D., & Borge, A. I. H. (2007). The timing of middle-childhood peer rejection and friendship: Linking early behavior to early-adolescent adjustment. *Child Development, 78*(4), 1037–1051.

Piaget, J. (1932). *The moral judgment of the child.* London: Kegan Paul, Trench, Trübner.

Poulin, F., Dishion, T. J., & Burraston, B. (2001). 3-year iatrogenic effects associated with aggregating high-risk adolescents in cognitive-behavioral preventive interventions. *Applied Developmental Science, 5*(4), 214–224.

Powers, C. J., Bierman, K. L., & Conduct Problems Prevention Research Group. (2013). The multifaceted impact of peer relations on aggressive disruptive behavior in early elementary school. *Developmental Psychology, 49*(6), 1174–1186.

Prinstein, M. J., & Cillessen, A. H. N. (2003). Forms and functions of adolescent peer aggression associated with high levels of peer status. *Merrill–Palmer Quarterly, 49,* 310–342.

Prinstein, M. J., & Giletta, M. (2016). Peer relations and developmental psychopathology. In D. Cicchetti (Ed.), *Developmental psychopathology* (3rd ed., pp. 527–579). Hoboken, NJ: Wiley.

Prinstein, M. J., & La Greca, A. M. (2004). Childhood peer rejection and aggression as predictors of adolescent girls' externalizing and health risk behaviors: A 6-year longitudinal study. *Journal of Consulting and Clinical Psychology, 72*(1), 103–112.

Rabiner, D. L., Coie, J. D., Miller-Johnson, S., Boykin, A. S. M., & Lochman, J. E. (2005). Predicting the persistence of aggressive offending of African American males from adolescence into young adulthood: The importance of peer relations, aggressive behavior, and ADHD symptoms. *Journal of Emotional and Behavioral Disorders, 13*(3), 131–140.

Reijntjes, A., Kamphuis, J. H., Prinzie, P., & Telch, M. J. (2010). Peer victimization and internalizing problems in children: A meta-analysis of longitudinal studies. *Child Abuse and Neglect, 34*(4), 244–252.

Rubin, K. H., Bukowski, W. M., & Bowker, J. (2015). Children in groups. In R. Lerner (Series Ed.) & M. Bornstein (Vol. Ed.), *The handbook of child psychology* (7th ed., pp. 175–222). New York: Wiley.

Rubin, K. H., Bukowski, W. M., & Parker, J. G. (2006). Peer interactions, relationships and groups. In W. Damon (Series Ed.) & N. Eisenberg (Vol. Ed.), *The handbook of child psychology* (6th ed., pp. 571–645). New York: Wiley.

Rubin, K. H., Lynch, D., Coplan, R. J., Rose-Krasnor, L., & Booth, C. L. (1994). "Birds of a feather . . . ": Behavioral concordances and preferential personal attraction in children. *Child Development, 65,* 1778–1785.

Rubin, K. H., Oh, W., Menzer, M., & Ellison, K. (2011). Dyadic relationships from a cross-cultural perspective: Parent–child relationships and friendship. In X. Chen & K. H. Rubin (Eds.), *Socioemotional development in cultural context* (pp. 208–237). New York: Guilford Press.

Rubin, K., Wojslawowicz, J., Burgess, K., Rose-Krasnor, L., & Booth-LaForce, C. (2006). The friendships of socially withdrawn and competent young adolescents. *Journal of Abnormal Child Psychology, 34,* 139–153.

Salmivalli, C., & Isaacs, J. (2005). Prospective relations among victimization, rejection, friendlessness, and children's self- and peer-perceptions. *Child Development, 76*(6), 1161–1171.

Salvas, M.-C., Vitaro, F., Brendgen, M., & Cantin, S. (2016). Prospective links between friendship and early physical aggression: Preliminary evidence supporting the role of friendship quality through a dyadic intervention. *Merrill–Palmer Quarterly, 62*(3), 285–305.

Salvas, M.-C., Vitaro, F., Brendgen, M., Lacourse, E., Boivin, M., & Tremblay, R. E. (2011). Interplay between friends' aggression and friendship quality in the development of child aggression during the early school years. *Social Development, 20*(4), 645–663.

Snyder, J., McEachern, A., Schrepferman, L., Just, C., Jenkins, M., Roberts, S., et al. (2010). Contribution of peer deviancy training to the early development of conduct problems: Mediators and moderators. *Behavior Therapy, 41*(3), 317–328.

Snyder, J., Prichard, J., Schrepferman, L., Patrick, M. R., & Stoolmiller, M. (2004). Child impulsiveness–inattention, early peer experiences, and the development of early onset conduct problems. *Journal of Abnormal Child Psychology, 32*(6), 579–594.

Snyder, J., Schrepferman, L., McEachern, A., Barner, S., Johnson, K., & Provines, J. (2008). Peer deviancy training and peer coercion: Dual processes associated with early-onset conduct problems. *Child Development, 79,* 252–268.

Stormshak, E. A., Bierman, K. L., Bruschi, C., Dodge, K. A., Coie, J. D., & Conduct Problems Prevention Research Group. (1999). The relation between behavior problems and peer preference in different classroom contexts. *Child Development, 70*(1), 169–182.

Sturaro, C., van Lier, P. A. C., Cuijpers, P., & Koot, H. M. (2011). The role of peer relationships in the development of early school-age externalizing problems. *Child Development, 82*(3), 758–765.

Tseng, W. L., Banny, A. M., Kawabata, Y., Crick, N. R., & Gau, S. S. F. (2013). A cross-lagged structural equation model of relational aggression, physical aggression, and peer status in a Chinese culture. *Aggressive Behavior, 39*(4), 301–315.

Tudge, J. (1992). Processes and consequences of peer collaborations: A Vygotskian analysis. *Child Development, 63,* 1364–1379.

Vaillancourt, T., Hymel, S., & McDougall, P. (2013). The biological underpinnings of peer victimization: Understanding why and how the effects of bullying can last a lifetime. *Theory into Practice, 523*(4), 241–248.

van Lier, P. A. C., & Koot, H. M. (2010). Developmental cascades of peer relations and symptoms of externalizing and internalizing problems from kindergarten to fourth-grade elementary school. *Development and Psychopathology, 22*(3), 569–582.

Vaughn, B. E., Vollenweider, M., Bost, K. K., Azria-Evans, M. R., & Snider, J. B. (2003). Negative interactions and social competence for preschool children in two samples: Reconsidering the interpretation of aggressive behavior for young children. *Merrill-Palmer Quarterly, 49,* 245–278.

Vitaro, F., Boivin, M., & Bukowski, W. M. (2009). The role of friendship in child and adolescent psychosocial development. In K. H. Rubin, W. M. Bukowski, & B. Laursen (Eds.), *Handbook of peer interactions, relationships and groups* (pp. 568–588). New York: Guilford Press.

Vitaro, F., Brendgen, M., Boivin, M., Cantin, S., Dionne, G., Tremblay, R. E., et al. (2011). A monozygotic twin difference study of friends' aggression and children's adjustment problems. *Child Development, 82,* 617–632.

Vitaro, F., Brendgen, M., Girard, A., Boivin, M., Dionne, G., & Tremblay, R. E. (2015). The expression of genetic risk for aggressive and non-aggressive antisocial behavior is moderated by peer group norms. *Journal of Youth and Adolescence, 44*(7), 1379–1395.

Vitaro, F., Pedersen, S., & Brendgen, M. (2007). Children's disruptiveness, peer rejection, friends' deviancy, and delinquent behaviors: A process-oriented approach. *Development and Psychopathology, 19*(2), 433–453.

Vitaro, F., Tremblay, R. E., Kerr, M., Pagani, L. S., & Bukowski, W. M. (1997). Disruptiveness, friends' characteristics, and delinquency: A test of two competing models of development. *Child Development, 68*(4), 676–689.

Vygotsky, L. (1978). *Mind in society.* London: Harvard University Press.

Werner, N. E., & Crick, N. R. (2004). Maladaptive peer relationships and the development of relational and physical aggression during middle childhood. *Social Development, 13*, 495–514.

Wood, M. A., Bukowski, W. M., & Santo, J. B. (2017). Friendship security, but not friendship intimacy, moderates the stability of anxiety during preadolescence. *Journal of Clinical Child and Adolescent Psychology, 46*(6), 798–809.

Zimmer-Gembeck, M. J., Geiger, T. C., & Crick, N. R. (2005). Relational and physical aggression, prosocial behavior, and peer relations: Gender moderation and bidirectional associations. *Journal of Early Adolescence, 25*(4), 421–452.

CHAPTER 11

Aggression and Morality
in Childhood and Adolescence

TINA MALTI, TYLER COLASANTE, and MARC JAMBON

Brief Introduction

The far-reaching, negative consequences of childhood aggression have been scruti-nized for decades (for reviews, see Eisner & Malti, 2015; Tremblay, 2000). Likewise, the topic of morality has a long history in both philosophy and psychology (e.g., Freud, 1930/2002; Hume, 1777/1992; Kant, 1788/2009; Sen, 2009). Although both aggression and morality revolve around the just and (un)caring treatment of oth-ers, inquests into each of these respective domains have rarely intersected over the years (Arsenio & Lemerise, 2004). In this chapter, we begin by briefly introduc-ing key terminology and discussing the normative development of moral emotions and moral cognitions (i.e., judgments and reasoning; for normative developmental trends of aggression, see Malti & Rubin, Chapter 1, and Ostrov, Perry, & Blakely-McClure, Chapter 3, this volume). We then introduce theoretical frameworks that have been used to link aggression with the development of emotions and cognitions in the moral domain. Next, we discuss the relatively limited research on the roles of moral emotions and moral cognitions in aggressive behavior across development. We conclude by highlighting directions for future study that will further our under-standing of the interrelations between moral functioning and aggression across development.

Main Issues

Aggression

Due to the significant comorbidity of externalizing behaviors, researchers com-monly use the term *aggression* to refer to a wide range of problem behaviors, such as defiance, disruption, hyperactivity, and impulsivity (see Eisner & Malti, 2015; Malti & Rubin, Chapter 1, this volume). In line with the conceptualization of aggression put forth by developmental scholars (Dodge, Coie, & Lynam, 2006), we adopt a more precise definition: Volitional behaviors that intend, threaten, or cause physical or psychological harm or distress to others (see Malti & Rubin, Chapter 1, this volume). This definition accounts for both the intentions of the individual and the nature of the act, allowing aggression to be distinguished from antisocial (e.g., drug use), undesirable (e.g., rule breaking), and phenotypically similar yet functionally distinct behaviors (e.g., rough-and-tumble play). Thus we do not cover links between moral development and other related problematic or antisocial behaviors (e.g., lying: Evans & Lee, 2014; delinquency: Stams et al., 2006) in this chapter.

Moral Development

There is heterogeneity in how researchers across various disciplines conceptualize and define morality. Developmental scientists generally agree that morality involves social norms and issues related to how individuals ought to behave toward and treat others (Killen & Malti, 2015). In line with philosophical (Dworkin, 1977) and psychological definitions, we focus on morality as it pertains to obligatory issues involving others' welfare, caring, fairness, and rights. Although different theoretical traditions emphasize distinct aspects of moral functioning (e.g., affect vs. reasoning; Jambon & Smetana, 2015), contemporary scholars have begun to highlight the interdependence of moral emotions and cognitions in relation to children's social behavior (Malti & Ongley, 2014). Nevertheless, historical divisions in the field have resulted in a paucity of empirical research concerning how emotions and cognitions *jointly* contribute to children's aggressive behavior. We therefore discuss moral emotions and judgments separately but offer thoughts on—and some recent empirical evidence for—how these psychological processes may be integrated and how they relate to aggressive behavior in children and adolescents.

Moral Emotions

Moral emotions are emotional responses that reflect norms concerning caring, justice, and harm—such as guilt after harming another—or indicate concern for the welfare of others, such as sympathy for others in need (Eisenberg, 2000; Malti, 2016; Tangney, Stuewig, & Mashek, 2007). Similar to basic emotions, feelings in the context of moral events arise in response to evaluating or appraising an incoming stimulus against one's own concerns—the goals and standards one holds important (Lazarus, 1991). Emotions in moral contexts are distinct from emotions in other contexts (e.g., guilt over stealing a desired object vs. guilt over not performing well on a test; see Malti, Dys, Colasante, & Peplak, 2018). Moral emotions are considered complex emotions because they involve coordinating and balancing one's own and others' emotions, perspectives, and concerns (Malti et al., 2018; Malti & Latzko, 2017). As such, they require greater social-cognitive skills than basic emotions. Emotions and cognitions likely influence one another in a recursive fashion, with judgments preceding emotions in some cases (e.g., feeling guilty after careful deliberation about one's misconduct) and "gut" feelings preceding judgments in other cases (e.g., empathic sadness prompting the moral consideration of how the other's feelings were hurt). This notion is supported by neuroscientific findings indicating that moral emotions recruit the complex coordination of brain regions implicated in affect and cognition (e.g., Decety, Michalska, & Kinzler, 2012).

One common method of assessing moral emotions in an experimental setting is to ask children to imagine themselves committing hypothetical transgressions and to report how they would feel and why (e.g., Keller, Lourenco, Malti, & Saalbach, 2003; Malti, Gummerum, Keller, & Buchmann, 2009). Although this paradigm is perhaps most well known for elucidating guilt feelings (broadly defined as regret over wrongdoing; Malti, 2016), research using this methodology has also identified the so-called happy victimizer phenomenon, or the tendency to focus on the hedonistic gains of transgressions. Children between 3 and 5 years of age tend to report positively valenced emotions after victimizing others (Barden, Zelko, Duncan, & Masters, 1980; Nunner-Winkler & Sodian, 1988). Due to advances in perspective taking and other social-cognitive skills, happy victimizing decreases by 6–7 years of age as children begin to associate negative or mixed emotions with immoral conduct (for reviews, see Arsenio, 2014; Malti & Ongley, 2014). Theoretically, the happy victimizer phenomenon has been detailed as a normative conflict between hedonistic desires and moral concerns that children predominantly resolve in favor of the latter as they develop relevant social–emotional and social-cognitive skills, such as the ability to down-regulate positive emotions associated with desirable objects and adopt the victim's perspective (Krettenauer, Malti, & Sokol, 2008).

Despite the well-documented normative age-related declines in happy victimizing (Arsenio, 2014; Malti & Keller, 2010), some individuals continue to express positive emotion expectancies in response to transgressing well into adolescence and adulthood (Krettenauer, Colasante, Buchmann, & Malti, 2014). Thus, whereas happy victimizing in early childhood may represent delays in perspective taking or the ability to coordinate one's own and others' mental states, happy victimizing in later childhood/adolescence may represent a failure to incorporate moral concerns into one's identity (Malti, 2016).

The other-oriented, negatively valenced emotion of sympathy has also received considerable attention. Sympathy refers to a feeling of care or concern for others in need. It is frequently confused with empathy, which involves sharing another's emotional state (Eisenberg, 2000). Unlike empathy, sympathy involves sorrow or concern for others, which is likely to motivate children to reconcile and later avoid transgressing against others. Empathy, on the other hand, may lead to personal distress and a focus on the self at the expense of others (Eisenberg, 2000). For these reasons, sympathy is considered a morally relevant emotion, whereas empathy is conceptualized as a relatively amoral emotional capacity. Feelings of other-oriented concern appear to increase in frequency from early to late childhood (Eisenberg, Spinrad, & Knafo-Noam, 2015). The affective precursors of sympathy, such as shared negative affect, exist from the first year of life (Davidov, Zahn-Waxler, Roth-Hanania, & Knafo, 2013; Hoffman, 2000). Facial and vocal signs of sympathy in response to others' distress (e.g., furrowed brows, cooing) increase in frequency from 14 and 20 months of age (Zahn-Waxler, Radke-Yarrow, Wagner, & Chapman, 1992), whereas comforting behavior becomes more prevalent during the third and fourth years of life (Phinney, Feshbach, & Farver, 1986; Svetlova, Nichols, & Brownell, 2010). Malti,

Eisenberg, Kim, and Buchmann (2013) further found that, ages 6–9, the majority of children followed increasing (47%) or high-stable (43%) trajectories of sympathy, whereas the remainder showed consistently low (10%) levels.

Researchers have organized moral emotions along the dimensions of valence (positive vs. negative) and orientation (self vs. other; Malti & Noam, 2016), which, in addition to sympathy and guilt, reveal positive self- and other-oriented moral emotions that are relevant to aggression, such as feeling proud about prosocial behavior (Ongley & Malti, 2014; Tangney et al., 2007) or feeling respect for another's moral virtues or behaviors (Peplak & Malti, 2017). To date, however, few studies have directly linked experiences of positive moral emotions to aggression in childhood and adolescence.

Moral Cognitions

Moral cognitions refer to children's prescriptive judgments and reasoning regarding others' welfare, justice, and rights (Killen & Smetana, 2015; Smetana, Jambon, & Ball, 2014). Due to the intrinsic consequences that moral transgressions (e.g., hitting) have for others, moral obligations are considered universally applicable to everyone regardless of context, explicit rules, or personal preferences. This differs from children's conceptions of *social conventions,* which reflect their understanding of societal arrangements, social organization, and contextually relative norms and customs (e.g., etiquette, forms of address). Social conventions facilitate group functioning by providing context-specific expectations for behavior in different social settings (e.g., raising one's hand to speak at school, but not at home).

To assess whether children differentiate between moral norms and other social rules, researchers present them with simple, hypothetical vignettes depicting examples of everyday moral transgressions (e.g., harming or acting unfairly toward an innocent victim) and other transgressions, such as conventional ones (e.g., calling a teacher by his or her first name; getting out of one's seat without asking permission). Children are then asked to evaluate the acceptability or wrongness of the acts in different circumstances (*criterion judgments*)—such as whether it would be permissible to do so if an adult figure allowed the behavior or there were no rules prohibiting it—to determine whether they use different criteria (e.g., authority and rule independence) to evaluate the events. Older children and adolescents are also asked to explain the reasons for their evaluations (*justifications*).

Numerous studies utilizing these interview methods have shown that children as young as 3–4 years of age differentiate between moral and social conventional events in their judgments and reasoning (for a review, see Smetana et al., 2014). Children evaluate moral violations to be wrong across different contexts, even in the absence of rules and authority prohibitions, based on a concern for others' well-being. Although children also consider violations of social conventions to be wrong, these evaluations are limited to specific social contexts and depend on the existence of prohibitive rules, authority commands, and consensual agreement. As such, children judge conventional violations to be more acceptable than moral transgressions if these external constraints and expectations are removed. Assessing criterion judgments and (in older youth) justifications is essential because all rule violations are, by definition, wrong. It therefore allows researchers to disentangle whether children's evaluations are based on obligatory moral concerns for others' welfare and rights or conventional concerns regarding rules, authority, or fear of punishment.

Although a basic understanding of moral norms as prescriptive and obligatory emerges early in development (see Hamlin, 2013), how children apply this knowledge in everyday social situations depends on a multitude of factors. Moral judgment researchers have focused on sources of variability that have relevance for understanding children's aggressive behavior. The first is that real-life situations are inherently *multifaceted* and may therefore present children with situations involving conflicts between competing moral concerns or moral and personal concerns (or between moral and nonmoral issues). For instance, although children judge straightforward, prototypical transgressions to be categorically wrong, they are more likely to consider harming others to be acceptable and justified when it is necessary for self-defense or to protect loved ones (Jambon & Smetana, 2014). The ability to notice, attend to, and coordinate competing concerns in multifaceted situations (e.g., hurting others vs. protecting oneself from harm) increases with age (Smetana et al., 2014), but individual differences in how children encode, interpret, and process social information can influence which concerns are salient in a given context (Arsenio & Lemerise, 2004). A second factor to consider is how children's factual or *informational assumptions* about a situation can influence their interpretation of morally relevant events (Turiel, Killen, & Helwig, 1987). For instance, beliefs regarding whether an act of harm was performed intentionally or accidentally are a major factor in children's assignment of blame and responsibility (Killen, Mulvey, Richardson, Jampol, & Woodward, 2011).

Theoretical Considerations

Understanding how and why children apply norms of justice, fairness, and care to the conflicts that inevitably occur in everyday life—and how children's feelings and thinking about these issues develop—can inform our understanding of why some children behave more aggressively than others, why aggression increases or decreases over time and/or in specific contexts, and how these trajectories affect health outcomes. Given the clear conceptual overlap of how children feel and think about harming others and their actual harmful behavior, researchers have called for a more integrative approach to the study of morality and aggression (e.g., Arsenio & Lemerise, 2004; Killen & Malti, 2015). Expanding on (1) affective development models, (2) social-cognitive models, and (3) clinical approaches to the study of moral emotions, an integrated clinical–developmental framework has been proposed (for a more detailed description of these models, see Malti, 2016; Malti & Keller, 2010). This approach systematically incorporates both situation–affect links and cognitive coordination skills and elaborates on potential implications for aggression, violence, and related problem behaviors across development.

A basic premise of this model is that moral emotions play a key motivational role in resolving social conflicts. They highlight the negative consequences of aggression and victimization for the self and others. Thus whether children show or lack moral emotions can provide insight into their motivations to engage in, or refrain from, aggression (Malti, 2016; Malti & Ongley, 2014). Specifically, the protective aspects of self-conscious moral emotions (guilt) and other-oriented moral emotions (sympathy and respect) help children link their immoral behavior to related emotional consequences for themselves and others (e.g., anticipating feeling guilty about hitting another child or that their victim will feel sad) and alert them to the severity of these events (e.g., hitting another child may have more serious consequences for that child than those that would result from not helping a child finish homework; Arsenio, 2014; Arsenio & Lemerise, 2004).

The anticipation of moral emotions also involves the coordination of affective experiences with judgments, justifications, and one's understanding of others' intentions (Malti & Ongley, 2014). With increasing social-cognitive skills, children are able to coordinate their emotions with their judgments of, and reasoning about, multifaceted events. For example, the anticipation of moral guilt indicates that children have successfully coordinated their feelings that the act is wrong with fairness considerations (e.g., it is not fair to hit someone to get what you want), which may produce fairness-induced guilt. As such, this integrative clinical–developmental model accounts for interactive processes between affect and cognition in children's responses to moral events, allowing for both independent and combined effects on aggression. In line with this theorizing, lower levels of anticipated guilt following one's own wrongdoing are associated with higher levels of aggression in community-based and clinical samples (i.e., across samples with varying levels of affective and cognitive deficits; Malti & Krettenauer, 2013).

Moral emotions have typically been conceptualized as consequential, occurring in response to a transgression or another's suffering that already happened (Malti & Ongley, 2014). However, consequential moral emotions may also spur future instances of anticipatory moral emotions over similar transgressions *before* they occur (Arsenio, 2014). Thus moral emotions can serve as a social–emotional barometer for children to determine the extent to which a past *or* prospective aggressive act misaligns with their principles and/or distresses others. This consequential-versus-anticipatory distinction further underscores the interaction of emotions and cognitions in the moral domain. For example, a consequential emotion may be largely affective given its reactionary nature, but the mental simulation processes characteristic of anticipatory emotions likely require more sophisticated cognitive input.

In sum, this integrated theoretical model allows the systematic study of affective and cognitive moral development in relation to aggression, bullying, and victimization in childhood and adolescence. The model integrates across past traditions that have focused on the development of moral emotions or moral reasoning in the context of social conflict. It should also be noted that emotions and judgments about aggression and victimization are embedded in peer-group dynamics, and peer social status influences how children feel and think about aggression (Killen & Malti, 2015). The peer relationship literature typically utilizes sociometric status as an indicator of being popular or unpopular (i.e., social status). Children who are identified as involved in aggression and children who are being victimized tend to differ in terms of social status (e.g., Olthof, Goossens, Vermande, Aleva, & van der Meulen, 2011). Specifically, victimizers tend to score higher on social status (if conceptualized as power) compared with children who are being victimized. Yet this status comes with high costs because these children often tend to be disliked (Cillessen & Rose, 2005). This has considerable implications for these children's social–emotional development, future propensity to engage in aggression, and related mental health outcomes (see Killen & Malti, 2015). For example, children with severe levels of aggression may become disliked and, as a consequence, rejected by their peers. They may also face a lack of support from friends and/or may be excluded from the peer group. Thus status in peer groups affect children's anticipation of emotions and judgments about victimization in various ways, and recent integrative approaches have accounted for the role of social status on judgments and emotions regarding victimization.

Central Research Findings

Aggression and the Development of Moral Emotions

Perhaps the most adaptive characteristic of moral emotions—and the reason they have received so much interest from philosophers and psychologists—is their ability to deter aggressive conduct (Malti, 2016). This property has received an abundance of empirical support over the past few decades. A meta-analysis found that negatively valenced self-reported moral emotions, such as guilt, were negatively associated with aggressive behavioral outcomes (d = .39), and this effect was not moderated by age despite a range of 4–20 years across studies (Malti & Krettenauer, 2013). Developmentally, expressions of guilt typically emerge around 6–7 years of age. Precursors to guilt, however, have been observed as early as 2 years of age (see Kochanska, Gross, Lin, & Nichols, 2002). At 3 years of age, children who harmed others (e.g., by accidentally breaking their toys) were found to show greater reparative behavior than children who had not caused harm (Vaish, Carpenter, & Tomasello, 2016). By mid-childhood, children develop a more complete concept of guilt (Malti, 2016). Feelings of guilt are thought to inhibit aggressive tendencies through highlighting the negative emotional consequences of wrongdoing. Moreover, the aggression-reducing properties of guilt-related emotions have been observed in both normative and clinical populations and across samples with different socioeconomic backgrounds (Arsenio, Adams, & Gold, 2009; Orobio de Castro, Merk, Koops, Veerman, & Bosch, 2005).

Similar to guilt and related emotions concerning one's *own* wrongdoing, an early foundation of *other-oriented* sympathy is critical for inhibiting aggressive acts and promoting the formation and maintenance of positive social connections. The ability to sympathize allows children to connect harmful actions to the misfortunes of others (Eisenberg, 2000). Such states likely motivate children to refrain from aggression, and, over time, iterations of this sympathetic process may contribute to the development of standards against harming others (Malti & Ongley, 2014). It is also possible that sympathy shifts children's attention away from the perceived benefits of aggressive behavior to the morally salient aspects of such acts and spurs related protective emotions such as guilt (Hoffman, 2000; Malti, 2016; Malti & Ongley, 2014).

There is cross-sectional and longitudinal evidence for an inverse relationship between other-oriented concern and aggressive behavior (e.g., Caravita, Di Blasio,

& Salmivalli, 2009; Jolliffe & Farrington, 2006; Miller & Eisenberg, 1988; van Noorden, Haselager, Cillessen, & Bukowski, 2015). A review of 17 studies on the relation between sympathy and aggression across development, however, concluded that findings for children tend to be mixed, with many studies showing no relation or even positive links between sympathy and aggression (Lovett & Sheffield, 2007). From early adolescence onward, however, low self-reported sympathy is reliably linked to higher levels of aggression (Lovett & Sheffield, 2007). A recent longitudinal study further demonstrated that decreases in children's sympathy in ages 6–12 were systematically linked to increases in their aggression over the same period (Zuffianò, Colasante, Buchmann, & Malti, 2018). The more consistent negative link between sympathy and aggression in adolescence compared with childhood may be due to enhanced regulatory skills (Eisenberg, Spinrad, & Morris, 2014).

Aggression and the Development of Moral Cognitions

A small body of research has consistently shown that, compared with their nonaggressive peers, aggressive children and adolescents are less concerned with and more approving of harmful acts in affectively charged situations involving responses to provocation, threat, or in retaliation for a perceived injustice (Astor, 1994; Gasser, Malti, & Gutzwiller-Helfenfinger, 2012; Orobio de Castro, Verhulp, & Runions, 2012). In contrast, virtually all children consider straightforward, unprovoked acts of harm against innocent others to be categorically wrong and deserving of punishment, and judgments of prototypical moral violations are not associated with individual differences in aggression (Astor, 1994; Gasser & Keller, 2009; Gasser et al., 2012; Malti et al., 2009). Longitudinal research has further demonstrated that more accepting attitudes toward provoked (but not unprovoked) harm are associated with relative increases in aggressive behavior over time (Huesmann & Guerra, 1997).

A similar pattern of findings has been found in studies involving youth exposed to violence (Posada & Wainryb, 2008). For instance, Ardila-Rey, Killen, and Brenick (2009) found that 6- to 12-year-old Colombian children with and without previous exposure to extreme political violence differed in their evaluations of multifaceted events involving provocation and retaliation. Compared with youth with minimal exposure, violence-exposed children were more accepting of causing harm and denying resources to others when provoked (e.g., hitting back after being hit), based on the need for retribution and self-protection (e.g., "she has to defend herself"). In contrast, nearly all children in both samples considered unprovoked acts of aggression as wrong.

These findings indicate that aggressive children (and those exposed to violence) are particularly likely to consider harm an acceptable behavioral response in complex situations involving provocation and retribution, but there is little evidence suggesting they lack a basic understanding of moral norms. As noted earlier, even typically developing children are more approving of harm that is defensive, protective, or provoked compared with selfishly motivated harm (Gutzwiller-Helfenfinger, Gasser, & Malti, 2010; Jambon & Smetana, 2014). Whereas virtually all children believe that it is morally wrong to harm others, biases in how aggressive children encode and process social events make them more likely to evaluate potentially heated interactions as hostile or threatening (Arsenio & Lemerise, 2004). This interpretation aligns with social information-processing research demonstrating that aggressive children are more likely to (mis)attribute hostile intentions to peers in ambiguous conflict situations, but not when their peers' intentions are clear (Dodge et al., 2006). Thus aggressive children's social-cognitive biases contribute to an informational assumption that others represent a threat to their well-being, leading them to prioritize their own personal safety at the expense of harming others (a multifaceted event involving competing concerns; Arsenio & Lemerise, 2004).

This conceptualization helps to clarify why some children consider hurting others to be an acceptable and justified behavioral response to conflict, yet there is emerging evidence that this interpretation may not be applicable to all aggressive youth. In particular, research has demonstrated the importance of distinguishing between reactive and proactive functions or motivations underlying children's aggressive behavior (Hubbard, McAuliffe, Morrow, & Romano, 2010; see Leventhal, Dupéré, & Elliott, Chapter 14, this volume). Reactive aggression involves impulsive, "hot-blooded" responses to perceived threat, whereas proactive aggression refers to more deliberate, "cold-blooded" behaviors aimed at obtaining rewards and accomplishing goals. Despite significant overlap between the two subtypes, studies have consistently found that the psychosocial deficits commonly associated with antisocial behavior (e.g., hostile attribution biases) are more strongly linked to reactive compared with proactive aggression (Card & Little, 2006). In contrast, studies that control for reactively aggressive tendencies have found proactive aggression to be unrelated to indicators of maladjustment or positively associated with measures of social competence, such as peer acceptance (Poulin & Boivin, 2000; Renouf et al., 2010). Compared with reactively aggressive and nonaggressive youth, children exhibiting proactively aggressive tendencies are more confident in their ability to use aggression to get what they want (Dodge, Lochman, Harnish, Bates, & Pettit, 1997), are more likely to fixate on their own desires at the expense of others (Crick & Dodge, 1996), and are less likely to show concern or remorse for those they have hurt (Arsenio et al., 2009; Kerig & Stellwagen, 2010).

The finding that some children deliberately harm others to fulfill their own selfish desires at the expense of others, rather than because they interpret peers' intentions as threatening or have difficulty controlling their emotions and behavior, contrasts with the large body of research showing that nearly all children believe that harming others is morally wrong. This contradiction has led some developmental theorists to conclude that moral judgments and reasoning are unimportant for understanding why children behave aggressively (Hawley, 2003).

An alternative explanation for this apparent "judgment–action" gap is that children who callously use aggression and coercion for self-gain *do not* share the same basic understanding of moral norms as other children but may nevertheless possess the cognitive sophistication to appear morally advanced when questioned by an adult. Indeed, a number of studies have found that proactive aggression is associated with more advanced verbal and cognitive abilities (Arsenio et al., 2009; Renouf et al., 2010). Children exhibiting proactively aggressive tendencies may therefore understand that harming others is considered wrong and may respond in a socially desirable manner. However, if some children fail to appreciate the obligatory status of moral violations as being intrinsically wrong, regardless of explicit sanctions or prohibitions, they may evaluate all rule violations in a similar manner. In support of this hypothesis, Jambon and Smetana (2017) found that teacher-reported proactive aggression was uniquely associated with deficits in children's ability to distinguish between moral and conventional norms along different criteria (e.g., whether the acts were wrong independent of rules and authority restrictions). However, children exhibiting proactively aggressive tendencies also rated moral violations to be more generally wrong (i.e., when asked in the abstract) than other children. A subsequent study using a similar methodological approach (Jambon & Smetana, 2018) further demonstrated that deficits in 4- to 7-year-olds' moral/conventional distinction ability was associated with relative increases in physical aggression over a period of 9 months, but only for children high in callous–unemotional tendencies—a construct closely linked to proactive aggression (Frick, Ray, Thornton, & Kahn, 2014). In addition, a recent longitudinal study by Cui, Colasante, Malti, Ribeaud, and Eisner (2016) found that youth exhibiting high, stable levels of proactive and reactive aggression from first to seventh grades were less likely than reactive-only and non-aggressive youth to reference empathic concern when reasoning about prototypical transgressions.

Future Directions

In the following paragraphs, we briefly discuss promising directions for future research on aggression and moral development in children and adolescents. We focus on interrelations between moral emotions, other domains of social–emotional development, and aggression.

Social events involve a complex array of competing factors, and adaptively responding to such encounters requires striking a balance of affective arousal or regulation (Eisenberg et al., 1989). Whereas moral emotions have typically been conceptualized as protective factors against aggression (Malti, 2016), developmental research on regulation and aggression has revolved around risk (Shields & Cicchetti, 2001), which, in the regulatory domain, tends to manifest in two ways: underarousal and overarousal.

The risks of underarousal are evident in the literature linking low autonomic arousal to aggression. Specifically, low resting heart rate (HR) is the best replicated biological risk factor for childhood aggression (Lorber, 2004; Ortiz & Raine, 2004; Portnoy & Farrington, 2015) and is one of the primary physiological risk factors for conduct disorder recognized by the fifth edition of the *Diagnostic and Statistical Manual of Mental Disorders* (American Psychiatric Association, 2013). If paired with the anticipated negative consequences of an aggressive act (or with the recall of such consequences), physiological arousal can serve as a repellent signal against aggressive behavior (Damasio, Everitt, & Bishop, 1996). On the other hand, children with low resting HRs are thought to be more likely to see aggressive acts through because they lack the arousal to fear their negative consequences and/ or because they enjoy their associated thrills (Raine, 2013). The cognitive components of moral emotions (e.g., understanding that one has violated a moral principle against harm) may compensate for affective underarousal to help children with low resting HRs navigate social conflicts. A recent study tested whether the aggravating link between low resting HR and aggression was offset for children with high levels of guilt or sympathy (Colasante & Malti, 2017). It found that lower resting HR was significantly associated with higher physical aggression in 5-year-olds who reported low—but not medium and high—levels of guilt and in 8-year-olds with low—but not medium and high—ratings of sympathy. In lieu of a strong physiological response, cognitive anticipation, evaluation, and/or reflection may represent important pathways to guilt and sympathy for children with low resting HRs. Guilt, for example, can arise from evaluating an aggressive act as incongruent with one's moral standards (Malti, 2016)—a scenario that requires neither empathy nor fear (both of which children with low resting HRs tend to lack; Raine, 2013; Zahn-Waxler, Cole, Welsh, & Fox, 1995). Similarly, understanding others' perspectives may promote sympathetic concern for victims of physical harm when a physiological response is lacking (Eisenberg, 2000). In line with these explanations, Ball, Smetana, and Sturge-Apple (2017) found that empathy (an affective capacity) was positively related to moral judgments in a sample of preschoolers, but only for those with low theory of mind (a cognitive capacity; higher theory of mind was associated with higher moral judgments regardless of empathy). Hence advanced cognitive capacities may provide a sufficient basis for moral functioning in children who lack affective arousal.

The risks of overarousal are perhaps best exemplified by research on anger and aggression. The frustration–aggression hypothesis (i.e., the notion that unharnessed anger and related arousal are expressed through overt aggressive behavior; Berkowitz, 1989) has been supported by studies with infants, children, and adolescents (Hay, 2005; Lochman, Barry, Powell, & Young, 2010). In their everyday lives, children encounter multifaceted social conflict situations that elicit a diverse range of emotions (Cooley, Elenbaas, & Killen, 2012), including some—such as guilt and anger—that conflict with one another. Feelings of guilt in anticipation of intentionally harming others may outweigh feelings of anger that would otherwise lead to aggression. Instead of externalizing anger toward others (e.g., via aggressive retaliation), children with high levels of guilt may be more inclined to internalize angry feelings in anticipation of violating their moral norms. It is also possible that children's guilt feelings shift their attention away from anger-inducing stimuli by highlighting the moral salience of situations and decreasing the attractiveness of aggressive reactions (Eisenberg, 2000; Malti & Latzko, 2017). Finally, the personal relevance of guilt may enhance its role in guiding behavioral outcomes (see Hoffman, 2000), as it could be argued that guilt feelings hold more intrinsic value than situational anger. In another recent study, Colasante, Zuffianò, and Malti (2016) addressed these possibilities, in part, by testing whether children's tendencies for guilt offset their day-to-day anger-related aggression. Multilevel modeling indicated that within-child spikes in daily anger were associated with more aggression, above and beyond between-child differences in average anger levels. However, this association was weaker for children who reported higher levels of guilt. This corroborates previous findings demonstrating that guilt feelings in conflict situations and sympathetic tendencies counteracted the positive link between dispositional anger and aggression in children and adolescents (Colasante, Zuffianò, & Malti, 2015), which collectively suggests that guilt feelings in social conflict situations protect children from developing stable tendencies of anger-related aggression and help them navigate *daily* spikes in anger. Nonetheless, some researchers suggest that amoral anger should be distinguished from moral anger, which may actually impede aggression. Moral anger is a specific case of anger, which can be experienced when individuals perceive disrespect or injustice to others (Kurzban, DeScioli, & O'Brien, 2007; Montada & Schneider, 1989). It is viewed as moral because identifying acts as right or wrong, even when one has not been harmed directly, precedes it (Brown, 1991).

Overall, these recent studies underscore the importance of studying moral emotions alongside related domains of social-emotional development, such as regulation, to better understand how they fit into managing aggressive behavior.

Implications and Conclusions

In this chapter, we provided a selective review of the literature on aggression and moral development in childhood and adolescence. We described a recent clinical–developmental account that attempts to integrate existing theoretical models from aggression and moral development research. We then reviewed lines of research on aggression and moral emotions, aggression and moral cognitions, and the intersection of moral emotions, moral cognitions, and other domains of social–emotional development. These integrative lines are particularly helpful for identifying promising avenues for future research and application. It has become clear that research is increasingly considering affective experiences in peer interactions that involve issues of fairness, caring, and harm, as well as evaluations of and reasoning about such events. Future work that utilizes longitudinal designs and comprehensive methodological approaches to the study of aggression and morality appear particularly useful to generate deeper knowledge on links between aggression and morality across development. In addition, more research that integrates work on the development of moral emotions with work on related domains of social–emotional development, such as emotion regulation, is necessary to generate a deeper understanding of the mechanisms that link children's affective experiences in moral encounters with their aggressive behaviors.

Research on aggression and moral development has already generated insights for educational practice and intervention approaches to reduce aggression in children and adolescents. For example, measures to assess moral emotions and moral cognition that have evolved in developmental research have shown strong reliability and validity across various cultural contexts. As such, these measures could be used to assess the development of moral emotions and moral reasoning at the child and/or group level (see Malti, Chaparro, Zuffianò, & Colasante, 2016). This knowledge, in turn, can be beneficial for the design, planning, and implementation of strategies that aim to promote social–emotional development and behavioral health, and reduce aggression and violence. Steps toward this goal have been made, as some social–emotional learning programs (see Malti & Song, Chapter 7, this volume) already integrate dimensions of moral development, such as empathy, as cornerstones of their respective curricula. As such, more integration of research on social–emotional development and morality appears useful to refine existing—and develop novel—strategies to prevent and reduce aggression in childhood and adolescence.

ACKNOWLEDGMENTS

This research was supported by the Social Sciences and Humanities Research Council of Canada and a Canadian Institutes of Health Research Foundation Scheme Grant awarded to Tina Malti (Grant No. FDN-148389).

REFERENCES

American Psychiatric Association. (2013). *Diagnostic and statistical manual of mental disorders* (5th ed.). Arlington, VA: Author.

Ardila-Rey, A., Killen, M., & Brenick, A. (2009). Moral reasoning in violent contexts: Displaced and non-displaced Colombian children's evaluations of moral transgressions, retaliation, and reconciliation. *Social Development, 18,* 181–209.

Arsenio, W. F. (2014). Moral emotion attributions and aggression. In M. Killen & J. Smetana (Eds.), *Handbook of moral development* (2nd ed., pp. 235–256). New York: Psychology Press.

Arsenio, W. F., Adams, E., & Gold, J. (2009). Social information processing, moral reasoning, and emotion attributions: Relations with adolescents' reactive and proactive aggression. *Child Development, 80*(6), 1739–1755.

Arsenio, W. F., & Lemerise, E. A. (2004). Aggression and moral development: Integrating social information processing and moral domain models. *Child Development, 75*(4), 987–1002.

Astor, R. (1994). Children's moral reasoning about family and peer violence: The role of provocation and retribution. *Child Development, 65*(4), 1054–1067.

Ball, C. L., Smetana, J. G., & Sturge-Apple, M. L. (2017). Following my head and my heart: Integrating preschoolers' empathy, theory of mind, and moral judgments. *Child Development, 88*(2), 597–611.

Barden, R. C., Zelko, F. A., Duncan, S. W., & Masters, J. C. (1980). Children's consensual knowledge about the experiential determinants of emotion. *Journal of Personality and Social Psychology, 39*(5), 968–976.

Berkowitz, L. (1989). Frustration–aggression hypothesis: Examination and reformulation. *Psychological Bulletin, 106,* 59–73.

Brown, D. E. (1991). *Human universals.* New York: McGraw-Hill.

Caravita, S. C. S., Di Blasio, P., & Salmivalli, C. (2009). Unique and interactive effects of empathy and social status on involvement in bullying. *Social Development, 18,* 140–163.

Card, N. A., & Little, T. D. (2006). Proactive and reactive aggression in childhood and adolescence: A meta-analysis of differential relations with psychosocial adjustment. *International Journal of Behavioral Development, 30*(5), 466–480.

Cillessen, A. H. N., & Rose, A. J. (2005). Understanding popularity in the peer system. *Current Directions in Psychological Science, 14*(2), 102–105.

Colasante, T., & Malti, T. (2017). Resting heart rate, guilt, and sympathy: A developmental psychophysiological study of physical aggression. *Psychophysiology, 54*(11), 1770–1781.

Colasante, T., Zuffianò, A., & Malti, T. (2015). Do moral emotions buffer the anger–aggression link in children and adolescents? *Journal of Applied Developmental Psychology, 41,* 1–7.

Colasante, T., Zuffianò, A., & Malti, T. (2016). Daily deviations in anger, guilt, and sympathy: A developmental diary study of aggression. *Journal of Abnormal Child Psychology, 44*(8), 1515–1526.

Cooley, S., Elenbaas, L., & Killen, M. (2012). Moral judgments and emotions: Adolescents' evaluations in intergroup social exclusion contexts. *New Directions for Youth Development, 2012*(136), 41–57.

Crick, N. R., & Dodge, K. A. (1996). Social information-processing mechanisms in reactive and proactive aggression. *Child Development, 67*(3), 993–1002.

Cui, L., Colasante, T., Malti, T., Ribeaud, D., & Eisner, P. (2016). Dual trajectories of reactive and proactive aggression from mid-childhood to early adolescence: Relations to sensation seeking, risk taking, and moral reasoning. *Journal of Abnormal Child Psychology, 44*(4), 663–675.

Damasio, A. R., Everitt, B. J., & Bishop, D. (1996). The somatic marker hypothesis and the possible functions of the prefrontal cortex. *Philosophical Transactions of the Royal Society B: Biological Sciences, 351*(1346), 1413–1420.

Davidov, M., Zahn-Waxler, C., Roth-Hanania, R., & Knafo, A. (2013). Concern for others in the first year of life: Theory, evidence, and avenues for research. *Child Development Perspectives, 7,* 126–131.

Decety, J., Michalska, K. J., & Kinzler, K. D. (2012). The contribution of emotion and cognition to moral sensitivity: A neurodevelopmental study. *Cerebral Cortex, 22*(1), 209–220.

Dodge, K. A., Lochman, J. E., Harnish, J. D., Bates, J. E., & Pettit, G. S. (1997). Reactive and proactive aggression in school children and psychiatrically impaired chronically assaultive youth. *Journal of Abnormal Psychology, 106,* 37–51.

Dodge, K. A., Coie, J. D., & Lynam, D. (2006). Aggression and antisocial behavior in youth. In W. Damon (Series Ed.) & N. Eisenberg (Vol. Ed.), *Handbook of child psychology: Vol. 3. Social, emotional, and personality development* (6th ed., pp. 719–788). New York: Wiley.

Dworkin, R. (1977). *Taking rights seriously.* Cambridge, MA: Harvard University Press.

Eisenberg, N. (2000). Emotion, regulation, and moral development. *Annual Review of Psychology, 51,* 665–697.

Eisenberg, N., Fabes, R. A., Miller, P. A., Fultz, J., Shell, R., Mathy, R. M., et al. (1989). Relation of sympathy and personal distress to prosocial behavior: A multimethod study. *Journal of Personality and Social Psychology, 57*(1), 55–66.

Eisenberg, N., Spinrad, T. L., & Knafo-Noam, A. (2015). Prosocial development. In M. Lamb (Ed.) & R. M. Lerner (Vol. Ed.), *Handbook of child psychology and developmental science: Vol. 3. Socioemotional processes* (7th ed., pp. 610–656). New York: Wiley

Eisenberg, N., Spinrad, T. L., & Morris, A. (2014). Empathy-related responding in children. In M. Killen & J. Smetana (Eds.), *Handbook of moral development* (2nd ed., pp. 184–207). New York: Psychology Press.

Eisner, M. P., & Malti, T. (2015). Aggressive and violent behavior. In M. E. Lamb (Vol. Ed.) & R. M. Lerner (Series Ed.), *Handbook of child psychology and developmental science: Vol. 3. Socioemotional processes* (7th ed., pp. 794–841). New York: Wiley.

Evans, A., & Lee, K. (2014). Lying, morality, and development. In M. Killen & J. Smetana (Eds.), *Handbook of moral development* (2nd ed., pp. 361–384). New York: Psychology Press.

Freud, S. (2002). *Civilization and its discontents* (D. McLintock, Trans.). London: Penguin. (Original work published in German 1930)

Frick, P., Ray, J., Thornton, L., & Kahn, R. (2014). Can callous-unemotional traits enhance the understanding, diagnosis, and treatment of serious conduct problems in children and adolescents?: A comprehensive review. *Psychological Bulletin, 140,* 1–57.

Gasser, L., & Keller, M. (2009). Are the competent the morally good?: Perspective taking and moral motivation of children involved in bullying. *Social Development, 18,* 798–816.

Gasser, L., Malti, T., & Gutzwiller-Helfenfinger, E. (2012). Aggressive and non-aggressive children's moral judgments and moral emotion attributions in situations involving retaliation and unprovoked aggression. *Journal of Genetic Psychology, 173,* 417–439.

Gutzwiller-Helfenfinger, E., Gasser, L., & Malti, T. (2010). Moral emotions and moral judgment in children's narratives: Comparing real-life and hypothetical transgressions. *New Directions for Child and Adolescent Development, 129,* 11–32.

Hamlin, K. J. (2013). Moral judgment and action in preverbal infants and toddlers: Evidence for an innate moral core. *Current Directions in Psychological Science, 22,* 186–193.

Hawley, P. H. (2003). Strategies of control, aggression, and morality in preschoolers: An evolutionary perspective. *Journal of Experimental Child Psychology, 85,* 213–235.

Hay, D. F. (2005). The beginnings of aggression in infancy. In R. Tremblay, W. W. Hartup, & J. Archer (Eds.), *Developmental origins of aggression* (pp. 107–132). New York: Guilford Press.

Hoffman, M. L. (2000). *Empathy and moral development: Implications for caring and justice.* New York: Cambridge University Press.

Hubbard, J., McAuliffe, M., Morrow, M., & Romano, L. (2010). Reactive and proactive aggression in childhood and adolescence: Precursors, outcomes, processes, experiences, and measurement. *Journal of Personality, 78,* 95–118.

Huesmann, L. R., & Guerra, N. G. (1997). Children's normative beliefs about aggression and aggressive behavior. *Journal of Personality and Social Psychology, 72*(2), 408–419.

Hume, D. (1992). *Enquiries concerning human understanding and concerning the principles of morals* (L. A. Selby-Bigge & P. H. Nidditch, Eds., 3rd ed.). Oxford, UK: Clarendon Press. (Original work published 1777)

Jambon, M., & Smetana, J. G. (2014). Moral complexity in middle childhood: Children's evaluations of necessary harm. *Developmental Psychology, 50,* 22–33.

Jambon, M., & Smetana, J. G. (2015). Theories of moral development. In J. Wright (Ed.), *International encyclopedia of social and behavioral sciences* (2nd ed., Vol. 15, pp. 788–795). Oxford, UK: Elsevier.

Jambon, M., & Smetana, J. G. (2017). Individual differences in prototypical moral and conventional judgments and children's proactive and reactive aggression. *Child Development.* [Epub ahead of print]

Jambon, M., & Smetana, J. G. (2018). Callous–unemotional traits moderate the association between children's early moral understanding and aggression: A short-term longitudinal study. *Developmental Psychology, 54,* 903–915.

Jolliffe, D., & Farrington, D. P. (2006). Examining the relationship between low empathy and bullying. *Aggressive Behavior, 32*(6), 540–550.

Kant, I. (2009). *The critique of practical reason.* Wellington, NZ: Floating Press. (Original work published 1788)

Keller, M., Lourenco, O., Malti, T., & Saalbach, H. (2003). The multifaceted phenomenon of "happy victimizers": A cross-cultural comparison of moral emotions. *British Journal of Developmental Psychology, 21,* 1–18.

Kerig, P. K., & Stellwagen, K. K. (2010). Roles of callous–unemotional traits, narcissism, and Machiavellianism in childhood aggression. *Journal of Psychopathology and Behavioral Assessment, 32,* 343–352.

Killen, M., & Malti, T. (2015). Moral judgments and emotions in contexts of peer exclusion and victimization. *Advances in Child Development and Behavior, 48,* 249–276.

Killen, M., Mulvey, K. L., Richardson, C., Jampol, N., & Woodward, A. (2011). The accidental transgressor: Morally-relevant theory of mind. *Cognition, 119*(2), 197–215.

Killen, M., & Smetana, J. (2015). Origins and development of morality. In R. Lerner (Editor-in-Chief) & M. Lamb (Vol. Ed.), *Handbook of child psychology and developmental science: Vol. 3. Socioemotional processes* (7th ed., pp. 701–749). New York: Wiley-Blackwell.

Kochanska, G., Gross, J. N., Lin, M., & Nichols, K. E. (2002). Guilt in young children: Development, determinants, and relations with a broader system of standards. *Child Development, 73*(2), 461–482.

Krettenauer, T., Colasante, T., Buchmann, M., & Malti, T. (2014). The development of moral emotions and decision-making from adolescence to early adulthood: A 6-year longitudinal study. *Journal of Youth and Adolescence, 43*(4), 583–596.

Krettenauer, T., Malti, T., & Sokol, B. (2008). The development of moral emotion expectancies and the happy victimizer phenomenon: A critical review of theory and applications. *European Journal of Developmental Science, 2,* 221–235.

Kurzban, R., DeScioli, P., & O'Brien, E. (2007). Audience effects on moralistic punishment. *Evolution and Human Behavior, 28*(2), 75–84.

Lazarus, R. S. (1991). Progress on a cognitive–motivational–relational theory of emotion. *American Psychologist, 46,* 819–834.

Lochman, J. E., Barry, T., Powell, N., & Young, L. (2010). Anger and aggression. In D. W. Nangle, D. J. Hansen, C. A. Erdley, & P. J. Norton (Eds.), *Practitioner's guide to empirically based measures of social skills* (pp. 155–166). New York: Springer.

Lorber, M. F. (2004). Psychophysiology of aggression, psychopathy, and conduct problems: A meta-analysis. *Psychological Bulletin, 130*(4), 531–552.

Lovett, B. J., & Sheffield, R. A. (2007). Affective empathy deficits in aggressive children and adolescents: A critical review. *Clinical Psychology Review, 27,* 1–13.

Malti, T. (2016). Toward an integrated clinical–developmental model of guilt. *Developmental Review, 39,* 16–36.

Malti, T., Chaparro, M. P., Zuffianò, A., & Colasante, T. (2016). School-based interventions to promote empathy-related responding in children and adolescents: A developmental analysis. *Journal of Clinical Child and Adolescent Psychology, 45*(6), 718–731.

Malti, T., Dys, S. P., Colasante, T., & Peplak, J. (2018). Emotions and morality: New developmental perspectives. In M. Harris (Series Ed.) & C. Helwig (Vol. Ed.), *Current issues in developmental psychology: New perspectives on moral development* (pp. 55–72). New York: Psychology Press.

Malti, T., Eisenberg, N., Kim, H., & Buchmann, M. (2013). Developmental trajectories of sympathy, moral emotion attributions, and moral reasoning: The role of parental support. *Social Development, 22*(4), 773–793.

Malti, T., Gummerum, M., Keller, M., & Buchmann, M. (2009). Children's moral motivation, sympathy, and prosocial behavior. *Child Development, 80,* 442–460.

Malti, T., & Keller, M. (2010). Development of moral emotions in cultural context. In W. Arsenio & E. Lemerise (Eds.), *Emotions, aggression, and morality in children: Bridging development and psychopathology* (pp. 177–198). Washington, DC: American Psychological Association.

Malti, T., & Krettenauer, T. (2013). The relation of moral emotion attributions to prosocial and antisocial behavior: A meta-analysis. *Child Development, 84*(2), 397–412.

Malti, T., & Latzko, B. (2017). Moral emotions. In J. Stein (Ed.), *Reference module on neuroscience and biobehavioral psychology.* Oxford, UK: Elsevier.

Malti, T., & Noam, G. G. (2016). Social-emotional development: From theory to practice. *European Journal of Developmental Psychology, 13*(6), 652–665.

Malti, T., & Ongley, S. F. (2014). The development of moral emotions and moral reasoning. In M. Killen & J. Smetana (Eds.), *Handbook of moral development* (2nd ed., pp. 163–183). New York: Psychology Press.

Miller, P. A., & Eisenberg, N. (1988). The relation of empathy to aggressive and externalizing/antisocial behavior. *Psychological Bulletin, 103*(3), 324–344.

Montada, L., & Schneider, A. (1989). Justice and emotional reactions to the disadvantaged. *Social Justice Research, 3*(4), 313–344.

Nunner-Winkler, G., & Sodian, B. (1988). Children's understanding of moral emotions. *Child Development, 59*(5), 1323–1338.

Olthof, T., Goossens, F. A., Vermande, M. M., Aleva, E. A., & van der Meulen, M. (2011). Bullying as strategic behavior: Relations with desired and acquired dominance in the peer group. *Journal of School Psychology, 49*(3), 339–359.

Ongley, S. F., & Malti, T. (2014). The role of moral emotions in the development of children's sharing behavior. *Developmental Psychology, 50*(4), 1148–1159.

Orobio de Castro, B., Merk, W., Koops, W., Veerman, J. W., & Bosch, J. D. (2005). Emotions in social information processing and their relations with reactive and proactive aggression in referred aggressive boys. *Journal of Clinical Child and Adolescent Psychology, 34*(1), 105–116.

Orobio de Castro, B., Verhulp, E., & Runions, K. (2012). Rage and revenge: Highly aggressive boys' explanations for their responses to ambiguous provocation. *European Journal of Developmental Psychology, 9*, 331–350.

Ortiz, J., & Raine, A. (2004). Heart rate level and antisocial behavior in children and adolescents: A meta-analysis. *Journal of the American Academy of Child and Adolescent Psychiatry, 43*(2), 154–162.

Peplak, J., & Malti, T. (2017). "That really hurt, Charlie!": Investigating the role of sympathy and moral respect in children's aggressive behaviour. *Journal of Genetic Psychology, 178*(2), 89–101.

Phinney, J. S., Feshbach, N. D., & Farver, J. (1986). Preschool children's response to peer crying. *Early Childhood Research Quarterly, 1*(3), 207–219.

Portnoy, J., & Farrington, D. P. (2015). Resting heart rate and antisocial behavior: An updated systematic review and meta-analysis. *Aggression and Violent Behavior, 22*, 33–45.

Posada, R., & Wainryb, C. (2008). Moral development in a violent society: Colombian children's judgments in the context of survival and revenge. *Child Development, 79*, 882–898.

Poulin, F., & Boivin, M. (2000). Reactive and instrumental aggression: Evidence of a two-factor model. *Psychological Assessment, 12*, 115–122.

Raine, A. (2013). *The anatomy of violence: The biological roots of crime.* New York: Pantheon Books.

Renouf, A., Brendgen, M., Seguin, J., Vitaro, F., Boivin, M., Tremblay, R., et al. (2010). Interactive links between theory of mind, peer victimization, and reactive and proactive aggression. *Journal of Abnormal Child Psychology, 38*, 1109–1123.

Sen, A. K. (2009). *The idea of justice.* Cambridge, MA: Harvard University Press.

Shields, A., & Cicchetti, D. (2001). Parental maltreatment and emotion dysregulation as risk factors for bullying and victimization in middle childhood. *Journal of Clinical Child and Adolescent Psychology, 30*(3), 349–363.

Smetana, J. G., Jambon, M., & Ball, C. (2014). The social domain approach to children's moral and social judgments. In M. Killen & J. Smetana (Eds.), *Handbook of moral development* (2nd ed., pp. 23–45). New York: Psychology Press.

Stams, G. J., Brugman, D., Dekovic, M., van Rosmalen, L., van der Laan, P., & Gibbs, J. C. (2006). The moral judgment of juvenile delinquents: A meta-analysis. *Journal of Abnormal Child Psychology, 34*, 697–713.

Svetlova, M., Nichols, S., & Brownell, C. (2010). Toddlers' prosocial behavior: From instrumental to empathic to altruistic helping. *Child Development, 81*, 1814–1827.

Tangney, J. P., Stuewig, J., & Mashek, D. J. (2007). Moral emotions and moral behavior. *Annual Review of Psychology, 58*, 345–372.

Tremblay, R. (2000). The development of aggressive behavior during childhood: What have we learned in the past century? *International Journal of Behavioral Development, 24*, 129–141.

Turiel, E., Killen, M., & Helwig, C. (1987). Morality: Its structures, functions, and vagaries. In J. Kagan & S. Lamb (Eds.), *The emergence of morality in young children* (pp. 155–243). Chicago: University of Chicago Press.

Vaish, A., Carpenter, M., & Tomasello, M. (2016). The early emergence of guilt-motivated prosocial behaviour. *Child Development, 87*(6), 1772–1782.

van Noorden, T., Haselager, G., Cillessen, A., & Bukowski, W. (2015). Empathy and involvement in bullying in children and adolescents: A systematic review. *Journal of Youth and Adolescence, 44*(3), 637–657.

Zahn-Waxler, C., Cole, P., Welsh, J., & Fox, N. (1995). Psychophysiological correlates of empathy and prosocial behaviors in preschool children with behavior problems. *Development and Psychopathology, 7*(1), 27–48.

Zahn-Waxler, C., Radke-Yarrow, M., Wagner, E., & Chapman, M. (1992). Development of concern for others. *Developmental Psychology, 28,* 126–136.

Zuffianò, A., Colasante, T., Buchmann, M., & Malti, T. (2018). The co-development of sympathy and overt aggression from middle childhood to early adolescence. *Developmental Psychology, 54*(1), 98–110.

CHAPTER 12

Social Networks and Aggression

JELLE J. SIJTSEMA and TIINA J. OJANEN

The creature was a party of boys, marching . . .
—WILLIAM GOLDING, *Lord of the Flies* (1954)

Brief Introduction

As William Golding (1954) vividly describes in his book *Lord of the Flies,* youth are very receptive to the behaviors and pressures of the peer group and may sometimes display behaviors that they would not do otherwise. Research in developmental psychology shows that peer social networks, or social ties with peers within a specific group, are important for the behavioral development of children and adolescents (Fredricks & Simpkins, 2013). Hence it comes as no surprise that peer networks also play an important role in the development of aggressive behavior (Brechwald & Prinstein, 2011; Dishion & Tipsord, 2011). In this chapter, we discuss the emergence and development of social networks and their impact on childhood and adolescent aggression. We define aggression as any behavior that involves the domination or harm of another individual, or that has the intention to do so. Aggression can be direct, or overt, and indirect, or covert (Björkqvist, Lagerspetz, & Kaukiainen, 1992; Little et al., 2003). The different forms of aggression are often differently related to social networks across childhood and adolescence. In the following sections, we focus on the theoretical perspectives of peer influence on aggressive behaviors, review the current evidence, and provide directions for future research.

Main Issues

As children grow older, peers take up a more prominent role in their lives. Starting in middle childhood, children begin to form close-knit peer groups, or cliques

(Crockett, Losoff, & Petersen, 1984). By early adolescence, peer relationships gain more importance, and more time is spent with peers than in childhood (see Rubin, Bukowski, & Bowker, 2015, for a relevant review). Although parents continue to play an important role in youths' behavioral development, peers become increasingly important role models for behavior, including aggressive behaviors. As such, it is not surprising that peers are often similar to each other in aggressive behavior (Brechwald & Prinstein, 2011; Dishion & Tipsord, 2011). One of the biggest puzzles in the study of peer relationships has been to explain how this behavioral similarity comes about. In this chapter, we discuss the role of peer networks in the development of aggression by focusing on different forms of aggression, different developments in childhood and adolescence, and the role of gender. We also discuss these topics for two different forms of peer contexts, namely, small peer clusters, or cliques (i.e., close-knit peer groups), and larger peer networks (e.g., classrooms, grades, schools).

Peer Cliques and Networks

Triads, cliques, or clusters transcend dyadic relationships such as friendship and are defined as strong or intimate clusters of peer relationships (Wasserman & Faust, 1994). Although there are various ways to define such small clusters (see the section "Measures and Methods," later in this chapter), they typically refer to groups within which the ties between peers are stronger than those with peers outside the cluster. Beyond clusters, we can distinguish classroom or school grade networks that involve larger numbers of peers. In these groups there exists a so-called "complete network" in which all individuals are aware of their peers in the network and can potentially establish a relationship with the other individuals. In addition to such social networks, researchers often refer to *peer crowds,* which are reputation-based groups of youth who are not necessarily friends but share similar values, attitudes, and behaviors (Prinstein & La Greca, 2002). In practice, the difference between a peer crowd and a (larger) peer social network is difficult to make, and our discussion of the literature in this chapter involves both. At the highest level of peer networks, there are school networks and social networks that go beyond the school context, such as a whole region or city (so-called *outside school networks*; see Burk, Steglich, & Snijders, 2007; Kiesner, Kerr, & Stattin, 2004). Although there are also worldwide networks such as seen in social media (e.g., Facebook, Twitter), these are beyond the scope of this chapter.

Forms of Aggression

Aggression can be verbal, relational, and physical in form and can serve instrumental (or proactive, goal-driven) and reactive (hostile, emotionally laden) functions (see Ostrov, Perry, & Blakely-McClure, Chapter 3, this volume). Moreover, a distinction has been made between direct aggression (e.g., hitting someone) and indirect aggression (e.g., gossiping behind someone's back; Björkqvist et al., 1992). Bullying may be construed as a distinct form of proactive aggression that comprises repetitive behavior and a clear power imbalance between the victim and the bully (see Salmivalli, Chapter 19, this volume). Presently, we focus on forms and functions of aggression other than bullying due to different underlying group dynamics.

Forms of aggression differ over the lifespan in frequency, and they often have different psychosocial correlates. Because aggression is often interindividual, it can affect social relationships and one's social standing within the peer group. It is important to mention that there is a distinction between being perceived as popular and actually being liked or accepted by members of the group. These two forms of social status do not necessarily coincide and are differently related to aggression. That is, direct aggression is less strongly, or even negatively, associated with peer acceptance over time, whereas indirect aggression is positively associated with perceived popularity (e.g., Bowker, Rubin, Buskirk-Cohen, Rose-Krasnor, & Booth-LaForce, 2010; Cillessen & Mayeux, 2004). As a result, children and adolescents may differ in the extent to which they are similar to their peers in aggressive behavior, depending on the social rewards and punishments associated with aggression.

Gender Differences

Boys and girls typically differ in the expression and frequency of aggression (see Ostrov et al., Chapter 3, this volume), and their peer networks have different characteristics. For example, girls are thought to have smaller and more intimate peer networks (e.g., Björkqvist et al., 1992; Maccoby, 1998), yet others have found that social networks are similar in size and structure for boys and girls (Bagwell, Coie, Terry, & Lochman, 2000; Cairns, Leung, Buchanan, & Cairns, 1995; Urberg, Degirmencioglu, Tolson, & Hallidayscher, 1995). Because girls' peer networks comprise fewer and closer friendships compared with boys, who have more numerous and casual relationships (Furman & Rose, 2015), *indirect* aggression may cause more damage among girls because it affects their relationships directly (Crick, Bigbee, & Howes, 1996). Girls' peer relationships are characterized by greater disclosure, support, and closeness than boys' peer relationships, whereas boys typically engage more in joint activities. Hence, aggression may be differently related to, or function differentially in, peer networks depending on gender.

Theoretical Considerations

In childhood and adolescence, most friendships are formed based on the similarity of demographic characteristics, such as gender, ethnicity, and age (Rubin et al., 2015); this appears to be the case for the friendships of aggressive youth as well (see Bukowski & Vitaro, Chapter 10, this volume). This similarity or *homophily* (McPherson, Smith-Lovin, & Cook, 2001) is typically the result of social selection and/or influence processes (Dishion & Tipsord, 2011; Veenstra, Dijkstra, Steglich, & Van Zalk, 2013). *Social selection* refers to the choice of potential friends based on characteristics that are attractive to a given individual. Thus it should be the case that aggressive youth would be likely to appear attractive to peers who are similarly aggressive. In contrast to social selection, *social influence* refers to the extent to which social relationships with peers *shape* individual behaviors over time. It has thus been speculated that aggressive youth who affiliate with one another grow increasingly similar in aggression over time.

General Processes of Behavioral Similarity

With regard to selection processes, previous work has largely focused on *similarity attraction,* suggesting that youth select similar peers because the similarity itself is attractive. In the case of aggression, peers may select each other as friends because they are similar in their cognitions about, and attitudes toward, aggression and hence are more inclined to meet and get along with each other. Recently, increasing attention has been given to the role of social status among peers in these selection processes. Youth may not necessarily be attracted to those who are similar (in the first place), but to those who are perceived to be high in social status. In some cases, aggression may be associated with high perceived popularity in the peer group (cf. Dijkstra, Berger, & Lindenberg, 2011). Simply put, many adolescents want to befriend peers who are perceived to be popular, and similarity in antisocial behavior seems to be a by-product of this selection.

Moreover, choice of friends may sometimes be the result of a process referred to as *default selection.* Some youth may not be able to establish the relationships they prefer and may settle, instead, for relationships with less preferred peers. There is some theoretical and empirical support for this notion, insofar as aggressive behavior is concerned (Deptula & Cohen, 2004; Sijtsema, Lindenberg, & Veenstra, 2010). Likewise, youth may actively *de*select peers due to their aggressive behavior, suggesting that the friendships of aggressive youth may be fragile. Overall, social selection processes may differ depending on the social rewards associated with aggression, and these rewards may differ for different forms of aggression and the specific contexts within which the aggression takes place. For example, in groups within which aggression is associated with high social status, youth are more inclined to imitate and select friends based on this behavior compared with groups within which aggression is associated with low social status (cf., Dijkstra, Lindenberg, & Veenstra, 2008).

It has also been argued that selection may occur based on *complementarity* (Aboud & Mendelson, 1996); to date, however, data supporting complementary status within the friendships of aggressive children are rather limited (Güroglu, Van Lieshout, Haselager, & Scholte, 2007).

Contrasting or complementing social selection processes are processes of social influence. That is, peers can become more similar to each other through repeated interaction and may imitate each other's behaviors, attitudes, and opinions over time. One of the mechanisms through which this influence occurs is *social learning* (Bandura, 1986): Aggressive behaviors can be rewarding in terms of status or gaining access to valuable resources and hence are imitated. A related mechanism that has received much attention is *deviancy training.* Deviancy training pertains to "social interactions among peers during which deviant attitudes and values are promoted by means of positive reinforcement in the relationship" (Dishion & Tipsord, 2011, p. 190). As such, peers can promote aggressive behaviors and youth may display aggression either to fit in or to gain and maintain their position in the peer network (see also Cillessen & Mayeux, 2004).

However, all youth are not equally susceptible to social selection and influence processes. Likewise, some youth may exert more influence over others or may be more likely to be selected as friends. Although research focusing on such moderators of social selection and influence is relatively scarce, we discuss these findings when applicable.

Group Size and Developmental Differences

There are different views pertaining to behavioral similarity in small and large peer networks, but certain things should be noted in the context of aggression. First, behavioral similarity in aggression can be the result of interactions in intimate friendship networks (e.g., youth may learn aggressive behaviors from their friends—deviancy training; Dishion & Tipsord, 2011) and/or processes related to conforming to group norms (e.g., Dijkstra et al., 2008) or the admiration of aggressive peers (e.g., Moffitt, 1993).

Second, developmental trends are important to consider. Conformity to antisocial peer behavior, but not to neutral peer behavior, increases from childhood to adolescence (Berndt, 1979). In addition, the prevalence and social influence of cliques typically peaks during early adolescence (Thompson, O'Neill Grace, & Cohen, 2001), and it has been suggested that associations between social status and clique dynamics are particularly important during this stage of development (see Closson, 2009). Finally, direct and indirect aggression are differently associated with social status during childhood and adolescence. Indirect aggression becomes more strongly associated with social prominence but more weakly associated with social preference. On the other hand, direct aggression becomes less disliked but is a weaker predictor of social prominence (Cillessen & Mayeux, 2004). In other words, the social rewards associated with direct and indirect aggression change during childhood and adolescence, and this has potential consequences for social selection and socialization effects (Dishion & Tipsord, 2011).

Differences in Gender

The structure and development of social networks defined by aggression may differ for boys and girls. In terms of frequency, boys are more likely to use direct and indirect aggression than girls and may have a preference for direct forms of aggression. When girls use aggression, it is more likely to be indirect (Card, Stucky, Sawalani, & Little, 2008). These differences may also have an impact on social relationships. Girls typically endorse communal needs and thus value intimacy and affection, whereas boys endorse agentic needs and hence value status and getting ahead (see Maccoby, 1998). One goal of boys' aggressive behavior may be to achieve social status; girls may use aggressive behavior to strengthen relationships within the peer group (e.g., by gossiping about an outgroup member). Thus the social rewards for aggression may differ between the genders, which in turn can explain differential effects of behavioral similarity in aggression displayed by girls and boys. For instance, direct aggression may be rewarded with status in boys' peer networks but punished with social rejection in girls' networks. Only a few researchers have examined these sex differences in relation to social networks, but we discuss them where possible (see also Ostrov et al., Chapter 3, this volume).

Measures and Methods

Many researchers rely on the identification of dyadic relationships (e.g., friend-ships) to assess peer clusters and peer networks. Typically, based on peer nomina-tions, aggregates of friendship dyads within a given group (e.g., a classroom, a grade) have been used as peer network data. Alternatively, some researchers have identified peer affiliation networks (e.g., "With whom do you hang out?"), which are typically larger in size and more stable over time compared with friendship net-works (Rodkin & Ahn, 2009). Next we discuss the most commonly used techniques to identify peer clusters and peer networks.

Small Clusters and Cliques

Although there are different ways to define a clique, it is typically viewed as a small cluster of peers who have strong social ties (Wasserman & Faust, 1994). The *social cognitive map* (SCM) procedure is the most commonly used technique to identify clusters or cliques of peers (Cairns, Perrin, & Cairns, 1985; Watling-Neal & Neal, 2013). In this procedure, it is assumed that individuals are able to accurately recall the social relationships of their peers (e.g., classmates), including those relation-ships they are not directly involved in. Thus, typically, each child is asked with whom they hang around, or with whom others in their group hang around. Fur-thermore, a related procedure, *cognitive social structures (CSS)*, may be utilized. In this method, respondents are asked to report the presence or absence of a "hanging out" relationship between each pair of classmates (Krackhardt, 1990; Neal, 2008).

Additionally, researchers have relied on friendship nominations within a larger group (e.g., classroom or grade) to identify small peer clusters. To identify peer clusters from friendship nominations, most researchers use the *NEGOPY* soft-ware (Richards, 1995). Clique identification in NEGOPY is based on several cri-teria. First, a clique consists of at least three members. Second, using an iterative approach, NEGOPY determines whether clique members have more links with the other clique members than with nonmembers. Third, a direct or indirect path (i.e., via a common friendship) has to exist between each member of the clique and all other clique members. To determine the robustness of an identified clique, NEGOPY tests whether the group criteria are fulfilled even when a random 10% of the clique members are deleted from the clique.

Social Networks

Several researchers have focused on the association between aggression and the position of an individual in the social network (e.g., Xie, Farmer, & Cairns, 2003). One of the most commonly used measures to assess this position is *network centrality*, or related measures such as *betweenness* and *centrality betweenness* (i.e., the number of shortest paths between individuals). For example, youth with high betweenness levels are connected to many peers in their social network and thus have more *control* over the network, have a more central position, and are closer to the other individuals in the network.

Second, many researchers have traditionally examined the extent to which individuals are similar in aggression to the larger peer network. However, in most of the extant studies, social selection and influence processes have not been statistically separated from each other. That is, the observed similarity in aggression in peer groups can be the result of social ties (social selection), behavior (social influence), or a combination of both. Moreover, due to the dependencies in the data when working with social relationships (e.g., triadic or higher-level cluster structures in social networks), it is difficult to assess selection or influence processes using standard analytic procedures, such as regression analysis (Haynie, 2001).

To address these issues, researchers have focused on disentangling the different processes underlying behavioral similarity, while also accounting for the structure of the social network and related dependencies in the data. Many of these researchers use longitudinal social network analysis, such as actor-based *SIENA* (Simulation Investigation for Empirical Network Analysis) models (Snijders, Van de Bunt, & Steglich, 2010), which allow a statistical separation of social selection from social influence effects in the development of aggression, while also accounting for the structure of the peer network. The assumption underlying these actor-based models is that individuals choose their ties (e.g., friendship) and behaviors (e.g., aggression) based on calculations of individual costs and benefits. At any given moment, participants may change a social tie or their behavior in response to the current network structure and/or the current behavior of other individuals in the social network. Via statistical simulations, SIENA models a number of potential changes that may occur, based on the observed data.

Within the SIENA framework, social selection effects are used to measure the extent to which an individual-level trait (e.g., level of aggression) predicts one's social relationships over time (e.g., selecting a peer who is similar in aggression), whereas social influence effects are measured as the extent to which social relationships (e.g., aggressive friends) affect individual traits (e.g., level of aggression) over time. Furthermore, these selection and influence effects may be moderated or mediated by group- or individual-level variables, such as peer rejection and gender.

In the following review, we focus on literature in which one or more of the procedures outlined above have been used. Research on small groups and clusters has typically used SCM or NEGOPY procedures to identify peer clusters, whereas studies on larger peer groups have usually employed SIENA analyses to study the development of aggression and the peer network.

Central Research Findings

In the following, we discuss recent advances in the study of behavioral similarity in aggression by focusing on the role of peer clusters (or cliques) and networks, separately for childhood (ages 4–13 years) and adolescence (ages 13–20 years). When applicable, we also provide insights into differences regarding the forms of aggression and gender.

Findings in Childhood

Small Clusters or Cliques

Several researchers have shown that aggressive children are likely to select peer clusters and cliques that are marked by a high degree of similarity in aggression (Berger & Rodkin, 2012; Cairns, Cairns, Neckermann, Gest, & Gariépy, 1988; Snyder, Horsch, & Childs, 1997; Xie, Cairns, & Cairns, 1999). However, the degree of similarity in aggression is sometimes overestimated, especially when relying on peer clusters identified by teachers (Gest, 2006). Although cliques of aggressive children are already identified at age 7, membership in these cliques is less stable over time compared with better adjusted cliques (e.g., low on aggression, high on prosocial behavior; Witvliet, Van Lier, Cuijpers, & Koot, 2010). Also, cliques of aggressive children are typically smaller in size than those comprising nonaggressive children (e.g., Bagwell et al., 2000; Cairns et al., 1988; Kwon & Lease, 2009). Significantly, cultural differences have been noted; a study of Chinese children indicated generally large peer cliques of aggressive children (Xu, Farver, Schwartz, & Chang, 2004). Collectively, the aforementioned studies reveal that cliques of aggressive children are rated as the lowest on indices of social status, such as social prominence and social preference (e.g., Kwon & Lease, 2009; Xu et al., 2004). Additionally, aggression has been associated with not being part of any subgroup, although aggressive children have a high network centrality within the larger group (Gest, Graham-Bermann, & Hartup, 2001). Aggressive children are thus not part of small peer clusters because their aggression may lead to conflicts, yet they are well connected to the larger peer group, in which their behaviors may be less problematic.

Moreover, boys and girls do not seem to differ in the clustering and social correlates of aggressive cliques. Although few researchers have found, or tested for, gender differences, one study indicated that boys who showed aggression and conduct problems were more likely to change clique membership status, resulting in either isolation or clique estrangement (Witvliet et al., 2010). Boys are also more likely than girls to be members of cliques that are based on aggression (Xu et al., 2004). It should be noted that identification, stability, and social influence and selection effects of peer cliques may differ per type of aggression. However, studies of aggressive peer cliques have either only focused on direct forms of aggression or assessed broadband scales of aggression.

Social Networks

Studies in which social networks of children were examined have typically assessed mutual friendship nominations within a given classroom; some researchers, however, have examined gradewide social networks. Classrooms with a more hierarchical network structure (i.e., larger differences in the centrality of individual children) are more likely to be characterized by aggression, whereas in classrooms with denser friendship networks, the association between aggression and social status is likely to be weaker, but only for boys (Ahn & Rodkin, 2014). This finding suggests that the structure of the peer network at the classroom level affects individual aggression and the payoffs associated with aggression. For instance, in classrooms with larger differences in social position, aggression can be used as a means to gain and maintain status (cf., Hawley, 1999). Assessing *network power,* or the interaction between the total number of relationships (mutual friendship nominations) within a classroom and affiliation with poorly connected peers, researchers showed additional support for the relation between network hierarchy and aggression (Neal & Cappella, 2012). That is, children who were connected to many poorly connected peers displayed more indirect aggression than other children. These effects held after controlling for direct aggression, suggesting that aggressive children may use their aggression to gain status within their peer network by dominating peers who have a weak social position in the network.

Researchers distinguishing among specific forms of aggression have shown that children in peer groups with aggressive peers report increasing direct and indirect aggression 3 months later (Ellis & Zarbatany, 2007). However, in the same study, high group centrality magnified peer socialization in indirect aggression, suggesting that the socialization of indirect aggression was stronger in more popular peer groups. This effect was not found for direct aggression and resonates with other studies reporting that direct aggression in children is negatively related to social centrality in peer networks and positively related to social isolation (Gest et al., 2001; Rodkin & Ahn, 2009). Collectively, these findings suggest that direct and indirect aggression are differently socialized within children's peer networks, with stronger social influence effects for indirect aggression in popularity networks.

To date, three studies have examined the simultaneous development of behavior and peer networks during childhood, while also controlling for structural characteristics of the social network. These studies reveal socialization, but not selection effects, for childhood aggression. That is, children become more similar to their friends in aggression over time but do not select peers based on aggression, particularly regarding indirect aggression (Dijkstra et al., 2011; Logis, Rodkin, Gest, & Ahn, 2013; Molano, Jones, Brown, & Aber, 2013). Importantly, Dijkstra and colleagues (2011) initially revealed that children selected each other based on aggression; however, these selection effects disappeared after accounting for social status, age, and structural network effects. Consequently, their study indicated that gender and social prominence were more important for the selection of friends, suggesting that selection on aggression seem to be a by-product of other variables or processes during childhood. The findings of this study have since been supported by Logis and colleagues (2013). Together, it would appear as if children's peer networks may *influence* individual members' displays of aggression; however, social *selection* in aggression can best be explained by the choice of peers with a high social status.

Although most of the above-mentioned studies did not test gender differences in the relations between social networks and aggressive behavior, there is one exception: Xie and colleagues (2003) showed that directly aggressive boys had higher social network centrality than nonaggressive boys. Moreover, fourth-grade girls characterized by indirect aggression had higher social network centrality than nonaggressive girls. Thus aggression overall seems to be related to a higher network centrality, but boys and girls may use different forms of aggression to obtain or maintain a central network position.

Findings in Adolescence

Small Clusters or Cliques

Apart from showing a high degree of similarity in aggression between clique members (e.g., Cairns et al., 1988; Espelage, Holt, & Henkel, 2003), researchers typically report social influence effects in clusters of aggressive peers. Specifically, being in an aggressive clique is associated with increases in individual levels of direct and indirect aggression over time (Low, Polanin, & Espelage, 2013). Low and colleagues (2013) also revealed that there is more within-group similarity between peers for indirect aggression than for direct aggression, suggesting that social influence effects are somewhat stronger for indirect aggression. Importantly, social influence effects likely depend on the status distribution within the clique, as social influences on aggression are more likely in cliques with many high-status peers (Pattiselanno, Dijkstra, Steglich, Vollebergh, & Veenstra, 2015). Again, this suggests that in such cliques, aggression is associated with high social status and therefore is more likely to be imitated.

Within adolescent cliques, there is often aggression toward members within the clique. For example, high-status peers use more indirect aggression toward their own clique members in popular cliques, and dominant adolescents use aggression as a means to maintain their position within the clique (Closson, 2009). Together with other similar work (Ellis, Dumas, Mahdy, & Wolfe, 2012; Pattiselanno et al., 2015), these findings suggest that aggression can be used to maintain high peer status within cliques, relative to the other clique members.

Lastly, it has been shown that social influence processes appear to be more salient for direct aggression in male than female peer cliques (Low et al., 2013). Moreover, the use of aggression *within* cliques is usually negatively associated with likeability in female cliques, but not in male cliques (Closson, 2009).

Social Networks

In research assessing large peer groups in adolescence, it is typically found that youth within the same classroom or grade-based peer group are similar in aggression (e.g., Xie et al., 1999). In one of the first studies examining the simultaneous development of aggression and peer networks, researchers, while controlling for gender similarity and structural characteristics of the friendship network, showed that adolescents became more similar to their friends in delinquency (including aggression) across time (Burk et al., 2007). Similar findings have emerged in later work (Fortuin, Van Geel, & Vedder, 2015; Van Zalk & Van Zalk, 2015), although findings differ slightly when differentiating between forms of aggression. One study of over 12,000 adolescents found clear support for social influence processes with regard to direct aggression (Haynie, Silver, & Teasdale, 2006). However, *social influence* with regard to direct aggression appears to depend on the reporter of the aggression. Using peer reports, it was found that adolescents who had physically aggressive friends became more aggressive over time (Rulison, Gest, & Loken, 2013). However, using self-reports, this effect was not supported (Sijtsema, Ojanen, et al., 2010). The latter study only showed support for social influence with regard to indirect aggression (see also Low et al., 2013, for childhood), and reactive and proactive functions of aggression.

Although less prevalent, in several studies there is support for *selection processes* while examining the simultaneous development of aggression and peer networks (the SIENA procedure; Turanovic & Young, 2016). Yet again, the findings depend on the form of aggression. When distinguishing between forms (direct and indirect) and functions (instrumental and reactive) of aggression, researchers found that adolescents became mutual friends with peers who were similar in instrumental and indirect aggression (Sijtsema, Ojanen, et al., 2010).

In several studies, it is also suggested that status achievement is an important motivation in explaining both peer selection and influence effects in adolescent aggression. According to *resource control theory,* a position of power or social dominance grants access to more resources (Hawley, 1999), and hence youth behave in ways that are in line with popular peers or peer groups. As such, social selection and influence effects may be by-products of status attainment (Dijkstra et al., 2011). When peers in the social network place high value on social status, adolescents are more likely to increase in aggression (Faris & Ennett, 2012; Laninga-Wijnen et al., 2017). Similarly, peer influence on boys' direct aggression is stronger in higher-status groups compared with lower-status groups (Shi & Xie, 2014), and high-status peers exert greater influence on adolescent aggression compared with low-status peers (Shi & Xie, 2012).

In most social network studies on adolescent aggression, researchers do not find, or do not test, gender differences in selection and influence. However, with regard to direct aggression, girls are more likely to select similarly aggressive peers and to adopt aggression from peers (Haynie, Doogan, & Soller, 2014). Also, girls are more likely to select directly aggressive friends (Rulison et al., 2013). Moreover, peer influence processes with regard to direct aggression appear stronger in more cohesive peer networks for both boys and girls (and in indirect aggression, for girls' peer networks; Shi & Xie, 2014). In sum, there appear to be some significant gender differences in the roles that the peer network plays in the development of aggression. However, overall, this research is still scarce, and thus caution is warranted before drawing any firm conclusions pertaining to gender differences with regard to the role of peer networks on aggressive development.

Implications

Collectively, the existing evidence suggests that youth are generally similar to their same-network peers in aggression. Although different processes may be responsible for this behavioral similarity, researchers who have examined social selection and influence processes simultaneously typically provide stronger evidence for social influence. That is, youth are more likely to become similar to each other in aggression instead of selecting peers who are similar in aggression. Furthermore, the findings are largely similar for children and adolescents and across gender. Despite observed minor differences based on the form of aggression, these differences must be interpreted with caution in the context of social selection and influence in youth aggression. For instance, many studies of children have only focused on direct forms of aggression. Moreover, there is variability in the methods used to assess aggression beyond the specific form (e.g., self-, peer, or teacher report), and some forms of aggression (e.g., reactive vs. proactive aggression) are not typically distinguished in many of the extant studies.

Finally, in adolescence and to a lesser extent in childhood, there is some evidence that social selection and influence processes are the by-product of social status selection (see also Dishion & Tipsord, 2011). That is, youth appear to want to befriend peers with high social status, and, at the same time, it appears to be the case that peers who are perceived as popular are often aggressive (cf., Cillessen & Mayeux, 2004; Dijkstra et al., 2011). This conclusion aligns with recent studies assessing relations between dyadic relationships (friendship) and aggression. For example, in an Indian sample of adolescents, those who showed direct aggression were high in perceived popularity, especially when their friends were low on aggression (Bowker, Ostrov, & Raja, 2011). Moreover, using longitudinal social network techniques to study social influence, a recent study provided support for the role of popularity with regard to truancy (Rambaran et al., 2017). The authors found that adolescents were more likely to become truant when their truant friends were perceived to be popular. Together, these studies suggest that being perceived as popular is linked to controlling behaviors, and such behaviors are more likely to be imitated by lower-status peers, although perceived popular peers are not always safe bets for high-quality friendships (see also Ellis & Zarbatany, 2007).

Future Directions

The study of social networks in the context of aggression is relatively novel; yet it has attracted increasing attention in the social sciences. Largely, this is the result of the introduction of new statistical techniques to analyze longitudinal social network processes. Given these developments, there are a number of suggestions to further our understanding of the structure and function of social networks regarding the development of youth aggression.

First, researchers may focus on alternative processes with regard to social selection in aggression. Many researchers have examined behavioral similarity in aggression as the result of an active social selection process, in which selection refers to creating new relationships based on similarity or attraction. However, there are two alternative selection processes that are less well studied: *deselection* and *default selection*. The first refers to breaking off existing social relationships based on certain characteristics, whereas the latter refers to the process of forming social relationships due to a lack of viable alternatives (see Deptula & Cohen, 2004; Sijtsema, Lindenberg, & Veenstra, 2010). These processes are highly relevant in the context of aggressive behavior because increased status concerns and related antisocial behaviors can come at a considerable cost. For one, the pursuit of status may not always be compatible with the establishment of positive social relationships with peers. In fact, in one study, it was found that the friendships of adolescents with strong status orientations are more likely to dissolve over time (Ojanen, Sijtsema, & Rambaran, 2013), potentially because these youth are behaviorally arrogant (Bowker, Rubin, Buskirk-Cohen, Rose-Krasnor, & Booth-LaForce, 2010). Furthermore, regarding status-rewarding behaviors such as aggression, there is some empirical support for the notion that aggressive youth with poor prosocial skills have limited opportunities for establishing friendships and hence have to settle for less preferred friendships (Deptula & Cohen, 2004; Ellis & Zarbatany, 2007; Hektner, August, & Realmuto, 2000; Sijtsema, Lindenberg, & Veenstra, 2010). Such default selection processes have also been observed in related behaviors, such as peer victimization (Sijtsema, Rambaran, & Ojanen, 2013) and may well extend to aggressive behaviors in rejected or unpopular youth.

Second, as our overview of empirical studies has illustrated, there is a need for more studies that test and explain developmental and gender differences in behavioral similarity processes. About half of the presently reviewed studies tested for gender differences, but often these tests were either omitted or conducted in an exploratory fashion. Hence, more concrete hypotheses and theories about potential gender differences should be formulated and tested. Moreover, the field is lacking studies that focus on the role of peer networks in early and middle childhood. It is obviously challenging to assess these networks at very young ages, but there are studies that have done this in 4- and 5-year olds using traditional peer nominations (Vermande, Van den Oord, Goudena, & Rispens, 2000). Also, computerized peer-nomination procedures via the use of pictures of the children in the peer network have been used in 5- to 10-year-olds (Verlinden et al., 2014).

Third, the role of moderators in behavioral similarity processes is attracting increasing research interest. At the individual level, youth can differ in the extent to which they are able to resist negative peer influences. For example, youth with traits that compromise consequential thinking (e.g., impulsivity) or with insufficient support from external significant others, such as teachers and parents, may be more susceptible to the lures of deviant peers and peer groups (Dishion & Tipsord, 2011). To date, little is known about the role of such individual-level moderators in social selection and influence processes, but recent studies have examined the extent to which cognitions affect social influence. Two studies have tested whether certain cognitions predispose youth to a heightened susceptibility to antisocial influences (Molano et al., 2013; Sijtsema, Rambaran, Caravita, & Gini, 2014). In both studies, the findings provided modest or marginal support for this hypothesis but suggested that youth higher on moral disengagement (i.e., justifying antisocial conduct) or hostile attribution biases (i.e., ascribing hostile intention to neutral or ambiguous cues) were more likely to become similar to their aggressive or bullying friends than youth lower in these cognitions.

Another important moderator of behavioral similarity to consider is social status, including both the dimension of perceived popularity and likeability. The strength of peer influences on individual aggression may be contingent upon status, as youth may either be more susceptible to peer influences or be more influential themselves. Specifically, on the likeability dimension, youth with a marginalized status may have a greater need to fit in and hence behave antisocially either to gain status or approval from peers (see also Dishion & Tipsord, 2011; Rudolph et al., 2014). Yet approval seeking can easily backfire when youth affiliate with aggressive peers who are unable to provide affection, leading to an even more severe detachment from the larger peer group. On the perceived popularity dimension, high-status youth may be more likely to set the norm with regard to antisocial behavior (Laninga-Wijnen et al., 2017).

Clearly, more research is needed for a thorough understanding of how factors such as social status and antisocial cognitions may moderate social selection and influence in the development of aggression and potentially result in either a heightened susceptibility to peer behavior or a heightened influence on peers.

Finally, this chapter focused on research in which peer networks have been assessed as friendship networks. In several studies, it is suggested that including nonfriendship relationships in the study of aggression would be fruitful. Indeed, some researchers have focused on mutual antipathies (Rambaran, Dijkstra, Munniksma, & Cillessen, 2015) and bullying relationships (Huitsing, Snijders, Van Duijn, & Veenstra, 2014). Also, youth typically have multiple simultaneous relationships within the peer network. For example, they can be friends with some group members (a friendship tie) and at the same time have a negative relationship (a dislike tie) with others within the same network. These different relationships may affect each other. For instance, liking or disliking someone (a network tie based on liking) is an important predictor of a future friendship (a friendship tie). Recent advances in social network analyses have allowed researchers to consider these complex multiple relationships, or so-called multiplex ties, between youth within a social network. For example, regarding bullying, over time defenders of victims (a defending tie) run the risk of becoming bullied (a victimization tie) by the bullies of the victims they defend (see Huitsing et al., 2014). Studying such processes with regard to aggression may thus yield valuable insights into aggression between subgroups of peers and the extent to which aggression affects the development of multiple relationships, or vice versa.

Conclusions

In conclusion, social networks play an important role in the development of both direct and indirect forms of aggression. In the past decades, researchers have clearly shown that there is behavioral similarity in aggression between youth and their social networks, be it a small close-knit clique or a large social network with weaker ties. Although in recent studies it is suggested that social influence processes lie at the basis of this behavioral similarity, more detailed analyses of both social influence and (alternative) selection processes is needed in order to fully understand this similarity. Returning to the peer processes described in *Lord of the Flies*, in this chapter we covered some main perspectives on the social selection and influence processes among peers with regard to the development of aggression. Often, these processes exist as a function of social status pursuit, and most of them can be observed in both childhood and adolescence, in small cliques and larger social networks, and they are mostly robust across gender and direct and indirect forms of aggression.

REFERENCES

Aboud, F. E., & Mendelson, M. J. (1996). Determinants of friendship selection and quality: Developmental perspectives. In W. M. Bukowski, A. F. Newcomb, & W. W. Hartup (Eds.), *The company they keep: Friendship in childhood and adolescence* (pp. 87–112). Cambridge, UK: Cambridge University Press.

Ahn, H.-J., & Rodkin, P. C. (2014). Classroom-level predictors of the social status of aggression: Friendship centralization, friendship density, teacher–student attunement, and gender. *Journal of Educational Psychology, 106*(4), 1144–1155.

Bagwell, C. L., Coie, J., Terry, R. A., & Lochman, J. E. (2000). Peer clique participation and social status in preadolescence. *Merrill–Palmer Quarterly, 46*(2), 280–305.

Bandura, A. (1986). *Social foundations of thought and action: A social cognitive theory.* Englewood Cliffs, NJ: Prentice Hall.

Berger, C., & Rodkin, P. C. (2012). Group influences on individual aggression and prosociality: Early adolescents who change peer affiliations. *Social Development, 21,* 396–413.

Berndt, T. J. (1979). Developmental changes in conformity to peers and parents. *Developmental Psychology, 15*(6), 608–616.

Björkqvist, K., Lagerspetz, K. M. J., & Kaukiainen, A. (1992). Do girls manipulate and boys fight?: Developmental trends in regard to direct and indirect aggression. *Aggressive Behavior, 18*(2), 117–127.

Bowker, J. C., Ostrov, J. M., & Raja, R. (2011). Relational and overt aggression in urban India: Associations with peer relations and best friends' aggression. *International Journal of Behavioral Development, 36*(2), 107–116.

Bowker, J. C., Rubin, K. H., Buskirk-Cohen, A., Rose-Krasnor, L., & Booth-LaForce, C. L. (2010). Behavioral changes predicting temporal changes in perceived popular status. *Journal of Applied Developmental Psychology, 31,* 126–133.

Brechwald, W. A., & Prinstein, M. J. (2011). Beyond homophily: A decade of advances in understanding peer influence processes. *Journal of Research on Adolescence, 21,* 166–179.

Burk, W., Steglich, C. E. G., & Snijders, T. A. B. (2007). Beyond dyadic interdependence: Actor-oriented models for co-evolving social networks and individual behaviors. *International Journal of Behavioral Development, 31,* 397–404.

Cairns, R. B., Cairns, B. D., Neckermann, H. J., Gest, S. D., & Gariépy, J. L. (1988). Social networks and aggressive behavior: Peer support or peer rejection. *Developmental Psychology, 24,* 815–823.

Cairns, R. B., Leung, M. C., Buchanan, L., & Cairns, B. D. (1995). Friendships and social networks in childhood and adolescence: Fluidity, reliability, and interrelations. *Child Development, 66,* 1330–1345.

Cairns, R. B., Perrin, J. E., & Cairns, B. D. (1985). Social structure and social cognition in early adolescence: Affiliative patterns. *Journal of Early Adolescence, 5,* 339–355.

Card, N. A., Stucky, B. D., Sawalani, G. M., & Little, T. D. (2008). Direct and indirect aggression during childhood and adolescence: A meta-analytic review of gender differences, intercorrelations, and relations to maladjustment. *Child Development, 79*(5), 1185–1229.

Cillessen, A. H. N., & Mayeux, L. (2004). From censure to reinforcement: Developmental changes in the association between aggression and social status. *Child Development, 75*(1), 147–163.

Closson, L. M. (2009). Aggressive and prosocial behaviors within early adolescent friendship cliques: What's status got to do with it? *Merrill–Palmer Quarterly, 55*(4), 406–435.

Crick, N. R., Bigbee, M. A., & Howes, C. (1996). Gender differences in children's normative beliefs about aggression: How do I hurt thee? Let me count the ways. *Child Development, 67*(3), 1003–1014.

Crockett, L., Losoff, M., & Petersen, A. C. (1984). Perceptions of the peer group and friendship in early adolescence. *Journal of Early Adolescence, 4*(2), 155–181.

Deptula, D. P., & Cohen, R. (2004). Aggressive, rejected, and delinquent children and adolescents: A comparison of their friendships. *Aggression and Violent Behavior, 9*(1), 75–104.

Dijkstra, J. K., Berger, C., & Lindenberg, S. (2011). Do physical and relational aggression explain adolescents' friendship selection?: The competing roles of network characteristics, gender, and social status. *Aggressive Behavior, 37*(5), 417–429.

Dijkstra, J. K., Lindenberg, S., & Veenstra, R. (2008). Beyond the class norm: Bullying behavior of popular adolescents and its relation to peer acceptance and rejection. *Journal of Abnormal Child Psychology, 36*(8), 1289–1299.

Dishion, T. J., & Tipsord, J. M. (2011). Peer contagion in child and adolescent social and emotional development. *Annual Review of Psychology, 62,* 189–214.

Ellis, W. E., Dumas, T. M., Mahdy, J. C., & Wolfe, D. A. (2012). Observations of adolescent peer group interactions as a function of within- and between-group centrality status. *Journal of Research on Adolescence, 22*(2), 252–266.

Ellis, W. E., & Zarbatany, L. (2007). Peer group status as a moderator of group influence on children's deviant, aggressive, and prosocial behavior. *Child Development, 78,* 1240–1254.

Espelage, D. L., Holt, M. K., & Henkel, R. R. (2003). Examination of peer-group contextual effects on aggression during early adolescence. *Child Development, 74,* 205–220.

Faris, R., & Ennett, S. (2012). Adolescent aggression: The role of peer group status motives, peer aggression, and group characteristics. *Social Networks, 34,* 371–378.

Fortuin, J., Van Geel, M., & Vedder, P. (2015). Peer influences on internalizing and externalizing problems among adolescents: A longitudinal social network analysis. *Journal of Youth and Adolescence, 44,* 887–897.

Fredricks, J. A., & Simpkins, S. D. (2013). Organized out-of-school activities and peer relationships: Theoretical perspectives and previous research. In J. A. Fredricks & S. D. Simpkins (Eds.), *New directions for child and adolescent development: No. 140. Organized out-of-school activities: Settings for peer relationships* (pp. 1–17). Hoboken, NJ: Wiley.

Furman, W., & Rose, A. (2015). Friendships, romantic relationships, and peer relationships. In R. Lerner (Series Ed.) & M. E. Lamb (Vol. Ed.), *Handbook of child psychology and developmental science: Vol. 3. Socioemotional development* (7th ed., pp. 932–974). Hoboken, NJ: Wiley.

Gest, S. D. (2006). Teacher reports of children's friendships and social groups: Agreement with peer reports and implications for studying peer similarity. *Social Development, 15,* 248–259.

Gest, S. D., Graham-Bermann, S. A., & Hartup, W. W. (2001). Peer experience: Common and unique features of number of friendships, social network centrality, and sociometric status. *Social Development, 10,* 23–40.

Golding, W. (1954). *Lord of the flies.* London: Faber & Faber.

Güroglu, B., Van Lieshout, C. F. M., Haselager, G. J. T., & Scholte, R. H. J. (2007). Similarity and complementarity of behavioral profiles of friendship types and types of friends: Friendships and psychosocial adjustment. *Journal of Research on Adolescence, 17*(2), 357–386.

Hawley, P. H. (1999). The ontogenesis of social dominance: A strategy-based evolutionary perspective. *Developmental Review, 19*(1), 97–132.

Haynie, D. L. (2001). Delinquent peers revisited: Does network structure matter? *American Journal of Sociology, 106,* 1013–1057.

Haynie, D., Doogan, N. J., & Soller, B. (2014). Gender, friendship networks, and delinquency: A dynamic network approach. *Criminology, 52,* 688–722.

Haynie, D., Silver, E., & Teasdale, B. (2006). Neighborhood characteristics, peer networks, and adolescent violence. *Journal of Quantitative Criminology, 22,* 147–169.

Hektner, J. M., August, G. J., & Realmuto, G. M. (2000). Patterns of temporal changes in peer affiliation among aggressive and nonaggressive children participating in a summer school program. *Journal of Clinical Child Psychology, 29,* 603–614.

Huitsing, G., Snijders, T. A. B., Van Duijn, M. A. J., & Veenstra, R. (2014). Victims, bullies, and their defenders: A longitudinal study of the coevolution of positive and negative networks. *Development and Psychopathology, 26*(3), 645–659.

Kiesner, J., Kerr, M., & Stattin, H. (2004). "Very important persons" in adolescence: Going beyond in-school, single friendships in the study of peer homophily. *Journal of Adolescence, 27,* 545–560.

Krackhardt, D. (1990). Assessing the political landscape: Structure, cognition and power in organizations. *Administrative Science Quarterly, 35,* 342–369.

Kwon, K., & Lease, A. M. (2009). Examination of the contribution of clique characteristics to children's adjustment: Clique type and perceived cohesion. *International Journal of Behavioral Development, 33,* 230–242.

Laninga-Wijnen, L., Harakeh, Z., Steglich, C., Dijkstra, J. K., Veenstra, R., & Vollebergh, W. (2017). The norms of popular peers moderate friendship dynamics of adolescent aggression. *Child Development, 88,* 1265–1283.

Little, T. D., Brauner, J., Jones, S. M., Nock, M. K., & Hawley, P. H. (2003). Rethinking aggression: A typological examination of the functions of aggression. *Merrill–Palmer Quarterly, 49,* 343–369.

Logis, H. C., Rodkin, P. C., Gest, S. D., & Ahn, H.-J. (2013). Popularity as an organizing factor of preadolescent friendship networks: Beyond prosocial and aggressive behavior. *Journal of Research on Adolescence, 23,* 413–423.

Low, S., Polanin, J. R., & Espelage, D. L. (2013). The role of social networks in physical and relational aggression among young adolescents. *Journal of Youth and Adolescence, 42,* 1078–1089.

Maccoby, E. E. (1998). *The two sexes: Growing up apart, coming together.* Cambridge, MA: Harvard University Press.

McPherson, M., Smith-Lovin, L., & Cook, J. M. (2001). Birds of a feather: Homophily in social networks. *Annual Review of Sociology, 27,* 415–444.

Moffitt, T. E. (1993). Adolescence-limited and life-course-persistent antisocial behavior: A developmental taxonomy. *Psychological Review, 100*(4), 674–701.

Molano, A., Jones, S. K., Brown, J., & Aber, J. L. (2013). Selection and socialization of aggressive and prosocial behavior: The moderating role of social-cognitive processes. *Journal of Research on Adolescence, 23,* 424–436.

Neal, J. W. (2008). "Kracking" the missing data problem: Applying Krackhardt's cognitive social structures to school-based social networks. *Sociology of Education, 81,* 140–162.

Neal, J. W., & Cappella, E. (2012). An examination of network position and childhood relational aggression: Integrating resource control and social exchange theories. *Aggressive Behavior, 38,* 126–140.

Ojanen, T., Sijtsema, J. J., & Rambaran, A. (2013). Social goals and adolescent friendships: Do power and affiliation motives evidence different friendship selection and influence processes? *Journal of Research on Adolescence, 23*(3), 550–562.

Pattiselanno, K., Dijkstra, J. K., Steglich, C., Vollebergh, W., & Veenstra, R. (2015). Structure matters: The role of clique hierarchy in the relationship between adolescent social status and aggression and prosociality. *Journal of Youth and Adolescence, 44,* 2257–2274.

Prinstein, M. J., & La Greca, A. M. (2002). Peer crowd affiliation and internalizing distress in childhood and adolescence: A longitudinal follow-back study. *Journal of Research on Adolescence, 12*(3), 325–351.

Rambaran, J. A., Dijkstra, J. K., Munniksma, A., & Cillessen, A. H. N. (2015). The development of adolescents' friendships and antipathies: A longitudinal multivariate network test of balance theory. *Social Networks, 43,* 162–176.

Rambaran, J. A., Hopmeyer, A., Schwartz, D., Steglich, C., Badaly, D., & Veenstra, R. (2017). Academic functioning and peer influences: A short-term longitudinal study of network-behavior dynamics in middle adolescence. *Child Development, 88,* 523–543.

Richards, W. D. (1995). *NEGOPY 4.30 manual and user's guide.* Burnaby, BC, Canada: Simon Fraser University School of Communications.

Rodkin, P. C., & Ahn, H. (2009). Social networks derived from affiliations and friendships, multi-informant and self-reports: Stability, concordance, placement of aggressive and unpopular children, and centrality. *Social Development, 18,* 557–576.

Rubin, K. H., Bukowski, W. M., & Bowker, J. C. (2015). Children in peer groups. In R. M. Lerner (Ed.), *Handbook of child psychology and developmental science* (Vol. 4, pp. 1–48). Hoboken, NJ: Wiley.

Rudolph, K. D., Lansford, J. E., Agoston, A. M., Sugimura, N., Schwartz, D., Dodge, K. A., et al. (2014). Peer victimization and social alienation: Predicting deviant peer affiliation in middle school. *Child Development, 85*(1), 124–139.

Rulison, K. L., Gest, S. D., & Loken, E. (2013). Dynamic social networks and physical aggression: The moderating role of gender and social status among peers. *Journal of Research of Adolescence, 23,* 437–449.

Shi, B., & Xie, H. (2012). Socialization of physical and social aggression in early adolescents' peer groups: High-status peers, individual status, and gender. *Social Development, 21,* 170–194.

Shi, B., & Xie, H. (2014). Moderating effects of group status, cohesion, and ethnic composition on socialization of aggression in children's peer groups. *Developmental Psychology, 50*(9), 2188–2198.

Sijtsema, J. J., Lindenberg, S. M., & Veenstra, R. (2010). Do they get what they want or are they stuck with what they can get?: Testing homophily against default selection for friendships of highly aggressive boys: The TRAILS study. *Journal of Abnormal Child Psychology, 38*(6), 803–813.

Sijtsema, J. J., Ojanen, T. J., Veenstra, R., Lindenberg, S. M., Hawley, P. H., & Little, T. D. (2010). Forms and functions of aggression in adolescent friendship selection and influence: A longitudinal social network analysis. *Social Development, 19*(3), 515–534.

Sijtsema, J. J., Rambaran, J. A., Caravita, S. C. S., & Gini, G. (2014). Friendship selection and influence in bullying and defending: Effects of moral disengagement. *Developmental Psychology, 50*(8), 2093–2104.

Sijtsema, J. J., Rambaran, J. A., & Ojanen, T. J. (2013). Overt and relational victimization and adolescent friendships: Selection, de-selection, and social influence. *Social Influence, 8*(2–3), 177–195.

Snijders, T., Van de Bunt, G., & Steglich, C. E. (2010). Introduction to stochastic actor-based models for network dynamics. *Social Networks, 32*(1), 44–60.

Snyder, J., Horsch, E., & Childs, J. (1997) Peer relationships of young children: Affiliative choices and the shaping of aggressive behavior. *Journal of Clinical Child Psychology, 26*(2), 145–156.

Thompson, M., O'Neill Grace, C., & Cohen, L. J. (2001). *Best friends, worst enemies: Understanding the social lives of children.* New York: Ballantine.

Turanovic, J. J., & Young, J. T. N. (2016). Violent offending and victimization in adolescence: Social network mechanisms and homophily. *Criminology, 54,* 487–519.

Urberg, K. A., Degirmencioglu, S. M., Tolson, J. M., & Hallidayscher, K. (1995). The structure of adolescent peer networks. *Developmental Psychology, 31,* 540–547.

Van Zalk, M. H. W., & Van Zalk, N. (2015). Violent peer influence: The roles of self-esteem and psychopathic traits. *Development and Psychopathology, 27,* 1077–1088.

Veenstra, R., Dijkstra, J. K., Steglich, C., & Van Zalk, M. (2013). Network–behavior dynamics. *Journal of Research on Adolescence, 23,* 399–412.

Verlinden, M., Veenstra, R., Ghassabian, A., Jansen, P. W., Hofman, A., Jaddoe, V. W. V., et al. (2014). Executive functioning and non-verbal intelligence as predictors of bullying in early elementary school. *Journal of Abnormal Child Psychology, 42,* 953–966.

Vermande, M. M., Van den Oord, E. J. C. G., Goudena, P. P., & Rispens, J. (2000). Structural characteristics of aggressor–victim relationships in Dutch school classes of 4- to 5-year-olds. *Aggressive Behavior, 26*(1), 11–31.

Wasserman, S., & Faust, K. (1994). *Social network analysis: Methods and applications.* Cambridge, UK: Cambridge University Press.

Watling-Neal, J. W., & Neal, Z. P. (2013). The multiple meanings of peer groups in social cognitive mapping. *Social Development, 22*(3), 580–594.

Witvliet, M., Van Lier, P. A. C., Cuijpers, P., & Koot, H. M. (2010). Change and stability in childhood clique membership, isolation from cliques, and associated child characteristics. *Journal of Clinical Child and Adolescent Psychology, 39*(1), 12–24.

Xie, H., Cairns, R. B., & Cairns, B. D. (1999). Social networks and social configuration in inner-city schools: Aggression, popularity, and implications for students with EBD. *Journal of Emotional and Behavioral Disorders, 7,* 147–155.

Xie, H., Farmer, T. W., & Cairns, B. D. (2003). Different forms of aggression among inner-city African–American children: Gender, configurations, and school social networks. *Journal of School Psychology, 41,* 355–375.

Xu, Y., Farver, J. A. M., Schwartz, D., & Chang, L. (2004). Social networks and aggressive behaviour in Chinese children. *International Journal of Behavioral Development, 28*(5), 401–410.

CHAPTER 13

Cyberbullying

MARION K. UNDERWOOD and SHERI A. BAUMAN

Brief Introduction

Adolescents are heavily engaged in text messaging (Lenhart, 2012) and social media (boyd, 2014); their social lives move seamlessly between online and offline interactions. Adolescents embrace digital communication as a way to connect with friends, peers and social networks, and family members and to create and display their developing identities. Not surprisingly, adolescents also use digital communication to express their anger and pursue their social goals. Cyberbullying refers to "any behavior performed through electronic or digital media by individuals or groups intended to inflict harm or discomfort on others" (Tokunaga, 2010, p. 278).

Although there is clearly some continuity between face-to-face bullying and cyberaggression, we cannot assume these are one and the same, for several reasons. First, digital platforms are unique in that they allow users to disseminate aggressive content to hundreds of friends and followers instantaneously, and digital platforms break down social boundaries in ways that may raise adolescents' exposure to hurtful experiences. In addition, each different digital platform offers particular features, affordances that may foster cyberbullying (e.g., Snapchat users may set a time after which the image they send disappears) but that also may reduce negative online behavior (Facebook has a "like" button but not a "dislike" option and allows users to designate friends but not enemies). Another reason that understanding cyberbullying may require different approaches is that the digital world may be a place in which high-status youth who would never sully their hands with physical aggression engage in the occasional act of cyberaggression, which could result in a terribly painful experience for the victim because the humiliation is so public.

Main Issues

Although cyberbullying is a recent phenomenon, more than 30,000 scholarly papers have been published on this topic. A comprehensive review of this large literature is beyond the scope of this chapter. This chapter begins with theoretical frameworks to guide research on cyberbullying. Next, methodological issues are considered; this new field is plagued by reliance on self-report measures and the challenge of shared method variance, and it is important to consider other ways of measuring cyberbullying. An overview of central research findings will focus on current knowledge of the forms cyberbullying takes, possible causes of cyberbullying (though most research to date is correlational), and how cyberbullying relates to psychosocial adjustment for victims as well as perpetrators. This review of central research findings will focus on studies of adolescents because most research has been conducted with adolescent participants, perhaps in part because adolescents are so heavily engaged in digital communication (Lenhart, 2015). The chapter concludes by highlighting implications for prevention and intervention and future directions.

Theoretical Considerations

Theories provide a lens through which a phenomenon such as cyberbullying can be examined and should generate pertinent research questions, as well as helping with integrating and interpreting research findings. In the broader field of traditional bullying research, several theoretical perspectives have gained prominence. It is tempting to assume that these theories apply to cyberbullying, as well, but the unique aspects of cyberbullying may not be adequately addressed in those theories. In this section, we review several theories that have been proposed as frameworks for cyberbullying research. Although many articles in the literature mention a theory, few of the theories have been tested empirically, although in some cases components of the theory have been evaluated; these are noted when applicable.

Social–Ecological Theory

The social–ecological theory of bullying, promoted by Espelage and Swearer (2004; Swearer & Espelage, 2011), is based on the theory of Uri Bronfenbrenner (1979, 2005). This theory emphasizes the influence of context in human development and behavior. The individual is at the center of overlapping layers of influence, defined as the microsystem (the immediate environment, including family, school, and peers); the mesosystem (the interactions among microsystems, as when parents meet with teachers), the exosystem (systems outside the individual that affect them indirectly, such as a parent's workplace), and the macrosystem (the societal and cultural context). It is appropriate for cyberspace to be placed in the microsystem because of its pervasive immediate presence in our lives, especially for youth (Eaton, 2014; Johnson & Puplampu, 2008; Renn & Arnold, 2003). Eaton argues that each platform (e.g., Instagram, Twitter) could be considered an individual microsystem because each involves different aspects of self and influences the individual in different ways. The companies that create social media sites are part of the exosystem; the individual is not involved, but the decisions made by software engineers provide the platforms used by individuals. Laws and policies in schools and workplaces are also part of the exosystem. Cyberspace might be considered a macrosystem because society as a whole has embraced new technologies, and the ubiquitous presence of digital technology permeates the environment. This updated theory places digital technology in the innermost layer, accurately reflecting the importance of the digital system in individual development and behavior, while recognizing the impact of larger systems.

Although social–ecological theory is often cited as the basis for cyberbullying research, studies have not directly tested the theory as a whole; rather, researchers have generally focused on the separate layers. For example, the individual is at the center of the model, and many individual characteristics have been examined with respect to their influence on cyberbullying dynamics (e.g., age, gender, race/ethnicity, sexual orientation). At the microsystem level, peer and family influences on aggression have been documented. Much less attention has been paid to the outer layers of the model. Arguably, the digital world and media are components of the exosystem, and the integration of the individual, microsystem, and mesosystem elements in studies have provided some validation of this theory. The macrosystem, or cultural layer, is difficult to measure, although perhaps some of the cross-national investigations are steps in this direction. The chronosystem—historical periods—is essentially absent from scholarly inquiry, although anecdotal reports suggest that in the current historical period in the United States, there are reasons to believe that cyberbullying would increase due to the use of social media by powerful political figures to disparage opponents. A daunting but important research endeavor would seek to understand the relative influence of the various layers on individual behavior. For example, are some young people more susceptible to macrosystem or chronosystem influences than others? What characteristics serve as risk or protective factors for those influences? Investigations that test the relative influence of the various systems and describe the mechanisms by which that influence occurs would provide support for this theory as an appropriate framework for cyberbullying research. Hong and Espelage (2012) provide a thorough review of this theory and related research.

The Online Disinhibition Effect: A Useful Model

The online disinhibition effect describes the tendency to behave differently in cyberspace than in offline settings (Suler, 2004) and is considered a primary feature that distinguishes cyberbullying from traditional bullying. This effect is typically offered as an explanation for excessive cruelty or vulgarity in online interactions, especially in cyberbullying. However, Suler's explication of online behavior is more nuanced than this most relevant proposition. Suler proposes that the online setting generates two kinds of disinhibition: The first is benign disinhibition, which can be seen in the majority of text messaging exchanges, which are positive and supportive interactions (Underwood, Ehrenreich, More, Solis, & Brinkley, 2015) or contain more self-disclosure than in-person conversation (Davis, 2012). For some people, such messages are easier to deliver online than in person. The kind of disinhibition that is found in cyberbullying, however, Suler calls toxic disinhibition, which refers to the tendency to say more cruel and vulgar things online than in person.

Suler (2004) described features of the digital environment that seem to encourage this disinhibition. Those include anonymity, physical invisibility (of both sender and receiver of content), asynchronicity of communication, solipsistic introjection (the feeling that the "others" one encounters and communicates with online are part of the self), dissociative imagination (the sense that the online world is not real, so ordinary rules of interaction do not apply), minimization of status and authority, individual differences in personality and intensity of feelings, and shifts among intrapsychic constellations (revealing one's "true" self online). Suler suggested that some online environments might be more likely to promote these processes than others. Relatively few studies have tested these factors. Swiss adolescents rated public and anonymous cyberbullying to be worse than private and known senders (Sticca & Perren, 2013). Type of cyberbullying and the degree of publicity of the event are crucial factors in the degree of distress experienced by targets of cyberbullying (Pieschl, Kuhlmann, & Porsch, 2015). More research that tests the other hypothesized components of online disinhibition could determine which of these mechanisms operates in which settings and for which individuals. It would also be helpful to examine differences in digital platforms (e.g., social media and apps) that may more readily encourage toxic inhibition.

The Theory of Planned Behavior

The theory of planned behavior (TPB; Ajzen, 1991) focuses on the precursors to enacting a behavior. Three factors are posited to influence the enactment (or not) of a particular action (Barkoukis, Lazuras, & Tsorbatzoudis, 2013). One is behavioral beliefs, or attitudes toward the behavior. Regarding cyberbullying, this refers to how the individual appraises or judges cyberbullying actions (are they harmless, funny, harmful, inappropriate?). These attitudes are formed by observational learning, direct instruction, and social interactions with valued others.

The second factor is normative beliefs, or one's beliefs about what others think and do, that is, what is "normal" or acceptable behavior in cyberspace or on social media sites. Such norms can be subjective, formed by the individual in response to his or her need for approval, so that the individual has an opinion about how much approval he or she will gain by enacting a behavior. Descriptive norms, however, refer to the individual's perception of the prevalence of the behavior in a given group (friends, classmates, schoolmates, society, etc.). Descriptive norms may operate at both conscious and unconscious levels to influence behavior (Barkoukis et al., 2013). When the behavior is believed to be common, one is more likely to engage in that behavior. This approach has been used in efforts to reduce substance abuse behavior in young people by presenting data showing that binge drinking, for example, is not as normal as many think. A study of young adults found that participants who endorsed statements about the acceptability and typicality of cyberaggression were more likely to engage in cyberaggression 6 months later (Wright & Li, 2013).

Finally, moral norms, which are the individual's moral code about the particular behavior (is it right or wrong?), contribute to the individual decision about whether or not to engage in cyberbullying or to take action when cyberbullying is observed. If an individual believes that cyberbullying is morally wrong (based on his or her moral development), he or she is much less likely to engage in the behavior. However, Bandura (1999) described the cognitive process of moral disengagement, whereby a person is able to behave in ways contrary to his or her moral code without suffering from guilt. This theory has been tested regarding cyberbullying (see Bussey, Fitzpatrick, & Raman, 2015; Menesini, Nocentini, & Camodeca, 2013; Perren & Gutzwiller-Helfenfinger, 2012; Robson & Witenberg, 2013; Wachs, 2012).

The third component of the TPB is self-efficacy, a component of Bandura's (1989) social-cognitive theory. When an individual is confronted with cyberbullying, self-efficacy, that is, confidence in one's ability to handle it effectively or to intervene effectively or to exercise self-control to resist pressure to engage in cyberbullying, is the final factor affecting the decision to enact a behavior. Even if one has attitudes that oppose cyberbullying and believes that most people disapprove of cyberbullying and that few actually engage in it, one may still be faced with a situation in which cyberbullying seems to be an option. One must have self-efficacy to withstand pressure from others in order to resist the temptation or pressure to cyberbully.

The advantage of this theory as a guide for research is that it describes malleable factors that can be influenced via formal and informal experiences. Attitudes can change when a critical mass of evidence or personal experience has accumulated. In a similar vein, normative beliefs can be revised in the face of persuasive evidence. For example, a belief that "everyone does it" can be disputed with scientific data showing the actual percentage of people who are involved in cyberbullying. Moral beliefs may be overridden by moral disengagement, noted above. For example, a person who cyberbullies another by impersonating him or her online and sending offensive content to others may justify the action by thinking, "they deserved that because they gave me their password and that's a stupid thing to do." Those disengaged beliefs are subject to influence, perhaps by one's own moral values. That is, when juxtaposed with one's moral principles, morally disengaged cognitions may be discarded. However, if one believes strongly that cyberbullying is absolutely wrong, and if that belief is reinforced via such avenues as anticyberbullying websites and speakers, the individual may develop the ability to recognize when his or her thinking drifts toward moral disengagement and catch him- or herself before succumbing to those disengaged thoughts.

All of these ideas about the usefulness of TPB as a prevention tool for cyberbullying can be empirically tested. They are also malleable factors that could be targeted for intervention and the effects evaluated.

Choice Theory as a Theoretical Perspective

Tanrikulu (2014) proposed that cyberbullying can be explained by the tenets of choice theory (Glasser, 1998), a counseling approach that evolved from reality therapy to control theory to choice theory in its most recent iteration. Choice theory posits that humans are motivated by five genetically encoded needs: survival, belonging, power, freedom, and fun. This theory emphasizes that individuals choose their own behaviors and are responsible for those choices and that a basic problem common to all unhappy people is that they do not have satisfying relationships in their lives. The counseling process helps people identify their unmet needs, evaluate whether their current behavior is helping them meet these needs, and design specific plans to more effectively meet those needs. When Glasser (1998) uses the term *behavior*, he refers to "total behavior," which includes action, emotion, cognition, and physiology. Choice theory conceives of a "quality world," a mental image of the people and things one sees as ideal and to which the person aspires.

Tanrikulu (2014) proposed that given that cyberbullying peaks in adolescence, choice theory is a useful explanatory framework, especially because Glasser (1998) developed his theories from his work with adolescents. Tanrikulu argued that cyberbullying behaviors are efforts to satisfy a person's needs for fun and power. It also may be that in the absence of a strong sense of belonging, one will engage in cyberbullying in an effort to fulfill that basic need (e.g., gain approval from friends). Empirical support for this is seen in the results of a study finding that those children who engaged in cyberbullying were more likely to be lonely and had fewer reciprocal friendships, lower social acceptance, and popularity (Schoffstall & Cohen, 2011). Although the study was cross-sectional and causality cannot be inferred, it suggests that further investigation of this theory could provide relevant findings with implications for practice.

Measures and Methods

Research to date on cyberbullying has utilized self-report survey methodology in the vast majority of studies. Questions included in such surveys are generally one of two types: a global item, such as "How often have you been cyberbullied in the last two months?," or behaviorally specific items, such as "How often in the last two months has someone shared private information about you using digital technology?" Some surveys include a definition of cyberbullying, and others do not use the term at all. Although such research has been informative, particularly in the beginning stages of this line of inquiry, the limitations are well known. Self-report is subject to social desirability and mischievous responding, and many results are limited by shared method variance. The small proportion of qualitative studies (e.g., Mishna, Saini, & Solomon, 2009; Mishna, Schwan, Lefebvre, Bhole, & Johnston, 2014) have added depth and nuance to the quantitative findings. A very few researchers (e.g., Bellmore, Calvin, Xu, & Zhu, 2015; Calvin, Bellmore, Xu, & Zhu, 2015; Underwood, Rosen, More, Ehrenreich, & Gentsch, 2012) have used innovative methods that utilize the technological tools that are available, often by partnering with researchers in other fields. Underwood and colleagues (2012) provided BlackBerry devices to young people; all data from those devices were captured for analysis. Thus their findings are based on authentic data. Spears and colleagues (2016) have tested using social media to reduce cyberbullying and have involved youth as coresearchers, ensuring that their views were incorporated into research design. Youth are more aware of current practices, apps, and social media that are widely used and can inform researchers of important items to include. They can also ensure that terminology is appropriate for the target population. Thus the studies are likely to be more thorough and useful than those in which scholars are the only ones conceptualizing a study. More of these authentic studies will allow direct testing of hypotheses about cyberbullying that are derived from the theoretical perspectives reviewed here.

Because survey research is so prominent in the field of cyberbullying, it bears mention that the surveys used should be the subject of careful scrutiny. Few researchers undertake careful psychometric analyses, often reporting only internal consistency statistics (Card, 2013). Exploratory and confirmatory factor analyses are needed, and evidence of validity should be presented. In addition, when measures are translated, efforts to ensure that the same properties hold for the original and translated versions should be documented (Strohmeier, Aoyama, Gradinger, & Toda, 2013). Without such analyses, the findings must be viewed with caution.

Many studies have used single-item indicators, whereas others use multiple behavioral indicators (Ybarra, boyd, Korchmaros, & Oppenheim, 2012) thought to represent the universe of cyberbullying behaviors. The challenge is that the universe of behaviors is constantly expanding, with new platforms and devices creating additional venues for cyberbullying. Thus a survey with behavioral descriptors may be quickly out of date when new platforms are omitted.

Ybarra and colleagues (2012) tested the effects of various wording and survey formats and found that the most accurate results are obtained when the word *bully* (or *cyberbully*) is used in the survey and when follow-up questions about differential power are answered by those who endorse a bullying experience. It would be helpful if researchers could agree on standard measures to ensure that all used the most accurate, psychometrically sound measures available. We also applaud those researchers who are exploring innovative research strategies that are particularly suited to the study of a digital phenomenon.

Central Research Findings

This overview of this burgeoning research literature focuses on three central questions: (1) What forms does cyberbullying take? (2) What are predictors of engaging in cyberbullying? (3) What are the psychosocial consequences of being a victim of cyberbullying?

Forms and Prevalence

Cyberbullying takes many forms, which continue to evolve as adolescents embrace new platforms with different affordances for social contact. Common cyberbullying behaviors include:

> hacking into another person's online accounts (Facebook, email, school account), unwanted sexual advances through the Internet or mobile device (sexting, explicit messages, or emails), embarrassing or threatening messages sent via text message, posting degrading comments or hate speech, sending embarrassing or threating emails, posting explicit or unwanted pictures without consent or knowledge, creating false profiles and using the imposter to post embarrassing comments, harassing other players during live online gaming, outing someone's sexual status or health status (e.g. STI status) online,

and creating group or website to harass another student or group of students."
(Selkie, Kota, Chan, & Moreno, 2015, p. 81)

Although research has yet to identify specific motives for forms of cyberbullying, it is not difficult to imagine that these are behaviors that serve several needs
proposed according to choice theory (Tanrikulu, 2014): power (to harm others),
freedom (to express these behaviors in a context monitored less by adults), and
fun (the sheer enjoyment of constant connectedness with peers, not to mention the
reinforcement from likes and comments).

On the basis of a large and comprehensive meta-analysis, Kowalski, Giumetti,
Schroeder, and Lattaner (2014) reported that prevalence rates for perpetrating
cyberbullying average about 10%, with a range of 1–79% across studies, and that
approximately 10–40% of adolescents report having been victims of cyberbullying.
Those who are victimized by cyberaggression are almost always also involved in
perpetrating cyberbullying; a latent class analysis with more than 6,000 European
adolescents found that there seems not to be a group that is only victimized by
cyberbullying (Schultze-Krumbholz et al., 2015). Perhaps this happens because of
the online disinhibition effect (Suler, 2004)—that, in the online context, victims are
more likely to retaliate because they are protected by anonymity, invisibility, and
lack of concern about physical size. Sadly, victims of cyberbullying are most often
hurt by those they know. In a large survey study of U.S. adolescents, of those who
had been cyberbullied, 33% reported having been bullied by a friend, and 28% by
someone they know from their schools (Waasdorp & Bradshaw, 2015). Research
has yet to examine the development of cyberbullying and cybervictimization; it will
be important to examine when these behaviors begin and how stable they may be
across developmental time.

Antecedents and Possible Causal Factors

Although most research to date is correlational, the large body of work on correlates may suggest some factors that could predict who will engage in cyberbullying, although, of course, determining causality remains challenging. Again on the
basis of a comprehensive meta-analysis, Kowalski and colleagues (2014) concluded
that perpetrating cyberbullying was positively related to being a victim of cyberbullying, frequency of Internet use, risky online behavior, normative beliefs about
aggression, moral disengagement, and anger, and that perpetrating cyberbullying
was negatively related to parental monitoring, empathy, school safety, and school
climate. A subsequent narrative review of 53 studies of possible antecedents concluded that perpetrating cyberbullying is related to being a boy, technology use,
personality factors, values, peer norms, and school risk factors (Baldry, Farrington,
& Sorrentino, 2015). The different levels of risk factors fit well with the propositions
of social–ecological theories of bullying (Espelage & Swearer, 2004) that a child's
behavior is influenced by microsystem factors in the immediate environment, as
well as by exosystem factors such as peer norms and school environments.

An important risk factor for engaging in cyberbullying appears to be intense
involvement with the Internet. Cyberbullying has been shown to be related to
higher use of mobile phones (Arsène & Raynaud, 2014; Shin & Ahn, 2015) and

to frequency of Internet use (Aricak & Ozbay, 2016). For a U.S. sample of third to eighth graders, engaging in cyberbullying was related to involvement with multiple social network sites and also with sharing passwords (Meter & Bauman, 2015). Perpetrating cyberbullying is related to Internet use and using social networking sites more than 2 hours daily (Tsitsika et al., 2015), to intensity of Facebook use (Pabian, De Backer, & Vandebosch, 2015), and to number of Facebook connections who are not friends in real life (Wegge, Vandebosch, Eggermont, & Walrave, 2015). For a large sample of Canadian middle and high school students, engagement with social network sites was related to cyberbullying in a dose–response relationship, though this was fully mediated by being victimized by cyberbullying (Sampasa-Kanyinga & Hamilton, 2015).

Recent evidence also suggests that difficulties in relationships with parents may contribute to risk for perpetrating cyberbullying. In a study of adolescents from Cyprus, perceived parental psychological control predicted cyberbullying directly, and perceived parental support of autonomy protected from perpetrating cyberbullying indirectly via its relation to empathy and recognition of the humanity of victims (Fousiani, Dimitropoulou, Michaelides, & Van Petegem, 2016). For an adolescent sample from the Czech Republic, poor parental attachment predicted membership in a cyberbully-victim group (Bayraktar, Machackova, Dedkova, Cerna, & Ševčíková, 2015).

Recent research confirms that several personality factors predict cyberbullying involvement: low self-esteem (Brewer & Kerslake, 2015), low empathy (Brewer & Kerslake, 2015), anger (Aricak & Ozbay, 2016; Lonigro et al., 2015), and moral disengagement (Bussey, Fitzpatrick, & Raman, 2015). Cyberbullying has been shown to be associated with psychopathy (Pabian et al., 2015), borderline personality features (this relationship was mediated by jealousy; Stockdale, Coyne, Nelson, & Erickson, 2015), and with depression and suicidality (Merrill & Hanson, 2016).

Newer studies suggest additional environmental risk factors: exposure to antisocial media (defined as television, Internet, DVD, and games depicting antisocial behavior, such as fighting, drug use, stealing, and destroying property; den Hamer & Konijn, 2015), being bullied on school property (Merrill & Hanson, 2016), and playing video games for more than 3 hours a day (Merrill & Hanson, 2016). Other environmental factors may be more protective: eating breakfast daily, playing on sports teams, being physically active (Merrill & Hanson, 2016), and having positive bonds with teachers (Pabian & Vandebosch, 2016). In a rare longitudinal study of risks for cyberbullying, Barlett (2015) suggests that each episode of cyberbullying serves as a learning trial for the perpetrator, serving to consolidate positive attitudes toward cyberbullying. Peer support may reinforce cyberbullying behavior; cyberbullying was associated with perceiving that peers approve of cyberaggression and with perceiving that bystanders join cyberbullying (Bastiaensens et al., 2016).

Although great progress has been made in a short time toward understanding possible developmental antecedents of cyberbullying, the list of possible risk factors to date is disjointed. This research area would benefit from theory, either theories developed to explain the developmental origins of cyberbullying or even borrowing developmental theories from the literature on traditional bullying. In addition, it will be important to investigate possible protective factors in future research.

Psychosocial Outcomes

Cyberbullying is associated with poor psychological adjustment, for victims but also for perpetrators (Kowalski et al., 2014). According to the most recent, comprehensive meta-analytic review, perpetrating cyberbullying was associated with several negative outcomes: drug and alcohol use, anxiety, depression, low life satisfaction, low self-esteem, and poor academic achievement (Kowalski et al., 2014). Being the victim of cyberbullying was associated with high stress levels, suicidal ideation, depression, anxiety, loneliness, somatic problems, conduct and emotional problems, drug and alcohol use, low life satisfaction, lower self-esteem, and reduced prosocial behavior (Kowalski et al., 2014). Because of space limitations, the overview below highlights adjustment outcomes related to victimization, but given that there seems not to be a victim-only group for cyberbullying (Schultze-Krumbholz et al., 2015), many of these outcomes are also be associated with perpetrating cyberbullying.

More recent research confirms that cybervictimization is associated with poor psychological adjustment. Most studies to date have been cross-sectional, in which cybervictimization and adjustment have been measured at the same point in time. For a large U.S. sample of adolescents, cybervictimization predicted internalizing and externalizing problems above and beyond being the victim of traditional bullying (Waasdorp & Bradshaw, 2015). Similarly, for a large sample of Italian 13-year-olds, cybervictimization predicted psychological and somatic problems, even after controlling for computer use and for experiencing traditional bullying (Vieno et al., 2014). A study of cybervictimization with children ages 14–17 from six European countries found that cybervictimization was associated with internalizing, externalizing, and academic problems (Tsitsika et al., 2015).

Other recent studies support the relation between cybervictimization and mental health difficulties, but also suggest possible protective factors. A Swedish population-based study found that cyberharassment was related to health complaints, but that for boys, this relation was moderated by parent/friend support (Fridh, Lindström, & Rosvall, 2015). A large U.S. survey study found that cybervictimization was associated with 11 mental health and substance use problems, but that these associations were weaker for adolescents who reported having frequent dinners with their families (Elgar et al., 2014).

Several recent longitudinal studies confirm the relation between cybervictimization and psychological problems. For a sample of U.S. 13-year-olds, cybervictimization predicted poor academic functioning 1 year later according to school records: poor grades, absenteeism, and behavior problems (Wright, 2015a, 2015b). A 1-year longitudinal study confirmed that cybervictimization predicts negative cognitions and depressive symptoms for a U.S. sample ages 8–13 (Cole et al., 2016). For a U.S. sample ages 16–18, cybervictimization predicted subsequent depression more strongly when adolescents perceived high levels of stress from parents, peers, and academics and when they also perpetrated cyberbullying. A study with Spanish adolescents found that stable cybervictimization across 1 year was associated with depressive symptoms and alcohol problems at Time 2 (Gámez-Guadix, Gini, & Calvete, 2015).

Recent research confirms that cybervictimization may be associated with suicide, for both typically developing and clinical samples. A large survey study of a representative sample of U.S. adolescents found that for this normative sample, cybervictimization was related to suicidal thinking, planning, and attempts but that these relations were mediated by violent behavior, substance abuse, and depression (Reed, Nugent, & Cooper, 2015). In this same study, girls who were cybervictims reported more depression and suicidal behaviors than boys who were cybervictims. Several studies of psychiatric samples have found that cybervictimization is associated with suicidal ideation (Alavi, Roberts, Sutton, Axas, & Repetti, 2015; Roberts, Axas, Nesdole, & Repetti, 2016; Roh et al., 2015).

Implications for Prevention and Intervention

Given the serious psychosocial consequences of cybervictimization, programs to prevent and reduce cyberbullying are urgently needed. Cyberaggression poses serious challenges for prevention and intervention because the behaviors occur on diverse digital platforms, outside the scope of monitoring of many parents and other concerned adults. Although completely eradicating cyberaggression may be unrealistic, programs should be designed with that goal in mind because even a single experience may cause prolonged pain, perhaps in part because of the often highly public nature of cyberbullying and the fact that the person can reexperience it repeatedly by reading the hurtful digital content (Underwood & Ehrenreich, 2017). These programs could be informed by existing evidence-based bullying interventions but will likely be more effective if they are tailored to specific features of cyberbullying: the facts that perpetrators do not have to look their victims in the eye but can instead hide behind a screen, that physical size and strength is less relevant than skill and creativity in using technology, and that the harm done by cyberbullying is so immediately public and the humiliation long-lasting.

Effective programs to prevent and reduce cyberbullying will likely be guided by the burgeoning research literature on antecedents and risk factors, but translating the numerous findings into effective strategies will be challenging. Just as research in this area would be strengthened by theory to guide hypotheses, research on intervention would benefit from the guidance of theories to help in setting priorities. Social–ecological theories of cyberbullying suggest that successful prevention and intervention approaches will have to address risk factors at multiple levels (Cross et al., 2015), by addressing individual risk factors (such as empathy, moral engagement), family factors (parenting engagement with children's online lives), peer influences (peer attitudes toward cyberbullying and the extent to which peers engage in cyberbullying), online influences (access to technology), and community-level factors (school transitions, whether laws prohibit cyberbullying). All of these may be highly suitable targets for intervention (Ang, 2015). The disinhibition effect strongly suggests that interventions to reduce cyberbullying will need to address perceptions of anonymity, dissociative imagination, and the desire to reveal one's true self online. The TPB proposes that intervention programs should target perpetrator's attitudes and normative beliefs and bolster the self-efficacy of victims

(Ajzen, 1991). Choice theory suggests that cyberbullying satisfies individuals' needs for fun and power (Tanrikulu, 2014), which poses serious challenges for prevention and intervention because it is difficult for interventionists to reduce the extent to which adolescents enjoy and receive peer reinforcement for cyberbullying.

Although few interventions to date have been guided by these theoretical perspectives, some programs show promise of success (for an overview, see Zych, Ortega-Ruiz, & Del Rey, 2015). Following a school-based prevention program with 16- to 18-year-olds in Greece that included group-based discussions to raise awareness of the harm caused by cyberbullying, participants' moral engagement scores increased (Barkoukis, Lazuras, Ourda, & Tsorbatzoudis, 2016). German adolescents (ages 11–17) who participated in a 10-week intervention to increase empathy showed decreases in cyberbullying and increases in empathy, though increases in empathy were not found to be associated with decreases in cyberbullying (Schultze-Krumbholz, Schultze, Zagorscak, Wölfer, & Scheithauer, 2016).

However, other well-designed, even theoretically motivated programs seem to have less impact. One such program using a social–ecological framework was called Cyber-Friendly Schools and addressed the five C's of cyberbullying (online contexts, online controls, confidentiality, conduct, and content; Cross et al., 2015). After 18 months of intervention, self-reported cyberbullying had decreased, but this positive effect had dissipated by 1 year later. A 3-year, randomized control trial of the effectiveness of the Second Step program (a year-long classroom-based intervention to teach social skills) with a large sample of U.S. sixth graders found no direct effects of the intervention on rates of cyberbullying (Espelage, Low, Van Ryzin, & Polanin, 2015).

One strong hope for preventing and reducing cyberbullying might be motivating peers to intervene with each other, especially given that cyberbullying happens on digital platforms that may be outside the realm of adult supervision. Studies with university students suggest that bystanders notice cyberbullying only about 68% of the time; of those who notice, only 10% intervene directly, but 68% intervene indirectly after the event (Dillon & Bushman, 2015). In a clever experimental study, empathy training had a short-term effect on adolescents' forwarding a mean message mocking a peer, but the long-term impact of the empathy training was small (Barlińska, Szuster, & Winiewski, 2015). Whether and how adolescents are willing to intervene with peers to stop cyberbullying may depend on their own victimization experiences; adolescents who had been victims of cyberbullying reported more negative bystander responses than those who had not been victimized, though girls who had been cyberbullied reported more positive, prosocial bystander behaviors than male victims (Cao & Lin, 2015). Here again, although interventions to reduce cyberbullying might borrow strategies from interventions to reduce traditional bullying, the specific guidance offered may have to be tailored to the unique features of the digital context; the risk of physical harm is low but the risks of long-lasting reputational harm and inviting attacks are great.

Because cyberbullying is by its very nature a digital phenomenon, perhaps prevention and intervention programs could be strengthened by taking advantage of the fun and appeal of digital technology for youth. Thirteen different prevention and intervention programs have used information and computer technologies (ICTs) to deliver the intervention in the form of serious games, virtual reality, and other digital activities (Nocentini, Zambuto, & Menesini, 2015), but only four of these showed any evidence of effectiveness. One example of an effective program, Cyberprogram 2.0, resulted in reduced cyberbullying and increased empathy for 13- to 15-year-olds in Spain (Garaigordobil & Martinez-Valderry, 2015a) and also increased positive conflict-solving strategies and self-esteem (Garaigordobil & Martinez-Valderry, 2015b). An especially promising digital approach to prevention of cyberbullying may be serious game design. Serious game design could be guided by an intervention mapping protocol, beginning with surveys and focus groups with adolescents and parents and educators, meta-analyses of research literature, and moving toward game design, implementation, and assessment of effectiveness (DeSmet et al., 2016).

Future Directions

Future research on cyberbullying would benefit from being guided by theory. Theory would be helpful in generating hypotheses that build on previous work, integrating the massive number of recent research findings in some meaningful way, or perhaps in illuminating results that demand new theories.

Future research on cyberbullying will also need to fully consider the challenge that cyberaggression may be extremely low-base-rate behavior but so lethally hurtful that even a single experience of victimization could cause long-term pain. This poses serious challenges for all forms of measurement. Surveys often focus on frequency, but someone who reports having experienced cyberbullying rarely may still have been harmed by an agonizing experience. Studies that capture content may miss the few key episodes of cyberbullying, in part because of the tremendous volume of many adolescents' digital communication. To understand the extent to which rare experiences of cyberbullying may be intensely painful, experience sampling or diary-type methods could be helpful, in which participants receive daily text messages asking them a few short questions about online experiences and then are directed to more detailed online questionnaires if they have experienced cyberaggression. More qualitative approaches may also be fruitful: simply asking youth to describe their most painful online experiences, then following up with questions to assess important dimensions of those episodes.

Asking youth about their worst online experiences may force researchers to expand our definitions of cyberaggression. When asked about "the worst thing that ever happened to you online," a sample of U.S. 13-year-olds reported the following: "Being excluded to some parties"; "I figured out a girl that I knew and we were friends blocked me"; "My best friends hung out without me, and posted it on Instagram"; "My friends went out without me and posted pictures on Instagram then denied they were out together"; "Not anything specific, but I don't like when people post pictures or tweet about a party that I wasn't invited to" (Underwood & Faris, 2015). In this same study, 47% of 13-year-olds reported feeling excluded by their friends at least sometimes because of posts they saw on social media. Over a third of this sample admitted to posting pictures online for the purpose of making others feel excluded. Posting pictures of small-group gatherings on social media could be a highly subtle form of cyberaggression, one that poses serious challenges for victims. Peers might be reluctant to confront each other about this behavior because it could be viewed as nothing but fun and friendly sharing, though youth clearly understand that it hurts others (Underwood & Faris, 2015). Even the most vigilant parent who might try to monitor adolescents' social media for cyberbullying might not be able to detect this behavior that young adolescents report to be hurtful.

Present definitions of cyberbullying may not include online behaviors that are a frequent source of pain for many youth. Fully understanding cyberaggression will require asking youth to help us understand what hurts them most in particular types of digital communication, what types of peer responses are more helpful and effective, and how caring adults could best support them.

Conclusions

As we continue to try to understand the phenomenon of cyberbullying, it will be important to be mindful that adolescents move seamlessly between offline and online social contexts (boyd, 2014); a clear distinction between the online and offline social worlds may exist only in adults' minds. Adolescents co-construct their offline and online identities (Subrahmanyam, Smahel, & Greenfield, 2006). Adolescents who engage in bullying offline are more likely to engage in cyberbullying (Kowalski et al., 2014), and adolescents are most likely to be hurt online by peers they know (Waasdorp & Bradshaw, 2015).

As we continue to try to understand cyberbullying, researchers will need to test existing developmental theories in this new context, develop new theories as needed, and engage in ongoing conversations with adolescents to help us understand what online experiences distress them the most.

REFERENCES

Ajzen, I. (1991). The theory of planned behavior. *Organizational Behavior and Human Decision Processes, 50,* 179–211.

Alavi, N., Roberts, N., Sutton, C., Axas, N., & Repetti, L. (2015). Bullying victimization (being bullied) among adolescents referred for urgent psychiatric consultation: Prevalence and association with suicidality. *Canadian Journal of Psychiatry, 60,* 427–431.

Ang, R. P. (2015). Adolescent cyberbullying: A review of characteristics, prevention, and intervention strategies. *Aggression and Violent Behavior, 25,* 35–42.

Aricak, O. T., & Ozbay, A. (2016). Investigation of the relationship between cyberbullying, cybervictimization, alexithymia and anger expression styles among adolescents. *Computers in Human Behavior, 55,* 278–285.

Arsène, M., & Raynaud, J. P. (2014). Cyberbullying (ou cyber harcèlement) et psychopathologie de l'enfant et de l'adolescent: État actuel des connaissances [Cyberbullying (or cyber harassment) and psychopathology of children and adolescents: Current state of knowledge]. *Neuropsychiatrie de l'Enfance et de l'Adolescence [Neuropsychiatry of Childhood and Adolescence], 62,* 249–256.

Baldry, A. C., Farrington, D. P., & Sorrentino, A. (2015). "Am I at risk of cyberbullying"?: A narrative review and conceptual framework for research on risk of cyberbullying and cybervictimization: The risk and needs assessment approach. *Aggression and Violent Behavior, 23,* 36–51.

Bandura, A. (1989). Human agency in social cognitive theory. *American Psychologist, 44,* 1175–1184.

Bandura, A. (1999). Moral disengagement in the perpetration of inhumanities. *Personality and Social Psychology Review, 3*(3), 193–209.

Barkoukis, V., Lazuras, L., Ourda, D., & Tsorbatzoudis, H. (2016). Tackling psychosocial risk factors for adolescent cyberbullying: Evidence from a school-based intervention. *Aggressive Behavior, 42,* 114–122.

Barkoukis, V., Lazuras, L., & Tsorbatzoudis, H. (2013). A social cognitive perspective in cyberbullying prevention [in Italian]. In M. L. Genta, A. Brighi, & A. Guarini (Eds.), *Cyberbullismo: Ricerche e strategie di intervento* (pp. 122–135). Milan, Italy: Franco Angeli.

Barlett, C. P. (2015). Predicting adolescent's cyberbullying behavior: A longitudinal risk analysis. *Journal of Adolescence, 41,* 86–95.

Barlińska, J., Szuster, A., & Winiewski, M. (2015). The role of short- and long-term cognitive empathy activation in preventing cyberbystander reinforcing cyberbullying behavior. *Cyberpsychology, Behavior, and Social Networking, 18,* 241–244.

Bastiaensens, S., Pabian, S., Vandebosch, H., Poels, K., Van Cleemput, K., DeSmet, A., et al. (2016). From normative influence to social pressure: How relevant others affect whether bystanders join in cyberbullying. *Social Development, 25,* 193–211.

Bayraktar, F., Machackova, H., Dedkova, L., Cerna, A., & Ševčíková, A. (2015). Cyberbullying: The discriminant factors among cyberbullies, cyber victims, and cyberbully-victims in a Czech adolescent sample. *Journal of Interpersonal Violence, 30,* 3192–3216.

Bellmore, A., Calvin, A. J., Xu, J. M., & Zhu, X. (2015). The five W's of "bullying" on Twitter: Who, what, why, where, and when. *Computers in Human Behavior, 44,* 305–314.

boyd, d. (2014). *It's complicated: The social lives of networked teens.* New Haven, CT: Yale University Press.

Brewer, G., & Kerslake, J. (2015). Cyberbulling, self-esteem, empathy and loneliness. *Computers in Human Behavior, 48,* 255–260.

Bronfenbrenner, U. (1979). Contexts of child rearing: Problems and prospects. *American Psychologist, 34,* 844–850.

Bronfenbrenner, U. (2005). *Making human beings human: Bioecological perspectives on human development.* Thousand Oaks, CA: SAGE.

Bussey, K., Fitzpatrick, S., & Raman, A. (2015). The role of moral disengagement and self-efficacy in cyberbullying. *Journal of School Violence, 14,* 30–46.

Calvin, A. J., Bellmore, A., Xu, J. M., & Zhu, X. (2015). #bully: Uses of hashtags in posts about bullying on Twitter. *Journal of School Violence, 14,* 133–153.

Cao, B., & Lin, W. Y. (2015). How do victims react to cyberbullying on social networking sites?: The influence of previous cyberbullying victimization experiences. *Computers in Human Behavior, 52,* 458–465.

Card, N. A. (2013). Psychometric considerations for cyberbullying research. In S. Bauman, D. Cross, & J. Walker (Eds.), *Principles of cyberbullying research: Definitions, measures, and methodology* (pp. 166–180). New York: Routledge.

Cole, D. A., Zelkowitz, R. L., Nick, E., Martin, N. C., Roeder, K. M., Sinclair-McBride, K., et al. (2016). Longitudinal and incremental relation of cybervictimization to negative self-cognitions and depressive symptoms in young adolescents. *Journal of Abnormal Child Psychology, 44,* 1321–1332.

Cross, D., Barnes, A., Papageorgiou, A., Hadwen, K., Hearn, L., & Lester, L. (2015). A social–ecological framework for understanding and reducing cyberbullying behaviours. *Aggression and Violent Behavior, 23,* 109–117.

Davis, K. (2012). Friendship 2.0: Adolescents' experiences of belonging and self-disclosure online. *Journal of Adolescence, 35,* 1527–1536.

den Hamer, A. H., & Konijn, E. A. (2015). Adolescents' media exposure may increase their cyberbullying behavior: A longitudinal study. *Journal of Adolescent Health, 56*(2), 203–208.

DeSmet, A., Van Cleemput, K., Bastiaensens, S., Poels, K., Vandebosch, H., Malliet, S., et al. (2016). Bridging behavior science and gaming theory: Using the Intervention Mapping Protocol to design a serious game against cyberbullying. *Computers in Human Behavior, 56,* 337–351.

Dillon, K. P., & Bushman, B. J. (2015). Unresponsive or un-noticed?: Cyberbystander intervention in an experimental cyberbullying context. *Computers in Human Behavior, 45,* 144–150.

Eaton, P. W. (2014, May 11). Viewing digital space(s) through Bronfenbrenner's ecological model. Retrieved from *https://profpeaton.com/2014/05/11/viewing-digital-spaces-through-bronfenbrenners-ecological-model.*

Elgar, F. J., Napoletano, A., Saul, G., Dirks, M. A., Craig, W., Poteat, V. P., et al. (2014). Cyberbullying victimization and mental health in adolescents and the moderating role of family dinners. *JAMA Pediatrics, 168,* 1015–1022.

Espelage, D. L., Low, S., Van Ryzin, M. J., & Polanin, J. R. (2015). Clinical trial of Second Step middle school program: Impact on bullying, cyberbullying, homophobic teasing, and sexual harassment perpetration. *School Psychology Review, 44,* 464–479.

Espelage, D. L., & Swearer, S. M. (2004). *Bullying in American schools.* Mahwah, NJ: Erlbaum.

Fousiani, K., Dimitropoulou, P., Michaelides, M. P., & Van Petegem, S. (2016), Perceived parenting and adolescent cyber-bullying: Examining the intervening role of autonomy and relatedness need satisfaction, empathic concern and recognition of humanness. *Journal of Child and Family Studies, 25,* 2120–2129.

Fridh, M., Lindström, M., & Rosvall, M. (2015). Subjective health complaints in adolescent victims of cyber harassment: Moderation through support from parents/friends—A Swedish population-based study. *BMC Public Health, 15,* 1–11.

Gámez-Guadix, M., Gini, G., & Calvete, E. (2015). Stability of cyberbullying victimization among adolescents: Prevalence and association with bully–victim status and psychosocial adjustment. *Computers in Human Behavior, 53,* 140–148.

Garaigordobil, M., & Martínez-Valderrey, V. (2015a). The effectiveness of cyberprogram 2.0 on conflict resolution strategies and self-esteem. *Journal of Adolescent Health, 57,* 229–234.

Garaigordobil, M., & Martínez-Valderrey, V. (2015b). Effects of cyberprogram 2.0 on "face-to-face" bullying, cyberbullying, and empathy. *Psicothema, 27,* 45–51.

Glasser, W. (1998). *Choice theory: A new psychology of personal freedom.* New York: HarperCollins.

Hong, J. S., & Espelage, D. L. (2012). A review of research on bullying and peer victimization in school: An ecological system analysis. *Aggression and Violent Behavior, 17,* 311–322.

Johnson, M. J., & Puplampu, K. P. (2008). Internet use during childhood and the ecological techno-subsystem. *Canadian Journal of Learning and Technology, 34,* 19–28.

Kowalski, R. M., Giumetti, G. W., Schroeder, A. N., & Lattaner, M. R. (2014). Bullying in the digital age: A critical review and meta-analysis of cyberbullying among youth. *Psychological Bulletin, 140,* 1072–1137.

Lenhart, A. (2012). Teens, smartphones, and texting. Retrieved from *http://pewinternet. org/~/media//Files/Reports/2012/PIP_Teens_Smartphones_and_Texting.pdf.*

Lenhart, A. (2015). Teens, social media and technology overview. Retrieved from *www. pewinternet.org/2015/04/09/teens-social-media-technology-2015.*

Lonigro, A., Schneider, B. H., Laghi, F., Baiocco, R., Pallini, S., & Brunner, T. (2015). Is cyberbullying related to trait or state anger? *Child Psychiatry and Human Development, 46,* 445–454.

Menesini, E., Nocentini, A., & Camodeca, M. (2013). Morality, values, traditional bullying, and cyberbullying in adolescence. *British Journal of Developmental Psychology, 31*(1), 1–14.

Merrill, R. M., & Hanson, C. L. (2016). Risk and protective factors associated with being bullied on school property compared with cyberbullied. *BMC Public Health, 16,* 1–10.

Meter, D. J., & Bauman, S. (2015). When sharing is a bad idea: The effects of online social network engagement and sharing passwords with friends on cyberbullying involvement. *Cyberpsychology, Behavior, and Social Networking, 18,* 437–442.

Mishna, F., Saini, M., & Solomon, S. (2009). Ongoing and online: Children and youth's perceptions of cyberbullying. *Children and Youth Services Review, 31,* 1222–1228.

Mishna, F., Schwan, K. J., Lefebvre, R., Bhole, P., & Johnston, D. (2014). Students in distress: Unanticipated findings in a cyberbullying study. *Children and Youth Services Review, 44,* 341–348.

Nocentini, A., Zambuto, V., & Menesini, E. (2015). Anti-bullying programs and information and communication technologies (ICTs): A systematic review. *Aggression and Violent Behavior, 23,* 52–60.

Pabian, S., De Backer, C. J., & Vandebosch, H. (2015). Dark triad personality traits and adolescent cyber-aggression. *Personality and Individual Differences, 75,* 41–46.

Pabian, S., & Vandebosch, H. (2016). Short-term longitudinal relationships between adolescents' (cyber) bullying perpetration and bonding to school and teachers. *International Journal of Behavioral Development, 40,* 162–172.

Perren, S., & Gutzwiller-Helfenfinger, E. (2012). Cyberbullying and traditional bullying in adolescence: Differential roles of moral disengagement, moral emotions, and moral values. *European Journal of Developmental Psychology, 9*(2), 195–209.

Pieschl, S., Kuhlmann, C., & Porsch, T. (2015). Beware of publicity!: Perceived distress of negative cyber incidents and implications for defining cyberbullying. *Journal of School Violence, 14,* 111–132.

Reed, K. P., Nugent, W., & Cooper, R. L. (2015). Testing a path model of relationships between gender, age, and bullying victimization and violent behavior, substance abuse, depression, suicidal ideation, and suicide attempts in adolescents. *Children and Youth Services Review, 55,* 128–137.

Renn, K. A., & Arnold, K. D. (2003). Reconceptualizing research on college student peer culture. *Journal of Higher Education, 74,* 261–291.

Roberts, N., Axas, N., Nesdole, R., & Repetti, L. (2016). Pediatric emergency department visits for mental health crisis: Prevalence of cyber-bullying in suicidal youth. *Child and Adolescent Social Work Journal, 33,* 469–472.

Robson, C., & Witenberg, R. T. (2013). The influence of moral disengagement, morally based self-esteem, age, and gender on traditional bullying and cyberbullying. *Journal of School Violence, 12*(2), 211–231.

Roh, B. R., Yoon, Y., Kwon, A., Oh, S., Lee, S. I., Ha, K., et al. (2015). The structure of co-occurring bullying experiences and associations with suicidal behaviors in Korean adolescents. *PLOS ONE, 10,* 1–14.

Sampasa-Kanyinga, H., & Hamilton, H. A. (2015). Social networking sites and mental health problems in adolescents: The mediating role of cyberbullying victimization. *European Psychiatry, 30,* 1021–1027.

Schoffstall, C. L., & Cohen, R. (2011). Cyber aggression: The relation between online offenders and offline social competence. *Social Development, 20,* 587–604.

Schultze-Krumbholz, A., Göbel, K., Scheithauer, H., Brighi, A., Guarini, A., Tsorbatzoudis, H., et al. (2015). A comparison of classification approaches for cyberbullying and traditional bullying using data from six European countries. *Journal of School Violence, 14,* 47–65.

Schultze-Krumbholz, A., Schultze, M., Zagorscak, P., Wölfer, R., & Scheithauer, H. (2016). Feeling cyber victims' pain: The effect of empathy training on cyberbullying. *Aggressive Behavior, 42,* 147–156.

Selkie, E. M., Kota, R., Chan, Y. F., & Moreno, M. (2015). Cyberbullying, depression, and problem alcohol use in female college students: A multisite study. *Cyberpsychology, Behavior, and Social Networking, 18,* 79–86.

Shin, N., & Ahn, H. (2015). Factors affecting adolescents' involvement in cyberbullying: What divides the 20% from the 80%? *Cyberpsychology, Behavior, and Social Networking, 18,* 393–399.

Spears, B. A., Taddeo, C., Barnes, A., Kavanagh, P., Webb-Williams, J., Stretton A., et al. (2016, June). *Safe and well online: A social marketing-styled approach to intervention.* Paper presented at the National Anti-Bullying Research and Resource Centre, Dublin City University, Dublin, Ireland.

Sticca, F., & Perren, S. (2013). Is cyberbullying worse than traditional bullying?: Examining the differential roles of medium, publicity, and anonymity for the perceived severity of bullying. *Journal of Youth and Adolescence, 42,* 739–750.

Stockdale, L. A., Coyne, S. M., Nelson, D. A., & Erickson, D. H. (2015). Borderline personality disorder features, jealousy, and cyberbullying in adolescence. *Personality and Individual Differences, 83,* 148–153.

Strohmeier, D., Aoyama, I., Gradinger, P., & Toda, Y. (2013). Cybervictimization and cyber-aggression in eastern and western countries: Challenges of constructing a cross-culturally appropriate scale. In S. Bauman, D. Cross, & J. Walker (Eds.), *Principles of cyberbullying research: Definitions, measures, and methodology* (pp. 202–221). New York: Routledge.

Subrahmanyam, K., Smahel, D., & Greenfield, P. (2006). Connecting developmental constructions to the Internet: Identity presentation and sexual exploration in online teen chat rooms. *Developmental Psychology, 42,* 395–406.

Suler, J. (2004). The online disinhibition effect. *CyberPsychology and Behavior, 7,* 321–326.

Swearer, S. M., & Espelage, D. L. (2011). Expanding the social-ecological framework of bullying among youth: Lessons learned from the past and directions for the future. In D. L. Espelage & S. M. Swearer (Eds.), *Bullying in North American schools* (2nd ed., pp. 3–10). New York: Routledge.

Tanrikulu, T. (2014). Cyberbullying from the perspective of choice theory. *Educational Research and Reviews, 9,* 660–665.

Tokunaga, R. S. (2010). Following you home from school: A critical review and synthesis of research on cyberbullying victimization. *Computers in Human Behavior, 26,* 277–287.

Tsitsika, A., Janikian, M., Wójcik, S., Makaruk, K., Tzavela, E., Tzavara, C., et al. (2015). Cyberbullying victimization prevalence and associations with internalizing and externalizing problems among adolescents in six European countries. *Computers in Human Behavior, 51,* 1–7.

Underwood, M. K., & Ehrenreich, S. E. (2017). The power and the pain of adolescents' digital communication: Cyber victimization and the perils of lurking. *American Psychologist, 72,* 144–158.

Underwood, M. K., Ehrenreich, S. E., More, D., Solis, J. S., & Brinkley, D. Y. (2015). The BlackBerry project: The hidden world of adolescents' text messaging and relations with internalizing symptoms. *Journal of Research on Adolescence, 25,* 101–117.

Underwood, M. K., & Faris, R. (2015). #Being thirteen: Social media and the hidden world of young adolescents' peer culture. Retrieved from *https://assets.documentcloud.org/documents/2448422/being-13-report.pdf.*

Underwood, M. K., Rosen, L. H., More, D., Ehrenreich, S. E., & Gentsch, J. K. (2012). The

BlackBerry project: Capturing the content of adolescents' text messaging. *Developmental Psychology, 48,* 295–302.

Vieno, A., Gini, G., Lenzi, M., Pozzoli, T., Canale, N., & Santinello, M. (2014). Cybervictimization and somatic and psychological symptoms among Italian middle school students. *European Journal of Public Health, 25,* 433–437.

Waasdorp, T. E., & Bradshaw, C. P. (2015). The overlap between cyberbullying and traditional bullying. *Journal of Adolescent Health, 56,* 483–488.

Wachs, S. (2012). Moral disengagement and emotional and social difficulties in bullying and cyberbullying: Differences by participant role. *Emotional and Behavioural Difficulties, 17*(3–4), 347–360.

Wegge, D., Vandebosch, H., Eggermont, S., & Walrave, M. (2015). The strong, the weak, and the unbalanced: The link between tie strength and cyberaggression on a social network site. *Social Science Computer Review, 33,* 315–342.

Wright, M. F. (2015a). Adolescents' cyber aggression perpetration and cyber victimization: The longitudinal associations with school functioning. *Social Psychology of Education, 18,* 653–666.

Wright, M. F. (2015b). Cyber victimization and perceived stress linkages to late adolescents' cyber aggression and psychological functioning. *Youth and Society, 47,* 789–810.

Wright, M. F., & Li, Y. (2013). Normative beliefs about aggression and cyber aggression among young adults: A longitudinal investigation. *Aggressive Behavior, 39,* 161–170.

Ybarra, M. L., boyd, d., Korchmaros, J. D., & Oppenheim, J. K. (2012). Defining and measuring cyberbullying within the larger context of bullying victimization. *Journal of Adolescent Health, 51,* 53–58.

Zych, I., Ortega-Ruiz, R., & Del Rey, R. (2015). Systematic review of theoretical studies on bullying and cyberbullying: Facts, knowledge, prevention, and intervention. *Aggression and Violent Behavior, 23,* 1–21.

CHAPTER 14

Poverty, Social Inequality, and Aggression

TAMA LEVENTHAL, VÉRONIQUE DUPÉRÉ,
and MARGARET C. ELLIOTT

Brief Introduction

. . . .

Social inequality is a defining feature of the world in which many children are growing up today (Currie, 2012). The unequal distribution of wealth and related resources (e.g., quality educational opportunities, stable employment, safe neighborhoods, accessible health care) exists across multiple contexts of children's lives, including their families, communities, and countries (Bornstein & Leventhal, 2015). In the United States, just under 20% of children in 2015 came from families who were considered poor based on their income and household composition (U.S. Census Bureau, 2015), making the U.S. child poverty rate among the highest of all developed countries (UNICEF, 2012). Poor children in the United States are often doubly disadvantaged because, not only do they experience poverty at the family level, but they are also more likely than children who are not poor to live in neighborhoods marked by high concentrations of poverty (i.e., poverty rates of 40% or higher; Kneebone & Holmes, 2016). Roughly 15% of the poor population fell into this double-disadvantage category, according to federal data from 2010 to 2014. The convergence of multiple forms of social inequality, along with other demographic and global trends, has had dire consequences for children's economic mobility among recent generations (Chetty, Hendren, & Katz, 2016).

Not only does social inequality play a role in children's economic mobility, but it also has ramifications for other aspects of their lives, including their social, emotional, and behavioral functioning. In the case of children's aggression, socioeconomic disparities are manifested in a variety of ways. Children from disadvantaged backgrounds have more confrontations with the education system (e.g., expulsions), as well as encounters with the juvenile justice system and ultimately the criminal justice system, than their more advantaged peers. For instance, low-income youth are more likely to commit violent and property crimes than higher-income youth (Harris & Kearney, 2014). Clearly, not only are the individual costs of social inequality great, but so, too, are the costs to society.

The goal of this chapter is to address the role of social inequality in the development of children's aggression across the first two decades of life. For purposes of this chapter, we focus on social inequality with respect to family and neighborhood socioeconomic status (SES). As such, the chapter begins with a discussion of how these key concepts of aggression, poverty, and SES are defined. We then turn to theoretical considerations linking poverty and SES to children's aggression, followed by an overview of major methodological challenges when studying this topic. After covering issues of theory and method, we present central findings on the associations between family and neighborhood poverty/SES and children's aggression. Finally, we draw implications from the work presented, followed by concluding remarks.

Main Issues

In this section we provide a brief description of aggression in childhood and adolescence, followed by a conceptualization of poverty and SES, differentiated at the family and neighborhood levels.

Aggression

We take a comprehensive view of children's aggression not limited to physical aggression because research on social inequality tends to examine aggression by considering a wide range of behaviors related to aggression or the intent to harm other people or things (e.g., via property crimes such as shoplifting or vandalism); in the case of others, the harm can be either physical or psychological (see Malti & Rubin, Chapter 1, this volume, for a fuller discussion). Typically, research on social inequality focuses on subclinical forms of aggression (i.e., symptomatology that does not rise to the level of a clinical disorder such as oppositional defiant disorder or conduct disorder) and related behaviors (e.g., attention deficits and hyperactivity; Achenbach, 2001). Specifically, the literature tends to investigate behavior problems among children and adolescents, especially the former. With respect to aggression, behavior problems often are defined broadly as such externalizing behaviors as acting out and destroying property. These behaviors fall along a continuum, and at more extreme levels they may be associated with clinically elevated levels of problems. In adolescence, as youth increasingly assume adult responsibilities and expectations, the focus tends to shift to behaviors with potential legal implications, such as delinquency, crime, and violence, often distinguished by deviant behavior that may include destruction of property or infringing on the rights of others (Raudenbush, Johnson, & Sampson, 2003).[1]

---

[1] *Crime* and *delinquency* are legal, rather than clinical, terms related to behaviors, aggressive or otherwise, that violate the law and potentially lead to involvement with the criminal and juvenile justice systems, respectively.

Family Conditions

Poverty refers specifically to a family's income: The U.S. Census Bureau determines a federal income threshold, based on family size and current economic conditions, considered the minimum income necessary for taking care of a family's basic needs (traditionally food, shelter, and clothing, although sanitation and education are increasingly included as basic needs; Iceland, 2013). For instance, the poverty line for a U.S. family of four in 2016 was $24,300; a family of four living with an income under that amount would be deemed poor (U.S. Department of Health & Human Services, 2016).

By contrast, SES is a more comprehensive measure, with scholars most commonly taking into account family economic resources, parental education, and parental occupation (Duncan, Magnuson, & Votruba-Drzal, 2015). Each of these aspects is multifaceted and can be measured in different ways. For instance, family economic resources may be evaluated as a continuous measure of income or wealth or via dichotomous measures comparing families below the poverty threshold and families above the threshold. Further complications arise from the fact that family SES sometimes is approximated by considering only one of the three aspects, whereas in other circumstances multiple features are examined simultaneously. Even within studies investigating multiple characteristics, there are disagreements as to whether they should be combined into a single indicator of family SES or analyzed separately. Multiple measures of family SES may be relevant for the development of aggression, but so far the aspect of family SES that is most consistently linked with this outcome is poverty (Duncan et al., 2015; see also the section "Central Research Findings," later in this chapter). As such, this particular facet of family SES should not be ignored in the context of research exploring SES and aggression.

Neighborhood Conditions

Both poverty and SES are used to describe individual families or households but can be aggregated to the neighborhood level (e.g., percentage of families below the poverty line) to gain an understanding of the socioeconomic conditions of a given community. Studies linking neighborhood characteristics with children's outcomes have defined neighborhoods using different census-derived geographical units (e.g., tracts [approximately 3,000–8,000 people] or block groups [approximately 600–3,000 people]). Unlike family poverty, there is no official definition of neighborhood poverty. The U.S. Census Bureau uses poverty rates of 20% or higher to indicate poverty areas and rates of 40% or higher to designate extreme-poverty areas; this latter definition is often used in research as a marker of a high-poverty neighborhood (Bishaw, 2014; e.g., Wilson, 1987).

Like family SES, neighborhood SES is a combination of social and economic indicators; however, researchers often separate measures of neighborhood SES into qualitatively different conceptualizations of low SES (e.g., percentage of poor residents, percentage of female-headed households, percentage on public assistance, and percentage unemployed)—also referred to as *concentrated poverty* or *disadvantage*—and high SES (e.g., percentage of high-income residents, percentage of professionals/managers, and percentage college educated)—also called *concentrated affluence* or *advantage*—because the presence of poor and affluent neighbors may have differential associations with children's outcomes (Jencks & Mayer, 1990). These aspects of neighborhood SES are measured fairly consistently across studies, but specific definitions may differ somewhat (Leventhal, Dupéré, & Shuey, 2015). Echoing findings on family SES underscoring the relevance of poverty, it appears that concentrated disadvantage is the dimension of neighborhood SES that is most predictive of children's aggression (Leventhal, Dupéré, & Brooks-Gunn, 2009; see also the section "Central Research Findings," later in this chapter).

Theoretical Considerations

Given that this chapter focuses on the roles of both family and neighborhood poverty/SES in the development of children's aggression, we ground the chapter generally in relational developmental systems (RDS) theories. RDS theories view development as occurring through a bidirectional, mutually influential relationship between the individual and his or her contexts (e.g., Lerner, 2006; Overton, 2015). For the study of social inequality and aggression, these theories help us to understand how family and neighborhood SES are associated with children's development, but also how family and neighborhood SES are affected by each other (as well as other contexts, such as peers). These theories also explicate how family and neighborhood SES and associated conditions (e.g., access to services, exposure to violence) might interact with individual characteristics such as child age or personality in shaping development. Finally, these theories highlight both developmental and historical timing, underscoring the need to explore how family and neighborhood SES may be differentially associated with developmental pathways of aggression at different points in the life course or in different historical periods, respectively (Elder, Shanahan, & Jennings, 2015). Within the context of this broad conceptual framework, we now turn to more specific theories connecting family and neighborhood SES to children's aggression.

Family SES Theories

The main theoretical models proposed to explain the association between family SES and children's aggression fall into three broad categories related to family and environmental stress, parental investments, and cultural theories. They are briefly described next.

Family and Environmental Stress Models

These models propose that belonging to a poor or low-SES family is stressful for all family members, and that stress exposure in turn compromises children's development (Bradley & Corwyn, 2002; Conger, Conger, & Martin, 2010; Duncan et al., 2015; Shaw & Shelleby, 2014). According to this perspective, children can be harmed indirectly or directly by family stress. Indirect pathways operate primarily via parents; that is, parents under economic pressure, who are unable to meet their family's material needs, are likely to feel anxious and to exhibit behavioral and emotional manifestations of this anxiety. For instance, they may be impatient toward other family members and respond harshly in daily interactions, leading to conflicts with spouses and children. In turn, children exposed to harsh parenting and parental conflicts are thought to be at greater risk of developing new or more severe behavior problems than their peers who are not exposed to such family contexts (see also Dishion, Patterson, Stoolmiller, & Skinner, 1991). Similarly, parents may respond to the stress associated with economic pressure by self-medicating with alcohol or other drugs, which in turn makes them less responsive to their children's needs (see Shaw & Shelleby, 2014). Economically stressed parents who manage to avoid conflicts and substance abuse still may be less responsive than parents not under such pressures because poverty taxes parents' cognitive and emotional availability when their mental resources are focused on resolving problems related to the provision of basic, immediate needs (Mullainathan, 2012).

In contrast, direct pathways propose that children living in poverty are subject to a number of environmental stressors that increasingly have been found to influence their aggression and other outcomes (e.g., impaired cognitive and socioemotional development), not necessarily by means of parents' behavior but by the unhealthy, chaotic, and turbulent conditions poverty creates, such as substandard housing, chronic lead exposure, overcrowding, pollution, or noise (Evans & Stecker, 2004; Ferguson, Cassells, MacAllister, & Evans, 2013; Leech, Adams, Weathers, Staten, & Filippelli, 2016). Regardless of whether exposure is direct or indirect, accumulating findings in neuroscience indicate that children chronically exposed to more severe environmental stress, or "toxic stress," exhibit higher levels of physiological stress, which interferes with cognitive and executive functions such as self-regulation, raising their odds of developing behavior problems such as aggression (Lupien, McEwen, Gunnar, & Heim, 2009; Shonkoff et al., 2012; Steinberg, 2014). Children growing up in poverty are particularly at risk of exposure to excessive environmental stress, and this exposure may help explain the link between poverty and children's behavior (Shonkoff et al., 2012).

Parental Investment Theories

The investment perspective focuses not so much on the stressors experienced by poor or low-SES children, but rather on the advantages conferred by greater family SES (Bradley & Corwyn, 2002; Conger et al., 2010; Duncan et al., 2015; Shaw & Shelleby, 2014). Higher-SES parents have more economic resources than lower-SES parents to invest in their children's development; for instance, they have the means to pay for high-quality child care and schools, enriching summer camps and extracurricular activities, educational toys, healthy food, and so on. Although differential investments by lower- and higher-SES parents in enrichment activities and settings are thought to create gaps primarily related to educational and cognitive outcomes, they also are relevant for behavioral outcomes for at least two reasons. First, low verbal ability is one of the most powerful individual-level risk factors for aggression (e.g., see Obsuth, Eisner, Malti, & Ribeaud, 2015; Snyder et al., 2008). Second, high-quality out-of-school settings provide adult supervision, structure, and support, which have the potential to mitigate problematic behavior (Vandell,

Larson, Mahoney, & Watts, 2015; see also the section "Routine Activities Theory and Peer Deviance," later in this chapter).

Parental investment models appear increasingly relevant in the current context of growing income inequality. For instance, the gap between the top and bottom family income quintiles in expenditures on enrichment activities for children has almost tripled in recent decades (Duncan et al., 2015). Moreover, these models are a useful complement to family stress models for understanding potential differences across the economic spectrum, notably between middle-income families and affluent families, as children from these families are unlikely to experience the stressors characteristic of extreme poverty but may be reared with differential levels of parental investments and expectations (Duncan et al., 2015; Luthar & Barkin, 2012). Although parental investments generally are thought to be beneficial, in some instances they may be accompanied by competitive pressures for outstanding achievement that could increase children's risk of behavior problems such as substance abuse; however, this hypothesis has received comparatively little research attention (Luthar & Barkin, 2012).

Cultural Theories

Cultural perspectives highlight how social class shapes norms and values regarding child rearing that are reflected in parenting practices and, ultimately, in children's outcomes (see Duncan et al., 2015; Shaw & Shelleby, 2014). Early cultural theories proposed that deprivation and marginalization led to a "culture of poverty," characterized in part by feelings of helplessness and low impulse control, which in turn facilitated aggressive behaviors and involvement in crime (Small, Harding, & Lamont, 2010). Although cultural norms and beliefs were depicted as initially resulting from deprivation, they ultimately were thought to become a cause of poverty. These early theories were widely criticized because they created a sense that poor families were a monolithic group whose values were distinct from middle-class family values and were to blame for their poverty.

More recent cultural analyses address these issues in more nuanced ways than the early theories, focusing specifically on child rearing practices. Particularly influential is extensive ethnographic field work by Lareau (2011). This research shows that middle-class SES parents often see and experience child rearing as a cultivation project, in which they closely manage their children's time to maximize involvement in structured activities with learning objectives. In contrast to this "concerted cultivation" approach, working-class and poor families tend to be more aligned with a "natural growth" perspective, in which parents' primary role is to fulfill basic needs and provide boundaries within which children are then allowed to experiment and develop freely. These parents tend to encourage their children to be self-reliant and to take matters into their own hands. Such a child rearing approach sometimes translates into injunctions to "fight back" when necessary, which may put both parents and their children at odds with authority figures such as school personnel, who themselves typically come from, and endorse, middle-class attitudes toward child rearing (see Shaw & Shelleby, 2014). In other words, specific child rearing strategies used by lower-SES parents may facilitate aggressive behavior in ways that middle-class strategies do not. Despite differences between middle-class and working-class and poor families, other studies show that there is a great deal of heterogeneity within classes, as well as overlap between classes (Small et al., 2010).

Neighborhood SES Theories

There are several theories relevant to how neighborhood SES and related social conditions may be associated with the extent and manner in which children engage in aggressive behaviors. Given space constraints, we limit our discussion of neighborhood SES theories to social disorganization theory and some of its offshoots, as well as to conceptual approaches focused on the availability, accessibility, and quality of neighborhood-based institutional resources.

Social Disorganization Theory

Much of the literature on neighborhood characteristics and children's aggressive and delinquent behaviors stresses the significance of low neighborhood SES (e.g., Elliott et al., 1996). Most prominently, social disorganization theories (Bursik & Grasmick, 1992; Sampson, Raudenbush, & Earls, 1997; Shaw & McKay, 1942, 1969) posit that certain neighborhood characteristics, rather than characteristics of individual residents per se, are largely responsible for neighborhood crime and delinquency. In their seminal work on the spatial distribution of delinquency, Shaw and McKay (1942, 1969) found that it was concentrated in high-poverty neighborhoods over long spans of time, despite almost complete turnover in the racial and ethnic composition of neighborhood populations. Neighborhood poverty and accompanying structural characteristics, notably racial/ethnic heterogeneity and high residential mobility, are thought to undermine social connections and shared norms, creating conditions conducive to crime and disorder.

Neighborhood disorder can be defined both physically (e.g., broken windows and poorly maintained roads) and socially (e.g., public drug dealing and prostitution; see Sampson & Raudenbush, 2004). Social disorganization theory proposes that signs of disorder are consequential for antisocial behaviors, as they provide observable cues that delinquent behaviors are prevalent and to some degree tolerated (Sampson, 1997). Although there is significant heterogeneity among lower-SES neighborhoods (Brody et al., 2001), more disadvantaged neighborhoods may be susceptible to disorder as a result of compromised socioeconomic and social resources (see Elo, Mykyta, Margolis, & Culhane, 2009). Neighborhood disorder and violence may explain the relationship between neighborhood disadvantage and children's aggression (Sampson, Morenoff, & Gannon-Rowley, 2002). Studies find that neighborhood disorder is associated with children's exposure to criminal and antisocial individuals in their neighborhoods, who may act as role models (e.g. Haynie, Silver, & Teasdale, 2006). In turn, children exposed to neighborhood violence are more likely to commit aggressive acts themselves (Chauhan & Reppucci, 2009). Furthermore, adolescents living in neighborhoods in which violence and disorganization are common may come to perceive that there is not much they personally can do to shield themselves from confrontations, and, more generally, to succeed in the larger world. This lack of efficacy, fear, and/or powerlessness may contribute to their own engagement in violent and aggressive behavior (Ross, Mirowsky, & Pribesh, 2001; Sharkey, 2006).

Cultural Heterogeneity and Social Control

In addition to contributing to neighborhood disorder, phenomena such as high population turnover in higher-poverty neighborhoods make it difficult for residents to develop strong social connections and shared values. As such, a variety of norms and social groups have space to emerge within a single community (see the earlier subsection "Cultural Theories"). Without a general consensus about what is and is not acceptable conduct, children may begin to engage in aggressive and deviant acts because there is insufficient social control to prevent them from doing so (Berg & Loeber, 2011). More unfavorable norms, behaviors, and attitudes may spread and reproduce themselves within disadvantaged neighborhoods. For instance, the proximity of peers engaging in problematic behavior may increase the chances that other children from the same neighborhood will do the same. Harding's (2011) model of cultural heterogeneity suggests that children living in high-poverty neighborhoods are exposed to a wide range of cultural scripts, mostly mainstream ones, but also many unconventional variants. Accordingly, children in these neighborhoods have a wider set of models to choose from than do their peers in more advantaged neighborhoods, increasing the likelihood that they will take part in aggressive or antisocial behaviors.

Lower-income neighborhoods also may have a shortage of *formal* social control deriving from the presence of institutional resources such as youth programs, as well as *informal* social control, or community capacity and residents' willingness to monitor others' behavior and intervene when witnessing disruption in the neighborhood. Lower levels of social control, both formal and informal, are associated with children's likelihood of aggressive and delinquent behaviors (e.g., Elliott et al., 1996).

Conversely, positive social dynamics can contribute to the prevention of children's antisocial behaviors. High collective efficacy, entailing trust among neighbors that there are shared norms and expectations for behavior and a collective willingness to enforce such norms (e.g., when residents see youth participating in delinquent activities), can prevent children from engaging in aggression, both directly through actual interventions (e.g., a resident discouraging youth from littering) and indirectly through children's understanding that residents will not tolerate deviant behavior (Sampson et al., 1997). In fact, adolescents in neighborhoods with greater collective efficacy are less likely to display aggressive behaviors and to affiliate with deviant peers (e.g., Molnar, Miller, Azrael, & Buka, 2004; Sampson, Morenoff, & Raudenbush, 2005).

Routine Activities Theory and Peer Deviance

Whereas social disorganization theory focuses primarily on neighborhood factors, routine activities theory (RAT) adds individual and interpersonal dynamics into the explanation of crime, delinquency, and related behaviors. RAT posits that crime can be explained by the spatial and temporal intersection of potential offenders, potential victims, and opportunities (Cohen & Felson, 1979). Specifically, three elements must be present: (1) individuals who are motivated to offend; (2) individuals perceived as "suitable targets" for crime; and (3) the absence of controls or "capable guardians" that protect against the commission of criminal or delinquent acts (i.e., social disorganization). RAT assumes that individuals are rational actors who may be inclined to commit offenses against people or properties but that there must be sufficient opportunity within a given space (i.e., a neighborhood) and time to act on that inclination; in other words, there must be potential victims *and* limited protections against potential crimes. (In the case of "victimless" crimes, such as truancy or drug use, the first and third elements must be present.) In neighborhoods high in poverty and low in social control, individuals—and especially adolescents—may perceive that committing aggressive acts has few costs (low likelihood of getting caught[2]) and many benefits (e.g., convenience, satisfaction of impulses, peer acceptance).

Moreover, adolescents without structured activities during their free time are more likely to affiliate with deviant peers. Findings from a number of studies suggest that the association between characteristics common to disadvantaged neighborhoods (e.g., low SES, crime and violence, cultural heterogeneity) and adolescents' antisocial behavior is mediated through exposure to peer behaviors, particularly violence and delinquency (Fite et al., 2010; Haynie et al., 2006; Tolan, Gorman-Smith, & Henry, 2003; Zimmerman & Messner, 2011). In other words, neighborhood disadvantage increases the likelihood of adolescents' problematic behavior generally, which in turn raises the odds of individual adolescents' aggression and delinquency via contact with deviant peers. This finding holds even at relatively low levels of exposure to peer delinquency (Tolan et al., 2003). Epidemic models suggest that violence and crime tend to spread throughout a neighborhood because peers learn behaviors from each other (Glaeser & Scheinkman, 2001; Mennis & Harrison, 2011). In accordance with RAT, peers are more likely to engage in such behaviors if the risk is low (e.g., no stigma exists for antisocial behaviors) and opportunity is high (e.g., abandoned buildings or vacant lots are present; Cohen & Felson, 1979). Moreover, some scholars suggest that weakened social controls contribute to the development and dominance of deviant peer networks over prosocial networks in disadvantaged neighborhoods (e.g., Anderson, 1999).

Institutional Resources

Institutional resources—opportunities or services available to neighborhood residents that are typically intended to foster economic, educational, physical, and socioemotional well-being—represent another dimension of the neighborhood context that may underlie the association between neighborhood disadvantage and children's aggression (e.g., Leventhal & Brooks-Gunn, 2000). Institutional resources that are especially relevant to children and adolescents and potentially to the development of aggression include schools, community centers and youth

---

[2]On the contrary, some scholars argue that in relatively disadvantaged neighborhoods, the likelihood of getting caught is actually *higher* than in more advantaged neighborhoods because poorer neighborhoods are more heavily policed (e.g., Hannon, 2003).

programming, health and social services, and employment opportunities (e.g., Leventhal & Brooks-Gunn, 2000). Access, or lack of access, to such resources of adequate quantity and quality may be one of the ways social inequality at the neighborhood level plays a role in the opportunities afforded to children (Chetty, Hendren, Kline, & Saez, 2014). More disadvantaged neighborhoods may lack the financial, physical, and social capital necessary to introduce and sustain even the most needed services (Granger, 2008; Leventhal et al., 2015). In line with social disorganization theory and research on peer deviance, children with fewer structured activities to participate in, either conventional or prosocial, may be more likely to engage in aggressive and delinquent behaviors (Snyder & Sickmund, 2006). For example, adolescents who live near neighborhood resources tend to display less aggression than adolescents who live farther from institutions (Molnar, Buka, Brennan, Holton, & Earls, 2003).

Finally, high-quality institutional resources (defined by the appropriateness of services for their target populations and the extent to which they meet their stated goals; Jacobs & Kapuscik, 2000) generally are less common in more disadvantaged neighborhoods than in more affluent neighborhoods (e.g., Burchinal, Nelson, Carlson, & Brooks-Gunn, 2008), despite the fact that such resources may confer the most benefits to children in more disadvantaged neighborhoods (e.g., Pettit, Bates, Dodge, & Meece, 1999; Small & McDermott, 2006). High-quality institutions are easier to develop and sustain in more advantaged neighborhoods that have the financial and organizational capacity to hire and retain competent staff (Leventhal et al., 2015). Resources of poor quality may even engender aggressive behavior among the children they serve rather than prevent it, particularly when they serve at-risk youth (e.g., Dishion, McCord, & Poulin, 1999).

In sum, the theories on family and neighborhood SES should be viewed as complementary rather than competing because they operate at different levels and are typically investigated independently. For example, some cultural theories about family SES implicitly invoke differential access to community resources in parents' efforts to rear their children. Likewise, families who do not invest in their children's structured activities because of lack of resources may inadvertently contribute to social disorganization arising from unsupervised peer groups. Given rising inequality at both the family and neighborhood levels, it is likely that processes placing youth at risk for aggressive behavior are operating at both the family and neighborhood levels for many youth.

Measures and Methods

With that theoretical backdrop in mind, we now turn to a few important methodological issues that must be considered when assessing research on social inequality and children's aggression. A complete review of these issues is beyond the scope of this chapter; rather, we focus here on one area fundamental to this topic: selection bias. Then we briefly discuss study designs in relation to this challenge.

Selection bias, also called *omitted variable bias,* is routinely described as the main methodological challenge facing researchers trying to isolate the effect of family or neighborhood SES on children's outcomes (Duncan et al., 2015; Leventhal et al., 2015). This bias arises when the association between family and neighborhood SES and children's aggression reflects the influence of other factors that affect families' access to socioeconomic resources and that are also relevant to the development of children's aggressive behaviors. For instance, as compared with parents without such a history, parents with a history of incarceration for aggressive offenses may be particularly likely to raise their children in lower-SES environments because of barriers to employment for the formerly incarcerated; they may also respond more aggressively when their children are demanding or unruly and may transmit genetic predispositions for aggression to their children (Rhee & Waldman, 2002). Thus associations between family or neighborhood SES and children's aggression could, in fact, be due to parental aggression and its social and biological correlates.

To address these challenges, researchers employ various research designs and methodologies to account for selection mechanisms when examining associations between family or neighborhood SES and children's outcomes such as aggression. First and foremost, the "gold standard" research design to isolate the impact of a single factor, such as family or neighborhood SES, is the randomized experiment (Shadish, Cook, & Campbell, 2002). In these experiments, participants are randomly assigned to control and intervention groups, a process that in theory balances groups on measured and unmeasured background differences (e.g., genetic predispositions, histories of incarceration) that could create bias if they were not distributed equally across groups. In the neighborhood literature, this strategy is exemplified by the Moving to Opportunity for Fair Housing Demonstration (MTO) study funded by the U.S. Department of Housing and Urban Development (Goering & Feins, 2003). Through this program, families living in public housing in high-poverty neighborhoods (i.e., poverty rates of 40% or higher) were randomly assigned to an intervention group that received assistance to move to private housing in low-poverty neighborhoods (i.e., poverty rates of 10% or lower), a comparison group that received assistance to move to private housing in neighborhoods of their choice, or a control group that remained in place (the findings from MTO and the other studies described here are discussed in the next section). Similarly, other studies based on randomized designs evaluate the impact of welfare programs that increased family income (Morris, Duncan, & Clark-Kauffman, 2005).

Experimental studies are useful for minimizing threats related to selection bias, but they are also limited in several ways. Because experiments are expensive and extremely complicated, they are rarely conducted, and when they are, they tend to focus on very specific populations, raising potential generalizability problems. For instance, in terms of neighborhood and family SES, to address potential ethical challenges concerning treatment receipt and coercion, experimental studies often evaluate programs aimed at improving the living conditions of extremely poor families receiving welfare or living in public housing located in very poor neighborhoods (Duncan et al., 2015; Leventhal et al., 2015). Because of budget constraints, these programs typically cannot serve all interested or eligible families. Thus it is unclear whether the findings generated from this work apply to other families, poor or not poor, who were not included in the respective program.

As such, other types of studies are needed to complement the results of randomized studies. In that respect, studies based on quasi-experimental designs offer a useful alternative, with the potential to reduce selection bias quite effectively in cases in which treatment exposure is not determined randomly but nearly so (Shadish et al., 2002). These studies take advantage of the fact that some families are subjected to changes in their economic circumstances that are not a function of individual families' characteristics, choices, and/or preferences but rather as a result of mechanisms over which individual families have little or no control. The outcomes of children exposed to these changes can then be compared with those of similar children not exposed. For instance, the Great Smoky Mountains Study followed a regional sample composed of Native American and non–Native American rural youth before and after the inauguration of a casino on a local Native American reservation that redistributed profits to the Native American families, lifting many of them out of poverty but not changing non–Native American youths' family economic conditions (Costello, Compton, Keeler, & Angold, 2003).

In contrast with experimental and quasi-experimental studies, studies based on correlational designs are much more frequent. A large majority of research on both family and neighborhood poverty/SES relies on longitudinal, nationally representative studies (e.g., the Panel Study of Income Dynamics; Hill, 1991). In the neighborhood literature, city-based studies that sample children and families stratified by different neighborhood types have been influential in this area as well (e.g., Project on Human Development in Chicago Neighborhoods [PHDCN]; Sampson et al., 2002).

Studies using correlational designs typically employ various statistical techniques to minimize potential selection bias. These approaches range from regression analyses that control for individual and family background characteristics to more rigorous analytic strategies such as propensity score matching, instrumental variable analysis, or fixed effects (Hipp & Wickes, 2016; Leventhal & Brooks-Gunn, 2011; Sharkey & Sampson, 2010). Propensity score methods use a variety of strategies to match children who are otherwise similar on a wide range of observed background characteristics except, for example, the types of families or neighborhoods from which they come (e.g., Wodtke, Harding, & Elwert, 2011). Instrumental variable analyses minimize unmeasured correlations between family or neighborhood characteristics and children's outcomes by means of a two-stage regression approach (e.g., Foster & McLanahan, 1996). Finally, fixed effects analyses take advantage of variation in individuals' own exposure to different family or neighborhood characteristics over time, thus holding unmeasured family characteristics constant (Berger, Bruch, Johnson, James, & Rubin, 2009).

None of the approaches described, however, are without limitations of various sorts for controlling selection bias in correlational studies. For example, propensity score methods are dependent on adequate measurement of relevant covariates that, if omitted, could generate selection bias (Guo & Fraser, 2010). Importantly, in studies trying to isolate the role of neighborhood SES, it is imperative to have measures of family SES (e.g., income and parent education), and ideally studies of family SES should account for neighborhood SES and other key demographic factors, notably race/ethnicity (family or neighborhood composition), because they are generally key drivers of many omitted variables related to inequality–child outcome links (Duncan et al., 2015; Leventhal et al., 2015).

Central Research Findings

In this section, we take a comprehensive, but not exhaustive, approach to reviewing the literature on social inequality and children's aggression and related behaviors. Because the literatures linking children's development to family and neighborhood poverty/SES are extensive and reviewed more generally elsewhere (e.g., Duncan et al., 2015; Duncan & Murnane, 2011; Leventhal et al., 2015; Sampson et al., 2002), this section draws primarily on studies that meet certain standards of quality and rigor. Most notably, given the serious problem of selection or omitted variable bias as described in the previous section, we generally only review studies that account for individual and family background characteristics in their analyses, such as child gender, age, race/ethnicity, family composition, and the like, as well as family SES (e.g., income, parent education, and so on) in the case of neighborhood poverty/SES. In addition, we highlight longitudinal studies and ones using alternative analytic methods or experimental designs to address selection when possible. In doing so, our goal is to rely on the strongest evidence possible for making some general conclusions about what is currently known about social inequality and children's aggression. In the remainder of this section, we first cover family poverty/SES and then neighborhood poverty/SES. To the extent possible, we also discuss differences by children's age or developmental status (children vs. adolescents) and gender.

Family Poverty, SES, and Children's Aggression

A large majority of the studies on social inequality and children's aggression rely on measures of either family income or poverty status rather than broader SES measures or other indicators, such as parent education, leading to different, but complementary, conceptualizations about how SES functions, as described in the earlier section "Theoretical Considerations." Across a number of reviews, a general pattern is clear: Children from more economically disadvantaged families are at greater risk of displaying more aggression and a range of related behaviors, including broader externalizing problems, hyperactivity, antisocial behavior, violence, and substance use (for reviews, see Costa et al., 2015; Duncan & Brooks-Gunn, 1997; Duncan et al., 2015; Murray & Farrington, 2010; Shaw & Shelleby, 2014; Yoshikawa, Aber, & Beardslee, 2012). Despite a suggestion that the association between family SES and children's externalizing behaviors may be nonlinear—with affluent and poor children both demonstrating more problem behaviors, notably substance use, than their middle-income peers (Luthar & Barkin, 2012; Luthar & Latendresse, 2005)—the research evidence supporting this claim is quite limited, mixed in nature (e.g., Lund & Dearing, 2013), and strictly nonexperimental.

Not surprisingly, most of the research contributing to the general conclusion about family disadvantage and children's aggression is based on nonexperimental studies. A small number of studies, however, have employed advanced statistical methods, primarily fixed effects analyses, to improve causal estimation. For example, one study using data from the National Institute of Child Health and Human Development Study of Early Child Care and Youth Development, a multisite birth cohort, found that children whose families were chronically poor had more externalizing problems than children whose families were never poor and that increases in family income from 2 to about 6 years of age were related to decreases in such problems, especially among chronically poor children (Dearing, McCartney, & Taylor, 2006). These associations were more pronounced among children from chronically poor families compared with children from families who were never poor. Using a nationally representative sample, the National Longitudinal Survey of Youth–Child Supplement (NLSY-CS), other studies similarly found that increases in family income in early and middle childhood have immediate and enduring benefits for children's behavioral functioning (Votruba-Drzal, 2006). In contrast, another study using this same dataset and specifically focused on aggression-related behavior found that lower family incomes in early childhood, but not changes in income over time, were related to children displaying more antisocial behavior in early childhood and sharper growth in these behaviors through adolescence (Strohschein, 2005), whereas a different study using NLSY-CS data comparing siblings or cousins—a variant of fixed effects that holds unmeasured family characteristics constant—reported that lower average family incomes across childhood were associated only with boys' greater average conduct problems during this period (D'Onofrio et al., 2009). The prior study did not consider gender differences.

Perhaps the strongest evidence to date for a connection between socioeconomic inequality at the family level and children's aggression comes from the handful of experimental and quasi-experimental studies conducted in this area. Specifically, results from a randomized experiment of approximately 800 families who participated in the Minnesota Family Investment Program, a welfare demonstration program that improved maternal employment outcomes and reduced family poverty, indicated that program participation had beneficial effects on children's externalizing behaviors (Gennetian & Miller, 2002). Additional analyses revealed that these program effects were largely restricted to school-age and not preschool-age children; no gender differences were evident. The researchers hypothesized that developmental differences may arise because of the greater child care demands on families with younger children and the variable quality of care that children from poor families may receive.

The other experimental evidence comes from the Great Smoky Mountains Study described earlier in which income generated from casino revenues improved the fortunes of Native American families but not non–Native American families. A study of adolescents found that youth whose families moved out of poverty, Native American and non–Native American alike, had reductions in psychiatric symptoms related to conduct disorder and oppositional defiant disorder, and their symptom levels were comparable to those of youth who were never poor (Costello, Mustillo, Erkanli, Keeler, & Angold, 2003). The Native American youth whose families were lifted out of poverty also were 22% less likely to commit minor crimes than their non–Native American peers who remained poor (Akee, Copeland, Keeler, Angold, & Costello, 2010). A follow-up study of these adolescents at 21 years of age reported that Native American youth had fewer substance abuse disorders compared with their non–Native American peers, especially among the youngest cohort, which was 9 years of age at the study outset (vs. ages 11 or 13; Costello, Erkanli, Copeland, & Angold, 2010).

Together, the selected work reviewed supports the conclusions of the more general nonexperimental research on the link between family economic disadvantage and children's risk of aggression. In terms of whether differences exist based on developmental period or gender, the findings are more mixed. Although a consensus is emerging that family economic circumstances during early childhood have pronounced associations with children's educational and economic outcomes (e.g., Duncan, Ziol-Guest, & Kalil, 2010; Heckman, 2006; Shonkoff et al., 2012), no such compelling evidence exists for children's social functioning, including aggression (Duncan et al., 2015). For example, results from a Quebec-based study specifically investigating children's aggression from early to middle childhood found that poor children were more aggressive than children who were not poor in very early childhood, and this difference remained stable through middle childhood (i.e., "effects" were comparable over time; Mazza et al., 2016). Admittedly, few studies have investigated developmental differences across the first two decades of life, but results across various studies do not support developmental sensitivities in the link between family social inequality and children's aggression. That is not to say that family SES in early childhood is not associated with subsequent behavior or that early childhood adjustment problems are not related to later problematic behavior, but rather that early childhood may not be a sensitive period for this class of outcomes (Duncan et al., 2015; Shaw & Shelleby, 2014). Nor is there sufficient evidence to conclude that adolescence is a sensitive period for family SES exposure and aggression or other social, emotional, or behavioral outcomes. Finally, like developmental or age differences, findings on gender differences are inconclusive because most studies do not examine them.

Neighborhood Poverty, SES, and Children's Aggression

In contrast to the research on family social inequality and children's aggression, many studies on neighborhood social inequality consider broad measures of neighborhood SES, particularly low SES or disadvantage, as well as more narrow measures of neighborhood poverty. Like the family poverty/SES research, several reviews indicate a consistent pattern: Living in neighborhoods marked by greater socioeconomic disadvantage is associated with children's aggressive and other problematic behaviors, particularly conduct problems, delinquency, and violence (for reviews, see Chang, Wang, & Tsai, 2016; Diez-Roux & Mair, 2010; Ingoldsby & Shaw, 2002; Leventhal et al., 2015; Sampson et al., 2002; Shaw & Shelleby, 2014). Across this general body of research, the "effect" of neighborhood disadvantage is generally small to modest (Leventhal & Brooks-Gunn, 2000). Given the nature of the outcomes considered, much of this research is based on samples of older children and adolescents as opposed to young children (Moffitt, 1993). This situation is not entirely surprising because neighborhoods are thought to play a more prominent role as children get older, are granted more autonomy than in earlier childhood, and spend increasing amounts of time with peers and outside the home (Leventhal et al., 2015; Steinberg & Morris, 2001). The growing salience of peers during adolescence, coupled with the peer-oriented nature of many of the behaviors, especially delinquency, are also likely contribute to a focus on adolescent problem behaviors and neighborhood social inequality (Dodge, Coie, & Lynam, 2008).

A vast majority of studies on neighborhood disadvantage and children's aggression are nonexperimental. Although many of them are longitudinal, neighborhood SES is often assessed at a single point in time, unlike the research on family income, which takes a more dynamic approach (Leventhal et al., 2015). Perhaps the most convincing support for a link between neighborhood disadvantage and physical aggression to emanate from this work comes from a meta-analysis of 43 such studies on physical aggression and neighborhood disadvantage; all of the studies met certain quality standards (e.g., multilevel, controlled for individual covariates and neighborhood clustering; Chang et al., 2016). In line with the general conclusion about the neighborhood disadvantage–aggression link are results of a study that employed longitudinal data on both children's antisocial behavior and neighborhood disadvantage. Using the Environmental Risk (E-Risk) Longitudinal Twin Study, a national British cohort study, Odgers and colleagues (2012) found that 5-year-olds living in disadvantaged neighborhoods displayed more antisocial behaviors than their peers living in more advantaged ones; this gap widened from 5 to 12 years of age despite overall declines in antisocial behavior, except among boys in the most disadvantaged neighborhoods. That is, boys in the most disadvantaged neighborhoods demonstrated an earlier onset and persistence of antisocial behavior.

Somewhat surprisingly, few neighborhood studies on aggression per se have used more robust statistical methods that address selection problems. Rather, most such work centers on educational and economic outcomes. As an exception, a study using data from the National Longitudinal Study of Adolescent to Adult Health (Add Health), a nationally representative, school-based study, employed a behavior genetics approach to explore the link between neighborhood disadvantage and adolescents' aggression (Cleveland, 2003). Behavior genetics models compare siblings of different genetic relatedness (e.g., monozygotic and dizygotic twins) in an attempt to distinguish between genetic and environmental—shared and unshared—influences on children's development. Presumably, by controlling for genetic relatedness, such designs provide some purchase on estimating contextual effects such as neighborhood influences as part of the shared family environment (Caspi, Taylor, Moffitt, & Plomin, 2000). Employing this strategy, Cleveland (2003) found that living in a more disadvantaged neighborhood was associated with adolescents' displaying more aggressive behavior and that genetic influences on aggression were more likely to be expressed at higher levels of neighborhood disadvantage. Another study using a similar approach with the E-Risk sample found that environmental influences accounted for 20% of the variance in 2-year-olds' behavior problems, with neighborhood disadvantage explaining 5% of this variance (Caspi et al., 2000).

A few other studies have used propensity score methods, as described earlier, to account for mobility across different types of neighborhoods. One such study drew on data from the PHDCN, a neighborhood-based study, following several cohorts of children over approximately 6 years; in this specific study, three cohorts of children 9, 12, and 15 years of age were included (Leventhal & Brooks-Gunn,

2011). The researchers found that only boys' trajectories of violent behavior were worse if they lived in neighborhoods that either decreased or increased in poverty compared with their peers in stable neighborhoods. Youth in high- and moderate- poverty neighborhoods were more susceptible to these neighborhood poverty dynamics than youth in low-poverty neighborhoods. The findings were interpreted as possibly related to rises in social disorganization when neighborhood socioeconomic and related conditions are in flux.

Another study with this same sample but focused on mobility across neighborhoods reported that moving within the city of Chicago was associated with increases in youth's violent behavior compared with not moving, whereas moving outside of the city of Chicago, as opposed to staying in the city, was associated with reductions in youth's violent behavior (Sharkey & Sampson, 2010). Exploration of potential mediators suggested that neighborhood poverty and racial/ethnic composition did not explain changes in behavior, but neighborhood violence and school quality did. Across this nonexperimental work, there is a very preliminary suggestion that the relationship between children's aggression and neighborhood disadvantage may be nonlinear such that the link may be especially pronounced in the most disadvantaged neighborhoods.

As with family poverty/SES, there are a small number of experimental studies that contribute to this discussion. MTO, described earlier, is the most well known and only true experimental study of neighborhood mobility (see the section "Measures and Methods"). A 10-year evaluation of MTO revealed that adolescent boys who were assigned to move to low-poverty neighborhoods had higher rates of conduct disorder and posttraumatic stress disorder than their peers in the control group, who remained in public housing in high-poverty neighborhoods (Kessler et al., 2014). To the contrary, girls whose families were given the opportunity to move to low-poverty neighborhoods were less likely to have serious behavioral–emotional problems or to use alcohol than their peers in the control group, who stayed in high-poverty neighborhoods (Gennetian et al., 2012; Sanbonmatsu et al., 2011). It is worth noting two additional findings. First, no program effects were reported for youths' delinquent or criminal behavior at the 10-year evaluation. Second, a longer term follow-up of MTO using administrative data from the Social Security Administration found that children who were 13 years or younger when their families moved to low-poverty neighborhoods, and who presumably were exposed to more advantaged neighborhoods earlier and longer than their older counterparts, were more likely to attend college and have higher earnings and less likely to be single parents in young adulthood compared with the control group (Chetty et al., 2016). No such benefits were seen among MTO children who were older than 13 years of age when they moved.

Aside from MTO, some quasi-experimental studies address neighborhood context and aggression-related behaviors. One is based on a court-ordered desegregation effort in Yonkers, New York, in 1985 in which 200 units of low-rise publicly funded townhouses were constructed in eight primarily white middle-class areas of the city. A quasi-experimental study followed approximately 220 low-income minority families 7 years after a group of them were randomly assigned via lottery to relocate to the new housing. As with the 10-year MTO evaluation, program effects were mixed. Among adolescents who were 15–18 years of age at the follow-up, youth who had moved to the new housing in middle-income neighborhoods reported more hyperactive behavior problems and substance use than their peers from the original high-poverty neighborhood, about half of whom had families who were on the waiting list for the new public housing (Fauth, Leventhal, & Brooks-Gunn, 2007). There was some evidence that children 8–11 years of age who moved to middle-income neighborhoods had fewer hyperactivity problems than their counterparts in high-poverty neighborhoods, but differences were more modest than ones seen among older youth.

Another notable study is a natural experiment and does not examine neighborhood SES or children and adolescents per se but is worth mentioning because of its relevance to aggression. It examined how changes in neighborhood residence resulting from the devastation of Hurricane Katrina were associated with prisoners' recidivism (Kirk, 2009). This study took advantage of changes in offenders' residential locations after release from prison in the aftermath of Hurricane Katrina. It found that not returning to one's former place of residence was associated with inmates' lower chances of recidivism and reincarceration compared with their counterparts who returned to their former residences. One potential explanation for the pattern of findings is that relocation likely disrupted deviant peer networks. In a similar vein, qualitative research on MTO suggests that some of the adverse program effects on boys' behavior may be due, at least in part, to the fact that boys in the program were not effectively separated from peers in their old neighborhoods because of the proximity of their new neighborhoods to their original ones (Clampet-Lundquist, 2011).

In sum, the highlighted research is consistent with the more general nonexperimental work on neighborhood disadvantage and children's aggression but is somewhat more complex. This complexity arises because studies trying to capture changes in neighborhood socioeconomic conditions as a way to limit selection bias often are confounded with other factors, such as mobility or shifts in other neighborhood conditions. Although changes in family SES typically are driven by other transitions (e.g., employment, marriage), sorting out these factors at the neighborhood level can be more challenging because many of the potential sources of change are often unmeasured.

In terms of developmental and gender differences, the findings are inconclusive. Because so much of the neighborhood research focuses on adolescents, comparisons across studies are difficult to make, and few studies explicitly test for age differences. The work reviewed suggests some gender differences, but results across studies are too mixed to make any general conclusions (for a full discussion of these findings, see Leventhal et al., 2015). It is also worth noting that some evidence suggests that biological or psychological characteristics may interact with neighborhood disadvantage such that individual risk factors amplify problematic outcomes. For example, the link between impulsivity or self-control and delinquency-related outcomes was strongest in disadvantaged neighborhoods in both city-based and national samples (Gibson, 2012).

Implications and Conclusions

Social inequality is a pervasive and growing problem for today's children (Massey & Denton, 1993; Proctor, Semega, & Kollar, 2016), with ramifications for many facets of their lives. What seems clear from the research reviewed in this chapter is that both family and neighborhood socioeconomic disadvantage raise the odds that children will display aggression and related behaviors. The causal nature of these associations remains debatable because of the lack of experimental research, of studies using advantaged statistical techniques to address selection bias, and—in the case of neighborhood research—of studies following both children and their neighborhood conditions over time. In addition, further narrowing down the question of for whom (e.g., boys or girls) or at what age (e.g., children vs. adolescents) socioeconomic inequality may have the most profound consequences is difficult because findings from the few studies that address these issues are quite mixed. All of these shortcomings suggest future directions for research on social inequality and children's aggression.

To draw implications for policy and practice, it is necessary to understand the processes through which social inequality may give rise to children's aggression. Although we did not systematically review research on pathways from inequality to aggressive behaviors, as it was beyond the scope of this broad chapter (for a review, see Shaw & Shelleby, 2014), we reference the previously discussed theoretical models because they are based in part on empirical work, though more such work is needed. With respect to family poverty and SES, all of the conceptual models point to the central role of parenting (e.g., behaviors, practices, and values) and family interactions. Some argue, however, that these family processes can be difficult to manipulate by external means, which makes translating them into action challenging (Huston, 2008). Rather, intervention efforts that target family social inequality directly may be more effective than indirect strategies aimed at altering family processes. More direct approaches might include bolstering existing policies that raise poor families' incomes, such as the Earned Income Tax Credit or Temporary Assistance for Needy Families, as well as other programs that support poor families' basic needs, such as Medicaid, food stamps, and housing assistance (Duncan et al., 2015).

At the neighborhood level, it is unclear whether targeting social inequality directly or indirectly (e.g., through social processes and institutional resources) might be most effective at preventing children's aggression. No single policy targets neighborhood social inequality per se, but two types of policy demonstrations are relevant to improving the socioeconomic conditions of neighborhoods in which families reside. First, mobility programs such as MTO increase poor families' residential options, giving them opportunities to move out of disadvantaged neighborhoods to more advantaged ones. Despite the mixed results of such efforts, as reviewed, public housing authorities across the United States are trying a variety of strategies to achieve this goal (e.g., pegging the amount of rent covered by housing subsidies to the local market, thereby allowing lower-income families to reside in neighborhoods that are more socioeconomically advantaged). The second strategy comprises comprehensive community initiatives (CCIs), which invest in poor neighborhoods to improve the living conditions of current residents (e.g., Zaff, Donlan, Pufall Jones, Lin, & Anderson, 2016). A notable example of a CCI is the Harlem Children's Zone (HCZ; Harlem Children's Zone, 2009). The program uses a "pipeline" approach, spanning the life course from before birth to college and involving coordinated community-based services in the educational, health, and social domains. Although social and behavioral outcomes have not been examined, research demonstrates the program is beneficial for children's achievement, particularly for older children (Dobbie & Fryer, 2011). It remains unclear, however, whether the complete bundle of HCZ services is necessary, over and above the charter schools, to obtain achievement benefits (Dobbie & Fryer, 2011). In any case, HCZ's success has been well received, and replication efforts are occurring in many communities through the federal government's Promise Neighborhoods Initiative.

Attempts to address indirect pathways also are a promising avenue for breaking the connection between neighborhood social inequality and children's aggression. A sizeable research base links neighborhood disadvantage and violent crime rates (e.g., Friedson & Sharkey, 2015). Neighborhood violence, disorganization, disorder, and low collective efficacy, in turn, are related to children's aggression, notably adolescent delinquency, and may explain, at least in part, the association between neighborhood disadvantage and children's problem behaviors (Leventhal et al., 2015; Sampson et al., 2002). Just as family processes may be hard to change, targeting neighborhood social dynamics can be challenging, too, but efforts such as community policing, which often entails a collaboration between local residents and police officers in fighting crime, can be fruitful (Cordner, 2014). In addition, the use of restorative justice in schools, or the attempt to repair harm done to one young person by another through communication and engagement of all involved parties (students, teachers and administrators, parents), can promote trust and strengthen ties within a given community by encouraging greater social control (e.g., more authority figures responding sensitively to children's misbehavior) and social cohesion (e.g., members of families whose children were in conflict getting to connect with one another; e.g., Bazemore, 2001; Bazemore & Schiff, 2015; see also Raby & Roisman, Chapter 9, and Salmivalli, Chapter 19, this volume). Restorative justice also can mitigate the direct consequences of aggression and delinquency for young people in low-income schools, rather than set them on a track to juvenile and criminal justice involvement, as in the "school-to-prison" pipeline (Bazemore, 2001; Bazemore & Schiff, 2015; e.g., González, 2012).

Ensuring that neighborhood institutional resources, notably child care, schools, and youth programs (especially after-school programming), are present and of high quality also may help weaken the link between neighborhood disadvantage and children's aggression. There is suggestive evidence that lack of these community resources or ones that are of low quality are a vehicle through which neighborhood inequality confers risks to children's behavior (Elliott, Dupéré, & Leventhal, 2015; Leventhal et al., 2015). In addition, enhancing the community resources available in impoverished neighborhoods may serve to improve children's outcomes by strengthening social organization.

In closing, this chapter provided a review of theory, methods, and empirical research on the relation between social inequality at the family and neighborhood levels and children's aggressive behaviors. Although much headway has been made with regard to documenting connections between social inequality and children's aggression and delineating potential pathways through which they emerge, more high-quality work—namely, research using experimental design or rigorous statistical approaches, such as propensity score matching or instrumental variable analysis—is needed to understand the best ways to address social inequality and its ramifications for children's aggression. As we have noted throughout this chapter, growing up in a poor family or neighborhood (or both) pervades all aspects of children's well-being and remains a fundamental challenge to prevention and intervention efforts targeting children's aggression.

ACKNOWLEDGMENT

We would like to acknowledge Julius Anastasio for assistance with this chapter.

REFERENCES

Achenbach, T. M. (2001). *Child Behavior Checklist for ages 6 to 18*. Burlington: University of Vermont, Research Center for Children, Youth, and Families.

Akee, R. K., Copeland, W., Keeler, G. P., Angold, A., & Costello, E. J. (2010). Parents' incomes and children's outcomes: A quasi-experiment. *American Economic Journal: Applied Economics, 2*(1), 86–115.

Anderson, E. (1999). *The code of the street: Decency, violence, and the moral life of the inner city*. New York: Norton.

Bazemore, G. (2001). Young people, trouble, and crime: Restorative justice as a normative theory of informal social control and social support. *Youth and Society, 33*(2), 199–226.

Bazemore, G., & Schiff, M. (2015). *Restorative community justice: Repairing harm and transforming communities*. Abingdon, UK: Routledge.

Berg, M. T., & Loeber, R. (2011). Examining the neighborhood context of the violent offending–victimization relationship: A prospective investigation. *Journal of Quantitative Criminology, 27*(4), 427–451.

Berger, L. M., Bruch, S. K., Johnson, E. I., James, S., & Rubin, D. (2009). Estimating the "impact" of out-of-home placement on child well-being: Approaching the problem of selection bias. *Child Development, 80*(6), 1856–1876.

Bishaw, A. (2014). *Changes in areas with concentrated poverty: 2000 to 2010*. Washington, DC: U.S. Department of Commerce Economics and Statistics Administration, U.S. Census Bureau.

Bornstein, M. H., & Leventhal, T. (2015). Children in bioecological landscapes of development. In M. H. Bornstein & T. Leventhal (Eds.) & R. M. Lerner (Ed.-in-Chief), *Handbook of child psychology and developmental science: Vol. 4. Ecological settings and processes* (7th ed., pp. 1–5). Hoboken, NJ: Wiley.

Bradley, R. H., & Corwyn, R. F. (2002). Socioeconomic status and child development. *Annual Review of Psychology, 53*, 371–399.

Brody, G. H., Ge, X., Conger, R., Gibbons, F. X., Murry, V. M., Gerrard, M., et al. (2001). The influence of neighborhood disadvantage, collective socialization, and parenting on African American children's affiliation with deviant peers. *Child Development, 72*(4), 1231–1246.

Burchinal, M., Nelson, L., Carlson, M., & Brooks-Gunn, J. (2008). Neighborhood characteristics and child care type and quality. *Early Education and Development, 19*, 702–725.

Bursik, R. J., & Grasmick, H. G. (1992). Longitudinal neighborhood profiles in delinquency: The decomposition of change. *Journal of Quantitative Criminology, 8*, 247–263.

Caspi, A., Taylor, A., Moffitt, T. E., & Plomin, R. (2000). Neighborhood deprivation affects children's mental health: Environmental risks identified in a genetic design. *Psychological Science, 11*, 338–342.

Chang, L.-Y., Wang, M.-Y., & Tsai, P.-S. (2016). Neighborhood disadvantage and physical aggression in children and adolescents: A systematic review and meta-analysis of multilevel studies. *Aggressive Behavior, 42*(5), 441–454.

Chauhan, P., & Reppucci, N. D. (2009). The impact of neighborhood disadvantage and exposure to violence on self-report of antisocial behavior among girls in the juvenile justice system. *Journal of Youth and Adolescence, 38*(3), 401–416.

Chetty, R., Hendren, N., & Katz, L. F. (2016). The effects of exposure to better neighborhoods on children: New evidence from the Moving to Opportunity experiment. *American Economic Review, 90*(4), 855–902.

Chetty, R., Hendren, N., Kline, P., & Saez, E. (2014). Where is the land of opportunity?: The geography of intergenerational mobility in the United States. *Quarterly Journal of Economics, 129*(4), 1553–1623.

Clampet-Lundquist, S. (2011). Teens, mental health, and Moving to Opportunity [Slide show]. Retrieved from *www.slideshare.net/PennUrbanResearch/teens-mental-health-and-moving-to-opportunity.*

Cleveland, H. H. (2003). Disadvantaged neighborhoods and adolescent aggression: Behavioral genetic evidence of context effects. *Journal of Research on Adolescence, 13,* 211–238.

Cohen, L. E., & Felson, M. (1979). Social change and crime rate trends: A routine activity approach. *American Sociological Review, 44*(4), 588–608.

Conger, R., Conger, K. J., & Martin, M. J. (2010). Socioeconomic status, family processes, and individual development. *Journal of Marriage and Family, 72*(3), 685–704.

Cordner, G. (2014). Community policing. In M. D. Reisig & R. J. Kane (Eds.), *The Oxford handbook of police and policing* (pp. 148–171). New York: Oxford University Press.

Costa, B. M., Kaestle, C. E., Walker, A., Curtis, A., Day, A., Toumbourou, J. W., et al. (2015). Longitudinal predictors of domestic violence perpetration and victimization: A systematic review. *Aggression and Violent Behavior, 24,* 261–272.

Costello, E. J., Compton, D. L., Keeler, G. P., & Angold, A. (2003). Relationships between poverty and psychopathology: A natural experiment. *Journal of the American Medical Association, 290*(15), 2023–2029.

Costello, E. J., Erkanli, A., Copeland, W., & Angold, A. (2010). Association of family income supplements in adolescence with development of psychiatric and substance use disorders in adulthood among an American Indian population. *Journal of the American Medical Association, 303*(19), 1954–1960.

Costello, E. J., Mustillo, S., Erkanli, A., Keeler, G., & Angold, A. (2003). Prevalence and development of psychiatric disorders in childhood and adolescence. *Archives of General Psychiatry, 60*(8), 837–844.

Currie, J. (2012). Antipoverty programs for poor children and families. In P. N. Jefferson (Ed.), *The Oxford handbook of the economics of poverty* (pp. 277–315). New York: Oxford University Press.

Dearing, E., McCartney, K., & Taylor, B. A. (2006). Within-child associations between family income and externalizing and internalizing problems. *Developmental Psychology, 46,* 237–252.

Diez-Roux, A. V., & Mair, C. (2010). Neighborhoods and health. *Annals of the New York Academy of Sciences, 1186,* 125–145.

Dishion, T. J., McCord, J., & Poulin, F. (1999). When interventions harm: Peer groups and problem behavior. *American Psychologist, 54,* 755–764.

Dishion, T. J., Patterson, G. R., Stoolmiller, M., & Skinner, M. L. (1991). Family, school, and behavioral antecedants to early adolescent involvement with antisocial peers. *Developmental Psychology, 27,* 172–180.

Dobbie, W., & Fryer, R. G., Jr. (2011). Are high-quality schools enough to increase achievement among the poor?: Evidence from the Harlem Children's Zone. *American Economic Journal: Applied Economics, 3,* 158–187.

Dodge, K. A., Coie, J. D., & Lynam, D. (2008). Aggression and antisocial behavior in youth. In W. Damon & R. M. Lerner (Eds.), *Child and adolescent development: An advanced course* (pp. 437–472). Hoboken, NJ: Wiley.

D'Onofrio, B. M., Goodnight, J. A., Van Hulle, C. A., Rodgers, J. L., Rathouz, P. J., Waldman, I. D., et al. (2009). A quasi-experimental analysis of the association between family income and offspring conduct problems. *Journal of Abnormal Child Psychology, 37*(3), 415–429.

Duncan, G. J., & Brooks-Gunn, J. (Eds.). (1997). *Consequences of growing up poor.* New York: Russell Sage Foundation Press.

Duncan, G. J., Magnuson, K., & Votruba-Drzal, E. (2015). Children and socioeconomic status. In M. H. Bornstein & T. Leventhal (Eds.) & R. M. Lerner (Ed.-in-Chief), *Handbook of child psychology and developmental science: Vol. 4. Ecological settings and processes* (7th ed., pp. 534–573). Hoboken, NJ: Wiley.

Duncan, G. J., & Murnane, R. J. (Eds.). (2011). *Whither opportunity?: Rising inequality, schools, and children's life chances.* New York: Russell Sage Foundation.

Duncan, G. J., Ziol-Guest, K. M., & Kalil, A. (2010). Early-childhood poverty and adult attainment, behavior, and health. *Child Development, 81*(1), 306–325.

Elder, G. H., Shanahan, M. J., & Jennings, J. A. (2015). Human development in time and place. In M. H. Bornstein & T. Leventhal (Eds.) & R. M. Lerner (Ed.-in-Chief), *Handbook of child psychology and developmental science: Vol. 4. Ecological settings and processes* (7th ed., pp. 6–54). Hoboken, NJ: Wiley.

Elliott, D. S., Wilson, W. J., Huizinga, D., Sampson, R. J., Elliott, A., & Rankin, B. (1996). The effects of neighborhood disadvantage on adolescent development. *Journal of Research in Crime and Delinquency, 33*(4), 389–426.

Elliott, M. C., Dupéré, V., & Leventhal, T. (2015). Neighborhood context and the development of antisocial and criminal behavior. In J. Morizot & L. Kazemian (Eds.), *The development of criminal and antisocial behavior: Theoretical foundations and practical implications* (pp. 253–266). New York: Springer.

Elo, I. T., Mykyta, L., Margolis, R., & Culhane, J. F. (2009). Perceptions of neighborhood disorder: The role of individual and neighborhood characteristics. *Social Science Quarterly, 90*(5), 1298–1320.

Evans, G. W., & Stecker, R. (2004). Motivational consequences of environmental stress. *Journal of Environmental Psychology, 24,* 143–165.

Fauth, R. C., Leventhal, T., & Brooks-Gunn, J. (2007). Welcome to the neighborhood?: Long-term impacts of moving to low-poverty neighborhoods on poor children's and adolescents' outcomes. *Journal of Research on Adolescence, 17*(2), 249–284.

Ferguson, K. T., Cassells, R. C., MacAllister, J. W., & Evans, G. W. (2013). The physical environment and child development: An international review. *International Journal of Psychology, 48*(4), 437–468.

Fite, P. J., Vitulano, M., Wynn, P., Wimsatt, A., Gaertner, A., & Rathert, J. (2010). Influence of perceived neighborhood safety on proactive and reactive aggression. *Journal of Community Psychology, 38*(6), 757–768.

Foster, E. M., & McLanahan, S. (1996). An illustration of the use of instrumental variables: Do neighborhood conditions affect a young person's chance of finishing high school? *Psychological Methods, 1*(3), 249–260.

Friedson, M., & Sharkey, P. T. (2015). Violence and neighborhood disadvantage after the crime decline. *Annals of the American Academy of Political and Social Science, 660,* 341–358.

Gennetian, L. A., & Miller, C. (2002). Children and welfare reform: A view from an experimental welfare program in Minnesota. *Child Development, 73*(2), 601–620.

Gennetian, L. A., Sanbonmatsu, L., Katz, L. F., Kling, J. R., Sciandra, M., Ludwig, J., et al.

(2012). The long-term effects of Moving to Opportunity on youth outcomes. *Cityscape, 14*(2), 137–167.

Gibson, C. L. (2012). An investigation of neighborhood disadvantage, low self-control, and violent victimization among youth. *Youth Violence and Juvenile Justice, 10*(1), 41–63.

Glaeser, E., & Scheinkman, J. (2001). Measuring social interactions. In S. N. Durlaf & H. P. Young (Eds.), *Social dynamics* (pp. 83–132). Cambridge, MA: MIT Press.

Goering, J., & Feins, J. D. (2003). *Choosing a better life:? Evaluating the Moving to Opportunity social experiment*. Washington, DC: Urban Institute Press.

González, T. (2012). Keeping kids in schools: Restorative justice, punitive discipline, and the school to prison pipeline. *Journal of Law and Education, 41*, 281–335.

Granger, R. C. (2008). After-school programs and academics: Implications for policy, practice, and research. *Social Policy Report, 22*, 1–19.

Guo, S., & Fraser, M. W. (2010). *Propensity score analysis: Statistical methods and applications*. Thousand Oaks, CA: SAGE.

Hannon, L. (2003). Poverty, delinquency, and educational attainment: Cumulative disadvantage or disadvantage saturation? *Sociological Inquiry, 73*(4), 575–594.

Harding, D. J. (2011). Rethinking the cultural context of schooling decisions in disadvantaged neighborhoods: From deviant subculture to cultural heterogeneity. *Sociology of Education, 84*, 322–339.

Harlem Children's Zone. (2009). The HCZ project. Retrieved from *www.hcz.org/index.php/about-us/the-hcz-project*.

Harris, B. H., & Kearney, M. S. (2014). *The unequal burden of crime and incarceration on America's poor*. Washington, DC: Brookings Institution.

Haynie, D. L., Silver, E., & Teasdale, B. (2006). Neighborhood characteristics, peer influence, and adolescent violence. *Journal of Quantitative Criminology, 22*, 147–169.

Heckman, J. J. (2006). Skill formation and the economics of investing in disadvantaged children. *Science, 312*, 1900–1902.

Hill, M. (1991). *The panel study of income dynamics: A user's guide.*. Newbury Park, CA: SAGE.

Hipp, J. R., & Wickes, R. (2016). Violence in urban neighborhoods: A longitudinal study of collective efficacy and violent crime. *Journal of Quantitative Criminology, 33*(4), 1–26.

Huston, A. C. (2008). From research to policy and back. *Child Development, 79*, 1–12.

Iceland, J. (2013). *Poverty in America: A handbook*. Berkeley: University of California Press.

Ingoldsby, E. M., & Shaw, D. S. (2002). Neighborhood contextual factors and early-starting antisocial pathways. *Clinical Child and Family Psychology Review, 5*(1), 21–55.

Jacobs, F., & Kapuscik, J. (2000). *Making it count: Evaluating family preservation services*. Medford, MA: Tufts University, Department of Child Development, Family Preservation Evaluation Project.

Jencks, C., & Mayer, S. (1990). The social consequences of growing up in a poor neighborhood. In L. E. Lynn & M. F. H. McGeary (Eds.), *Inner-city poverty in the United States* (pp. 111–186). Washington, DC: National Academy Press.

Kessler, R. C., Duncan, G. J., Gennetian, L. A., Katz, L. F., Kling, J. R., Sampson, N. A., et al. (2014). Associations of housing mobility interventions for children in high-poverty neighborhoods with subsequent mental disorders during adolescence. *Journal of the American Medical Association, 311*(9), 937–947.

Kirk, D. S. (2009). A natural experiment on residential change and recidivism: Lessons from Hurricane Katrina. *American Sociological Review, 74*, 484–505.

Kneebone, E., & Holmes, N. (2016). U.S. concentrated poverty in the wake of the Great Recession. Retrieved from *www.brookings.edu/research/u-s-concentrated-poverty-in-the-wake-of-the-great-recession*.

Lareau, A. (2011). *Unequal childhoods: Class, race and family life*. Berkeley: University of California Press.

Leech, T. G. J., Adams, E. A., Weathers, T. D., Staten, L. K., & Filippelli, G. M. (2016). Inequitable chronic lead exposure. *Family and Community Health, 39*(3), 151–159.

Lerner, R. M. (2006). Developmental science, developmental systems, and contemporary theories of human development. In W. Damon & R. M. Lerner (Eds.) & R. M. Lerner (Ed.-in-Chief), *Handbook of child psychology: Vol. 1. Theoretical models of human development* (6th ed., pp. 1–17). Hoboken, NJ: Wiley.

Leventhal, T., & Brooks-Gunn, J. (2000). The neighborhoods they live in: The effects of neighborhood residence on child and adolescent outcomes. *Psychological Bulletin, 126*(2), 309–337.

Leventhal, T., & Brooks-Gunn, J. (2011). Changes in neighborhood poverty from 1990 to 2000 and youth's problem behaviors. *Developmental Psychology, 47*(6), 1680–1698.

Leventhal, T., Dupéré, V., & Brooks-Gunn, J. (2009). Neighborhood influences on adolescent development. In R. M. Lerner & L. Steinberg (Eds.), *Handbook of adolescent psychology: Vol. 2. Contextual influences on adolescent development* (3rd ed., pp. 411–443). Hoboken, NJ: Wiley.

Leventhal, T., Dupéré, V., & Shuey, E. A. (2015). Children in neighborhoods. In M. H. Bornstein & T. Leventhal (Eds.) & R. M. Lerner (Ed.-in-Chief), *Handbook of child psychology and developmental science: Vol. 4. Ecological settings and processes* (7th ed., pp. 493–533). Hoboken, NJ: Wiley.

Lund, T. J., & Dearing, E. (2013). Is growing up affluent risky for adolescents or is the problem growing up in an affluent neighborhood? *Journal of Research on Adolescence, 23*(2), 274–282.

Lupien, S. J., McEwen, B. S., Gunnar, M. R., & Heim, C. (2009). Effects of stress throughout the lifespan on the brain, behaviour and cognition. *Nature Reviews Neuroscience, 10*(6), 434–445.

Luthar, S. S., & Barkin, S. H. (2012). Are affluent youth truly "at risk"?: Vulnerability and resilience across three diverse samples. *Development and Psychopathology, 24,* 429–449.

Luthar, S. S., & Latendresse, S. J. (2005). Comparable "risks" at the SES extremes: Preadolescents' perceptions of parenting. *Development and Psychopathology, 17,* 207–230.

Massey, D. S., & Denton, N. (1993). *American apartheid: Segregation and the making of the underclass.* Cambridge, MA: Harvard University Press.

Mazza, J. R. S., Boivin, M., Tremblay, R. E., Michel, G., Salla, J., Lambert, J., et al. (2016). Poverty and behavior problems trajectories from 1.5 to 8 years of age: Is the gap widening between poor and non-poor children? *Social Psychiatry and Psychiatric Epidemiology, 51*(8), 1083–1092.

Mennis, J., & Harrison, P. A. (2011). Contagion and repeat offending among urban juvenile delinquents. *Journal of Adolescence, 34,* 951–963.

Moffitt, T. E. (1993). Adolescence-limited and life-course-persistent antisocial behavior: A developmental taxonomy. *Psychological Review, 100*(4), 674–701.

Molnar, B. E., Buka, S. L., Brennan, R. T., Holton, J. K., & Earls, F. (2003). A multilevel study of neighborhoods and parent-to-child physical aggression: Results from the Project on Human Development in Chicago Neighborhoods. *Child Maltreatment, 8*(2), 84–97.

Molnar, B. E., Miller, M. J., Azrael, D., & Buka, S. L. (2004). Neighborhood predictors of concealed firearm carrying among children and adolescents: Results from the Project on Human Development in Chicago Neighborhoods. *Archives of Pediatrics and Adolescent Medicine, 158,* 657–664.

Morris, P. A., Duncan, G. J., & Clark-Kauffman, E. (2005). Child well-being in an era of welfare reform: The sensitivity of transitions in development to policy change. *Developmental Psychology, 41*(6), 919–932.

Mullainathan, S. (2012). Decision making and policy in contexts of poverty. In E. Shafir (Ed.), *The behavioral foundations of public policy* (pp. 281–297). Princeton, NJ: Princeton University Press.

Murray, J., & Farrington, D. P. (2010). Risk factors for conduct disorder and delinquency: Key findings from longitudinal studies. *Canadian Journal of Psychiatry, 55*(10), 633–642.

Obsuth, I., Eisner, M. P., Malti, T., & Ribeaud, D. (2015). The developmental relation between aggressive behaviour and prosocial behaviour: A 5-year longitudinal study. *BMC Psychology, 3*(1). Retrieved from *https://bmcpsychology.biomedcentral.com/articles/10.1186/s40359-015-0073-4*.

Odgers, C. L., Caspi, A., Russell, M. A., Sampson, R. J., Arseneault, L., & Moffitt, T. E. (2012). Supportive parenting mediates neighborhood socioeconomic disparities in children's antisocial behavior from ages 5 to 12. *Development and Psychopathology, 24*(3), 705–721.

Overton, W. F. (2015). Processes, relations, and relational–developmental–systems. In F. Overton & P. C. M. Molenaar (Eds.) & R. M. Lerner (Ed.-in-Chief), *Handbook of child psychology and developmental science: Vol. 1. Theory and method* (7th ed., pp. 9–62). Hoboken, NJ: Wiley.

Pettit, G. S., Bates, J. E., Dodge, K. A., & Meece, D. W. (1999). The impact of after-school peer contact on early adolescent externalizing problems is moderated by parental monitoring, perceived neighborhood safety, and prior adjustment. *Child Development, 70*(3), 768–778.

Proctor, B. D., Semega, J. L., & Kollar, M. A. (2016). *Income and poverty in the United States: 2015* (Report No. P60-256). Washington, DC: U.S. Census Bureau.

Raudenbush, S. W., Johnson, C., & Sampson, R. J. (2003). Rasch model with application to self-reported criminal behavior. *Sociological Methodology, 33*(1), 169–211.

Rhee, S. H., & Waldman, I. D. (2002). Genetic and environmental influences on antisocial behavior: A meta-analysis of twin and adoption studies. *Psychological Bulletin, 128*(3), 490–529.

Ross, C. E., Mirowsky, J., & Pribesh, S. (2001). Powerlessness and the amplification of threat: Neighborhood disadvantage, disorder, and mistrust. *American Sociological Review, 66*, 568–591.

Sampson, R. J. (1997). Collective regulation of adolescent misbehavior: Validation results from eighty Chicago neighborhoods. *Journal of Adolescent Research, 12*, 227–244.

Sampson, R. J., Morenoff, J. D., & Gannon-Rowley, T. (2002). Assessing "neighborhood effects": Social processes and new directions in research. *Annual Review of Sociology, 28*, 443–478.

Sampson, R. J., Morenoff, J. D., & Raudenbush, S. (2005). Social anatomy of racial and ethnic disparities in violence. *American Journal of Public Health, 95*(2), 224–232.

Sampson, R. J., & Raudenbush, S. W. (2004). Seeing disorder: Neighborhood stigma and the social construction of "broken windows." *Social Psychology Quarterly, 67*(4), 319–342.

Sampson, R. J., Raudenbush, S. W., & Earls, F. (1997). Neighborhoods and violent crime: A multilevel study of collective efficacy. *Science, 277*, 918–924.

Sanbonmatsu, L., Ludwig, J., Katz, L. F., Genettian, L. A., Duncan, G. J., Kessler, R. C., et al. (2011). *Moving to Opportunity for Fair Housing Demonstration Program: Final impacts evaluation*. Washington, DC: U.S. Department of Housing and Urban Development.

Shadish, W. R., Cook, T. D., & Campbell, D. T. (2002). *Experimental and quasi-experimental designs for generalized causal inference*. Boston: Houghton Mifflin.

Sharkey, P. T. (2006). Navigating dangerous streets: The sources and consequences of street efficacy. *American Sociological Review, 71*, 826–846.

Sharkey, P. T., & Sampson, R. J. (2010). Destination effects: Residential mobility and trajectories of adolescent violence in a stratified metropolis. *Criminology, 48*, 639–672.

Shaw, C. R., & McKay, H. D. (1942). *Juvenile delinquency and urban areas*. Chicago: University of Chicago Press.

Shaw, C. R., & McKay, H. D. (1969). *Juvenile delinquency and urban areas* (rev. ed.). Chicago: University of Chicago Press.

Shaw, D. S., & Shelleby, E. C. (2014). Early-starting conduct problems: Intersection of conduct problems and poverty. *Annual Review of Clinical Psychology, 10,* 503–528.

Shonkoff, J. P., Garner, A. S., Siegel, B. S., Dobbins, M. I., Earls, M. F., Garner, A. S., et al. (2012). The lifelong effects of early childhood adversity and toxic stress. *Pediatrics, 129*(1), e232–e246.

Small, M. L., Harding, D., & Lamont, M. (2010). Reconsidering culture and poverty. *Annals of the American Academy of Political and Social Science, 629,* 6–27.

Small, M. L., & McDermott, M. (2006). The presence of organizational resources in poor urban neighborhoods: An analysis of average and contextual effects. *Social Forces, 84*(3), 1697–1724.

Snyder, H. N., & Sickmund, M. (2006). *Juvenile offenders and victims: 2006 national report.* Washington, DC: Office of Juvenile Justice and Delinquency Prevention.

Snyder, J., Schrepferman, L., McEachern, A., Barner, S., Johnson, K., & Provines, J. (2008). Peer deviancy training and peer coercion: Dual processes associated with early-onset conduct problems. *Child Development, 79*(2), 252–268.

Steinberg, L. (2014). *Age of opportunity: Lessons from the new science of adolescence.* New York: Houghton Mifflin Harcourt.

Steinberg, L., & Morris, A. S. (2001). Adolescent development. *Annual Review of Psychology, 52*(1), 83–110.

Strohschein, L. (2005). Household income histories and child mental health trajectories. *Journal of Health and Social Behavior, 46*(4), 359–375.

Tolan, P. H., Gorman-Smith, D., & Henry, D. B. (2003). The developmental ecology of urban males' youth violence. *Developmental Psychology, 39,* 274–291.

UNICEF. (2012). Measuring child poverty: New league tables of child poverty in the world's rich countries. Retrieved from *www.unicef-irc.org/publications/660.*

U.S. Census Bureau. (2015). *Geographical mobility: 2014 to 2015.* Washington, DC: U.S. Census Bureau. Retrieved from *www.census.gov/data/tables/2015/demo/geographic-mobility/cps-2015.html.*

U.S. Department of Health and Human Services. (2016). Poverty guidelines. Retrieved February 9, 2017, from *https://aspe.hhs.gov/poverty-guidelines.*

Vandell, D. L., Larson, R. W., Mahoney, J. L., & Watts, T. W. (2015). Children's organized activities. In M. H. Bornstein & T. Leventhal (Eds.) & R. M. Lerner (Ed.-in-Chief), *Handbook of child psychology and developmental science: Vol. 4. Ecological settings and processes* (7th ed., pp. 305–344). Hoboken, NJ: Wiley.

Votruba-Drzal, E. (2006). Economic disparities in middle childhood development: Does income matter? *Developmental Psychology, 42*(6), 1154–1167.

Wilson, W. J. (1987). *The truly disadvantaged: The inner city, the underclass, and public policy.* Chicago: University of Chicago Press.

Wodtke, G. T., Harding, D. J., & Elwert, F. (2011). Neighborhood effects in temporal perspective: The impact of long-term exposure to concentrated disadvantage on high school graduation. *American Sociological Review, 76*(5), 713–736.

Yoshikawa, H., Aber, J. L., & Beardslee, W. R. (2012). The effects of poverty on the mental, emotional, and behavioral health of children and youth: Implications for prevention. *American Psychologist, 67*(4), 272.

Zaff, J. F., Donlan, A. E., Pufall Jones, E., Lin, E. S., & Anderson, S. (2016). Comprehensive community initiatives creating supportive youth systems: A theoretical rationale for creating youth-focused CCIs. In J. F. Zaff, E. Pufall Jones, A. E. Donlan, & S. Anderson (Eds.), *Community initiatives for positive youth development* (pp. 1–16). New York: Routledge.

Zimmerman, G. M., & Messner, S. F. (2011). Neighborhood context and nonlinear peer effects on adolescent violent crime. *Criminology, 49*(3), 873–903.

PART III

INTERVENTIONS AND POLICY IMPLICATIONS

CHAPTER 15

Measuring Social–Emotional Correlates of Aggression in Children and Adolescents

TINA MALTI, ANTONIO ZUFFIANÒ, and CONNIE CHEUNG

Brief Introduction

Social–emotional understanding is a core construct of human development. Not only are social–emotional skills related to better outcomes later in life, such as academic achievement and mental well-being (e.g., Jones, Greenberg, & Crowley, 2015), but they have been shown to counteract aggression and antisocial behaviors in children and youth (Durlak, Weissberg, Dymnicki, Taylor, & Shellinger, 2011; Malti, Chaparro, Zuffianò, & Colasante, 2016). Therefore, clinicians, practitioners, and educators have become interested in promoting social–emotional development in children and adolescents. In recent years, it has been acknowledged that it is essential to know how to support children's specific developmental needs and challenges in designing and implementing intervention programs that target aggression and antisocial behaviors. As such, there has been an increasing emphasis on the systematic use of screening and assessments that focus on indicators of social–emotional development. Utilizing this information allows not only the advancement of developmentally tailored intervention strategies informed by the social–emotional strengths and needs of the child (Malti et al., 2016), but also the determination of the quality of intervention programs and their effectiveness. The social–emotional evaluation can involve the use of screening and assessment tools from both a population and an individual perspective; thus it has the potential to inform policy by providing road maps that guide strategic planning and intervention services.

In this chapter, we review existing social–emotional assessment tools that can be used to inform the development, implementation, and evaluation of intervention approaches to prevent and reduce aggression in children and adolescents. First, we discuss population-based assessments and some of the advantages related to policy development and strategic planning. We also provide examples of commonly implemented population-based assessment tools to illustrate the utility of these measures in understanding the social–emotional developmental profiles of different communities. We then discuss individual-based *screening* and *assessment*, distinguishing between these two approaches. A select review of screening and assessment tools with demonstrated psychometric properties is presented. Lastly, we conclude with a discussion of the utility of using social–emotional assessment information to inform aggression intervention approaches and program evaluation.

Assessment of Social–Emotional Development

Social–emotional assessment instruments can be used to monitor and understand children's social–emotional development across different contexts. From a methodological point of view, they can be distinguished into population-based instruments and individual-based assessments. Population-based evaluations focus on collecting and analyzing data from a sample of children living in the same geographical location (e.g., neighborhood, communities) to inform the areas of development that differ among children and where these discrepancies exist. Individual- and group-based screening and assessment, on the other hand, aim to identify individual or specific subgroups of children who are at risk for aggression or related social–emotional difficulties (e.g., low empathy/sympathy) and provide an overall summary of where challenges may lie (e.g., Carter, Briggs-Gowan, & Davis, 2004). Distinct from population-based instruments, individual-based screening and assessments are aimed to inform individual service planning and intervention.

Population-Based Assessments of Social–Emotional Development

Population-based assessments of social–emotional development provide an understanding of children's growth in various spheres of social–emotional capacities. The main advantage of population-level tools is the ability to capture developmental profiles at different macrolevels (e.g., neighborhood, school, and country levels), while also assessing the value of community-level interventions (e.g., wide social–emotional screening in kindergarten children to identify those at greatest risk for aggressive problems). Furthermore, population sampling ensures that all individuals are potentially assessable, minimizing the risk of underrepresenting certain subgroups of children and families (e.g., ethnic minorities; Anderman et al., 1995). Establishing a population-based profile allows the identification of neighborhoods or communities in which children and/or adolescents could be at greater risk for developing aggression and related maladaptive outcomes. For instance, mandatory social–emotional screening of all children in kindergarten can identify neighborhoods with children at greatest risk for developing later behavioral concerns. From a population health perspective, this information can be used to strategically allocate appropriate resources to implement aggression prevention actions and mitigate the risk of later violence within specific communities or neighborhoods.

Population-based assessments are also important for measuring and evaluating the effectiveness of universal intervention programs for reducing aggression among children and adolescents. Universal interventions are those that target all children within the community by preventing symptoms or exposure to risk, regardless of vulnerability (e.g., Costello, 2016). The use of population-based screening tools can help monitor change in key outcomes, such as aggression and associated social–emotional challenges, following the implementation of community-level interventions. By establishing a baseline and monitoring change over time through standardized assessment tools, it is possible to detect population-level differences across neighborhoods, provinces, states, or countries. Related to our previous example above, once appropriate resources and intervention strategies have been introduced, the implementation of population-based measures over time can allow for the monitoring of change in social–emotional risk profiles within and between communities.

Ultimately, the intent of population-based assessments is to describe the profile of the community as a whole. Therefore, community trends can also inform disproportionality of risk of certain subgroups of children within different neighborhoods, enabling policy makers to advocate for specific needs of a community (for a more detailed discussion of the benefit of population-based assessments, refer to Mustard & Young, 2007). In subsequent sections, we present and illustrate the utility of two population-based assessments in understanding social–emotional development: the Early Development Instrument and the Middle Years Development Instrument.

The Early Development Instrument: A Population-Based Measure for Communities

To date, there is a scarcity of instruments assessing social–emotional development from a population perspective. A widely used tool is the Early Development Instrument: A Population-Based Measure for Communities (EDI). The EDI is an example of a population-based tool that provides an overall snapshot of child development, including social–emotional competency in kindergarten children. The EDI was developed in Canada in the late 1990s by Drs. Dan Offord and Magdalena Janus of the Offord Centre for Child Studies at McMaster University, in response to the need for a population-based instrument that incorporates both cognitive and social–emotional indicators of school readiness (e.g., Janus & Offord, 2007). The EDI consists of 103 items that measure development across five developmental domains (i.e., physical health and well-being, social competence, emotional maturity, language and communication, and cognitive development and general knowledge). Two domains—social competence and emotional maturity—measure key social–emotional constructs. Specifically, the social competence domain examines children's ability to engage with others and contains 26 items that assess areas, such as competence and cooperation in working with others, ability to remember and follow rules, and approaches to learning and problem solving. The emotional maturity domain examines children's aggression and other problem behaviors, as well as prosocial behavior (see Janus & Duku, 2007, for a review).

Widely used in Canada, the EDI has also been adapted for use in seven other countries—Australia, Chile, Jamaica, Kosovo, the Netherlands, New Zealand, and the United States. The EDI has good psychometric properties with acceptable levels of interrater reliability and concurrent and convergent validity (Janus & Offord, 2007). Mean domain and domain-based vulnerability scores are provided by the EDI to help identify children who may be vulnerable for developmental concerns (i.e., falling below the 10th percentile of a normative distribution on at least one domain). Depending on the country of implementation, vulnerability cutoff scores are defined provincially (e.g., Canada) or nationally (e.g., Australia; Janus, Harrison, Goldfield, Guhn, & Brinkman, 2016).

The Middle Years Development Instrument

Similar to the EDI, the Middle Years Development Instrument (MDI) is a population-based screening tool that assesses social–emotional development. However, the MDI examines domains of social–emotional development and well-being in 6- to 12-year-olds rather than kindergarten-age children. The MDI consists of 71 items that measure outcomes across five dimensions: (1) social and emotional development, (2) connectedness to peers and adults at school, home, and in the neighborhood, (3) school experiences, (4) physical health and well-being, and (5) constructive use of time after school (Schonert-Reichl et al., 2013). Analysis of MDI's psychometric properties indicates high internal consistency and theoretically coherent convergent and discriminant validity patterns (see Schonert-Reichl et al., 2013, for a review).

Utility of the EDI and MDI

To date, the EDI and MDI have been used to inform policy planning and structuring for cities and provinces. For instance, in Canada, the EDI is used to identify priority neighborhoods across the country. In the province of Ontario, this information has been used to help the City of Toronto plan child care centers, with the aim of rendering this service more accessible for children and families ("Early Development Instrument," 2017). There is also some emerging evidence to suggest that both the EDI and MDI can be used to predict individual outcomes. For instance, EDI measures across physical, social, emotional, language, and cognitive domains were significantly associated with later grade 3 reading, writing, and math standardized achievement scores in a sample of 45,000 kindergarten students in Ontario, Canada (Davies, Janus, Duku, & Gaskin, 2016). Data linkages between EDI and MDI have also been possible, allowing researchers to examine longitudinal population patterns in social–emotional development across early and middle childhood. Emerging evidence suggests that there is within-domain convergence across these two tools. For instance, in a sample of more than 7,000 children, teacher-rated social competence in kindergarten, as assessed by the EDI, predicted children's subsequent self-report of their connectedness to peers in grade 4 on the MDI. Similarly, early emotional maturity predicted children's rating of their later emotional well-being (Guhn, Gadermann, Almas, Schonert-Reichl, & Hertzman, 2016).

   In sum, population-based assessment tools such as the EDI provide insight into the average social–emotional functioning of children across different neighborhoods and communities. This information is particularly useful in the area of policy development and can provide policy makers with data to promote more evidence-informed decision making when designing plans of intervention and allocating resources.

Individual-Based Assessment of Social–Emotional Development

Understanding the social–emotional needs or strengths of individual children is critical, as it allows the implementation of tailored interventions to prevent and reduce aggression that consider developmental differences between children (e.g., Malti, 2016; Malti et al., 2016; Malti & Noam, 2016). As such, a number of individual-based social–emotional tools have been developed that provide a snapshot of child functioning. From a practical perspective, they can be categorized into social–emotional instruments for *screening* purposes and social–emotional instruments for *assessment* purposes. Unlike individual-based assessment tools, individual-based screening tools utilize cutoff scores to identify children who can benefit from further social–emotional assessments. This is particularly important because service and health care professionals and parents often have difficulty detecting social–emotional concerns in young children (e.g., Alakortes et al., 2017). For instance, systematic screening using the Ages and Stages: Social–Emotional questionnaire (ASQ-SE; Squires, Bricker, & Twombly, 2002) can improve the detection rate for social–emotional risk among vulnerable groups of young children (i.e., children in foster care vs. surveillance alone; Jee et al., 2010). In sum, the goal of a social–emotional screening tool is to identify a subset of children who can benefit the most from intervention given their social–emotional profiles.

Conversely, social–emotional assessment tools assess the maximum skill level of social–emotional functioning for a child at any given age. In other words, they provide a comprehensive assessment of children's developmental levels both within and across social–emotional domains (Malti et al., 2016; Malti & Noam, 2016). Most measures provide scores that are standardized and continuous, making it possible to compute a developmental quotient (e.g., Fernald, Kariger, Engle, & Raikes, 2009). Social–emotional assessment tools allow consistent, long-term monitoring of behaviors over time, tracking the developmental trajectory of social–emotional understanding. Combined, the use of individual-based social–emotional screening and assessment tools is integral for understanding the unique needs of children and the subsequent planning and implementation of individualized intervention strategies. For instance, children at risk for aggressive problems can be identified with questionnaire-based screening tools that measure their social–emotional capacities and aggressive behaviors (e.g., ASQ-SE). Of the children identified as being at greatest risk for aggression and related social–emotional factors (e.g., those low on empathy), specialized intervention strategies that enhance children's empathy-related responding—an important protective factor against the onset of aggressive problems (e.g., Durlak et al., 2011; Eisenberg, Eggum, & Di Giunta, 2010; Zuffianò, Colasante, Buchmann, & Malti, 2018)—can be implemented. Further assessments with developmentally sensitive tools can subsequently be used to inform on a child's social–emotional functioning and evaluate prevention and treatment efficacy and effectiveness by monitoring change before and after intervention.

Despite the potential application of strengths-based social–emotional screening and assessments, many of the existing tools commonly used in applied intervention research, particularly in the school setting, do not have a conceptual background that clearly aligns with social–emotional developmental theory and research (Malti et al., 2016). There also appears to be a general trend of providing a partial evaluation by favoring a psychopathological or deficit-based assessment (Haggerty, Elgin, & Woolley, 2011). Furthermore, commonly used assessment instruments often lack an in-depth analysis of the psychometric properties related to factor structure and developmental sensitivity (see Cordier et al., 2015). This is quite surprising, as the implementation of ad hoc intervention strategies at school (e.g., counteracting aggressive behaviors and bullying, improving children's emotion regulation) depends on the reliable, sensitive, and theoretically based assessment of children's resilience factors, including social–emotional strengths.

In the following sections, we review a select number of social–emotional screening and assessment tools with robust psychometric properties that are predominately strength-based, with the exception of the Child Behavior Checklist (CBCL). The CBCL is included in the current review given its widespread use in research and practice.

Individual-Based Social–Emotional Screening Tools

Individual-based social–emotional screening tools are those that identify children who may be vulnerable to delays in social–emotional development and/or at risk for aggression. However, despite the potential utility of social–emotional screening tools (e.g., identifying children at risk who will require further assessment), there are relatively few social–emotional screening instruments that have an in-depth analysis of their psychometric properties. Therefore, the purpose of the following section is to describe four promising screening tools that have been shown through research to be valid and reliable measures of social–emotional functioning: (1) the ASQ-SE, (2) the Brief Infant–Toddler Social–Emotional Assessment, (3) the Devereux Student Strengths Assessment Mini, and (4) the Strengths and Difficulties Questionnaire.

Ages and Stages Questionnaire: Social–Emotional

The ASQ-SE is a 30-item social–emotional screening tool designed for infants and children between birth (starting at 1 month of age) and 5 years of age. The ASQ-SE consists of nine age-appropriate parent-version questionnaires that screen for self-regulation, compliance, communication, adaptive behaviors, autonomy, affect, and interaction with people. Higher scores suggest greater levels of difficulty. Based on receiver operating characteristic procedures, cutoff scores for each of the eight questionnaires are identified (Yovanoff & Squires, 2006). Psychometric properties suggest good internal consistency, high test–retest reliability with satisfactory levels of sensitivity and specificity (refer to Squires, Bricker, Heo, & Twombly, 2001, for a review). To date, the ASQ-SE has been widely implemented in multiple countries around the world, including Korea (Heo & Squires, 2011), China (Bian, Xie, Squires, & Chen, 2017), and Brazil (Chen et al., 2017), across multiple service sectors (e.g., public health, child welfare). Although there are some concerns regarding the consistency of the ASQ-SE's psychometric properties in clinical samples (Salomonsson & Sleed, 2010) and across ages and languages (Velikonja et al., 2016), the ASQ-SE represents an easy-to-use instrument that can be applied across different contexts and practice settings.

Brief Infant–Toddler Social–Emotional Assessment

The Brief Infant–Toddler Social–Emotional Assessment (BITSEA) is a 42-item parent-completed questionnaire for 12- to 36-month-olds that screens for both social-emotional/behavior problems (e.g., aggression, defiance; 31 items) and social–emotional understanding (e.g., empathy, prosocial behaviors; 11 items). The BITSEA identifies children with either elevated levels of problem behaviors or low levels of social competence. The BITSEA has good overall psychometric properties with demonstrated test–retest reliability, interrater reliability, and internal consistency. These psychometric patterns have been demonstrated in community samples (e.g., Briggs-Gowan, Carter, Irwin, Wachtel, & Cicchetti, 2004) and clinical samples (e.g., Briggs-Gowan et al., 2013). Lastly, the BITSEA has been adapted for use across several countries, including Turkey (Karabekiroglu, Briggs-Gowan, Carter, Rodopman-Arman, & Akbas, 2010), and the Netherlands (Kruizinga et al., 2012).

The BITSEA uses cutoff scores to help identify children who may be experiencing social–emotional difficulties. A cutoff score of the 75th percentile on the BITSEA problem scale and a cutoff score of the 15th percentile on the BITSEA competence scale suggest the risk of problem behaviors and low social–emotional understanding, respectively (see Briggs-Gowan et al., 2004, for a review). There is evidence that these cutoff scores are predictive of later difficulties during middle childhood. In a sample of more than 1,000 socially and ethnically diverse children living in the United States, more than 50% of those children identified by their parents and/or teachers as having emotional/behavioral problems in elementary school were identified by the BITSEA (at 12–36 months) as being vulnerable to social–emotional/behavioral problems (Briggs-Gowan & Carter, 2008).

Devereux Student Strengths Assessment Mini

The Devereux Student Strengths Assessment (DESSA) Mini is a brief, 8-item social-emotional screener that provides a snapshot of a child's social–emotional competence for children between 5 and 12 years of age. DESSA-Mini norms were developed from the DESSA (reviewed in the following section) standardization sample of 1,249 children and youth rated by teachers and program staff. The sample was selected to be representative of gender, grade, geographical region, race, Hispanic origin, and socioeconomic status. Drawing from the larger 72-item DESSA (LeBuffe, Shapiro, & Naglieri, 2009), four different versions of the DESSA-Mini were developed. After accounting for overlapping items, four forms of the DESSA-Mini showed significant correlation with the DESSA, as well as significant correlation between all four DESSA-Mini forms. The DESSA-Mini demonstrates good test-retest reliability (ranging between .88 and .94) and interrater reliability (ranging from .70 to .81) across all four forms. Concurrent criterion validity studies have estimated DESSA-Mini sensitivity rates between 62 and 81% and specificity rates between 83 and 98% (for a review, see LeBuffe, Shapiro, & Robitaille, 2017; Naglieri, LeBuffe, & Shapiro, 2014). Lastly, some emerging evidence suggests that the DESSA-Mini can accurately predict later academic difficulty. Specifically, students identified as having a need for social–emotional learning instruction at the beginning of the year were 4½ times more likely to have a record of serious disciplinary infraction at the end of the school year compared with those who were not identified (Shapiro, Kim, Robitaille, & LeBuffe, 2016).

Strengths and Difficulties Questionnaire

The Strengths and Difficulties Questionnaire (SDQ; Goodman, 1997) is a short, multirater (teacher, parent, and student reports) screening tool for children and adolescents from 4 to 17 years of age. The SDQ consists of 25 items tapping into one protective factor (prosocial behavior) and four risk factors (emotional symptoms, conduct problems, hyperactivity, and peer relationship problems; Goodman, 1997). The psychometric properties of the SDQ have been extensively examined in several studies with large samples (e.g., Goodman & Goodman, 2012), showing good to excellent results in terms of both reliability and validity. Importantly, the factor structure of the SDQ has been found to be invariant across grades and sex, thereby fully attesting to the developmental sensitivity of the instrument (e.g., Caci, Morin, & Tran, 2015). Finally, the utility of the SDQ as a screening tool has been corroborated in cross-cultural studies (e.g., Shojaei, Wazana, Pitrou, & Kovess, 2009) and in clinical populations (e.g., Lambie & Krynen, 2017; Moriwaki & Kamio, 2014).

Summary

The current review of social–emotional screening tools highlights several gaps in the literature and practice. First, compared to the high number of social–emotional assessment instruments, the availability of social–emotional screening tools is limited. Although there are a number of promising social–emotional screening tools with demonstrated psychometric properties, many of them are developed for children under the age of 5, with only the DESSA-Mini designed for screening during middle childhood. Social–emotional screening tools for adolescents are virtually nonexistent. The limited availability of appropriate screening tools that span all developmental periods limits our ability to universally identify children and youth who can benefit from additional assessment. Moreover, further examination is warranted to ensure consistency of psychometric properties across different practice contexts and cultures. Particularly for the ASQ, evidence related to the stability of the tool's psychometric properties for clinical samples have been mixed.

Individual-Based Social–Emotional Assessment Tools

Once a child has been identified as being vulnerable for social–emotional concerns and/or aggressive behavior, an individual-based assessment instrument can help determine whether these concerns are clinical in nature. A commonly used individual-based assessment tool is the CBCL. However, despite its strong psychometric properties (Achenbach & Rescorla, 2001), one limitation of the CBCL is its exclusive focus on psychopathology (e.g., Haggerty et al., 2011; psychometric properties of the CBCL are reviewed below). Indeed, developmental research has strongly urged the use of reliable strength-based screening and assessment tools to evaluate children's resilience factors, such as their social–emotional skills (Koller & Verma, 2017; Malti, Zuffianò, Cui, Colasante, Peplak, & Bae, 2017). Particularly because screening and assessment of social–emotional development have traditionally focused on the assessment of risk, a strengths-based perspective can complement the developmental profile of the child. Similar to how a mechanic is required to determine what is working and what is faulty to understand and identify the origin of squeaky brakes, screening and assessment of risk and resilience provides us with a more detailed road map that can be used to inform intervention strategies that are tailored to the specific needs of the child. This focus on screening and assessment is particularly relevant in the field of social–emotional learning programs (Durlak et al., 2011), as the central tenet of most social–emotional learning curricula is the promotion of social–emotional strength factors (Collaborative for Academic, Social, and Emotional Learning [CASEL], 2013; Malti, Sette, & Dys, 2016). As such, there is the need for strengths-based developmentally sensitive screening and assessment tools to measure and monitor individual differences across children (Cordier et al., 2015; Frydenberg, Liang, & Muller, 2017).

As it is beyond the scope of this chapter to review all existing social–emotional assessment tools, we focus on individual-based assessment instruments that are predominantly strength-based with demonstrated psychometric properties.

Behavioral and Emotional Rating Scale–2

The Behavioral and Emotional Rating Scale–2 (BERS-2; Buckley & Epstein, 2004) is a 52-item strengths-based questionnaire for children and youth (from ages 5 to 18) available for teacher, parent, and youth reports. The BERS-2 is aimed at assessing five core developmental dimensions: (1) interpersonal strength (e.g., the ability to properly interact in social situations), (2) family involvement (e.g., the relationships within the family environment, (3) intrapersonal strength (e.g., levels of competence and success), (4) school functioning (e.g., academic skills), and (5) affective strength (e.g., emotional skills). Both parent and youth reports include an additional 5-item career strength scale that assesses children's work or community-related involvement. Psychometric analyses (e.g., exploratory factor analysis [EFA] and confirmatory factor analysis [CFA]) attested to the accuracy of the hypothesized factor structure and reliability of the BERS-2 (e.g., Buckley, Ryser, Reid, & Epstein, 2006). Furthermore, validity analyses showed expected moderate negative relations with both internalizing and externalizing problems (e.g., Epstein, Mooney, Ryser, & Pierce, 2004). Notably, the psychometric properties of the BERS-2 have been also confirmed in various cultural contexts, such as Finland (e.g., Sointu, Savolainen, Lambert, Lappalainen, & Epstein, 2014).

Child Behavior Checklist

The CBCL (Achenbach & Rescorla, 2001) is an adult report of children's behavioral and emotional problems. The CBCL has a 100-item version for preschool children (from 1½ to 5 years of age; CBCL/1½–5) and a 118-item version for school-age children (from 6 to 18 years of age; CBCL/6–18). The CBCL assesses six areas including affective problems, anxiety problems, somatic problems, attention-deficit/hyperactivity problems, oppositional defiant problems, and conduct problems. To date, numerous studies have demonstrated CBCL's strong psychometric properties, including good levels of reliability, as well as convergent and discriminative validity (Nakamura, Ebesutani, Bernstein, & Chorpita, 2008; see Achenbach & Rescorla, 2001, for a review). Despite CBCL's strong psychometric properties and utility, one of its main drawbacks is its exclusive focus on psychopathology. Indeed, many researchers and clinicians argue the importance of also considering a child's strengths when understanding social–emotional development (e.g., Haggerty et al., 2011; Hoffman, 2009).

Communities That Care Survey

The Communities That Care Survey (CTC; Arthur, Hawkins, Pollard, Catalano, & Baglioni, 2002) is 121-item self-report questionnaire aimed at measuring both risk and protective factors among adolescents from 11 to 18 years of age. Twenty-one risk factors (e.g., low commitment to school, low neighborhood attachment, rebelliousness) and nine protective factors (e.g., opportunities for prosocial involvement, social skills) were identified across four domains (community, family, school, and peer/individual) based on literature reviews on adolescent drug use and violence in the field of prevention science (see Arthur et al., 2002). The CTC dimensions showed expected relations with substance use and delinquent behavior outcomes (see Arthur et al., 2002). The factor structure of a slightly revised version of the CTC survey (consisting of 133 items) was also analyzed in depth in a large sample of 172,628 U.S. students (Glaser, Van Horn, Arthur, Hawkins, & Catalano, 2005). CFA analyses attested to the good psychometric properties of the CTC, as well as to its strong measurement invariance across five ethnic groups (African Americans, Asians/Pacific Islanders, Caucasians, Hispanic Americans, and Native Americans) and sex (boys vs. girls), but not across grades (item thresholds were different across grades 6, 8, 10, and 12).

Developmental Assets Profile

The Developmental Assets Profile (DAP; Search Institute, 2005) is 58-item, self-report strengths-based tool that assesses four external-oriented assets (i.e., support from others, empowerment, boundaries and expectations, and constructive use of time) and four internal-oriented assets (i.e., commitment to learning, positive values, social competencies, and positive identity) among adolescents from 11 to 18 years of age. The DAP showed good psychometric properties in terms of reliability and construct validity, both in cross-sectional (Search Institute, 2005), and longitudinal studies (Scales, Benson, Roehlkepartain, Sesma, & van Dulmen, 2006). Although Scales (2011) reported good CFA results in his cross-cultural study of the DAP across five countries (i.e., Albania, Bangladesh, Japan, Lebanon, and the Philippines), an in-depth analysis of the factor structure of the instrument (e.g., measurement invariance across grades and sex) is still missing in the literature.

Devereux Student Strengths Assessment

The Devereux Student Strengths Assessment (DESSA; LeBuffe, Shapiro, & Naglieri, 2009) is a 72-item, adult-report (i.e., teachers and parents) strengths-based questionnaire that assesses eight distinct social–emotional dimensions (i.e., self-awareness, social awareness, self-management, goal-directed behavior, relationship skills, personal responsibility, decision making, and optimistic thinking) among children and adolescents (from 5 to 14 years of age). The eight dimensions can be also used to create an overall score of social–emotional competency (LeBuffe et al., 2009). The dimensions of the DESSA showed expected relations with both positive (e.g., adaptive skills; see Nickerson & Fishman, 2009) and negative (e.g., ADHD problems) outcomes, thereby attesting to its construct validity (see LeBuffe et al., 2017). Although the DESSA has consistently shown excellent internal reliabilities, results confirming its factor structure and measurement invariance are less evident. The DESSA has also been adapted for young children, with specific measures for infants (Devereux Early Childhood Assessment [DECA] for Infants), toddlers (DECA for Toddlers) and preschoolers (DECA for Preschoolers).

Holistic Student Assessment

The Holistic Student Assessment (HSA; Malti, Zuffianò, & Noam, 2017) is a recently developed, short strengths-based assessment tool for children and adolescents from 9 to 18 years of age. Based on social–emotional theory and research, the HSA consists of 25 items tapping into four self-oriented skills (emotion control, optimism, action orientation, and self-reflection) and three other-oriented skills (trust, empathy, and assertiveness). The hypothesized 7-dimension factor structure of the HSA has been corroborated in a large sample (5,946) of U.S. students, and its measurement invariance has been confirmed across late childhood, early adolescence, and middle to late adolescence, thereby attesting to the developmental sensitivity of the self-report version of the instrument. Construct validity analyses indicated expected relations with prosocial behavior, externalizing problems, and internalizing problems in each developmental phase considered (Malti et al., 2017).

School Social Behaviors Scale–2

The School Social Behaviors Scale–2 (SSBS-2; Merrell, 2002) is a 65-item teacher and parent report questionnaire that measures both risk and protective factors in children and adolescents from 5 to 18 years of age (Merrell, 2002). The SSBS-2 consists of an Antisocial Behavior scale (33 items), which measures students' hostile, aggressive, and defiant behaviors, and a Social Competence scale (32 items), which measures students' interpersonal, self-regulative, and academic skills. Although the SSBS-2 can be considered one of the best instruments in terms of psychometric properties (e.g., reliability and validity) to be used in school assessment (Cordier et al., 2015), some methodological aspects (e.g., measurement invariance and developmental sensitivity across grades) need further investigation. Notably, there is some evidence of the cross-cultural validity of the Social Competence scale in Portuguese school contexts (Raimundo et al., 2012).

Social–Emotional Assets and Resilience Scale

The Social–Emotional Assets and Resilience Scale (SEARS; Merrell, 2011) is a multirater strengths-based tool aimed at assessing four core social–emotional skills (self-regulation, social competence, empathy, and responsibility) that can be combined to create an overall score of social–emotional competency in children and adolescents (from 5 to 18 years of age). The SEARS consists of three versions that can be filled out by parents (SEARS-P, 39 items; Merrell, Felver-Gant, & Tom, 2011), teachers (SEARS-T, 41 items; Merrell, Cohn, & Tom, 2011), and students (SEARS-A, 35 items; Romer & Merrell, 2013).[1] The three versions consistently reported good levels of reliability (see Cordier et al., 2015), and convergent validity analyses of the SEARS showed expected positive correlations with other measures of social–emotional development (e.g., Merrell et al., 2011). Although both EFA and CFA results corroborated the hypothesized factor structure of the instrument, an in-depth analysis of its developmental sensitivity (e.g., measurement invariance across grades, sex) is still missing.

Social Skills Improvement System Rating Scales

The Social Skills Improvement System Rating Scales (SISS-RS; Gresham & Elliott, 2008) is a multirater social–emotional tool for children and adolescents from 3 to 18 years of age. The SISS-RS is available for teacher (83 items), parent (79 items), and student reports (75 items) and evaluates children's social skills (e.g., empathy, self-control, engagement), problem behaviors (e.g., externalizing and internalizing problems, autism spectrum disorders), and academic competence (only for teacher reports). Although the SISS-RS has been found to have excellent psychometric properties in terms of reliability and construct validity in relation to both positive and negative outcomes (see Cordier et al., 2015), its factor structure and measurement invariance have been confirmed to some extent (see Schneider, 2012). Notably, in line with its multirater focus, a moderate degree of informant convergence has been reported across the three versions (teacher, parent, and student reports) of the SISS-RS (Gresham, Elliott, Cook, Vance, & Kettler, 2010).

Summary

Although a systematic analysis of the existing individual-based social–emotional assessment tools is beyond the scope of this chapter, we identified a collection of strengths-based social–emotional assessment tools that can help clinicians, practitioners, teachers, and school principals evaluate children's social–emotional profiles. This is important to inform the planning, implementation, and evaluation of aggression interventions for the following reasons. First, traditional assessment tools focus primarily on psychopathology. Given that high levels of social–emotional development can reduce and prevent aggression (e.g., Zuffianò et al., 2018), the inclusion of a strength-based assessment approach allows the identification and

---

[1]A self-report version for children (SEARS-C; 35 items) has been also developed by Romer and Merrell (2013). Yet the SEARS-C only provides an overall score of social–emotional competence.

monitoring of social–emotional correlates prior to the onset of later difficulties. This has important implications for practice, as the early and reliable identification of children with elevated risk allows the opportunity to intervene in a more timely and efficacious manner. Second, from a measurement perspective, assessment of both social–emotional risk and strengths mitigates against respondent bias (e.g., Carter, Briggs-Gowan, & Davis, 2004), where consistency across multiple measures allows the triangulation of information. This also ensures accuracy of ratings across multiple domains of social–emotional development. Third, in line with recent findings attesting to the codevelopment of social–emotional variables and aggression (e.g., Zuffianò et al., 2018), the assessment of children's strengths can facilitate the development of intervention strategies that rely on children's social–emotional potentials (a child with low emotion control may still have potential for a proper empathic development) while simultaneously decreasing their aggression problems.

Our selective review also identified a number of current gaps/challenges in the literature: First, although all the questionnaires examined were psychometrically sound instruments, not all of them underwent an in-depth examination of their factor structure in terms of measurement invariance and developmental sensitivity across grades or developmental phases. In this regard, the CCT, HSA, SSBS-2, SSIS-RS, and SDQ appeared to have stronger psychometric properties. Second, all the instruments reviewed varied in their lengths (from the 121 items of the CTC to the 25 items of the HSA and SDQ). Hence, the long format of some (e.g., CCT, SSIS-RS) may prevent their use in universal and/or large-scale school-based assessments. For this reason, the use of a social–emotional screening tool may be more effective in identifying a subgroup of children who may benefit from further assessment that monitors a broader, more extensive repertoire of social-emotional behaviors. Third, only some instruments reported a clear theoretical rationale underlying the selection of the constructs to be measured (e.g., CCT, HSA). This is particularly surprising because the planning and implementation of aggression and related intervention strategies, the ultimate goals of these screening tools, rely strongly on a clear nomological network that explains the interrelations among the constructs and how they can be simultaneously changed. Fourth, some scales included both risk and protective factors (i.e., CCT, SISS-RS, SSBS-2, SDQ, BITSEA, ASQ-SE), whereas other scales strictly focused on students' social-emotional strengths (i.e., BERS-2, DAP, DESSA, HSA, SEARS). Although the selection of the most appropriate instrument should be ultimately driven by the goal of the intervention and/or the needs of the school, strengths-based social–emotional assessment tools might easily complement universal screening, whereas scales that include both risk and protective factors may offer additional, relevant knowledge in selective screening contexts (e.g., youth at risk). Finally, although many of the reviewed instruments were translated into different languages and adapted in different cultural contexts (e.g., SSBS-2, SDQ, ASQ-SE), researchers and teachers working in non-English-speaking environments may need to conduct a further preliminary validation of the questionnaire before its use for screening purposes. Indeed, psychometric properties across various cultural and linguistic adaptions of social–emotional screening and assessment measures may vary (e.g., Velikonja et al., 2016).

Integrating Social–Emotional Screening and Assessment Information into Clinical Decision Making

Social–emotional screening and assessment tools provide a standardized assessment of a child's social–emotional functioning. This is particularly important because the process of decision making appears to be influenced by various contextual factors (e.g., case and organization factors) and practitioner or teacher characteristics such as training, knowledge, attitudes, and experience (e.g., Fluke, Baumann, Dalgleish, & Kern, 2014). As such, implementation of standardized tools can guard against potential biases that may result from contextual and individual-specific differences across decision makers. For instance, although two teachers may provide information on the same student, each may interpret and assess a child's aggressive behavior differently depending on differences in knowledge of social–emotional development, professional experience, and so forth. Therefore, the use of validated screening and assessment tools not only increases consistency, accountability, and transparency of decisions but can also promote better decision making. Ultimately, this can improve selection of intervention approaches and services aimed at reducing aggression (Jensen-Doss, McLeod, & Ollendick, 2013).

This is even more important in light of research showing that service professionals and parents are not always able to accurately identify social–emotional challenges in children. When asked to identify children with social–emotional concerns, professional health care providers and parents identified only 7–14% of all children who fell within the of-concern range as screened with the BITSEA (Alakortes et al., 2017). Similar patterns were also observed with child welfare workers; 24% of children receiving out-of-home care were identified by the ASQ-SE as having social–emotional problems relative to only 4% identified based on surveillance alone (Jee et al., 2010). Clearly, social–emotional screening and assessment information are essential in helping service providers and professionals make more evidence-informed decisions.

Once a child has been identified as being at risk for social–emotional delay, and more specific social–emotional assessments have identified areas of need, how does the practitioner or educator integrate this knowledge into service planning? Specifically, how can clinicians reasonably integrate multimethod, multi-informant information into critical decisions about their prevention approach and/or clinical practice? One promising approach that allows for the integration of assessment information and clinical wisdom is through evidence-based practice (EBP). EBP is a systematic process that integrates clinical state and circumstance, client preferences (whenever possible), and current best evidence, resulting in services that are both individualized and empirically sound. It involves the identification and appraisal of current research that can address a practice question that can be used to inform clinical decision making (e.g., see Shlonsky & Benbenishty, 2013, for a review). Related to the area of aggression, social–emotional assessment information can be used to inform the clinical state and circumstance domain of EBP. Combining assessment information and the clinician's own appraisal of the situation allows the triangulation of information across multiple informants and measures. Convergence of these different perspectives strengthens the conceptualization of the case. Similarly, it is also important to consider the client's preference, particularly as factors such as family history, culture, and socioeconomic circumstance can affect treatment implementation and efficacy (e.g., Carter et al., 2004). Lastly, considered in light of clinical state and circumstance and client preference, research and current best practices related to the area of aggression prevention can then be used to guide treatment decisions, identifying the best course of action based on the needs and contextual environment of the child.

The use of the EBP framework is helpful in that it provides a mechanism whereby clinicians are able to describe their decision-making process. Furthermore, by combining the decision-making process with standardized assessment information and research, arguably the influence of contextual factors such as clinician experience, training, and attitudes can be minimized. However, despite the promising approach of EBP, it is important to be mindful of a number of organization- and child-specific factors that can influence treatment efficacy, despite support from research and evidence. First, organizational climate, or the quality of the work environment, has been linked to child outcomes. Specifically, when compared to organizations with less engaged employees, organizations with employees who perceived their work as meaningful and worthwhile were also more likely to see better mental health outcomes in the children they worked with 84 months later (Glisson & Green, 2011). This suggests that, in addition to efforts to prevent aggression in individual children, long-term, sustained improvement also requires whole-system improvement (Ghate, 2016). Second, the extent to which a treatment approach is effective depends largely on the congruency between the needs of the client and what is addressed through intervention strategies. For instance, most coping strategies for youth depression were developed from the perspective of adults. Therefore, unless a therapeutic approach incorporates coping strategies that youth themselves identify as effective, the youth's ability to implement change may be difficult. Indeed, there is some evidence to suggest that when compared with youth with less depressive symptoms, those with more depressive symptoms were also less likely to report using coping strategies that matched evidence-based psychotherapy components they received (Ng, Eckshtain, & Weisz, 2016). These patterns of results are intriguing, suggesting that despite reported effectiveness, treatment efficacy may be largely dependent on the "goodness of fit" between the needs of the client and what is offered by treatment.

In sum, EBP is a promising approach that can be used by clinicians to systematically integrate standardized assessment information into clinical decision making. The main advantage of using the EBP framework is the potential to mitigate against the influence of contextual factors on decision making, therefore enhancing accountability, transparency, and consistency across different decision makers. However, it is important to acknowledge that regardless of evidence, treatment efficacy can be influenced by a number of implementation factors related to the organization and the child and young person.

Implications and Conclusions

Counteracting aggression before it develops into more severe pathological problems requires an in-depth understanding of its social–emotional precursors and correlates. To this aim, social–emotional developmental theory and associated research findings can help psychologists and practitioners design theoretically sound and empirically based intervention programs (see Malti, Sette, & Dys, 2016). A number of studies, for instance, have indicated the role of other-oriented and self-conscious emotional responses, such as sympathy (e.g., Zuffianò et al., 2018), and guilt (e.g., Colasante, Zuffianò, & Malti, 2016), as affective barriers against the onset of aggressive problems during childhood and adolescence. The role of social–emotional research in informing future practice of intervention cannot merely be based on identifying malleable factors to be manipulated in intervention programs (e.g., self-conscious and other-oriented emotions). Rather, researchers should also offer a series of valid, theoretically sound instruments of assessment that should be in the "toolbox" of each practitioner. As we have highlighted in this chapter, different tools serve distinct purposes (e.g., population-based vs. individual-based evaluation), and their combined use may help tailor intervention strategies to the social–emotional needs of each student (e.g., screening tools and assessment tools). Although all instruments reviewed here have evidence of validity and reliability, we identified five areas of concern for future development. First, only a few tools (e.g., CCT, HSA) were rooted in a clear theoretical social–emotional framework that informed the selection of the constructs and their nomological relations. As previously discussed, the strict link between theory and assessment is crucial for planning efficacious intervention strategies. Second, there is a clear paucity of social–emotional screening tools compared with the large number of assessment instruments. This is alarming because, very often, the implementation of timely intervention actions in high-risk children is based on screening data. Furthermore, many of them are developmentally appropriate for screening only from early to middle childhood (except for the DESSA-Mini and SDQ, which have been designed for screening from middle childhood to adolescence). Hence, more work is needed to develop screening instruments that reliably identify adolescents at risk of problem behaviors. Third, only two instruments (i.e., CBCL and SDQ) are part of a more comprehensive, multi-informant evaluation approach that covers the full transition from early childhood to late adolescence. Accordingly, CBCL and SDQ might be particularly useful for comparing scores across different ages in large-scale intervention programs. Fourth, although many of the reviewed tools include both parent and teacher versions, more empirical work is needed to establish the sensitivity of these instruments in capturing children's social–emotional development across different contexts of observation (e.g., home vs. school; De Los Reyes et al., 2015). Lastly, many assessment tools do not include qualitative questions. The combined use of quantitative and qualitative methodologies can offer a more accurate evaluation of the social–emotional potentials and needs of each student (see Frydenberg et al., 2017).

In sum, many ad hoc instruments have been designed to measure children's social–emotional development across different ages in the last 20 years. Moving forward, developmental researchers may need to devote their efforts to fill the five gaps previously identified. Only a stronger connection between social–emotional theory and its empirical assessment can reliably inform policy makers, practitioners, educators, and psychologists about which intervention strategies (and associated resources) are most likely to be effective in counteracting aggressive problems under specific conditions.

REFERENCES

Achenbach, T. M., & Rescorla, L. A. (2001). *Manual for the ASEBA School-Age Forms and Profiles*. Burlington: University of Vermont, Research Center for Children, Youth, and Families.

Alakortes, J., Kovaniemi, S., Carter, A. S., Bloigu, R., Moilanen, I. K., & Ebeling, H. E. (2017). Do child healthcare professionals and parents recognize social–emotional and behavioral problems in 1-year-old infants? *European Child and Adolescent Psychiatry, 26*(4), 481–495.

Anderman, C., Cheadle, A., Curry, S., Diehr, P., Shultz, L., & Wagner, E. (1995). Selection bias related to parental consent in school-based survey research. *Evaluation Review, 19*(6), 663–674.

Arthur, M. W., Hawkins, J. D., Pollard, J. A., Catalano, R. F., & Baglioni, A. J. (2002). Measuring risk and protective factors for substance use, delinquency, and other adolescent problem behaviors: The Communities That Care Youth Survey. *Evaluation Review, 26*, 575–601.

Bian, X., Xie, H., Squires, J., & Chen, C. Y. (2017). Adapting a parent-completed, social–emotional questionnaire in China: The Ages and Stages Questionnaires: Social–emotional. *Infant Mental Health Journal, 38*(2), 258–266.

Briggs-Gowan, M. J., & Carter, A. S. (2008). Social–emotional screening status in early childhood predicts elementary school outcomes. *Pediatrics, 121*, 957–962.

Briggs-Gowan, M. J., Carter, A. S., Irwin, J. R., Wachtel, K., & Cicchetti, D. V. (2004). The Brief Infant–Toddler Social and Emotional Assessment: Screening for social–emotional problems and delays in competence. *Journal of Pediatric Psychology, 29*(2), 143–155.

Briggs-Gowan, M. J., Carter, A. S., McCarthy, K., Augustyn, M., Caronna, E., et al. (2013). Clinical validity of a brief measure of early childhood social–emotional/behavioral problems. *Journal of Paediatric Psychology, 38*, 577–587.

Buckley, J. A., & Epstein, M. H. (2004). The behavioral and Emotional Rating Scale-2 (BERS-2): Providing a comprehensive approach to strength-based assessment. *California School Psychologist, 9*(1), 21–27.

Buckley, J. A., Ryser, G., Reid, R., & Epstein, M. H. (2006). Confirmatory factor analysis of the Behavioral and Emotional Rating Scale–2 (BERS-2) Parent and Youth Rating Scales. *Journal of Child and Family Studies, 15*(1), 27–37.

Caci, H., Morin, A. J., & Tran, A. (2015). Investigation of a bifactor model of the Strengths and Difficulties Questionnaire. *European Child and Adolescent Psychiatry, 24*(10), 1291–1301.

Carter, A. S., Briggs-Gowan, M. J., & Davis, N. O. (2004). Assessment of young children's social–emotional development and psychopathology: Recent advances and recommendations for practice. *Journal of Child Psychology and Psychiatry, 45*(1), 109–134.

Chen, C. Y., Xie, H., Filgueiras, A., Squires, J., Anunciacao, L., & Landeira-Femandez, J. (2017). Examining the psychometric properties of the Brazilian Ages and Stages Questionnaires—Social–Emotional: Use in public child daycare centers in Brazil. *Journal of Child and Family Studies, 26*, 2412–2425.

Colasante, T., Zuffianò, A., & Malti, T. (2016). Daily deviations in anger, guilt, and sympathy: A developmental diary study of aggression. *Journal of Abnormal Child Psychology, 44*(8), 1515–1526.

Collaborative for Academic, Social and Emotional Learning. (2013). Social and emotional learning core competencies. Retrieved from *https://casel.org/core-competencies*.

Cordier, R., Speyer, R., Chen, Y. W., Wilkes-Gillan, S., Brown, T., Bourke-Taylor, H., et al. (2015). Evaluating the psychometric quality of social skills measures: A systematic review. *PLOS ONE, 10*(7), e0132299.

Costello, E. J. (2016). Early detection and prevention of mental health problems:

Developmental epidemiology and systems of support. *Journal of Clincial Child and Adolescent Psychology, 45*(6), 710–717.

Davies, S., Janus, M., Duku, E., & Gaskin, A. (2016). Using the Early Development Instrument to examine cognitive and non-cognitive school readiness and elementary student achievement. *Early Childhood Research Quarterly, 35,* 63–75.

De Los Reyes, A., Augenstein, T. M., Wang, M., Thomas, S. A., Drabick, D. A., Burgers, D. E., et al. (2015). The validity of the multi-informant approach to assessing child and adolescent mental health. *Psychological Bulletin, 141*(4), 858–900.

Durlak, J. A., Weissberg, R. P., Dymnicki, A. B., Taylor, R. D., & Schellinger, K. B. (2011). The impact of enhancing students' social and emotional learning: A meta-analysis of school-based universal interventions. *Child Development, 82,* 405–432.

Early Development Instrument. (2017). Toronto: City of Toronto. Retrieved from *www1.toronto.ca/wps/portal/contentonly?vgnextoid=9e5a7bd135427510VgnVCM10000071d60f89RCRD.*

Eisenberg, N., Eggum, N. D., & Di Giunta, L. (2010). Empathy-related responding: Associations with prosocial behavior, aggression, and intergroup relations. *Social Issues and Policy Review, 4*(1), 143–180.

Epstein, M. H., Mooney, P., Ryser, G., & Pierce, C. D. (2004). Validity and reliability of the Behavior and Emotional Rating Scale—Second Edition: Youth Rating Scale. *Research on Social Work Practice, 14,* 358–367.

Fernald, L. C. H., Kariger, P., Engle, P., & Raikes, A. (2009). *Examining early child development in low-income countries: A toolkit for the assessment of children in the first five years of life.* Washington, DC: International Bank for Reconstruction and Development/World Bank.

Fluke, J., Baumann, D., Dalgleish, L., & Kern, D. H. (2014). Decisions to protect children: A decision-making ecology. In J. E. Korbin & R. D. Krugman (Eds.), *Handbook of child maltreatment* (pp. 463–476). Dordrecht, The Netherlands: Springer.

Frydenberg, E., Liang, R., & Muller, D. (2017). Assessing students' social and emotional learning: A review of the literature on assessment tools and related issues. In E. Frydenberg, A. Martin, & R. J. Collie (Eds.), *Social and emotional learning in Australia and the Asia–Pacific* (pp. 55–82). Singapore: Springer.

Ghate, D. (2016). From program to systems: Deploying implementation science and practice for sustained real world effectiveness in services for children and families. *Journal of Clinical Child and Adolescent Psychology, 45*(6), 812–826.

Glaser, R. R., Van Horn, M. L., Arthur, M. W., Hawkins, J. D., & Catalano, R. F. (2005). Measurement properties of the Communities That Care Youth Survey across demographic groups. *Journal of Quantitative Criminology, 21,* 73–102.

Glisson, C., & Green, P. (2011). Organizational climate, services, and outcomes in child welfare systems. *Child Abuse and Neglect, 35*(8), 582–591.

Goodman, A., & Goodman, R. (2012). Strengths and Difficulties Questionnaire scores and mental health in looked-after children. *British Journal of Psychiatry, 200*(5), 426–427.

Goodman, R. (1997). The Strengths and Difficulties Questionnaire: A research note. *Journal of Child Psychology and Psychiatry, 38*(5), 581–586.

Gresham, F. M., & Elliott, S. N. (2008). *SSIS Social Skills Improvement System: Rating Scales Manual.* Minneapolis, MN: Pearson.

Gresham, F. M., Elliott, S. N., Cook, C. R., Vance, M. J., & Kettler, R. (2010). Cross-informant agreement for ratings for social skill and problem behavior ratings: An investigation of the Social Skills Improvement System—Rating Scales. *Psychological Assessment, 22*(1), 157.

Guhn, M., Gadermann, A. M., Almas, A., Schonert-Reichl, K. A., & Hertzman, C. (2016). Associations of teacher-rated social, emotional, and cognitive development in kindergarten to self-reported well-being, peer relations, and academic test scores in middle childhood. *Early Childhood Research Quarterly, 35,* 76–84.

Haggerty, K., Elgin, J., & Woolley, A. (2011). *Social–emotional learning assessment measures for middle school youth.* Seattle: University of Washington, Social Development Research Group.

Heo, K. H., & Squires, J. (2011). Cultural adaptation of a parent-completed social–emotional screening instrument for young children: Ages and Stages Questionnaire—Social Emotional. *Early Human Development, 88*(3), 151–158.

Hoffman, D. M. (2009). Reflecting on social–emotional learning: A critical perspective on trends in the United States. *Review of Educational Research, 79*(2), 533–556.

Janus, M., & Duku, E. (2007). The school entry gap: Socioeconomic, family, and health factors associated with children's school readiness to learn. *Early Education and Development, 18*(3), 375–403.

Janus, M., Harrison, L. J., Goldfeld, S., Guhn, M., & Brinkman, S. (2016). International research utilizing the Early Development Instrument (EDI) as a measure of early child development: Introduction to the Special Issue. *Early Childhood Research Quarterly, 35,* 1–5.

Janus, M., & Offord, D. R. (2007). Development and psychometric properties of the Early Development Instrument (EDI): A measure of children's school readiness. *Canadian Journal of Behavioural Science/Revue canadienne des sciences du comportement, 39*(1), 1–22.

Jee, S. H., Conn, A. M., Szilagyi, P. G., Blumkin, A., Baldwin, C. D., & Szilagyi, M. A. (2010). Identification of social–emotional problems among young children in foster care. *Journal of Child Psychology and Psychiatry, 51,* 1351–1358.

Jensen-Doss, A., McLeod, B. D., & Ollendick, T. H. (2013). Diagnostic assessment. In B. D. McLeod, A. Jensen-Doss, & T. H. Ollendick (Eds.), *Diagnostic and behavioral assessment in children and adolescents: A clinical guide* (pp. 34–55). New York: Guilford Press.

Jones, D. E., Greenberg, M., & Crowley, M. (2015). Early social–emotional functioning and public health: The relationship between kindergarten social competence and future wellness. *American Journal of Public Health, 105*(11), 2283–2290.

Karabekiroglu, K., Briggs-Gowan, M. J., Carter, A. S., Rodopman-Arman, A., & Akbas, S. (2010). The clinical validity and reliability of the Brief Infant–Toddler Social and Emotional Assessment (BITSEA). *Infant Behavior and Development, 33,* 503–509.

Koller, S. H., & Verma, S. (2017). Commentary on cross-cultural perspectives on positive youth development with implications for intervention research. *Child Development, 88,* 1178–1182.

Kruizinga, I., Jansen, W., de Haan, C. L., van der Ende, J., Carter, A. S., & Raat, H. (2012). Reliability and validity of the Dutch version of the brief Infant–Toddler Social and Emotional Assessment. *PLOS ONE, 7*(6), e19326203.

Lambie, I., & Krynen, A. (2017). The utility of the Strengths and Difficulties Questionnaire as a screening measure among children and adolescents who light fires. *Journal of Forensic Psychiatry and Psychology, 28*(3), 313–330.

LeBuffe, P. A., Shapiro, V. B., & Naglieri, J. A. (2009). *Devereux Student Strengths Assessment.* Lewisville, NC: Kaplan.

LeBuffe, P. A., Shapiro, V. B., & Robitaille, J. L. (2017). The Devereux Student Strengths Assessment (DESSA) comprehensive system: Screening, assessing, planning, and monitoring. *Journal of Applied Developmental Psychology, 55,* 62–70.

Malti, T. (2016). Toward an integrated clinical developmental model of guilt. *Developmental Review, 39,* 16–36.

Malti, T., Chaparro, M. P., Zuffianò, A., & Colasante, T. (2016). School-based interventions to promote empathy-related responding in children and adolescents: A developmental analysis. *Journal of Clinical Child and Adolescent Psychology, 45*(6), 718–731.

Malti, T., & Noam, G. G. (2016). Social–emotional development: From theory to practice. *European Journal of Developmental Psychology, 13*(6), 652–665.

Malti, T., Sette, S., & Dys, S. P. (2016). Social–emotional responding: A perspective from developmental psychology. In R. A Scott & S. M. Kosslyn (Eds.), *Emerging trends in the social and behavioral sciences* (pp. 1–15). Hoboken, NJ: Wiley.

Malti, T., Zuffianò, A., Cui, L., Colasante, T., Peplak, J., & Bae, N. Y. (2017). Children's social–emotional development in contexts of peer exclusion. In N. J. Cabrera & B. Leyendecker (Eds.), *Handbook on positive development of minority children and youth.* (pp. 295–306). Cham, Switzerland: Springer.

Malti, T., Zuffianò, A., & Noam, G. G. (2017). Knowing every child: Validation of the Holistic Student Assessment (HSA) as a measure of social–emotional development. *Prevention Science.* [Epub ahead of print]

Merrell, K. W. (2002). *School Social Behavior Scales* (2nd ed.). Baltimore: Brookes.

Merrell, K. W. (2011). *SEARS: Social, emotional assets and resilience scales.* Lutz, FL: Psychological Assessment Resources.

Merrell, K. W., Cohn, B. P., & Tom, K. M. (2011). Development and validation of a teacher report measure for assessing social–emotional strengths of children and adolescents. *School Psychology Review, 40*(2), 226–241.

Merrell, K. W., Felver-Gant, J. C., & Tom, K. M. (2011). Development and validation of a parent report measure for assessing social–emotional competencies of children and adolescents. *Journal of Child and Family Studies, 20*(4), 529–540.

Moriwaki, A., & Kamio, Y. (2014). Normative data and psychometric properties of the Strengths and Difficulties Questionnaire among Japanese school-aged children. *Child and Adolescent Psychiatry and Mental Health, 8*(1), 1–12.

Mustard, F. J., & Young, M. E. (2007). Measuring child development to leverage ECD policy and investment. In M. E. Young (Ed.), *Early child development from measurement to action: A priority for growth and equity* (pp 193–218). Washington, DC: International Bank for Reconstruction and Development/World Bank.

Naglieri, J. A., LeBuffe, P. A., & Shapiro, V. B. (2014). *The Devereux Student Strengths Assessment–Mini (DESSA-Mini): Assessment, technical manual, and user's guide.* Charlotte, NC: Apperson.

Nakamura, B. J., Ebesutani, C., Bernstein, A., & Chorpita, B. F. (2008). A psychometric analysis of the Child Behavior Checklist DSM-oriented scales. *Journal of Psychopathology and Behavioral Assessment, 31*(3), 178–189.

Ng, M. Y., Eckshtain, D., & Weisz, J. R. (2016). Assessing fit between evidence-based psychotherapies for youth depression and real-life coping in early adolescence. *Journal of Clinical Child and Adolescent Psychology, 45*(6), 732–748.

Nickerson, A. B., & Fishman, C. (2009). Convergent and divergent validity of the Devereux Student Strengths Assessment. *School Psychology Quarterly, 24*(1), 48–59.

Raimundo, R., Carapito, E., Pereira, A. I., Pinto, A. M., Lima, M. L., & Ribeiro, M. T. (2012). School Social Behavior Scales: An adaptation study of the Portuguese version of the Social Competence scale from SSBS-2. *Spanish Journal of Psychology, 15*(3), 1473–1484.

Romer, N., & Merrell, K. W. (2013). Temporal stability of strength-based assessments: Test–retest reliability of student and teacher reports. *Assessment for Effective Intervention, 38*(3), 185–191.

Salomonsson, B., & Sleed, M. (2010). The ASQ:SE: A validation study of a mother-report questionnaire on a clinical mother–infant sample. *Infant Mental Health Journal, 31*(4), 412–431.

Scales, P. C. (2011). Youth developmental assets in global perspective: Results from international adaptations of the Developmental Assets Profile. *Child Indicators Research, 4*(4), 619–645.

Scales, P. C., Benson, P. L., Roehlkepartain, E. C., Sesma, A., Jr., & van Dulmen, M. (2006). The role of developmental assets in predicting academic achievement: A longitudinal study. *Journal of Adolescence, 29*(5), 691–708.

Schneider, B. P. (2012). *A structural analysis of the Social Skills Improvement System Rating Scales, Parent Form: Measurement invariance across race and language format.* Unpublished doctoral dissertation, Pennsylvania State University.

Schonert-Reichl, K. A., Guhn, M., Gadermann, A. M., Hymel, S., Sweiss, L., & Hertzman, C. (2013). Development and validation of the Middle Years Development Instrument (MDI): Assessing children's well-being and assets across multiple contexts. *Social Indicators Research, 114,* 345–369.

Search Institute. (2005). *Developmental Assets Profile technical manual.* Minneapolis, MN: Author.

Shapiro, V. B., Kim, B. K. E., Robitaille, J. L., & LeBuffe, P. A. (2016). Protective factor screening for prevention practice: Sensitivity and specificity of the DESSA-Mini. *School Psychology Quarterly, 32*(4), 449–464.

Shlonsky, A., & Benbenishty, R. (2013). From evidence to outcomes in child welfare. In A. Shlonsky & R. Benbenishty (Eds.), *From evidence to outcomes in child welfare: An international reader* (pp. 3–23). New York: Oxford University Press.

Shojaei, T., Wazana, A., Pitrou, I., & Kovess, V. (2009). The Strengths and Difficulties Questionnaire: Validation study in French school-aged children and cross-cultural comparisons. *Social Psychiatry and Psychiatric Epidemiology, 44*(9), 740–747.

Sointu, E. T., Savolainen, H., Lambert, M. C., Lappalainen, K., & Epstein, M. H. (2014). Behavioral and emotional strength-based assessment of Finnish elementary students: Psychometrics of the BERS-2. *European Journal of Psychology of Education, 29*(1), 1–19.

Squires, J., Bricker, D., Heo, K., & Twombly, E. (2001). Identification of social–emotional problems in young children using a parent-completed screening measure. *Early Childhood Research Quarterly, 16,* 405–419.

Squires, J., Bricker, D., & Twombly, E. (2002). *Ages and Stages Questionnaires: Social-Emotional (ASQ:SE): A parent completed, child-monitoring system for social-emotional behaviors.* Baltimore: Brookes.

Velikonja, T., Edbrooke-Childs, J., Calderon, A., Sleed, M., Brown, A., & Deighton, J. (2016). The psychometric properties of the Ages and Stages Questionnaires for use as population outcome indicators at 2.5 years in England: A systematic review. *Child: Care, Health and Development, 43,* 1–17.

Yovanoff, P., & Squires, J. (2006). Determining cutoff scores on a developmental screening measure: Use of receiver operating characteristics and item response theory. *Journal of Early Intervention, 29,* 48–62.

Zuffianò, A., Colasante, T., Buchmann, M., & Malti, T. (2018). The co-development of sympathy and overt aggression from childhood to early adolescence. *Developmental Psychology, 54*(1), 98–110.

CHAPTER 16

Youth-Focused
Intervention for
Severe Aggression

JOHN E. LOCHMAN, CAROLINE L. BOXMEYER,
BRENDAN ANDRADE, and PIETRO MURATORI

Brief Introduction

Children with serious levels of aggressive and disruptive behavior show numerous and severe short- and long-term difficulties (Burke, Loeber, & Birmaher, 2002). Impairments in social, academic, and family functioning are pronounced in the short term. In the longer term, children with early aggressive and disruptive behavior are at greater risk for delinquency, mood and anxiety disorders, substance use, and other severe mental health and life difficulties compared with nonaffected peers. An understanding of the factors that are associated with aggression and disruptive behavior has contributed to the development of targeted intervention to prevent and reduce the impacts of these behavioral disturbances (Lochman & Wells, 2003). Identifying effective developmentally appropriate interventions for these children that can be deployed at key points from early childhood through adolescence and that can prevent these numerous negative outcomes is a critically important task. This chapter first summarizes developmental and clinical research on risk factors for aggression and disruptive behavior, then considers implications of theoretical frameworks consistent with the pattern of risk factors identified, and finally describes targeted intervention elements and intervention outcomes for children with aggression and disruptive behavior.

Main Issues

Children who are aggressive show developmentally atypical levels of verbal and/or physical actions that create social, emotional, and behavioral disturbance for the child and individuals in their surroundings. Aggression has been classified using a number of theoretical frameworks. Very generally, aggression comes in the form of proactive and reactive subtypes (Dodge, Lochman, Harnish, Bates, & Pettit, 1997). Proactive aggressive behavior is purposeful and goal directed. The function of this type of aggression is typically to assert power, to obtain a desired object or goal. Reactive aggression, on the other hand, is in response to a perceived peer provocation and considered "hot blooded" and more emotional (de Castro, Welmoet, Koops, Veerman, & Bosch, 2005). Although highly correlated in many studies, reactive and proactive aggression seem to be associated with slightly different outcomes (Crick, 1996). Children who show relatively high levels of proactive aggression compared with their peer groups tend to show disproportionately higher rates of delinquency, conduct problems, and antisocial behavior in adulthood. Children who are high in reactive aggression tend to show disproportionately high levels of peer relationship problems and longer-term mood and anxiety problems (Price & Dodge, 1989). Both forms of aggression are associated with childhood disruptive behavior, including oppositional defiant disorder (ODD) and conduct disorder (CD).

ODD is characterized by a pattern of angry/irritable mood, argumentative/defiant behavior, and vindictiveness that emerges in childhood and creates impairment in the child's functioning. Symptoms of ODD include "often losing temper," "often arguing with authority figures," and being "spiteful or vindictive." Often, children with ODD show deficits in their ability to accurately interpret social situations and show high rates of emotional regulation and neurocognitive deficits. ODD occurs in about 3% of children and is somewhat more prevalent in males. In childhood, children with ODD show high rates of social, academic, and family problems. Irritability in the ODD symptom profile appears to be associated with the emergence of mood and anxiety difficulties in the longer term, whereas argumentative/defiant symptoms are associated with the emergence of CD (Stringaris, Maughan, & Goodman, 2010). ODD in many cases appears to be a precursor for CD (Burke et al., 2002).

CD is characterized in DSM-5 as a repetitive and persistent pattern of behavior that violates the rights of others and societal norms and rules (American Psychiatric Association, 2013). CD occurs in about 4% of children and adolescents and, like ODD, is more prevalent in males. Prevalence rates for CD rise during adolescence, and the gender difference becomes less pronounced. Symptoms of CD include bullying, threatening, intimidating others, deliberate fire setting, stealing items of nontrivial value, and school truancy. Persistent CD is associated with personality and adjustment difficulties in adulthood. Children and youth with CD show social-cognitive and neurocognitive deficits (Ogilvie, Stewart, Chan, & Shum, 2011), including impairments in problem solving and inhibiting behavioral responses. The diagnosis of CD is further subtyped by the presence of limited prosocial emotion, which is related to callous–unemotional (CU) traits (Frick, Ray, Thornton, & Kahn, 2014). Children with CD who display CU traits have a more stable pattern of behavior problems and more severe aggression than children without CU traits (Frick et al., 2014).

Theoretical Considerations

As is the case for many forms of childhood psychopathology, a number of factors are associated with the emergence and maintenance of aggressive and disruptive behavior. A biopsychosocial model of aggression, and much supporting research, provide evidence of biological, psychological, and social/family-based contributions to aggressive and disruptive behavior (Dodge & Pettit, 2003) and is evident in the contextual social-cognitive models of aggression that serve as a framework for intervention (Lochman & Wells, 2002). However, not all children with these risk factors develop aggressive behavior, and many children show a desisting trajectory of aggression (Cote, Vaillancourt, LeBlanc, Nagin, & Tremblay, 2006) because of protective factors they possess or that are in their social environment.

A number of biologically based and contextual factors (including family and peer contexts) are associated with aggressive behavior. First, a moderate degree of heritability of aggression is associated with family history of antisocial or aggressive behavior (Odgers et al., 2007). Paternal criminality is a significant predictive risk factor for a son's delinquency (Farrington, Jolliffe, Loeber, Stouthamer-Loeber, & Kalb, 2001). Maternal depression and related parenting challenges have been associated with an increased risk of physical aggression in youth (Nagin & Tremblay, 2001). In addition, adverse events during pregnancy, including in utero exposure to substances, particularly opiates or methadone, alcohol, marijuana, and cigarettes, confer increased risk of conduct problems in children up to 10 years later (de Cubas & Field, 2010).

At a contextual level, risk factors in the child's family, peer relationships, and community are associated with an increased risk of aggression. At the community level, growing up in a low-income neighborhood with higher rates of problems (e.g., drug selling) and exposure to community violence are associated with increased and, in some studies, persistent physical aggression (Evans, Davies, & DiLillo, 2008). Peer rejection, peer neglect, and associations with deviant peer groups are associated with higher rates of childhood aggression and delinquency (Price & Dodge, 1989). Adaptive social relationships and prosocial behavior (e.g., sharing readily with other children; volunteering to help others), on the other hand, may be protective for children (Andrade & Tannock, 2014; Crick, 1996). Within the family environment, children who are exposed to violence in the family or who are physically abused show higher levels of aggression compared with unaffected peers (Evans et al., 2008). Parenting behavior and parent–child attachment are associated with childhood aggression (Hoeve et al., 2009). Harsh, punitive-rejecting parenting styles and parents who are permissive in their approach or provide minimal supervision and monitoring of children's behaviors are associated with increased aggression and disruptive childhood behavior (Dishion & Patterson, 2016; Stormshak, Bierman, McMahon, Lengua, & the Conduct Problems Prevention Research Group, 2000).

Social-cognitive, neuropsychological, and emotional processes are associated with childhood aggression and disruptive behavior. First, children who have difficulties with social-cognitive processes often are involved in a vicious cycle whereby social-cognitive deficit, and negative reciprocal peer responses lead to further aggression (Lochman & Dodge, 1994), which in turn lead to poorer social-cognitive processing. From a social information-processing (SIP) perspective (Crick & Dodge, 1994), aggressive children have been found to be hypervigilant in encoding negative or problematic social cues and to have hostile attributional biases of others' intentions (de Castro, Veerman, Koops, Bosch, & Monshouwer, 2002), to have social goals that are dominance- and revenge-oriented, to generate disproportionate maladaptive solutions to perceived problems, and to have greater confidence in the likelihood of success of aggressive solutions compared with nonaggressive solutions (Matthys, Cuperus, & Van Engeland, 1999). Aggressive solutions are perceived by these children to lead to desired outcomes, such as attaining a social goal or object (Lochman & Dodge, 1994). It is theorized that each stage in the information-processing cycle occurs in conjunction with a database of stored memories and cognitions that facilitate automaticity of information processing. Second, a number of neuropsychological processes, including children's ability to inhibit a behavioral response, problem solving, spatial working memory, and language, have been associated with the emergence and persistence of aggression (Ellis, Weiss, & Lochman, 2009). Third, children's ability to regulate their emotions is related to their levels of behavioral reactivity, aggression, and disruptive behavior (Boylan, Vaillancourt, Boyle, & Szatmari, 2007). Not surprisingly, children with early emotional dysregulation are three times more likely to meet criteria for ODD in middle childhood (White, Jarrett, & Ollendick, 2013).

Measures and Methods

In this section, we describe the types of cognitive-behavioral strategies commonly used in intervention with children and their parents when the children have serious problems with aggressive and disruptive behaviors. The focus of this overview is on the types of therapeutic activities conducted with children and their parents, rather than focusing on broader interventions at the neighborhood or community levels. Research outcome findings for interventions that use these types of child and parent components are summarized in a subsequent section.

Sessions with Youth

Evidence-based programs employing cognitive-behavioral therapy (CBT) techniques have been shown to be efficacious in reducing serious externalizing behavior problems (severe aggressive and disruptive behaviors) in at-risk and clinic-referred youth, including examples such as the Coping Power Program (Lochman & Wells, 2003, 2004), the Life Skills Training program (Botvin & Griffin, 2004), multisystemic therapy (Henggeler & Schaeffer, 2016), and the Art of Self-Control (Feindler & Ecton, 1986). Youth-focused treatment components most common to these types of CBT-based programs include emotion awareness, perspective taking, anger management, social problem solving, and goal setting (Lochman, Powell, Boxmeyer, & Jimenez-Camargo, 2011). For the purpose of this chapter, each of these components is described using the Coping Power Program as an exemplar. Coping Power can be delivered as an individual intervention with a therapist or in a small-group format. Group-based intervention offers a number of advantages, including more efficient treatment of a larger number of children and families, opportunities to practice skills with peers and to give and receive support from peers, and normalization of children's and parents' experiences.

Emotion Awareness

Emotion awareness strategies typically allow children to learn to recognize the emotions that lead them to engage in externalizing behaviors. Recognition of negative emotions and the degree to which they are experienced enables children to determine the conditions under which they are most prone to act out. CBT-oriented clinicians utilize a range of techniques to teach emotion awareness in children. In Coping Power, child clients first learn to describe their emotions in terms of physiological sensations (e.g., heart racing, tight muscles, face flushing), behaviors (e.g., raising one's voice, making a threatening gesture, pushing or shoving), and cognitions (e.g., "I hate my mom"; "My teacher always picks on me"; "I am going to show that kid he can't mess with me"). Using a thermometer analogy, children are taught to identify varying intensities of particular emotions. Situational triggers and thought patterns associated with varying levels of such emotions are then identified (e.g., an extra homework assignment might make you a little bit upset, whereas someone making fun of a family member might make you enraged). In-session activities and self-monitoring homework assignments assist children to identify common situational triggers for their anger arousal. Clinicians must be aware of normative age-related changes in emotional awareness to determine whether a particular child is delayed in this area. Children become aware of their emotions in early childhood (Hietanen, Glerean, Hari, & Nummenmaa, 2016), but there are age-related changes in emotion understanding. Older children are more accurate in recognizing and labeling emotions in themselves and others and viewing their emotions from the perspective of others (Bajgar, Ciarrochi, Lane, & Deane, 2005). They are more accurate in understanding emotion dimensions such as intensity (Wintre & Vallance, 1994), and they develop more awareness of how their body sensations are related to specific emotions (Hietanen et al., 2016).

Perspective Taking

This component is designed to teach children the difficulty involved in accurately determining others' intentions. Children who exhibit externalizing behaviors tend to overly interpret others' intentions as hostile (Lochman & Dodge, 1994); thus it is necessary to teach children about other, more benign alternate explanations for others' behaviors. The clinician can have children role-play different characters in an ambiguous situation. Upon completion of the role play, children are encouraged to discuss the different viewpoints of each of the characters portrayed. Children are also asked to recall real-life incidents in which they later realized they had misinterpreted the reason for another person's actions in an overly hostile light. In school settings, clinicians may also wish to have children interview their teachers to allow children the opportunity to obtain a firsthand account of common student misconceptions regarding disciplinary procedures and classroom management.

Anger Management

Emotion regulation, specifically anger control, is one key to successfully decreasing conduct problems and is often introduced to children immediately after sessions addressing emotion awareness and just before sessions addressing perspective-taking skills. With a working knowledge of personal emotion awareness and perspective-taking skills, children are more likely to successfully implement anger management techniques before becoming inundated by an unmanageable level of anger arousal. A number of strategies can be taught to children to help them manage their anger arousal, including distraction, relaxation, and coping self-statements. With regard to relaxation, guided imagery and progressive muscle relaxation techniques may be taught to prevent escalation of low levels of anger. In terms of distraction, exercises through which the child is taught to divert his or her attention away from the anger-provoking stimulus can be conducted. By focusing on the task at hand, the child learns that he or she can prevent his or her anger from escalating by ignoring, or focusing attention away from, the anger-evoking stimulus. The use of coping self-statements can be taught through a series of graded exposure role plays, starting with puppets and progressing to more emotionally charged live role plays of anger-arousing situations. Initially children can be provided with a list of coping self-statements that they may find helpful to lower their anger (e.g., "It's not worth it to get angry"; "He is trying to make me mad, but I am not going to let him get to me"). Children are encouraged to generate their own coping statements, which may have a greater impact on their anger management.

Social Problem Solving

Children are encouraged to practice the anger-reducing techniques just described to allow them time to generate more adaptive solutions to anger-evoking problem situations. Variations on the antecedents–behavior–consequences (ABC) model, in which children identify the antecedents to a particular problem and how different behaviors in response to those antecedents can result in different outcomes, can be used to demonstrate problem-solving techniques. The PICC (Problem Identification, Choices, Consequences) model utilized in Coping Power, for example, teaches children how to first identify a problem by defining it in objective and behavioral terms. The children are then encouraged to generate a variety of choices in response to the problem that lead to both positive and negative outcomes. The children are then asked to discuss the consequences of each choice, evaluate all choices in terms of their benefits and disadvantages, and choose the outcome with the most positive consequences. This model can be applied to a variety of child problems, including peer or sibling conflict, teacher–student relations, parental conflict, and neighborhood problems. Children can practice and consolidate their problem-solving skills using several methods, such as role plays or creation of a video illustrating problem solving in action.

Goal Setting

Throughout the implementation of the above CBT components, clinicians can also help children learn to set personal goals. As a first step, clinicians can introduce the concept of personal goal setting and have each child identify one or two long-term goals that he or she would like to accomplish in the next 6 months to 1 year. The clinician can then work with the child to help him or her break the long-term goals into short-term goals that can be accomplished within a day or a week. Children and preadolescents often require more concrete assistance from the clinician in identifying relevant longer-term goals (using visual aids such as a set of stairs, with a long-term goal at the top and short-term goals on the steps), a task that comes more naturally to adolescents. Prior to initiating the goal-setting process, it is beneficial for clinicians to consult with parents and teachers to elicit their input on goals that may improve the child's functioning in the school or home setting. The clinician's role is to synthesize the ideas for goals generated by the child, parent, and teacher, as well as the goals on the treatment plan, and to work collaboratively with the child to generate a list and hierarchy of goals that the child is motivated to work to reach. This process can be executed using a weekly goal sheet. Upon mastering a goal, the child can move toward a more difficult goal to complete. Throughout the goal-setting process, clinicians seek to incorporate goals that allow children opportunities to practice the skills they are learning in the program. Goal setting works well when used in combination with a point–rewards system to motivate children to attain their goals.

Sessions with Parents

Because of the extensive research that has documented certain parenting practices as risk factors for the development and maintenance of children's aggressive behavior (Dishion & Patterson, 2016), most evidence-based cognitive-behavioral interventions for aggressive youth also include parent components based on well-established behavioral parent training programs (e.g., Patterson, Reid, Jones, & Conger, 1975) and focus on improving the parent–child bond and helping parents utilize positive parenting skills. Sessions include a focus on praise and improving the parent–child relationship, use of planned ignoring of minor disruptive behavior, antecedent control by giving clear instructions, and consistent use of consequences, using methods such as privilege removal and work chores. Additional sessions, which are more specific to Coping Power, focus on parents' own stress management, building family cohesion and communication, and family problem solving. An important objective of each parent session is also to inform parents about what their children are learning in the child intervention sessions and to discuss ways that the parents can reinforce these skills at home.

Parent group sessions follow a consistent sequence. Time is reserved at the beginning and end of each session to allow parents to visit with each other, which helps to develop group cohesion and supportive relationships among the group members. The session then opens with a review of prior content, including discussion of parents' utilization of new parenting strategies at home and the observed impact on their relationships with their children and on the children's behavior. New discussion topics are then introduced, and group activities are utilized to facilitate skill acquisition (e.g., interactive worksheets, role plays). Homework assignments are given at the end of each session to facilitate generalization of parenting skills outside of the intervention setting. Clinicians deliver the intervention content in a flexible manner, with a goal of adapting session activities to best address the specific problems and issues of the group members.

Central Research Findings

Empirically supported interventions for children with severe aggressive and conduct behavioral problems have been identified (Battagliese et al., 2015). This section focuses on several examples of selected evidence-based programs across the developmental range from preschool age through adolescence.

The Incredible Years

The Incredible Years (IY) training series (Webster-Stratton & Reid, 2010) encompasses a range of programs designed to prevent and treat aggressive and disruptive behaviors in children from birth to age 12. The programs include universal, targeted prevention and treatment protocols, with separate curricula available for implementation with children, parents, and teachers. The child component seeks to decrease aggressive and disruptive behaviors and to promote resilience through teaching concepts that include social skills, strategies for school success, emotional understanding, problem solving, and anger management. In the parenting program, parents are taught skills to interrupt the cycle of negative parent–child interactions, including positive attention and praise, establishing predictable rules and routines, and effective limit setting. The teacher component is designed to promote effective classroom management practices, including using praise and encouragement, providing incentives to address behavioral problems, and establishing positive teacher student relationships. Originally designed for implementation with 4- to 8-year-old children, a substantial body of literature now provides solid evidence for the program's effectiveness in preventing and treating conduct problems in the preschool and early elementary school years (Webster-Stratton & Reid, 2010).

Several randomized controlled studies showed that the IY parent, teacher, and child interventions have proven efficacious in reducing conduct problems in young children with the primary diagnosis of ODD or CD (Webster-Stratton, Reid, & Hammond, 2004). Studies have shown that adding the child and/or teacher program to the parent treatment program has resulted in greater improvement in children's conduct problems in the classroom setting and more sustained results at follow-up assessments (Webster-Stratton et al., 2004; Webster-Stratton, Reid, & Stoolmiller, 2008). In addition, findings from studies on the child component of the IY, delivered as universal or targeted prevention level, provide support for the efficacy of this curriculum for enhancing school protective factors and reducing child and classroom risk factors faced by socioeconomically disadvantaged children (Bywater, Hutchings, Whitaker, Evans & Parry, 2011; Webster-Stratton et al., 2008). The effectiveness of the IY parenting program for prevention of conduct problems in at-risk children has also been demonstrated in three randomized trials involving Head Start students (Reid, Webster-Stratton, & Baydar, 2004). Results of these studies support the program's effectiveness in improving parenting behaviors, preventing child conduct problems, and improving child prosocial behaviors.

Problem-Solving Skills Training plus Parent Management Training

The full problem-solving skills training (PSST) plus parent management training (PMT) program has a component addressing parent training and a component addressing prosocial problem-solving skills among children with disruptive behavior disorders. This program is targeted for school-age children with antisocial behaviors between 7 and 13 years old. PSST consists of weekly 30- to 50-minute sessions with the child. The core program (10–12 sessions) may be supplemented with optional sessions if the child requires additional help, for example, in grasping the problem-solving steps. Parent participation is a large component of the training, and parents attend their own training as well as watching the child sessions, serving as a coleaders, and supervising the child's use of the new skills at home (Kazdin, Siegel, & Bass, 1992).

Outcome studies suggest that PMT and PSST alone or in combination produce reliable and significant reductions in oppositional, aggressive, and antisocial behavior and increases in prosocial behavior among children. PSST significantly reduces antisocial behavior during 1-year follow-up periods (for a comprehensive review, see Kazdin, 2016). Although PSST has been found to do better than PMT at increasing children's social competence at school and reducing self-reports of aggression and delinquency, a combination of both treatments is optimal for most outcomes (Kazdin et al., 1992). The combination of PSST and PMT can produce significant change in severely disturbed children referred for inpatient or outpatient treatment. Child–therapist (in PSST) and parent–therapist (in PMT and PSST) alliances relate to several outcomes: The more positive the child–therapist and parent–therapist alliances are during treatment, the greater are the therapeutic change of the child and improvements of the parents in parenting practices (Kazdin & Durbin, 2012).

Coping Power Program

The Coping Power Program (CPP) was derived from earlier research on the child-focused Anger Coping Program, which produced lower rates of alcohol, marijuana, and other drug use at a follow-up period 3 years after the intervention, in comparison with a control condition (Lochman, 1992). Coping Power includes a 34-session child component and a 16-session parent component. Coping Power is a comprehensive, multicomponent intervention program that is based on the contextual social-cognitive model of risk for youth violence (Lochman & Wells, 2002).

In an initial efficacy study of the CPP, Lochman and Wells (2002, 2004) randomly assigned 183 aggressive boys (60% African American, 40% European

American non-Hispanic) to one of three conditions: a cognitive-behavioral Coping Power child component, combined Coping Power child and behavioral parent training components, and an untreated cell. The two intervention conditions took place during fourth and fifth grades or fifth and sixth grades, and the intervention lasted for 1½ school years. Screening of risk status took place in 11 elementary schools and was based on a multiple-gating approach using teacher and parent ratings of children's aggressive behavior (participants were in the top 20% on teacher ratings). At 1-year follow-up, the CPP conditions (child component only; child plus parent component) produced reductions in children's self-reported delinquent behavior, in parent-reported alcohol and marijuana use by the child, and improvements in their teacher-rated functioning at school during the follow-up year, in comparison with the high-risk control condition (Lochman & Wells, 2004). Coping Power intervention effects on parent-rated youth substance use and delinquent behavior were most apparent for participants who received the combined child and parent program, with effect sizes in the medium range. In contrast, boys' teacher-rated behavioral improvements in school during the follow-up year appeared to be primarily influenced by the child component. The intervention effects on delinquency, parent-reported substance use, and teacher-rated improvement at 1-year follow-up were mediated by intervention-produced improvements in child and parent mechanisms expected to influence child aggressive behavior, based on the contextual social-cognitive model (parents' consistency of discipline, children's attributional biases, children's social problem solving, children's expectations that aggression would not work for them, and children's internal locus of control; Lochman & Wells, 2002).

Coping Power was originally designed to be implemented with fourth- to sixth-grade children, but it has been successfully adapted for younger and older children. An abbreviated version was recently developed that can be readily completed in one academic year (24 child sessions, 10 parent sessions) and still produce significant reductions in children's aggressive behavior at a multiyear follow-up (Lochman et al., 2014) . Recently, a version of the program for individual delivery (rather than group delivery) has been evaluated (Lochman, Dishion, et al., 2015).

Coping Power has also been successfully adapted for other languages (e.g., Dutch, Spanish, Italian) and cultures. The CPP, in its original form, is a targeted prevention intervention. However, Dutch and Italian clinicians adjusted it for the more severely disturbed children and their parents seen in clinic settings. In both these adapted versions of the CPP, intervention sessions are more varied, with proportionally fewer discussions and more activities to suit the short attention span of the children. The version of the CPP for children with severe aggressive behavioral problems followed in a mental care unit includes 24 sessions for the child component during a period of 9 months, and there are 15 sessions for parents. Dutch researchers using the Utrecht-CPP (UCPP; the Dutch version of Coping Power) found a reduction in the overt aggression of children with conduct disorders in Dutch outpatient clinics, in comparison with children receiving care as usual (van de Wiel et al., 2007). Analyses of cost effectiveness of UCPP found that Coping Power produced reductions in children's conduct problems at the end of intervention for 49% less cost than a care-as-usual condition. Long-term follow-up analyses of the Dutch sample, 4 years after the end of intervention, indicated that the UCPP had preventive effects by reducing adolescent marijuana and cigarette use (but not alcohol use). The rates of substance use of the youth in UCPP were within the range of typically developing Dutch adolescents (Zonnevylle-Bender, Matthys, van de Wiel, & Lochman, 2007). Italian researchers found that the CPP was more effective than two other active treatment programs in reducing aggressive behaviors in children with disruptive behavior disorders (Muratori, Milone, et al., 2017), as well as improving children's CU traits and parenting practices. One comparison intervention was a generic multicomponent cognitive-behavioral treatment delivered in individual settings for children and parents that did not have structured modules that addressed specific active mechanisms associated with aggressive behavior as CPP does. In the second intervention model, children received weekly child therapy, and parents did not receive specific therapeutic interventions. Italian children in the CPP group showed also a lower rate of referrals to mental health services at 1-year follow-up. In addition, in an initial report of a project regarding the implementation of CPP in Italian community hospitals, preliminary findings indicated the program's ability to reduce externalizing behavioral problems in children treated in mental care services (Muratori, Milone, et al., 2017).

Multisystemic Therapy

Multisystemic therapy (MST) is an intensive family and community-based treatment program that has been implemented with chronic and violent juvenile offenders, and substance-abusing youth offenders. Adapted versions of the original MST model have since evolved and been successfully applied to youth and families with other serious clinical problems, including child maltreatment, psychiatric disturbance, problem sexual behavior, and pediatric chronic illness (Henggeler & Lee, 2003). MST optimizes outcomes by targeting risk factors within (e.g., parenting practices) and between (e.g., caregiver interactions with school) multiple domains. MST assumes that several contextual factors can create barriers to the effective functioning of proximal systems and must be addressed to increase the probability of favorable change. MST interventions are provided where problems occur and are delivered by key members of the ecological system of the youth. Strategies for changing the adolescent's behavior are developed in close collaboration with family members by identifying the major environmental drivers, identified in assessments and in interviews, that help maintain the adolescent's deviant behavior. Services can include a variety of treatment approaches, such as parent training, family therapy, school consultation, marital therapy, and individual therapy. Although the techniques used within these treatment strategies can vary, many of them are either behavioral or cognitive-behavioral in nature (e.g., contingency management, behavioral contracting). Clinicians are guided by a set of nine MST principles, which include concepts such as focusing on system strengths, delivering developmentally appropriate treatment, and improving effective family functioning. The nine MST treatment principles are applied using an analytical/decision-making process that structures the treatment plan, its implementation, and the evaluation of its effectiveness. Clinician adherence to these treatment principles is closely monitored through weekly consultation with MST experts.

Several investigations have shown that families who receive MST report lower levels of adolescent behavior problems and improvements in family functioning at posttreatment in comparison with alternative treatment conditions. In the first randomized clinical trial, MST was compared with treatment as usual with a sample of 84 serious juvenile offenders. Juveniles in the MST condition had significantly fewer arrests and weeks of incarceration at a 1-year follow-up and showed reduced recidivism at a 2-year follow-up. Results from a subsequent extensive evaluation of MST found lower recidivism rates in juvenile offenders assigned to MST, in comparison with youth who completed individual counseling at 4-year follow-up (Borduin et al., 1995) and outcomes were sustained though a 22-year follow-up (Sawyer & Borduin, 2011).

Several groups of European researchers have conducted MST randomized controlled trials (RCT) with youth presenting serious antisocial behavior and their families. In a multisite Norwegian study, Ogden and colleagues (Ogden & Hagen, 2006; Ogden & Halliday-Boykins, 2004) found that MST decreased youth externalizing and internalizing symptoms, as well as out-of-home placements; and some of these outcomes were sustained through a 24-month follow-up. Other European researchers (Butler, Baruch, Hickey, & Fonagy, 2011) observed that MST improved parenting and reduced youth offenses and out-of-home placements for British juvenile offenders, and such reductions in crime were associated with cost savings (Cary, Butler, Baruch, Hickey, & Byford, 2013). Asscher, Dekovic, Manders, van der Laan, and Prins (2013) found similar outcomes in a sample of Dutch youths with severe and violent antisocial behavior at posttreatment. Sundell and colleagues (2008) investigated the effectiveness of MST in Swedish youth with CD and their families; they failed to replicate favorable MST outcomes. In this RCT, treatment fidelity was very low and was associated inversely with youth improvements. Subsequently, Löfholm, Eichas, and Sundell (2014) found that therapist fidelity and corresponding youth outcomes were lowest during the time of the RCT and steadily improved as therapists and teams gained experience. Overall, MST is one of the most extensively evaluated family-based treatments (for a comprehensive review, see Henggeler & Schaeffer, 2016), and outcome research has yielded primarily favorable results for youth and families. However, the MST investigators also indicated that clinical trials should not begin until practitioners and programs have demonstrated satisfactory adherence to intervention protocols (Henggeler & Schaeffer, 2016).

Implications

The available evidence from RCTs indicates that cognitive-behavioral interventions can lead to significant reductions in youths' serious aggressive, criminal, and substance use behaviors. When assessing the implications of interventions for real-world use, it is especially important to consider an intervention's ability to be disseminated, or widely circulated to a broader audience. Interventions may display excellent indications of efficacy under controlled conditions, but then be unable to demonstrate those effects when delivered by typical clinicians in community clinics and schools. Although limited research has examined the dissemination process, it does appear that the type of training provided to clinicians is pivotal and that staff and work-setting characteristics affect the quality of the implementation of the intervention (Lochman, Boxmeyer, et al., 2009; Lochman, Powell, et al., 2009).

As an example of a prevention-oriented dissemination trial, counselors from 57 elementary schools in Alabama were randomly assigned to one of three conditions: Coping Power–Intensive Training, Coping Power–Basic Training, or care as usual (Lochman, Boxmeyer, et al., 2009). Counselors in both training conditions received 3 days of training prior to the intervention, as well as monthly additional trainings throughout the intervention. The Intensive Training group also had access to individualized problem solving via email or a telephone hotline, as well as received feedback based on audio recordings of individual sessions. Training intensity was found to have a significant impact on outcomes, with the Coping Power–Intensive Training group showing significantly greater reductions in teacher-, parent-, and self-reported externalizing behaviors and greater improvements in social and academic behaviors than the other groups (Lochman, Boxmeyer, et al., 2009). Significant improvements in behavior only occurred in the Intensive Training groups, emphasizing the importance of intensive training and availability of feedback to counselors throughout intervention. A follow-up study of this dissemination trial found that children with counselors who received the Coping Power–Intensive Training experienced smaller declines in language arts grades than children with counselors in the other groups after 2 years (Lochman et al., 2012).

Research examining characteristics of the counselors and their schools has found that counselors in this study who were in schools that granted more professional autonomy to staff and who scored higher on personality dimensions for conscientiousness and agreeableness implemented the sessions with greater quality (Lochman, Powell, et al., 2009) and continued on their own to use important elements of the program 2 years after the training period had ended (Lochman, Powell et al, 2015). Further research on the dissemination process is essential to gain the broad public health benefits of evidence-based interventions for serious youth aggression.

Future Directions

There are a number of important future research directions for the treatment of aggression in children and adolescents. Several emerging areas for future research are described below.

Clinician Behaviors

Intervening with youth with aggressive behavior can be challenging, as these youth may talk or act disrespectfully, resist engaging in treatment, and even present a safety risk if they become aggressive in session. Clinicians who work with aggressive youth need to be skilled in establishing and maintaining a positive therapeutic alliance, while also enforcing clear behavioral expectations. Research is needed to identify specific clinician characteristics and training approaches that lead to successful treatment engagement and outcomes for aggressive youth.

Lochman, Dishion, Boxmeyer, Powell, and Qu (2017) recently coded child and leader behavior in 938 video-recorded Coping Power intervention sessions for preadolescent children with aggressive behavior. They found that a specific set of clinical skills (e.g., ability to convey interpersonal warmth, low emotional reactivity even in the presence of challenging child behavior, having a mature and professional demeanor, and being able to implement a manualized intervention flexibly and responsively) predicted lower teacher-rated youth conduct problems at 1-year follow-up. Notably, this clinical skill construct had stronger effects on children's externalizing behavior outcomes than clinicians' behavior management skills. Other aspects of clinician characteristics can also influence the success of cognitive-behavioral treatment for children. For example, Muratori, Polidori, and colleagues (2017) found that therapists who had an anxious attachment style produced less change in the aggressive behavior of clients with disruptive behavior disorder than did other therapists, suggesting the importance of therapists being sensitive to their own attachment experiences.

Lochman and colleagues (2017) also found that high levels of negative child behavior and deviant talk predicted worse long-term child behavioral outcomes. These findings indicate that it is important for clinicians to closely monitor children's in-session behavior and that a clinician's ability to adapt his or her implementation style in response to observed child behavior is an important skill (and likely a trainable one). The clinicians in the Coping Power study received intensive training and supervision while the intervention was under way. Thus the range of clinical skills observed may not fully reflect the range of skills in community-based clinicians. In future studies, it will be important to examine how well community clinicians treating youth with aggressive behavior are trained to monitor and address children's in-session behavior, the extent to which they are able to adapt their intervention styles in response to observed child behaviors, and whether these factors have an impact on the long-term outcomes of children receiving community-based treatment.

Initial findings from Lochman and colleagues' (2017) study suggest that clinicians can adjust their therapeutic styles and behavior in response to children's in-session behavior, especially when they receive regular supervisory feedback. Thus a well-specified performance feedback approach (e.g., Ricciardi, 2005) may be particularly useful for training community clinicians to intervene effectively with youth with aggressive behavior. Further research is needed to develop and test such a training approach.

Intervention Delivery Models

Group versus Individual Intervention

Coping Power and other evidence-based interventions for aggressive behavior in youth are often implemented in a group format. Although individual intervention does not provide all of these benefits, it can allow for greater intervention tailoring to fit each child or family's needs. Individual intervention also avoids a central concern for group-based intervention for youth with aggressive behavior, which is that aggregating these youth increases the risk of peer deviancy training. Peer deviancy training involves children reinforcing deviant talk or behavior; children's relationships with deviant peers may also be strengthened as a result of being in a group together (e.g., Dodge, Dishion, & Lansford, 2006).

To assess for this, Lochman, Dishion, and colleagues (2015) directly compared the effects of group versus individual Coping Power using a randomized design. Children in both conditions exhibited fewer externalizing and internalizing behavior problems at 1-year follow-up. However, the degree of improvement in teacher-reported outcomes was significantly greater for children receiving individual intervention. Moderator analyses indicated that for children with poorer self-regulation, individualized interventions will likely yield the most significant reductions in externalizing behavior in the school setting. Although this is informative, these findings also report on interventions delivered by well-trained clinicians. Thus future studies are needed to compare the benefits of group versus individual intervention for youth with aggressive behavior, as implemented by community clinicians, as well as any impact of peer deviancy training.

Web-Based Intervention

New technologies are emerging that can be harnessed to provide intervention to youth with aggressive behavior and their families. A recent randomized trial with 96 child–parent dyads tested the feasibility and preliminary effects of a hybrid Web and in-person delivery format for CPP (Lochman, Boxmeyer, et al., 2017). This more efficient format allows the full content of the CPP intervention to be delivered in one-third the number of in-person sessions, while children and parents have access to the content of the full CPP through interactive Web and video content. This much briefer, hybrid version of the CPP was found to have beneficial effects on children's conduct problems compared with children in the control condition. Moreover, the size of these effects were comparable to the effects of the longer version of CPP. Children actively engaged with the website materials. Parents were more difficult to engage in the Web-based component, yet parents' use of the website predicted children's improvements in conduct problems. Thus it will be important to develop engaging Web-based intervention content.

Potential future research directions include conducting a large-scale trial of this hybrid Web and in-person intervention format, as well as developing and testing intervention content that can be delivered solely via the Web, in a way that is highly engaging to participants. One such model for Web-based intervention with young children with disruptive behavior problems is the Internet-delivered format of parent–child interaction therapy (I-PCIT; Comer et al., 2015).

Precision Medicine and Individually Tailored Treatment

Precision medicine is an emerging trend in health care that involves tailoring the treatments delivered to best meet individual patient needs. One way this has been offered to families of children with aggressive behavior is through the integration of the Family Check-Up (FCU; Dishion & Kavanagh, 2005) and the Coping Power parent program. In the FCU, families are formally assessed and then receive feedback on strengths and areas of concern that can be targeted for change. The Coping Power parent component was adapted for tailored, modular use to address only the specific areas of need identified for a family using the FCU (Herman et al., 2012). Seven parent modules have been created from the Coping Power parent curriculum, which can be used alone or in combination. This form of tailored, adaptive intervention is designed to offer parents only the modules relevant to them and may also reduce the overall length of intervention. The Coping Power child component can also be adapted for this type of modular use. Future studies are needed to examine the benefits of this type of tailored intervention derived from existing evidence-based interventions for youth aggression. As is the case with any manualized intervention, if the child or parent requires additional services beyond the scope of Coping Power, then the clinician assists with relevant referrals.

In other areas of health care, precision medicine often refers to the use of an individual's genetic information to diagnose or treat his or her disease. Glenn and colleagues (2017) are pursuing an innovative line of research examining whether genetic factors can be useful in identifying the optimal psychosocial treatment modality for a particular individual. For example, they recently found that the variant a child carries of the oxytocin gene (which is associated with attachment and social behavior) differentially predicts the child's response to group-based psychosocial intervention. In contrast, child genotype on this oxytocin gene does not differentially affect outcomes of individually delivered treatment. These findings suggest that it may be worthwhile to screen for the mechanisms (e.g., excessive social sensitivity, heightened orientation to social rewards from peers) associated with the oxytocin genotype before enrolling a child with aggressive behavior in group intervention. In a series of studies, other factors that help to predict weaker response to group interventions are very low levels of inhibitory control (Lochman, Dishion, et al., 2015), very poor emotional regulation (assessed with respiratory sinus arrhythmia; Glenn, Lochman, et al., in press), and high levels of negative behavior and deviant talk in sessions (Lochman, Dishion et al., 2017). Further research in this area is actively under way and likely to yield new innovations in the treatment of aggressive behavior in children and adolescents.

Program Enhancements and Developmental Adaptations

Other future directions include testing adaptations and enhancements to existing evidence-based interventions for aggressive behavior in children and adolescents. A number of cultural, content, and developmental adaptation studies are currently under way.

Integrating Mindfulness and Cognitive-Behavioral Intervention Approaches

To enhance intervention effects on children's reactive aggression, an ongoing study is testing the effects of integrating mindfulness, yoga, and compassion practices with the cognitive-behavioral practices in traditional Coping Power (CP) to increase children's emotional regulation. In this study, the enhanced Mindful Coping Power (MCP) program is being directly compared with CP in a randomized feasibility trial with 96 child–parent dyads. In the first cohort, which included half of the total expected sample, MCP was found to be well received by child and parent participants. Furthermore, group leaders reported that children in MCP became better at self-regulating during group sessions than children in CP, child conduct problems were lower at postintervention for children in MCP than CP, and parent intervention attendance was higher in MCP than CP (Boxmeyer & Miller, 2016).

Coping Power for Early Adolescents

There is a relative lack of evidence-based interventions for early to midadolescents with aggressive behavior, especially programs that include both youth and parent components. To fill this gap, a version of CP that extends the program through early adolescence (CP-EA) was recently developed and piloted. CP-EA includes increased focus on adolescent issues such as assertive communication, cyberbullying and social media use, and how to repair damaged relationships. The adapted sessions were constructed to be more appropriate for adolescents, using journaling and making greater use of video and media content. CP-EA is now being tested in an efficacy study in 40 middle schools in Alabama and Maryland. Preliminary analyses for the Alabama subsample for the first of three cohorts indicate that CP-EA produced reductions in youth teacher-rated aggression and conduct problems at a 1-year follow-up in comparison with the control condition (Lochman et al., 2016). Development and testing of a high school version of Coping Power is also under way in Baltimore.

Conclusions

Overall, research has supported cognitive-behavioral interventions for reducing aggressive children's presenting problems and their likelihood of developing more severe antisocial behaviors in later years. Clinical and prevention programs have been found to reduce children's conduct problems across the developmental spectrum from the preschool to early elementary school years (e.g., Incredible Years) to the preadolescent and early adolescent years (e.g., CP) and to later adolescent years (e.g., multisystemic therapy). Interventions have significantly reduced aggressive behaviors in children in rigorous efficacy studies using highly trained grant-funded staff, as well as in effectiveness and dissemination studies using "real-world" school and clinic staff and in adaptations to specialized populations and diverse international communities. Important future directions for research that can optimize intervention effects can involve key therapeutic skills that can facilitate intervention effects, different models and formats for delivering intervention, methods for tailoring interventions to specific subpopulations of youth, and new methods for extending interventions to new populations and for creating hybrid interventions by combining elements from different intervention models.

REFERENCES

American Psychiatric Association (2013). *Diagnostic and statistical manual of mental disorders* (5th ed.). Arlington, VA: Author.

Andrade, B. F., & Tannock, R. (2014). Sustained impact of inattention and hyperactivity–impulsivity on peer problems: Mediating roles of prosocial skills and conduct problems in a community sample of children. *Child Psychiatry and Human Development, 45,* 318–328.

Asscher, J. J., Dekovic, M., Manders, W. A., van der Laan, P. H., & Prins, P. J. M. (2013). A randomized controlled trial of the effectiveness of multisystemic therapy in the Netherlands: Post-treatment changes and moderator effects. *Journal of Experimental Criminology, 9,* 169–187.

Bajgar, J., Ciarrochi, J., Lane, R., & Deane, F. P. (2005). Development of the Levels of Emotional Awareness Scale for Children (LEAS-C). *British Journal of Developmental Psychology, 23,* 569–586.

Battagliese, G., Caccetta, M., Luppino, O. I., Baglioni, C., Cardi, V., Mancini, F., & Buonanno, C. (2015). Cognitive-behavioral therapy for externalizing disorders: A meta-analysis of treatment effectiveness. *Behaviour Research and Therapy, 75,* 60–71.

Borduin, C. M., Mann, B. J., Cone, L. T., Henggeler, S. W., Fucci, B. R., Blaske, D. M., et al. (1995). Multisystemic treatment of serious juvenile offenders: Long-term prevention of criminality and violence. *Journal of Consulting and Clinical Psychology, 63,* 569–578.

Botvin, G. J., & Griffin, K. W. (2004). Life skills training: Empirical findings and future directions. *Journal of Primary Prevention, 25,* 211–232.

Boxmeyer, C., & Miller, S. (2016, August). *Mindful Coping Power Program for emotionally reactive youth and their parents.* Paper presented at the National Center for Complementary and Integrative Health Workshop Research on Mind–Body Approaches to Improve Children's Health, Bethesda, MD.

Boylan, K., Vaillancourt, T., Boyle, M., & Szatmari, P. (2007). Comorbidity of internalizing disorders in children with oppositional defiant disorder. *European Child and Adolescent Psychiatry, 16,* 484–494.

Burke, J. D., Loeber, R., & Birmaher, B. (2002). Oppositional defiant disorder and conduct disorder: A review of the past 10 years: Part II. *Journal of the American Academy of Child and Adolescent Psychiatry, 41,* 1275–1293.

Butler, S., Baruch, G., Hickey, N., & Fonagy, P. (2011). A randomized controlled trial of MST and a statutory therapeutic intervention for young offenders. *Journal of the American Academy of Child and Adolescent Psychiatry, 50,* 1220–1235.

Bywater, T., Hutchings, J., Whitaker, C., Evans, C., & Parry, L. (2011). The Incredible Years therapeutic dinosaur programme to build social and emotional competence in Welsh primary schools: Study protocol for a randomised controlled trial. *Trials, 12,* 1. Retrieved from *https://trialsjournal.biomedcentral.com/articles/10.1186/1745-6215-12-39.*

Cary, M., Butler, S., Baruch, G., Hickey, N., & Byford, S. (2013). Economic evaluation of multisystemic therapy for young people at risk for continuing criminal activity in the UK. *PLOS ONE, 8*(4), e61070.

Comer, J. S., Furr, J. M., Cooper-Vince, C., Madigan, R. J., Chow, C., Chan, P. T., et al. (2015). Rationale and considerations for the internet-based delivery of parent–child interaction therapy. *Cognitive and Behavioral Practice, 22,* 302–316.

Cote, S. M., Vaillancourt, T., LeBlanc, J. C., Nagin, D. S., & Tremblay, R. E. (2006). The development of physical aggression from toddlerhood to pre-adolescence: A nation *wide* longitudinal study of Canadian children. *Journal of Abnormal Child Psychology, 34,* 71–85.

Crick, N. R. (1996). The role of overt aggression, relational aggression, and prosocial behavior in the prediction of children's future social adjustment. *Child Development, 67,* 2317–2327.

Crick, N. R., & Dodge, K. A. (1994). A review and reformulation of social information-processing mechanisms in children's social adjustment. *Psychological Bulletin, 115,* 74–101.

de Castro, B. O., Veerman, J. W., Koops, W., Bosch, J. D., & Monshouwer, H. J. (2002). Hostile attribution of intent and aggressive behavior: A meta-analysis. *Child Development, 73,* 916–934.

de Castro, B. O., Welmoet, M., Koops, W., Veerman, J. W., & Bosch, J. D. (2005). Emotions in social information-processing and their relations with reactive and proactive aggression in referred aggressive boys. *Journal of Clinical Child and Adolescent Psychology, 34,* 105–116.

de Cubas, M. M., & Field, T. (2010). Children of methadone dependent women: Developmental outcomes. *American Journal of Othopsychiatry, 63,* 266–276.

Dishion, T. J., & Kavanagh, K. (2005). *Intervening in adolescent problem behavior: A family-centered approach.* New York: Guilford Press.

Dishion, T. J., & Patterson, G. R. (2016). The development and ecology of antisocial behavior: Linking etiology, prevention, and treatment. In D. Cicchetti (Ed.), *Developmental psychopathology: Vol. 3. Maladaptation and psychopathology* (3rd ed., pp. 647–678). Hoboken, NJ: Wiley.

Dodge, K. A., Dishion, T. J., & Lansford, J. E. (2006). *Deviant peer influences in programs for youth: Problems and solutions.* New York: Guilford Press

Dodge, K. A., Lochman, J. E., Harnish, J. D., Bates, J. E., & Pettit, G. S. (1997). Reactive and proactive aggression in school children and psychiatrically impaired chronically assaultive youth. *Journal of Abnormal Psychology, 106,* 37–51.

Dodge, K. A., & Pettit, G. S. (2003). A biopsychosocial model of the development of chronic conduct problems in adolescence. *Developmental Psychology, 39,* 349–371.

Ellis, M. L., Weiss, B., & Lochman, J. E. (2009). Executive functions in children: Associations with aggressive behavior and appraisal processing. *Journal of Abnormal Child Psychology, 37,* 945–956.

Evans, S. E., Davies, C., & DiLillo, D. (2008). Exposure to domestic violence: A meta-analysis of child and adolescent outcomes. *Aggression and Violent Behavior, 13,* 131–140.

Farrington, D. P., Jolliffe, D., Loeber, R., Stouthamer-Loeber, M., & Kalb, L. M. (2001). The concentration of offenders in families, and family criminality in the prediction of boys' delinquency. *Journal of Adolescence, 24,* 579–596.

Feindler, E. L., & Ecton, R. B. (1986). *Adolescent anger control: Cognitive-behavior techniques.* New York: Pergamon Books.

Frick, P. J., Ray, J. V., Thornton, L. C., & Kahn, R. E. (2014). Can callous–unemotional traits enhance the understanding, diagnosis, and treatment of serious conduct problems in children and adolescents?: A comprehensive review. *Psychological Bulletin, 140*(1), 1–57.

Glenn, A. L., Lochman, J. E., Dishion, T., Powell, N. P., Boxmeyer, C., Kassing, F., et al. (in press). Toward tailored interventions: Sympathetic and parasympathetic functioning predicts responses to an intervention for conduct problems delivered in two formats. *Prevention Science.*

Glenn, A. L., Lochman, J. E., Dishion, T., Powell, N. P., Boxmeyer, C., & Qu, L. (2017). Oxytocin receptor gene variant interacts with intervention delivery format in predicting intervention outcomes for youth with conduct problems. *Prevention Science, 19*(1), 38–48.

Henggeler, S. W., & Lee, T. (2003). Multisystemic treatment of serious clinical problems. In A. E. Kazdin & J. R. Weisz (Eds.), *Evidence-based psychotherapies for children and adolescents* (pp. 301–322). New York: Guilford Press

Henggeler, S. W., & Schaeffer, C. M. (2016). Multisystemic therapy: Clinical overview, outcomes, and implementation research. *Family Process, 55,* 514–528.

Herman, K. C., Reinke, W. M., Bradshaw, C. P., Lochman, J. E., Boxmeyer, C. L., Powell, N. P., et al. (2012). Integrating the Family Check-Up and the parent Coping Power Program. *Advances in School Mental Health Promotion, 5,* 208–219.

Hietanen, J. K., Glerean, E., Hari, R., & Nummenmaa, L. (2016). Bodily maps of emotions across child development. *Developmental Science, 19,* 1111–1118.

Hoeve, M., Dubas, J. S., Eichelsheim, V. I., Van der Laan, P. H., Smeenk, W., & Gerris, J. R.

M. (2009). The relationship between parenting and delinquency: A meta-analysis. *Journal of Abnormal Child Psychology, 37,* 749–775.

Kazdin, A. E. (2016). Implementation and evaluation of treatments for children and adolescents with conduct problems: Findings, challenges, and future directions. *Psychotherapy Research, 28,* 3–17.

Kazdin, A. E., & Durbin, K. A. (2012). Predictors of child–therapist alliance in cognitive-behavioral treatment of children referred for oppositional and antisocial behavior. *Psychotherapy, 49,* 202–217.

Kazdin, A. E., Siegel, T. C., & Bass, D. (1992). Cognitive problem-solving skills training and parent management training in the treatment of antisocial behavior in children. *Journal of Consulting and Clinical Psychology, 60,* 733–747.

Lochman, J. E. (1992). Cognitive-behavioral intervention with aggressive boys: Three-year follow-up and preventive effects. *Journal of Consulting and Clinical Psychology, 60*(3), 426–432.

Lochman, J. E., Baden, R. E., Boxmeyer, C. L., Powell, N. P., Qu, L., Salekin, K. L., et al. (2014). Does a booster intervention augment the preventive effects of an abbreviated version of the Coping Power Program for aggressive children? *Journal of Abnormal Child Psychology, 42,* 367–381.

Lochman, J. E., Boxmeyer, C. L., Jones, S., Qu, L., Ewoldsen, D., & Nelson, W. M. (2017). Promoting parent and child engagement in school-based preventive intervention with aggressive children: A hybrid intervention with face-to-face and Internet components. *Journal of School Psychology, 62,* 33–50.

Lochman, J. E., Bradshaw, C. P., Powell, N., Debnam, K., Pas, E., & Ialongo, N. (2016, June). Preventing conduct problems in middle schoolers: Preliminary effects of the Early Adolescent Coping Power Program. In C. Bradshaw (Chair), *Parents as a protective influence in adolescence: A focus on aggression, bullying, and romantic relationships.* Symposium conducted at the 24th annual meeting of the Society for Prevention Research, San Francisco, CA.

Lochman, J. E., Boxmeyer, C. L., Powell, N., Qu, L., Wells, K., & Windle, M. (2009). Dissemination of the Coping Power Program: Importance of intensity of counselor training. *Journal of Consulting and Clinical Psychology, 77,* 397–409.

Lochman, J. E., Boxmeyer, C. L., Powell, N. P., Qu, L., Wells, K., & Windle, M. (2012). Coping Power dissemination study: Intervention and special education effects on academic outcomes. *Behavioral Disorders, 37,* 192–205.

Lochman, J. E., Dishion, T. J., Boxmeyer, C. L., Powell, N. P., & Qu, L. (2017). Variation in response to evidence-based group preventive intervention for disruptive behavior problems: A view from 938 Coping Power sessions. *Journal of Abnormal Child Psychology, 45*(7), 1271–1284.

Lochman, J. E., Dishion, T. J., Powell, N. P., Boxmeyer, C. L., Qu, L., & Sallee, M. (2015). Evidence-based preventive intervention for preadolescent aggressive children: One-year outcomes following randomization to group versus individual delivery. *Journal of Consulting and Clinical Psychology, 83,* 728–735.

Lochman, J. E., & Dodge, K. A. (1994). Social-cognitive processes of severely violent, moderately aggressive, and nonaggressive boys. *Journal of Consulting and Clinical Psychology, 62,* 366–374.

Lochman, J. E., Powell, N. P., Boxmeyer, C. L., & Jimenez-Camargo, L. A. (2011). Cognitive behavioral therapy for externalizing disorders in children and adolescents. *Psychiatric Clinics of North America, 20,* 305–318.

Lochman, J. E., Powell, N. P., Boxmeyer, C. L., Qu, L., Sallee, M., Wells, K. C., et al. (2015). Counselor-level predictors of sustained use of an indicated preventive intervention for aggressive children. *Prevention Science, 16,* 1075–1085.

Lochman, J. E., Powell, N. P., Boxmeyer, C. L., Qu, L., Wells, K. C., & Windle, M. (2009). Implementation of a school-based prevention program: Effects of counselor and school characteristics. *Professional Psychology: Research and Practice, 40,* 476–482.

Lochman, J. E., & Wells, K. C. (2002). Contextual social-cognitive mediators and child outcome: A test of the theoretical model in the Coping Power Program. *Development and Psychopathology, 14,* 945–967.

Lochman, J. E., & Wells, K. C. (2003). Effectiveness of the Coping Power Program and of classroom intervention with aggressive children: Outcomes at a 1-year follow-up. *Behavior Therapy, 34,* 493–515.

Lochman, J. E., & Wells, K. C. (2004). The Coping Power Program for preadolescent aggressive boys and their parents: Outcome effects at the 1-year follow-up. *Journal of Consulting and Clinical Psychology, 72,* 571–578.

Löfholm, C. A., Eichas, K., & Sundell, K. (2014). The Swedish implementation of multisystemic therapy for adolescents: Does treatment experience predict treatment adherence? *Journal of Clinical Child and Adolescent Psychology, 43,* 643–655.

Matthys, W., Cuperus, J. M., & Van Engeland, H. (1999). Deficient social problem-solving in boys with ODD/CD, with ADHD, and with both disorders. *Journal of the American Academy of Child and Adolescent Psychiatry, 38,* 311–321.

Muratori, P., Milone, A., Manfredi, A., Polidori, L., Ruglioni, L., Lambruschi, F., et al. (2017). Evaluation of improvement in externalizing behaviors and callous–unemotional traits in children with disruptive behavior disorder: A 1-year follow up clinic-based study. *Administration and Policy in Mental Health and Mental Health Services Research, 44,* 452–462.

Muratori, P., Polidori, L., Chiodo, S., Dovigo, V., Mascarucci, M., Milone, A., et al. (2017). A pilot study implementing Coping Power in Italian community hospitals: Effect of therapist attachment style on outcomes in children. *Journal of Child and Family Studies, 26,* 3093–3101.

Nagin, D. S., & Tremblay, R. E. (2001). Parental and early childhood predictors of persistent physical aggression in boys from kindergarten to high school. *Archives of General Psychiatry, 58,* 389–394.

Odgers, C. L., Milne, B. J., Caspi, A., Crump, R., Poulton, R., & Moffitt, T. E. (2007). Predicting prognosis for the conduct-problem boy: Can family history help? *Journal of the American Academy of Child and Adolescent Psychiatry, 46,* 1240–1249.

Ogden, T., & Hagen, K. A. (2006). Multisystemic treatment of serious behaviour problems in youth: Sustainability of effectiveness two years after intake. *Child and Adolescent Mental Health, 11,* 142–149.

Ogden, T., & Halliday-Boykins, C. A. (2004). Multisystemic treatment of antisocial adolescents in Norway: Replication of clinical outcomes outside of the US. *Child and Adolescent Mental Health, 9,* 77–83.

Ogilvie, J. M., Stewart, A. L., Chan, R. C. K., & Shum, D. H. K. (2011). Neuropsychological measures of executive function and antisocial behavior: A meta-analysis. *Criminology, 49,* 1063–1107.

Patterson, G. R., Reid, J. B., Jones, R. R., & Conger, R. E. (1975). *A social learning approach to family intervention: Vol. 1. Families with aggressive children.* Eugene, OR: Castalia.

Price, J. M., & Dodge, K. A. (1989). Reactive and proactive aggression in childhood: Relations to peer status and social context dimensions. *Journal of Abnormal Child Psychology, 17,* 455–471.

Reid, M. J., Webster-Stratton, C., & Baydar, N. (2004). Halting the development of conduct problems in Head Start children: The effects of parent training. *Journal of Clinical Child and Adolescent Psychology, 33,* 279–291.

Ricciardi, J. N. (2005). Achieving human service outcomes through competency-based training: A guide for managers. *Behavior Modification, 29,* 488–507.

Sawyer, A. M., & Borduin, C. M. (2011). Effects of multisystemic therapy through midlife: A 21.9-year follow-up to a randomized clinical trial with serious and violent juvenile offenders. *Journal of Consulting and Clinical Psychology, 79,* 643–652.

Stormshak, E. A., Bierman, K. L., McMahon, R. J., Lengua, L. J., & the Conduct Problems Prevention Research Group. (2000). Parenting practices and child disruptive behavior problems in early elementary school. *Journal of Clinical Child Psychology, 29,* 17–29.

Stringaris, A., Maughan, B., & Goodman, R. (2010). What's in a disruptive disorder?: Temperamental antecedents of oppositional defiant disorder: Findings from the Avon Longitudinal Study. *Journal of the American Academy of Child and Adolescent Psychiatry, 49,* 474–482.

Sundell, K., Hansson, K., Löfholm, C. A., Olsson, T., Gustle, L. H., & Kadesjö, C. (2008). The transportability of multisystemic therapy to Sweden: Short-term results from a randomized trial of conduct-disordered youths. *Journal of Family Psychology, 22,* 550–560.

van de Wiel, N. M., Matthys, W., Cohen-Kettenis, P. T., Maassen, G. H., Lochman, J. E., & van Engeland, H. (2007). The effectiveness of an experimental treatment when compared to care as usual depends on the type of care as usual. *Behavioral Modification, 31,* 298–312.

Webster-Stratton, C., & Reid, M. J. (2010). The Incredible Years parents, teachers and children training series: A multifaceted treatment approach for young children with conduct problems. In A. E. Kazdin & J. R. Weisz (Eds.), *Evidence-based psychotherapies for children and adolescents* (2nd ed., pp. 194–210). New York: Guilford Press.

Webster-Stratton, C., Reid, M. J., & Hammond, M. (2004). Treating children with early-onset conduct problems: Intervention outcomes for parent, child, and teacher training. *Journal of Clinical Child and Adolescent Psychology, 33,* 105–124.

Webster-Stratton, C., Reid, M. J., & Stoolmiller, M. (2008). Preventing conduct problems and improving school readiness: Evaluation of the Incredible Years teacher and child training programs in high-risk schools. *Journal of Child Psychology and Psychiatry, 49,* 471–488.

White, B. A., Jarrett, M. A., & Ollendick, T. H. (2013). Self-regulation deficits explain the link between reactive aggression and internalizing and externalizing behavior problems in children. *Journal of Psychopathology and Behavioral Assessment, 35,* 1–9.

Wintre, M. G., & Vallance, D. D. (1994). A developmental sequence in the comprehension of emotions: Intensity, multiple emotions. and valence. *Developmental Psychology, 30,* 509–514.

Zonnevylle-Bender, M. J., Matthys, W., van de Wiel, N. M., & Lochman, J. E. (2007). Preventive effects of treatment of disruptive behavior disorder in middle childhood on substance use and delinquent behavior. *Journal of the American Academy of Child and Adolescent Psychiatry, 46,* 33–39.

CHAPTER 17

Family-Based Treatments
for Aggressive Problem Behavior

ELIZABETH A. STORMSHAK and S. ANDREW GARBACZ

Brief Introduction

Problem behavior is a broad category used to define a variety of externalizing behaviors that emerge throughout the course of a child's development. Problem behavior may include aggression, attention-deficit/hyperactivity disorder (ADHD), oppositional behavior, attention problems, delinquency, risk behavior, or violence. Comorbidity of these behaviors is high, and they tend to cluster into a construct of risk behavior that changes as children develop more complex behaviors and respond differently to their environments (Moffitt, Caspi, Harrington, & Milne, 2002). Due to the comorbidity of problem behaviors, such as attention problems and oppositional behavior, this chapter focuses on aggression and related problem behaviors. In that deficits in prosocial behaviors can place children at risk for subsequent behavior problems, approaches and strategies to build prosocial behavior are addressed. After having been studied for more than 30 years and scrutinized through the lens of a developmental–ecological model, the pathways to the development and maintenance of problem behavior have become clear. Early risks, such as contextual risk factors, poverty, family mental health problems, and early learning difficulties, impinge upon families' ability to parent effectively, which can lead to their children's worsening behavior over time. When individual risk factors, such as early learning problems or poor self-regulation, are also present, the risk of problem behavior increases and becomes magnified in adolescence, when behaviors such as violence, substance abuse, and high-risk sexual behavior jeopardize individual development and the safety of the community (Conduct Problems Prevention Research Group [CPPRG], 2014).

Despite these contextual and individual predictors and risk factors, effective parenting and family management have been key targets of successful interventions aimed at reducing aggression and related problem behaviors. Research has long suggested that parenting skill deficits form the core of risk for both the development and maintenance of aggression and related problem behaviors. As such, parenting interventions are the most promising targets of prevention and intervention because they reduce risk behavior, support adaptation, build prosocial behavior, improve parenting skills, and enhance parenting education (Dishion & Stormshak, 2007; Knerr, Gardner, & Cluver, 2013; Sheridan et al., 2012; Spoth, Kavanagh, & Dishion, 2002). In fact, much of what we have learned about parenting skills and child behavior outcomes has been derived from intervention research. Developmental research suggests that skillful parenting predicts positive outcomes despite contextual risks, such as poverty and family hardship, and is a robust predictor of outcomes such as school readiness and problem behavior across various ages and cultural groups (Ackerman, Brown, & Izard, 2004; Raver, Gershoff, & Aber, 2007). This suggests that the tailored approach to assessment and intervention in family-centered models may be relevant for children and families of various backgrounds (Smith, Knoble, Zerr, Dishion, & Stormshak, 2014).

Even in the face of genetic risk, poverty, and high levels of neighborhood risk, warm and supportive parenting mediates the link between socioeconomic status and later antisocial behavior from early development to adolescence (Musci et al., 2014; Odgers et al., 2012). Parental monitoring can reduce the development of antisocial behavior over time, and antisocial behavior predicts parents' knowledge of their child's activities, suggesting bidirectionality in the relations between child behavior and parenting skills (Dishion & McMahon, 1998; Wertz et al., 2016). Parents are influenced by their child's behavior, and, in turn, parents' skill enhancement reduces children's and youths' problem behavior (Dishion, Nelson, & Kavanagh, 2003; Wang, Dishion, Stormshak, & Willett, 2011). The implication of the model is that motivation and support to improve parenting skills and reduce co-occurring child aggressive behavior can reduce the long-term negative impact of parenting skill deficits and children's behavior problems by enhancing self-regulation skills and behavioral competence indicators, thereby decreasing the risks of developing aggressive behavior problems at home and at school that can last a lifetime.

A review of all family-based treatments for aggression, which have been developed over decades of research and represent a wide range of disciplines and practices, from family systems approaches to individual therapy, is outside the scope of this chapter. It is essential to note, however, that the challenge common to many of these treatments involves reaching parents and families in the community to provide services, especially underserved populations who are less likely to have contact with medical professionals and community health services (Kazdin & Rabbitt, 2013). As a result, the most effective approaches to prevention and treatment with this population tend to include partnering with families and schools, either by delivering the treatment or by coordinating across contexts in which the treatment will occur (Paternite, 2005; Rones & Hoagwood, 2000) to create consistency across settings and engage key stakeholders (Crosnoe, 2015). In early childhood, effective prevention involves direct service to families either in the context of home visiting models or coordinated through early intervention programs, such as Head Start

(Culp, Hubbs-Tait, Culp, & Starost, 2000). Thus this chapter focuses on family-centered approaches for the treatment of aggression and related problem behaviors that link family-based treatment with school-based service delivery.

Main Issues

Challenges to Implementing School-Based Services for Families

Children and adolescents with problem behavior at school are at risk for a variety of difficulties, including poor academic achievement, poor school attendance, school dropout, depression, and substance use (DeShazo Barry, Lyman, & Klinger, 2002; Henry, Knight, & Thornberry, 2012), all of which can be challenging for teachers and school administrators to address. Unfortunately, most children do not receive the services they need in schools, and schools are not well equipped to handle the range and levels of problem behavior among typical children and adolescents. For example, the latest Youth Risk Behavior Survey suggests that among 10- to 17-year-olds, 30% report feeling sad or hopeless, 22% report having been in a physical fight, and 20% report being bullied at school (Kann et al., 2016). Conservative estimates suggest that about 20% of students at school have at least one mental health problem, with only 1 in 5 of these students receiving the services they need to succeed in school, delivered within either the school context or by community health providers (Kataoka, Zhang, & Wells, 2002). That said, schools are an ideal location in which to implement evidence-based prevention and intervention programs to address problem behaviors because youth spend a considerable amount of time at school and families tend to be connected to schools, especially in early childhood (Dishion, 2011). Furthermore, parent involvement in schools predicts a variety of positive outcomes for youth, including enhanced achievement and behavioral outcomes (Hill & Tyson, 2009). The World Health Organization Centre for Public Health (2009) and the Centers for Disease Control and Prevention (2012) promote school settings as particularly important for treatments that address and improve outcomes for child and adolescent health by engaging parents in their children's learning, behavior, and mental health. Moreover, using schools as service delivery settings may increase opportunities to provide health services to underserved populations, such as rural populations, low-income families, and ethnically diverse youth. As such, local, state, and federal policies have increasingly called for the use of evidence-based practices to reduce problem behavior in school settings. Because parents typically wait for schools to initiate contact (Christenson & Reschly, 2010; Davies, 1991), using the school setting as the primary avenue to engage parents in evidence-based prevention and intervention is appropriate. After parents and school faculty are engaged in problem solving, the design and delivery of coordinated, scoped, and sequenced implementation across settings can occur (Smolkowski et al., 2017).

Yet despite these clear benefits of school-based health programs, challenges remain. Schools often lack the infrastructure and technical assistance necessary to systematically and effectively support children and adolescents who have academic, behavioral, and mental health concerns (Flannery, Fenning, Kato, & McIntosh, 2014; Ringeisen, Henderson, & Hoagwood, 2003). Multiple barriers, such as time, money, staff turnover, and competing priorities, limit the ability of schools to implement interventions that involve families and sustain these interventions over time (Forman, Olin, Hoagwood, Crowe, & Saka, 2009; Fosco et al., 2014), making most interventions that target parenting practices unrealistic for many schools (Christenson, 2004), despite their proven efficacy. Given the difficult economic situation currently facing educational systems in the United States, a cost-effective means of improving student success rates that is efficient and effective, realistic, and does not require extensive school staff time to implement with fidelity is needed to enhance partnerships with schools. A family-centered approach to prevention and treatment with schools is effective (Power et al., 2012) and may yield cost savings if school personnel can be trained in the model and implement these programs with little resources or external support (Spoth, Guyll, & Day, 2002).

Conceptual Models: Home–School Connections

A judicious approach to treating aggression and related problem behaviors in childhood and adolescence is to foster connections across home and school (Crosnoe, 2015) so that children experience their key settings as consistent and predictable. There are many conceptual models that describe how to engage families and school staff together to address aggression and related problem behaviors and support children's appropriate behavior (Epstein, 1995; Fantuzzo, Tighe, & Childs, 2000; Garbacz et al., 2016), many of which have been validated across cultures (Garbacz & Sheridan, 2011) and school levels (Fosco et al., 2014; Manz, Fantuzzo, & Power, 2004). These models share a common framework that includes (1) using empirically validated parenting strategies at home that are connected with school systems, (2) supporting children's behavior at school, and (3) establishing connections across strategies used at home and at school.

Use of empirically validated parenting strategies at home is essential to effective family management (Patterson, 1982), and these strategies have been consistently associated with lower rates of aggression and antisocial behavior (Stormshak et al., 2011). Outcomes can be maximized for children when the empirically validated strategies adopted at home are connected with empirically validated strategies at school. Schoolwide positive behavioral interventions and supports (SWPBIS; Sugai & Horner, 2002) is a schoolwide system that closely resembles effective family management. In SWPBIS, the emphasis is on proactive support for children's behavior (Walker et al., 1996) delivered in a multilevel fashion so that children receive the level of support most closely matched with their needs. Through connecting the multilevel empirically validated SWPBIS strategies at school with effective family management at home, children in elementary school (Garbacz et al., 2016) and middle school (Fosco et al., 2014) will receive consistent and positive support to prevent and address behavior problems.

Engaging families and school staff together in schoolwide systems such as SWPBIS integrates family culture into the schoolwide systems, establishes shared governance in school decisions, and facilitates a connection to practices that families use at home (Garbacz et al., 2016). Many families may not be using empirically validated parenting strategies, but schoolwide behavioral support practices may easily transfer to homes. Thus engaging families in effective schoolwide systems may serve as a vehicle to implement effective family management at home (Garbacz et al., 2016). To facilitate connections across home and school, schoolwide systems that support children's behavior should reflect family cultural and linguistic values, beliefs, and preferences (Mapp & Hong, 2010). For example, schools can use two-way communication to examine and discuss behavior expectations across settings to make modifications based on family values (Leverson, Smith, McIntosh, Rose, & Pinkelman, 2016). This may be accomplished by using shared governance to include families in decision making (Walker, Shenker, & Hoover-Dempsey, 2010). For example, family members can be on school teams, a school can consistently communicate with the parent–teacher organization, and families can be polled at important decision points throughout the year.

Key considerations for engaging families in schoolwide systems are derived from family centeredness. *Family centeredness* suggests that schools use respectful, flexible, and responsive strategies with families (Dunst, 2002). It also indicates that families should be fully informed so that they can make appropriate decisions for their children (Dunst, 2002). For example, when addressing behavior concerns for an individual student, school staff should discuss with families all available options, their appropriateness, and possible outcomes. When families are made aware of options and possible outcomes, they are better equipped to partner with school faculty and make informed decisions about their children's education and behavior planning. At the schoolwide level, families should be active participants with school staff to create systems and practices that reflect family culture, values and beliefs, and language preferences. Furthermore, school staff will find it useful to use a strengths-based view of family capabilities and tailor practices to meet family needs (Dunst, Trivette, & Hamby, 2007).

Effective communication is the foundation for home–school connections to address aggression and related problem behaviors and to support children's positive behavior (Christenson & Sheridan, 2001). To ensure that all families are provided equal access (Mapp & Hong, 2010), multidirectional communication (Sheridan, Rispoli, & Holmes, 2014) should be used so families and school staff can each easily initiate contacts and information can flow back and forth. Informing families of a practice via a school newsletter would be insufficient, for example. Families should have an opportunity to respond to information in multiple ways, such as in person, by telephone, or through an email. When effective communication is used and families are included in school decisions, uptake of consistent, empirically validated practices across home and school can increase the likelihood that children and adolescents will be supported by consistent, predictable, and effective strategies.

Theoretical Considerations

The Ecological Model

The ecological theoretical model provides a foundation for the assessment and treatment of aggression and related problem behaviors. Ecological theory emphasizes the importance of a child's nested environments and the interactions between them as pivotal for child development (Bronfenbrenner, 1977). Overarching socio-cultural systems provide a vital lens through which to view and understand child development, but a child's immediate environments, such as home and school, influence his or her day-to-day learning and development. For example, changes in education policy can influence the design and implementation of practices to support children's behavior in school. Effective proximal support for children is necessary within each environment. In addition, if immediate environments are linked, children can experience consistency and congruence in behavior support practices across home and school.

Interconnections among Systems

In the ecological model, the mesosystem is of particular importance to treating behavior problems. The mesosystem consists of the interconnections among the microsystems in a child's life, which hold substantial relevance for the development of behavior problems (Bronfenbrenner, 1979). In this view a child's behavior is best considered within the broader interconnected set of systems that support it (Gutkin, 2012). This view underscores the usefulness of connecting behavior support systems at home and school and engaging families and school staff together as partners (Reschly & Christenson, 2012). By coordinating treatment across home and school, parents and teachers can align their practices so that children experience two of their primary settings as consistent and predictable. In fact, in the context of an intervention for children with behavior concerns, the parent–teacher relationship was found to be partially responsible for improvements in child behavior (Sheridan et al., 2012).

Parenting and Self-Regulation

It is clear that enhancing parenting skills has direct effects on sustained problem behavior and aggression and on a host of other related outcomes, such as depression, achievement, and social skills (Fosco, Van Ryzin, Connell, & Stormshak, 2016; Stormshak et al., 2011). However, the link between improved parenting skills and reduced child problem behavior involves multiple intermediate steps and targets. One important mechanism of change in children's behavior is self-regulation skills. Self-regulation is a core component of most health models and is a central feature of several early childhood problems that affect learning at school, including ADHD, impaired social relationships, and aggression and related problem behaviors (Blair & Raver, 2015; Blair, Ursache, Greenberg, & Vernon-Feagans, 2015). Research has made major advances in understanding the many developmental influences on self-regulation, including neurocognitive and biological mechanisms (Bryck & Fisher, 2012) and the family context in which self-regulation is promoted and supported by parents from early to middle childhood (Eisenberg et al., 2003, 2005). Extensive research has shown that early risk factors, such as poverty and contextual stress, affect parenting skills and long-term self-regulation, which are disrupted through cumulative stress across multiple contexts, including family and community (Evans & Kim, 2013). These studies have confirmed that contextual stress and parenting skill deficits are linked to youth behavioral outcomes via level of early self-regulation skills, such as sustained attention, memory, and planning, during the elementary school years.

Although the relationship between parenting skills and the development of self-regulatory skills has been well established, there are specific parenting skills that seem to be clearly associated with regulated behavior in children. For example, establishing behavioral routines at home by using limit setting, clear rules, parental control, and predictable family events helps solidify these skills in children (Karreman, van Tuijl, van Aken, & Deković, 2006). Parents' emotional regulation and modeling of appropriate emotional control also affect children's development of self-regulation (Bariola, Gullone, & Hughes, 2011). Parents who emphasize positive parenting through proactive structuring, identifying expectations, and positive support of their children enhance self-regulation and behavioral control (Bernier, Carlson, & Whipple, 2010). Parents can also work in partnership with school personnel to establish predictable cross-setting routines that encourage positive behavior, such as homework completion and positive social skills. These socialization strategies in the home support engagement in effortful attention control and promote the strengthening and refinement of self-regulation from childhood through adolescence (Bariola et al., 2011). Parent interventions have shown direct effects on self-regulation and related behavior in early childhood, including negative emotionality, inhibitory control, and behavioral control, all of which are directly related to a profile of aggressive behavior (Blair, 2002; Chang, Shaw, Dishion, Gardner, & Wilson, 2014; Fosco, Frank, Stormshak, & Dishion, 2013; Stormshak, DeGarmo, Chronister, & Caruthers, 2018). In the context of a family-centered approach to assessment and treatment, improvements in self-regulation are linked to a reduced risk for growth in antisocial behavior (Fosco et al., 2013).

Measures and Methods

Two important considerations for measuring and assessing behavior problems are that (1) family-based interventions to treat behavior problems are often implemented within a larger service delivery model, and (2) children and adolescents frequently exhibit behavior problems across settings. These considerations require a particular approach to assessment. Because family-based interventions are often implemented within a larger service delivery model (e.g., SWPBIS, the Family Check-Up), there are two components to assess (Sheridan et al., 2014): the process or procedures used and the actual intervention steps that are designed and implemented to decrease aggression and improve adaptive skills. Measuring the process used to identify intervention components to be used with children and the actual intervention steps is necessary to draw inferences about behavior change (Strickland-Cohen & Horner, 2014). The assessment of these two components provides treatment integrity data for the process and the intervention. *Treatment integrity* refers to the degree to which treatments are delivered as intended (Sechrest, West, Phillips, Redner, & Yeaton, 1979). Treatment integrity is critical to assess in applied settings, such as homes and schools, with respect to the environment and the interventionist (McIntyre, Gresham, DiGennaro, & Reed, 2007). Both components should be assessed using multiple dimensions, including adherence, dosage, quality, participant responsiveness, and program differentiation (Dane & Schneider, 1998; O'Donnell, 2008).

Children often exhibit behavior problems across settings, including their primary settings of home and school (Achenbach, McConaughy, & Howell, 1987). This pattern necessitates assessing treatment integrity, as well as outcomes across settings. A multisource, multisetting, multimethod data collection strategy (Pereplet-chikova, Hilt, Chereji, & Kazdin, 2009) ensures that all relevant data are tracked. Data sources can include family members, teachers, administrators, and other key stakeholders involved in the treatment process or the delivery of the intervention. Outcome data and treatment integrity for the intervention should be collected in all settings in which the intervention is implemented. Baseline (pretreatment) data are essential to establish a response pattern. Methods of data collection can include direct observations, permanent records and by-products of the intervention (e.g., sticker charts that show intervention steps completed; Sheridan, Swanger-Gagné, Welch, Kwon, & Garbacz, 2009), and parent and teacher ratings of the outcome.

It is also prudent to use a universal screening approach to assessment (Dowdy et al., 2015) to accurately identify children and adolescents with unmet mental health needs (Kataoka et al., 2002). Within a population-based system of prevention (Gutkin, 2012), systems such as schools use universal screening so that children and adolescents can be linked with appropriate interventions based on their need (Dowdy et al., 2015). Universal screening systems are increasingly common, but it is less common to include family members and the home setting. However, when family members provide information about their child's behavior, a more complete picture of the child's needs is established, which allows staff to provide ecologically based behavior supports and readily engage in proactive outreach (Moore et al., 2016).

Central Research Findings

Conjoint Behavioral Consultation

Conjoint behavioral consultation (CBC; Sheridan & Kratochwill, 2008) is an indirect service delivery model wherein a consultant works with a parent and teacher to address behavior problems within and across settings. Through CBC, a common and clear understanding of presenting concerns is reached; data are collected, reviewed, and analyzed; goals are set based on data; treatment plans are designed and implemented in homes and schools; and progress is evaluated relative to the data-based goals set at the outset of the process.

CBC includes four stages: needs identification, needs analysis, plan implementation, and plan evaluation. During needs identification, a parent, teacher, and consultant meet together to review strengths and presenting concerns, operationally define target behaviors for the home and school setting, and develop a plan for collecting data about the target behaviors. The parent, teacher, and consultant meet again during needs analysis to examine baseline data collected in the home and school, set data-based goals, discuss environmental contingencies (antecedents, sequential behaviors, consequences), and develop a function-based behavior support plan based on environmental contingencies reviewed during the meeting. In addition to discussing environmental contingencies during the meeting, data may also be gathered about environmental contingencies and plotted for the parent, teacher, and consultant to review (Eckert, Martens, & DiGennaro, 2005).

During plan implementation, the function-based behavior support plans are implemented in homes and schools. In addition, the home and school plans are connected to coordinate implementation (Kelley & McCain, 1995). Parents and teachers are the natural treatment agents who implement plans, but the consultant provides support to promote implementation at fidelity. For example, consultants model the plan (Catania, Almeida, Liu-Constant, & DiGennaro Reed, 2009), provide *in vivo* coaching while a parent or teacher implements the plan (LaFleur, Witt, Naquin, Harwell, & Gilbertson, 1998), and deliver performance feedback (Sanetti, Luiselli, & Handler, 2007). The parent, teacher, and consultant meet during the plan evaluation interview to review data collected about child behavior after implementation and examine those data in comparison with baseline data (Kratochwill et al., 2010) relative to goals. If goals are met, the intervention can be transferred to other settings or faded. If goals are not met, the parent, teacher, and consultant may make modifications to the plan, implement the revised plan, and reassess progress toward goals at a second plan evaluation meeting.

As described in the preceding "Measures and Methods" section, data collected during the CBC process pertain to the procedures of CBC, the intervention steps implemented in the home and school, and child behavior. Multimethod, multisource, and multisetting data (Perepletchikova et al., 2009) are gathered to provide a complete picture of the process, the intervention, and child outcomes. Research that has examined CBC indicates that the process is consistently implemented at fidelity and that parents and teachers typically implement behavior support plans in homes and schools at fidelity (Garbacz & McIntyre, 2016). An examination of CBC outcomes has indicated positive effects for children, parents, and the parent–teacher relationship. Relative to children in a control condition, children whose parents and teachers participated in CBC demonstrated reductions in behavior problems (Sheridan, Ryoo, Garbacz, Kunz, & Chumney, 2013) and improvements in appropriate behavior (Sheridan et al., 2012). Relative to parents in a control condition, parents in the CBC condition improved their competence in problem solving. Finally, teachers who participated in CBC reported improvements in the parent–teacher relationship (Sheridan et al., 2012). In fact, the teacher-rated parent–teacher relationship partially mediated the effects of CBC on child adaptive skills and social skills (Sheridan et al., 2012). In a follow-up study, communication, and in particular congruent communication across parents and teachers based on teacher report, was identified as particularly important in the context of CBC for children's social skills (Garbacz, Sheridan, Koziol, Kwon, & Holmes, 2015). This is important because inadequate social skills may place children at risk for peer rejection and subsequent problem behaviors (Patterson, DeBaryshe, & Ramsey, 1990).

The Family Check-Up and Positive Family Support Model

The Family Check-Up (FCU; Dishion & Stormshak, 2007) was originally developed as an intervention to reduce aggression and related problem behavior and to prevent the onset of substance use in middle school youth during the transition to high school. As a school-based, family-centered intervention, the FCU has been tested across a number of efficacy trials, primarily delivered in schools, to reduce the risk of problem behavior, aggression, substance use, and a variety of other risk outcomes that impair healthy adult development. Results have been widely published and suggest that the FCU reduces problem behavior, aggression, family conflict, depression, substance use, affiliation with deviant peers, and risky sexual behavior (Dishion, Kavanagh, Schneiger, Nelson, & Kaufman, 2002; Fosco et al., 2013; Stormshak et al., 2011; Van Ryzin, Stormshak, & Dishion, 2012). The FCU in early childhood enhances and supports parenting skills, and these skills lead to reductions in later risk behavior, positive school achievement, improved self-regulation, and reductions in maternal depression (Chang et al., 2014; Reuben, Shaw, Brennan, Dishion, & Wilson, 2015). As such, the FCU has been shown to be a successful, evidence-based intervention for the treatment of aggression and related problem behaviors across multiple efficacy trials during the past 20 years.

In 2009 the FCU was adapted into an intervention called Positive Family Support (PFS; Dishion, Fosco, Moore, Falkenstein, & Stormshak, 2015). PFS is an adapted version of behavioral parenting training for integration into the public middle school setting and potentially other service settings that have regular and repeated contact with families (Dishion & Stormshak, 2007). The goal was to support schools in dissemination and implementation of the FCU with a model of the intervention adapted to their contexts, resources, and needs. The PFS intervention model comprises three major components: (1) a family resource center housed in the school that provides information about schoolwide discipline, rules, parenting skills, and behavioral support; (2) a check-in, check-out schoolwide behavior planning intervention that connects student behavior at home and at school; and (3) a brief version of the FCU delivered by school staff. A key feature of PFS is that it is assessment driven, tailored to the needs of youth and families, and delivered by staff in the school (Dishion & Stormshak, 2007; Stormshak & Dishion, 2002). The FCU, a core component of the PFS approach, specifically targets family management and socialization practices in early adolescence to reduce and prevent the onset of problem behavior and to increase academic success.

To adapt the FCU model to schools, our research team simplified the FCU to support uptake by school personnel. First, videotaping of family interactions was removed from the protocol, and the parent and teacher ratings form used to provide feedback to parents was shortened. The PFS model used a modified and brief version of the family assessment appropriate to schools that included a focus on homework completion, achievement, and school behavior problems. The intervention could then be completed in one session with a parent by school staff, in contrast to the minimum 3 hours of contact of the FCU used in efficacy studies (initial interview, assessment session, and feedback session; see Dishion & Stormshak, 2007). Parent management training was reduced to include three sessions particularly relevant to school staff, with content that incorporated positive behavior support to increase academic engagement, limit setting and monitoring, and relationship building through negotiating conflict and family problem solving.

The PFS project (funded by the Institute of Education Sciences [IES] as a Goal 4 effectiveness study built upon prior evidence of efficacy) was successful in many ways and helped develop the FCU into a feasible intervention for delivery in schools. The PFS model was most successful with at-risk youths; among the top 15–25% of students at risk for behavior problems, those in intervention schools outperformed those in control schools on student-reported parental monitoring and emotional problems and on parent-reported negative school contacts (Smolkowski et al., 2017). When we examined fidelity of implementation, we found that schools with high fidelity had supportive administrators, stable staffing, and higher levels of family-centered support at the schools (Dishion et al., 2016). Unfortunately, our efforts to implement the PFS project in schools were hampered by a number of extraneous events, including the recession and school budget cuts, limited staffing, labor disputes between teachers and administrators, and a general lack of infrastructure in schools to support uptake of the model (Stormshak et al., 2016).

Implications

One of the biggest challenges to the field of prevention is the translation of research to practice, and the treatment of problem behavior and aggression is the most pervasive example reported in the literature. For the most part, studies have supported efficacy trials that examine outcomes associated with a variety of family-centered approaches to treatment. Many of these treatments were housed in schools, but once support from the research programs ended, very few continued to be successfully disseminated in schools. This led to a more systematic approach to dissemination and implementation of school-based programs that has been examined across several studies.

Literature pertaining to the diffusion, implementation, and sustainability of school-based, evidence-based interventions is sparse and leaves schools with little strategic support regarding their use (Feldstein & Glasgow, 2008). Additional research has found that evidence-based programs implemented outside of controlled trials are generally not executed to proficient levels of quality (Dusenbury, Brannigan, Hansen, Walsh, & Falco, 2005; Gottfredson & Gottfredson, 2002). This is unfortunate because program fidelity is strongly linked to positive intervention outcomes, including parenting skills and child behavior (Durlak & DuPre, 2008; Smith, Dishion, Shaw, & Wilson, 2013). A more systematic understanding of how to effectively and accurately implement evidence-based, family–school partnership interventions in school settings is needed to ensure successful student outcomes (Greenberg, Domitrovich, Graczyk, & Zins, 2001). The processes through which evidence-based practices are adopted, implemented, and sustained at the school level should be a priority for future funding and research efforts (Spoth et al., 2013). One example of this approach is exemplified by the PROSPER (Promoting School–Community–University Partnerships to Enhance Resilience) program, an evidence-based system for implementing family-focused and school-based interventions (Chilenski, Ang, Greenberg, Feinberg, & Spoth, 2014; Spoth et al., 2013). By linking evidence-based prevention with extension systems at land grant universities and public school systems, PROSPER provides a model for partnership that helps schools adapt and sustain prevention programs. The PROSPER model has enhanced community participation, cost-effectiveness, implementation of evidence-based programs, and sustainability of these programs over time, while reducing youth substance abuse (Chilenski et al, 2014; Spoth et al., 2013). As a consequence of PROSPER, community stakeholders have increased and expanded their knowledge of evidence-based programming, implementation of these programs in communities, and evaluation of implementation efforts (Crowley, Greenberg, Feinberg, Spoth, & Redmond, 2012).

Future Directions

Family-centered interventions to treat aggression and related problem behavior are at an important juncture. Theoretical models position homes and schools, and connections between them, as the immediate systems that can provide proximal support to prevent and address behavior problems (Bronfenbrenner, 1977, 1979). Experimental research underscores these theoretical models and demonstrates the strength of bringing together families and educators to implement evidence-based practices to prevent and address behavior problems and promote educational engagement (Dishion et al., 2002; Sheridan et al., 2012; Stormshak et al., 2011; Van Ryzin et al., 2012). Now is the time to invest in scalable family-centered efforts to improve systems-level adoption of these efficacious programs in schools and communities. Based on the lines of work reviewed in this chapter, the following future directions are offered.

At the macrosystem level, policy investments are needed to provide school districts with the resources necessary to embed family-centered programs within their existing systems. As Stormshak and colleagues (2016) showed, adoption, implementation, and maintenance (Feldstein & Glasgow, 2008) are linked with social and economic climates, as well as with educational policy. The Every Student Succeeds Act (2015) calls for an increase in efforts for schools to partner with families to support children. Leveraging policies such as this to establish capacity within school districts for family-centered priorities is critical. Figure 17.1 is a conceptual diagram of macrosystemic influences on the core components of family-centered treatments for behavior problems. Family management, home–school connections, and school and community engagement are components of family-centered treatment programs and are influenced by the broader systems.

In preservice training programs, an emphasis on ecological approaches and family-centered services is necessary. In response to decades of research demonstrating the importance of family-centered treatments, school staff have adopted and implemented a wide range of approaches to engage families in their children's care. However, many common school-based approaches (Manz et al., 2004), such as inviting families to volunteer in schools and chaperone class trips, are unlikely to lead to coordinated implementation of evidence-based practices across home and school. Furthermore, there are many barriers to adopting family engagement programs (Christenson, 2004; Forman et al., 2009). Some school staff and other service providers may not be equipped to handle challenges associated with implementing evidence-based, family-centered practices. By modifying preservice training programs with an orientation toward ecological systems of care, we can establish the capacity within systems to adopt and implement family-centered programs.

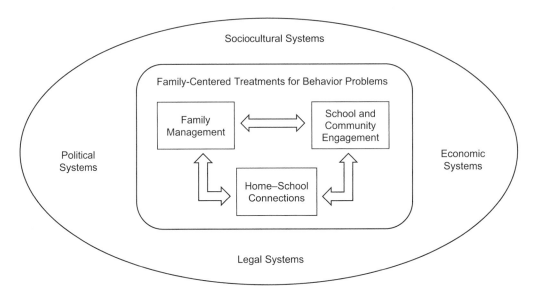

FIGURE 17.1. Ecological factors and components of family-centered treatments for behavior problems.

   Planning stages of implementation is central to a discussion of scalable efforts to improve adoption, implementation, and maintenance of family-centered efforts in schools. Stages of implementation include exploration and adoption, program installation, initial implementation, full operation, innovation, and sustainability (Fixsen, Naoom, Blase, Friedman, & Wallace, 2005). Defining exploration and adoption is a priority for family-centered services. For example, it is currently unknown what prerequisite conditions are necessary to support installation and initial implementation. Models such as the Practical, Robust, Implementation and Sustainability Model (Feldstein & Glasgow, 2008) can provide guidance, but increased specification is needed for family-centered treatments. For example, it is necessary to determine whether an organization has achieved readiness before proceeding with installation. The building blocks for family-centered program readiness are available (Christenson & Sheridan, 2001; Fosco et al., 2014), but the components of readiness have not been empirically identified. Research is needed to identify components of family-centered program readiness.
   Durlak and DuPre (2008) note that a balance of fidelity and adaptation is essential to implementing evidence-based practices in applied settings. Three key future directions thus emerge: First, implementation of the program must be comprehensively measured and reported. In the absence of implementation data, the nature of program delivery is unknown and impact is limited. Second, research is needed that identifies active ingredients, core elements, and mechanisms of change. For family-centered intervention research, improving parental monitoring and the parent–teacher relationship has emerged as a critical mechanism of change. More research is needed to ascertain core elements of programs to guide later adaptation. Third, incorporating data that measure usability and feasibility (Lane et al., 2009), as well as cultural fit, is necessary to inform future adoption and implementation efforts.

Conclusions

Engaging systems and stakeholders to support children is the cornerstone of family-based treatments to prevent and address behavior problems. Ecological theory provides a model to guide assessment and treatment. Decades of family-centered research demonstrate that we can prevent escalation in behavior problems and address current problems by engaging families and other key stakeholders to implement evidence-based practices. This juncture in family-centered research represents an important opportunity to invest in family-centered efforts in key domains, such as policy and preservice training, to support effectiveness research and scaled dissemination.

ACKNOWLEDGMENTS

We gratefully acknowledge research funding from the U.S. Department of Education, Institute of Education Sciences (Grant No. R305A140189), to Elizabeth A. Stormshak.

REFERENCES

Achenbach, T. M., McConaughy, S. H., & Howell, C. T. (1987). Child/adolescent behavioral and emotional problems: Implications of cross-informant correlations for situational specificity. *Psychological Bulletin, 101,* 213–232.

Ackerman, B. P., Brown, E. D., & Izard, C. E. (2004). The relations between contextual risk, earned income, and the school adjustment of children from economically disadvantaged families. *Developmental Psychology, 40,* 204–216.

Bariola, E., Gullone, E., & Hughes, E. K. (2011). Child and adolescent emotion regulation: The role of parental emotion regulation and expression. *Clinical Child and Family Psychology Review, 14*(2), 198–212.

Bernier, A., Carlson, S. M., & Whipple, N. (2010). From external regulation to self-regulation: Early parenting precursors of young children's executive functioning. *Child Development, 81,* 326–339.

Blair, C. (2002). School readiness: Integrating cognition and emotion in a neurobiological conceptualization of children's functioning at school entry. *American Psychologist, 57*(2), 111–127.

Blair, C., & Raver, C. C. (2015). School readiness and self-regulation: A developmental psychobiological approach. *Annual Review of Psychology, 66,* 711–731.

Blair, C., Ursache, A., Greenberg, M., & Vernon-Feagans, L. (2015). Multiple aspects of self-regulation uniquely predict mathematics but not letter–word knowledge in the early elementary grades. *Developmental Psychology, 51*(4), 459–472.

Bronfenbrenner, U. (1977). Toward an experimental ecology of human development. *American Psychologist, 32,* 513–531.

Bronfenbrenner, U. (1979). Contexts of child rearing: Problems and prospects. *American Psychologist, 34,* 844–850.

Bryck, R. L., & Fisher, P. A. (2012). Training the brain: Practical applications of neural plasticity from the intersection of cognitive neuroscience, developmental psychology, and prevention science. *American Psychologist, 67*(2), 87–100.

Catania, C. N., Almeida, D., Liu-Constant, B., & DiGennaro Reed, F. D. (2009). Video modeling to train staff to implement discrete-trial instruction. *Journal of Applied Behavior Analysis, 42,* 387–392.

Centers for Disease Control and Prevention. (2012). *Parent engagement: Strategies for involving parents in school health.* Atlanta, GA: U.S. Department of Health and Human Services.

Chang, H., Shaw, D. S., Dishion, T. J., Gardner, F., & Wilson, M. N. (2014). Direct and indirect effects of the Family Check-Up on self-regulation from toddlerhood to early school-age. *Journal of Abnormal Child Psychology, 42,* 1117–1128.

Chilenski, S. M., Ang, P. M., Greenberg, M. T., Feinberg, M. E., & Spoth, R. L. (2014). The impact of a prevention delivery system on perceived social capital: The PROSPER Project. *Prevention Science, 15,* 125–137.

Christenson, S. L. (2004). The family–school partnership: An opportunity to promote the learning competence of all students. *School Psychology Review, 33,* 83–104.

Christenson, S. L., & Reschly, A. R. (2010). Preface. In S. L. Christenson & A. L. Reschly (Eds.), *Handbook of school–family partnerships* (pp. xiii–xvii). New York: Routledge.

Christenson, S. L., & Sheridan, S. M. (2001). *Schools and families: Creating essential connections for learning.* New York: Guilford Press.

Conduct Problems Prevention Research Group. (2014). Trajectories of risk for early sexual activity and early substance use in the Fast Track prevention program. *Prevention Science, 15*(S1), S33–S46.

Crosnoe, R. (2015). Continuities and consistencies across home and school systems. In S. M. Sheridan & E. M. Kim (Eds.), *Processes and pathways of family–school partnerships across development* (pp. 61–80). New York: Springer.

Crowley, D., Greenberg, M., Feinberg, M., Spoth, R., & Redmond, C. (2012). The effect of the PROSPER partnership model on cultivating local stakeholder knowledge of evidence-based programs: A five-year longitudinal study of 28 communities. *Prevention Science, 13*(1), 96–105.

Culp, A. M., Hubbs-Tait, L., Culp, R. E., & Starost, H.-J. (2000). Maternal parenting characteristics and school involvement: Predictors of kindergarten cognitive competence among Head Start children. *Journal of Research in Childhood Education, 15*(1), 5–17.

Dane, A. V., & Schneider, B. H. (1998). Program integrity in primary and early secondary prevention: Are implementation effects out of control? *Clinical Psychology Review, 18,* 23–24.

Davies, D. (1991). Schools reaching out: Family, school, and community partnerships for student success. *Phi Delta Kappan, 72,* 376–382.

DeShazo Barry, T., Lyman, R. D., & Klinger, L. G. (2002). Academic underachievement and attention-deficit/hyperactivity disorder: The negative impact of symptom severity on school performance. *Journal of School Psychology, 40*(3), 259–283.

Dishion, T. J. (2011). Promoting academic competence and behavioral health in public schools: A strategy of systemic concatenation of empirically based intervention principles [Special issue]. *School Psychology Review, 40*(4), 590–597.

Dishion, T. J., Fosco, G. M., Moore, K., Falkenstein, C., & Stormshak, E. A. (2015). *Positive Family Support manual.* Unpublished manual, University of Oregon Prevention Science Institute.

Dishion, T. J., Garbacz, A., Seeley, J. R., Kim, H., Stormshak, B., Moore, K., et al. (2016). *Translational research on evidence-based parenting support within public schools: Strategies, challenges and potential solutions.* Manuscript submitted for publication.

Dishion, T. J., Kavanagh, K., Schneiger, A., Nelson, S., & Kaufman, N. (2002). Preventing early adolescent substance use: A family-centered strategy for public middle school [Special issue]. *Prevention Science, 3,* 191–201.

Dishion, T. J., & McMahon, R. J. (1998). Parental monitoring and the prevention of child and adolescent problem behavior: A conceptual and empirical formulation. *Clinical Child and Family Psychology Review, 1,* 61–75.

Dishion, T. J., Nelson, S. E., & Kavanagh, K. (2003). The Family Check-Up with high-risk young adolescents: Preventing early-onset substance use by parent monitoring [Special issue]. *Behavior Therapy, 34,* 553–571.

Dishion, T. J., & Stormshak, E. A. (2007). *Intervening in children's lives: An ecological, family-centered approach to mental health care.* Washington, DC: American Psychological Association.

Dowdy, E., Furlong, M., Raines, T. C., Bovery, B., Kauffman, B., Kamphaus, R. W., et al. (2015). Enhancing school-based mental health services with a preventive and promotive approach to universal screening for complete mental health. *Journal of Educational and Psychological Consultation, 25,* 178–197.

Dunst, C. J. (2002). Family-centered practices: Birth through high school. *Journal of Special Education, 36,* 139–147.

Dunst, C. J., Trivette, C. M., & Hamby, D. W. (2007). Meta-analysis of family-centered helpgiving practices research. *Mental Retardation and Developmental Disabilities Research Reviews, 13,* 370–378.

Durlak, J. A., & DuPre, E. P. (2008). Implementation matters: A review of research on the influence of implementation on program outcomes and the factors affecting implementation. *American Journal of Community Psychology, 41,* 327–350.

Dusenbury, L., Brannigan, R., Hansen, W. B., Walsh, J., & Falco, M. (2005). Quality of implementation: Developing measures crucial to understanding the diffusion of preventive interventions. *Health Education Research, 20*(3), 308–313.

Eckert, T. L., Martens, B. K., & DiGennaro, F. D. (2005). Describing antecedent–behavior–consequence relations using conditional probabilities and the general operant contingency space: A preliminary investigation. *School Psychology Review, 34,* 520–528.

Eisenberg, N., Zhou, Q., Losoya, S. H., Fabes, R. A., Shepard, S. A., Murphy, B. C., et al. (2003). The relations of parenting, effortful control, and ego control to children's emotional expressivity. *Child Development, 74,* 875–895.

Eisenberg, N., Zhou, Q., Spinrad, T. L., Valiente, C., Fabes, R. A., & Liew, J. (2005). Relations among positive parenting, children's effortful control, and externalizing problems: A three-wave longitudinal study. *Child Development, 76*(5), 1055–1071.

Epstein, J. L. (1995). School/family/community partnerships: Caring for the children we share. *Phi Delta Kappan, 76,* 701–712.

Evans, G. W., & Kim, P. (2013). Childhood poverty, chronic stress, self-regulation, and coping. *Child Development Perspectives, 7*(1), 43–48.

Every Student Succeeds Act of 2015, 20 U.S.C. § 1177 (2015).

Fantuzzo, J., Tighe, E., & Childs, S. (2000). Family involvement questionnaire: A multivariate assessment of family participation in early childhood education. *Journal of Educational Psychology, 9,* 367–376.

Feldstein, A. C., & Glasgow, R. E. (2008). A practical, robust implementation and sustainability model (PRISM). *Joint Commission Journal on Quality and Patient Safety, 34,* 228–243.

Fixsen, D. L., Naoom, S. F., Blase, K. A., Friedman, R. M., & Wallace, F. (2005). *Implementation research: A synthesis of the literature* (FMHI Publication No. 231). Tampa: Florida Mental Health Institute, National Implementation Research Network.

Flannery, K. B., Fenning, P., Kato, M. M., & McIntosh, K. (2014). Effects of school-wide positive behavioral interventions and supports and fidelity of implementation on problem behavior in high schools. *School Psychology Quarterly, 29*(2), 111–124.

Forman, S. G., Olin, S. S., Hoagwood, K. E., Crowe, M., & Saka, N. (2009). Evidence-based interventions in schools: Developers' views of implementation barriers and facilitators. *School Mental Health, 1*(1), 26–36.

Fosco, G. M., Frank, J. L., Stormshak, E. A., & Dishion, T. J. (2013). Opening the "black box": Family Check-Up intervention effects on self-regulation that prevents growth in problem behavior and substance use. *Journal of School Psychology, 51*(4), 455–468.

Fosco, G. M., Seeley, J. R., Dishion, T. J., Smolkowski, K., Stormshak, E. A., Downey-McCarthy, R., et al. (2014). Lessons learned from scaling up the ecological approach to family interventions and treatment (EcoFIT) program in middle schools. In M. Weist, N. Lever, C. Bradshaw, & J. Owens (Eds.), *Handbook of school mental health* (2nd ed., pp. 237–251). New York: Springer.

Fosco, G. M., Van Ryzin, M. J., Connell, A. M., & Stormshak, E. A. (2016). Preventing adolescent depression with the Family Check-Up: Examining family conflict as a mechanism of change. *Journal of Family Psychology, 30*(1), 82–92.

Garbacz, S. A., McIntosh, K., Eagle, J. W., Dowd-Eagle, S. E., Ruppert, T., & Hirano, K. (2016). Family engagement within schoolwide positive behavioral interventions and supports. *Preventing School Failure: Alternative Education for Children and Youth, 60,* 60–69.

Garbacz, S. A., & McIntyre, L. L. (2016). Conjoint behavioral consultation for children with autism spectrum disorder. *School Psychology Quarterly, 31*(4), 450–466.

Garbacz, S. A., & Sheridan, S. M. (2011). A multidimensional examination of New Zealand family involvement in education. *School Psychology International, 32,* 600–615.

Garbacz, S. A., Sheridan, S. M., Koziol, N. A., Kwon, K., & Holmes, S. R. (2015). Congruence in parent–teacher communication: Implications for the efficacy of CBC for students with behavioral concerns. *School Psychology Review, 44,* 150–168.

Gottfredson, D. C., & Gottfredson, G. D. (2002). Quality of school-based prevention programs: Results from a national survey. *Journal of Research on Crime and Delinquency, 39,* 3–35.

Greenberg, M. T., Domitrovich, C., Graczyk, P., & Zins, J. (2001). *The study of implementation in school-based preventive interventions: Theory, research, and practice.* Washington, DC: U.S. Department of Health and Human Services, Substance Abuse and Mental Health Administration, Center for Mental Health Services.

Gutkin, T. B. (2012). Ecological psychology: Replacing the medical model paradigm for school-based psychological and psychoeducational services. *Journal of Educational and Psychological Consultation, 22,* 1–20.

Henry, K. L., Knight, K. E., & Thornberry, T. P. J. (2012). School disengagement as a predictor of dropout, delinquency, and problem substance use during adolescence and early adulthood. *Youth Adolescence, 41,* 156–166.

Hill, N. E., & Tyson, D. F. (2009). Parental involvement in middle school: A meta-analytic assessment of the strategies that promote achievement. *Developmental Psychology, 45*(3), 740–763.

Kann, L., McManus, T., Harris, W. A., Shanklin, S. L., Flint, K. H., Hawkins, J., et al. (2016). Youth Risk Behavior Surveillance—United States, 2015. *Surveillance Summaries, 65*(6), 1–174.

Karreman, A., van Tuijl, C., van Aken, M. A. G., & Deković, M. (2006), Parenting and self-regulation in preschoolers: A meta-analysis. *Infant and Child Development, 15,* 561–579.

Kataoka, S. H., Zhang, L., & Wells, K. B. (2002). Unmet need for mental health care among US children: Variation by ethnicity and insurance status. *American Journal of Psychiatry, 159*(9), 1548–1555.

Kazdin, A. E., & Rabbitt, S. M. (2013). Novel models for delivering mental health services and reducing the burdens of mental illness. *Clinical Psychological Science, 1*(2), 170–191.

Kelley, M. L., & McCain, A. P. (1995). Promoting academic performance in inattentive children: The relative efficacy of school–home notes with and without response cost. *Behavior Modification, 19,* 357–375.

Knerr, W., Gardner, F., & Cluver, L. (2013). Improving positive parenting skills and reducing harsh and abusive parenting in low- and middle-income countries: A systematic review. *Prevention Science, 14*(4), 352–363.

Kratochwill, T. R., Hitchcock, J., Horner, R. H., Levin, J. R., Odom, S. L., Rindskopf, D. M., et al. (2010). Single-case designs technical documentation. Retrieved from *http://ies.ed.gov/ncee/wwc/Document/229*.

LaFleur, L., Witt, J. C., Naquin, G., Harwell, V., & Gilbertson, D. M. (1998). Use of coaching to enhance proactive classroom management by improvement of student transitioning between classroom activities. *Effective School Practices, 17,* 70–82.

Lane, K. L., Kalberg, J. R., Bruhn, A. L., Driscoll, S. A., Wehby, J. H., & Elliott, S. N. (2009). Assessing social validity of school-wide positive behavior support plans: Evidence for the reliability and structure of the primary intervention rating scale. *School Psychology Review, 38,* 135–144.

Leverson, M., Smith, K., McIntosh, K., Rose, J., & Pinkelman, S. (2016). PBIS cultural responsiveness field guide: Resources for trainers and coaches. Retrieved from *www.pbis.org/Common/Cms/files/pbisresources/PBIS%20Cultural%20Responsiveness%20Field%20Guide.pdf*.

Manz, P. H., Fantuzzo, J. W., & Power, T. J. (2004). Multidimensional assessment of family involvement among urban elementary students. *Journal of School Psychology, 42,* 461–475.

Mapp, K. L., & Hong, S. (2010). Debunking the myth of the hard-to-reach parent. In S. Christenson & A. Reschly (Eds.), *Handbook of school–family partnerships* (pp. 345–361). New York: Routledge.

McIntyre, L. L., Gresham, F. M., DiGennaro, F. D., & Reed, D. D. (2007). Treatment integrity in school-based interventions with children. *Journal of Applied Behavior Analysis, 40,* 659–672.

Moffitt, T. E., Caspi, A., Harrington, H., & Milne, B. J. (2002). Males on the life-course-persistent and adolescence-limited antisocial pathways: Follow-up at age 26 years. *Developmental Psychopathology, 14*(1), 179–207.

Moore, K. J., Garbacz, S. A., Gau, J. M., Dishion, T. J., Brown, K. L., Stormshak, E. A., et al. (2016). Proactive parent engagement in public schools: Using a brief strengths and needs assessment in a multiple gating risk management strategy. *Journal of Positive Behavior Interventions, 18*(4), 230–240.

Musci, R. J., Bradshaw, C. P., Maher, B., Uhl, G. R., Kellam, S. G., & Ialongo, N. S. (2014). Reducing aggression and impulsivity through school-based prevention programs: A gene-by-intervention interaction. *Prevention Science, 15*(6), 831–840.

Odgers, C. L., Caspi, A., Russell, M. A., Sampson, R. J., Arseneault, L., & Moffitt, T. E. (2012). Supportive parenting mediates neighborhood socioeconomic disparities in children's antisocial behavior from ages 5–12. *Development and Psychopathology, 24*(3), 705–721.

O'Donnell, C. L. (2008). Defining, conceptualizing, and measuring fidelity of implementation and its relationship to outcomes in K–12 curriculum intervention research. *Review of Educational Research, 78,* 33–84.

Paternite, C. E. (2005). School-based mental health programs and services: Overview and introduction to the special issue. *Journal of Abnormal Child Psychology, 33*(6), 657–663.

Patterson, G. R. (1982). *Coercive family process.* Eugene, OR: Castalia.

Patterson, G. R., DeBaryshe, B., & Ramsey, E. (1990). A developmental perspective on antisocial behavior. *American Psychologist, 44,* 329–335.

Perepletchikova, F., Hilt, L. M., Chereji, E., & Kazdin, A. E. (2009). Barriers to implementing treatment integrity procedures: Survey of treatment outcome researchers. *Journal of Consulting and Clinical Psychology, 77*(2), 212–218.

Power, T. J., Mautone, J. A., Soffer, S. L., Clarke, A. T., Marshall, S. A., Sharman, J., et al. (2012). A family–school intervention for children with ADHD: Results from a randomized clinical trial. *Journal of Consulting and Clinical Psychology, 80,* 611–623.

Raver, C. C., Gershoff, E. T., & Aber, J. L. (2007). Testing equivalence of mediating models of income, parenting, and school readiness for white, black, and Hispanic children in a national sample. *Child Development, 78*(1), 96–115.

Reschly, A. L., & Christenson, S. L. (2012). Moving from "context matters" to engaged partnerships with families. *Journal of Educational and Psychological Consultation, 22,* 62–78.

Reuben, J. D., Shaw, D. S., Brennan, L. M., Dishion, T. J., & Wilson, M. N. (2015). A family-based intervention for improving children's emotional problems through effects on maternal depressive symptoms. *Journal of Consulting and Clinical Psychology, 83*(6), 1142–1148.

Ringeisen, H., Henderson, K., & Hoagwood, K. (2003). Context matters: Schools and the "research to practice gap" in children's mental health. *School Psychology Review, 32*(2), 153–169.

Rones, M., & Hoagwood, K. (2000). School-based mental health services: A research review. *Clinical Child and Family Psychology Review, 3*(4), 223–241.

Sanetti, L. M. H., Luiselli, J. K., & Handler, M. W. (2007). Effects of verbal and graphic performance feedback on behavior support plan implementation in a public elementary school. *Behavior Modification, 31,* 454–465.

Sechrest, L. B., West, S. G., Phillips, M. A., Redner, R., & Yeaton, W. (1979). Some neglected problems in evaluation research: Strength and integrity of treatments. In L. B. Sechrest, S. G. West, M. A. Phillips, R. Redner, & W. Yeaton (Eds.), *Evaluation studies review annual* (Vol. 4, pp. 15–35). Beverly Hills, CA: SAGE.

Sheridan, S. M., Bovaird, J. A., Glover, T. A., Garbacz, S. A., Witte, A., & Kwon, K. (2012). A randomized trial examining the effects of conjoint behavioral consultation and the mediating role of the parent–teacher relationship. *School Psychology Review, 41,* 23–46.

Sheridan, S. M., & Kratochwill, T. R. (2008). *Conjoint behavioral consultation: Promoting family–school connections and interventions* (2nd ed.). New York: Springer Science+Business Media.

Sheridan, S. M., Rispoli, K., & Holmes, S. R. (2014). Treatment integrity in conjoint behavioral consultation: Conceptualizing active ingredients and potential pathways of influence. In L. Sanetti & T. Kratochwill (Eds.), *Treatment integrity: A foundation for evidence-based practice in applied psychology* (pp. 255–278). Washington, DC: American Psychological Association.

Sheridan, S. M., Ryoo, J. H., Garbacz, S. A., Kunz, G. M., & Chumney, F. L. (2013). The efficacy of conjoint behavioral consultation on parents and children in the home setting: Results of a randomized controlled trial. *Journal of School Psychology, 51,* 717–733.

Sheridan, S. M., Swanger-Gagné, M., Welch, G. W., Kwon, K., & Garbacz, S. A. (2009). Fidelity measurement in consultation: Psychometric issues and preliminary examination. *School Psychology Review, 38,* 476–495.

Smith, J. D., Dishion, T. J., Shaw, D. S., & Wilson, M. N. (2013). Indirect effects of fidelity to the Family Check-Up on changes in parenting and early childhood problem behaviors. *Journal of Consulting and Clinical Psychology, 81*(6), 962–974.

Smith, J. D., Knoble, N. B., Zerr, A. A., Dishion, T. J., & Stormshak, E. A. (2014). Family Check-Up effects across diverse ethnic groups: Reducing early-adolescence antisocial behavior by reducing family conflict. *Journal of Clinical Child and Adolescent Psychology, 43,* 400–414.

Smolkowski, K., Seeley, J. R., Gau, J. M., Dishion, T. J., Stormshak, E. A., Moore, K. J., et al. (2017). Effectiveness evaluation of the positive family support intervention: A three-tiered public health delivery model for middle schools. *Journal of School Psychology, 62,* 103–125.

Spoth, R. L., Guyll, M., & Day, S. X. (2002). Universal family-focused interventions in alcohol-use disorder prevention: Cost-effectiveness and cost-benefit analyses of two interventions. *Journal of Studies on Alcohol, 63,* 219–228.

Spoth, R. L., Kavanagh, K., & Dishion, T. J. (2002). Family-centered preventive intervention science: Toward benefits to larger populations of children, youth, and families. [Special issue]. *Prevention Science, 3,* 145–152.

Spoth, R., Redmond, C., Shin, C., Greenberg, M., Feinberg, M., & Schainker, L. (2013). PROSPER community–university partnership delivery system effects on substance misuse through 6½ years past baseline from a cluster randomized controlled intervention trial. *Preventive Medicine, 56,* 190–196.

Stormshak, E. A., Brown, K. L., Moore, K. J., Dishion, T. J., Seeley, J., & Smolkowski. K. (2016). Going to scale with family-centered, school-based interventions: Challenges and future directions. In S. M. Sheridan & E. Kim (Eds.), *Family–school partnerships in context* (pp. 25–44). New York: Springer.

Stormshak, E. A., Connell, A. M., Véronneau, M.-H., Myers, M. W., Dishion, T. J., Kavanagh, K., et al. (2011). An ecological approach to promoting early adolescent mental health and social adaptation: Family-centered intervention in public middle schools. *Child Development, 82,* 209–225.

Stormshak, E. A., DeGarmo, D. D., Chronister, K. M., & Caruthers, A. (2018). The impact of family-centered prevention on self-regulation and subsequent long-term risk in emerging adults. *Prevention Science, 19*(4), 549–558.

Stormshak, E. A., & Dishion, T. J. (2002). An ecological approach to clinical and counseling psychology. *Clinical Child and Family Psychology Review, 5,* 197–215.

Strickland-Cohen, M. K., & Horner, R. H. (2014). Typical school personnel developing and implementing basic behavior support plans. *Journal of Positive Behavior Interventions, 17,* 83–94.

Sugai, G., & Horner, R. H. (2002). The evolution of discipline practices: Schoolwide positive behavior supports. *Child and Family Behavior Therapy, 24,* 23–50.

Van Ryzin, M. J., Stormshak, E. A., & Dishion, T. J. (2012). Engaging parents in the Family Check-Up in middle school: Longitudinal effects on family conflict and problem behavior through the transition to high school. *Journal of Adolescent Health, 50*(6), 627–633.

Walker, H., Horner, R., Sugai, G., Bullis, M., Sprague, J., Bricker, D., et al. (1996). Integrated approaches to preventing antisocial behavior patterns among school age children and youth. *Journal of Emotional and Behavioral Disorders, 4,* 194–209.

Walker, J. M. T., Shenker, S. S., & Hoover-Dempsey, K. V. (2010). Why do parents become involved in their children's education?: Implications for school counselors. *Professional School Counseling, 14,* 27–41.

Wang, M.-T., Dishion, T. J., Stormshak, E. A., & Willett, J. B. (2011). Trajectories of family management practices and early adolescent behavioral outcomes. *Developmental Psychology, 47,* 1324–1341.

Wertz, J., Wright, K., Agnew-Blais, J., Matthews, T., Pariante, C. M., Moffitt, T. E., et al. (2016). Parental monitoring and knowledge: A test of bidirectional associations with youths' antisocial behavior. *Development and Psychopathology, 28,* 623–638.

World Health Organization Centre for Public Health. (2009). Preventing violence by developing life skills in children and adolescents. Retrieved from *http://apps.who.int/iris/bitstream/10665/44089/1/9789241597838_eng.pdf.*

CHAPTER 18

Preventing Aggression and Youth Violence in Schools

SHELLEY HYMEL and DOROTHY L. ESPELAGE

Brief Introduction

Youth violence is recognized as a major problem in countries around the world. Indeed, the World Health Organization (WHO; 2015) ranks youth homicide as the fourth leading cause of death among young people, with youth suicide ranked third. These international data also indicate that about 40% of youth were involved in a physical fight over the previous year and that 25% were bullied within the previous month, despite estimates that one in three victims never report the violence to which they are exposed. Although we recognize the value of an international perspective on youth violence (Benbenishty & Astor, 2012), this chapter focuses on youth violence in the United States and the role that schools can play in addressing such problems.

Schools are an ideal context in which to address youth violence, with the capacity to reach the majority of children and youth through prevention and intervention efforts undertaken over multiple years. Given that the three strongest predictors of continued delinquency are younger age at first offense, first contact with the legal system, and a history of nonsevere pathology (Cottle, Lee, & Heilbrun, 2001), addressing youth violence through schools can also help to reduce future criminal behavior. Moreover, many of the risk and protective factors that contribute to youth violence (see Bernat, Oakes, Pettingell, & Resnick, 2012; Herrenkohl, Lee, & Hawkins, 2012; Lösel & Farrington, 2012; WHO, 2015) emerge from and operate within school settings. Among other things, youth violence has been linked to individual characteristics (e.g., attention problems, hyperactivity, conduct disorder, early antisocial behavior, truancy, early delinquency, low intelligence, substance use), peer relationship factors (association with deviant peers, gang membership, bullying, victimization), and school factors (low school commitment or connectedness, low grade-point average, and poor achievement). Identified protective factors relevant to the school context include above-average intelligence, low impulsivity, prosocial attitudes and behaviors, strong ties to school, good achievement, positive class/school climate, association with prosocial peers, and later onset of alcohol and drug use. Given that risk of violence decreases as protective factors accrue (Lösel & Farrington, 2012), efforts to address early risk factors preventively and to promote protective factors in schools and communities that reduce the likelihood of aggression hold considerable promise in addressing delinquency and later criminal behavior.

Our chapter begins with an overview of major forms of youth violence and their prevalence. We then summarize theoretical arguments that have been offered to explain youth violence. Against this backdrop, we consider various approaches to addressing school violence, with emphasis on evidence-based practices and efforts to create safe school environments in which all students can thrive. As Olweus (1993) pointed out decades ago, every child has a right to attend schools without fear of harm or victimization.

Main Issues

Prevalence Rates

According to the National Center for Education Statistics in the U.S. (2017), overall victimization through school violence, including weapon carrying, threats, and fights on school property, declined by 82% from 1993 to 2015. The percentage of youth who reported taking a weapon to school in the preceding month dropped from 17.9% in 2013 to 4.1% in 2015 (Kann et al., 2014, 2016). Despite these declines, media attention given to school shootings (e.g., Columbine, Sandy Hook) has raised concerns about school violence at a national level. Although youth homicides at school have been less than 3% since the 1990s (Zhang, Musu-Gillette, & Oudekerk, 2016), it is sobering to recognize that, from July 2011 through June 2012, there were 45 school-associated violent deaths in the United States (Robers, Zhang, Morgan, & Musu-Gillette, 2015). Such extreme violence, although rare, not only affects perpetrators and victims but also the broader school community. In a 2013 national survey, 7% of high school students reported missing school at least once because they felt unsafe (Kann et al., 2014), and with good reason. The same survey revealed that in the preceding year over 5% of students reported carrying a weapon to school, 7% reported being threatened or injured with a weapon at school, and over 8% reported being in a physical fight at school. In that same year (2013), the rate of violent victimization was higher in school than away from school (Robers et al., 2015).

In the following sections, we consider some of the major forms of aggression and youth violence that take place in schools—youth gangs, weapon carrying, sexual harassment, bullying, dating violence, and emotional abuse, as well as violence against teachers.

Gangs at School

Youth gangs are a serious problem in the United States (Decker, Melde, & Pyrooz, 2013; Pyrooz & Sweeten, 2015). In 2013, 12% of U.S. public school students nationwide (ages 12–18) reported gang presence at their school, a decrease from 18% in 2011 (Zhang et al., 2016), with more gangs reported in urban than suburban schools. Although youth gangs are less prevalent in Canada than in the United States, results of the Canadian Police Survey on Youth Gangs and other sources suggest that youth gangs are a growing concern in many Canadian jurisdictions (Ezeonu, 2014). Further research is needed to explore differences in youth gangs and the risk and protective factors that affect their prevalence.

The presence of youth gangs can increase the likelihood of school violence and student aggression and adversely affect school climate (Forster, Grigsby, Unger, & Sussman, 2015; Laub & Lauritsen, 1998). With strong links between gang presence and availability of firearms and drugs in schools (Howell & Lynch, 2000), it is not clear whether gangs directly cause victimization in schools or are a self-protective response to threatening school climates (Howell & Lynch, 2000). Despite many gang prevention initiatives at local, state, and federal levels, there are few guidelines or training opportunities for professionals working with students at risk for gang affiliation (Brandt, Sidway, Dvorsky, & Weist, 2013).

Weapons at School

High-profile school shootings have been pivotal in developing policies and programs to ensure student safety in school, with efforts to curtail students' *carrying lethal weapons* to school. Survey data from the Centers for Disease Control (CDC; Kann et al., 2014) indicated that the prevalence of weapon carrying ranges from 3 to 10% across 34 states, with more weapons carried by male than female students. In one national survey (Yun & Hwang, 2011), 8% of secondary students reported being injured or threatened with a weapon in school. Other research has documented declines in overall reports of weapon carrying at school between the 1990s and 2013 (from 26 to 18%, Child Trends Databank, 2014; from 12 to 5%, Zhang et al., 2016), although rates increased among white students, from 17% in 2011 to 21% in 2013 (Child Trends Databank, 2014). As with gang membership, it is difficult to determine whether weapon carrying is intended to harm others or to protect oneself, although understanding the motives behind such behavior would help to direct efforts to prevent youth weapon carrying.

Sexual Harassment

Sexual harassment among students in educational settings is now recognized as a growing social concern (CDC, 2012). As a form of sexual discrimination, sexual harassment involves unwanted sexual conduct, including unwelcome verbal, nonverbal, and physical behaviors that interfere with an individual's right to an equal education (Hill & Kearl, 2011; U.S. Department of Education, Office for Civil Rights, 2010) by limiting a student's ability to participate in or benefit from educational programs or creating a hostile or abusive educational environment (Espelage

& De La Rue, 2013). In adolescence, sexual harassment tends to involve sexual commentary, spreading sexual rumors, and inappropriate touching (Espelage, Basile, & Hamburger, 2012). Such behavior is common among teens, with one national study reporting sexual harassment rates as high as 56% for females and 40% for males (Hill & Kearl, 2011), including being called "gay" (Rinehart & Espelage, 2016). Among sixth-grade students from 36 Midwest middle schools, 8% admitted to perpetrating at least one incident of sexual harassment, and 15% reported being victims of at least one form of sexual harassment in the preceding year (Rinehart & Espelage, 2016), with 34% reporting being targets of homophobic epithets and 31% identifying as victims of homophobic name calling.

Despite high rates of sexual harassment in our schools, school personnel feel ill equipped to address the problem, reporting little professional development or support within this area (Charmaraman, Jones, Stein, & Espelage, 2013). Making prevention of sexual harassment a priority in schools requires the efforts of teachers, staff, administrators, and other school personnel (e.g., counselors, school psychologists), as well as students. Educators first need to understand that sexual harassment comes in various forms, from physical (e.g., being "pantsed" or forced to do something sexual) to nonphysical (e.g., homophobic harassment or sexual commentary), and areas where sexual harassment is most likely to occur need to be monitored. Under Title IX (U.S. Department of Education, Office for Civil Rights, 2010), schools have a legal obligation to protect students from gendered harassment, with districts required to have consistently enforced policies about sexual harassment, and to provide training and guidelines on how to deal with such incidents and how to respond when students report sexual harassment.

School Bullying

The most common form of violence experienced by students is bullying, which can also take many forms (verbal, physical, social, electronic) and serve many functions (discrimination, sexism, sexual harassment, humiliation, exclusion, etc.). Although definitions vary across studies, scholars typically view *bullying* as a subcategory of aggression characterized by intentionality, repetition, and a power imbalance; perpetrators have some advantage over their victims (e.g., size, strength, status, competence, numbers), and victims have difficulty defending themselves (Juvonen, Graham, & Shuster, 2003; Olweus, 1993). According to the CDC, bullying is any unwanted aggressive behavior(s) by another youth or group of youths who are not siblings or current dating partners that involves an observed or perceived power imbalance and is repeated multiple times or is highly likely to be repeated. Bullying may inflict harm or distress on the targeted youth including physical, psychological, social, or educational harm (Gladden, Vivolo-Kantor, Hamburger, & Lumpkin, 2014).

Although prevalence rates vary across schools and across studies, boys typically report more bullying than girls, and girls report more victimization (e.g., Cook, Williams, Guerra, Kim, & Sadek, 2010; Olweus, 1993). Bullying increases across the elementary years, peaking during middle school and declining by the end of high school (e.g., Currie et al., 2012; Espelage & Swearer, 2003; Vaillancourt et al., 2010).

Victimization becomes increasingly stable with age (see Hymel & Swearer, 2015), with significant short- and long-term consequences for those who are targeted (see McDougall & Vaillancourt, 2015). Nationally, Nansel and colleagues (2001) found that 30% of adolescents reported moderate or frequent involvement in bullying. More recently, Robers and colleagues (2015) found that 28% of middle school students reported being bullied at school within the preceding year; sixth-grade students reported even higher rates (37%). Over the past decade, rates of bullying have started to decline. According to the Department of Education (Zhang et al., 2016), bullying decreased from 29% in 1999–2000 to 16% in 2013–2014, though decreases were not evident in schools with gangs or other crime or violence problems. Rates also vary across types of bullying, with rates of physical bullying on the decline (22% in 2003 vs. 15% in 2008; Finkelhor, Turner, Ormrod, & Hamby, 2010), but electronic bullying increasing from 6% in 2000 to 11% in 2010 (Jones, Mitchell, & Finkelhor, 2013).

Following a 2011 White House Conference on bullying, state governments have introduced policies requiring school districts to establish bully prevention programs in all K–12 settings, with accompanying efforts to evaluate their efficacy. In the most comprehensive meta-analysis of such efforts, Ttofi and Farrington (2011) found that, on average, antibullying programs yielded a 20–23% decrease in bullying perpetration and a 17–20% decrease in victimization. Although their review included more studies of European than U.S. antibullying programs (34%), findings demonstrate that decreased *victimization* was associated with use of nonpunitive discipline, cooperative group work, parent training/meetings, and use of videos. Reductions in bullying perpetration were more likely with improvements in playground supervision, classroom rules and management, teacher training, whole-school antibullying policies, school conferences, and information for parents.

Beyond prevention and intervention efforts aimed directly at school bullying, more broadly focused social–emotional learning and social-cognitive intervention programs have targeted common risk and protective factors for aggression, bullying, and violence, including social–emotional skills (e.g., anger, empathy, perspective taking, respect for diversity, attitudes supportive of aggression, coping, willingness to intervene to help others, communication and problem-solving skills; see Cook et al., 2010). Such efforts are aimed at providing students with the social and emotional skills needed to navigate the social world of schools *without* resorting to bullying or other forms of aggression. These programs have been found to reduce bullying and other forms of youth aggression (Espelage, Low, Polanin, & Brown, 2013, 2015), especially when implemented with fidelity (Polanin & Espelage, 2015). Unfortunately, most teacher education programs in the United States fail to provide educators with such training because of a reluctance to use professional development for this type of training and limited resources to purchase curricula (Schonert-Reichl, Hansen-Peterson, & Hymel, 2015).

Teen Dating Violence

Teen dating violence is recognized as a growing public health concern that has serious long-term mental health implications for both victims and perpetrators (CDC, 2016). The CDC (2016) defines dating violence as "the physical, sexual, psychological, or emotional violence within a dating relationship, including stalking." Such behavior reaches a peak in early adolescence and declines thereafter (Capaldi & Langhinrichsen-Rohling, 2012). On the 2013 Youth Risk Behavior Survey, about 10% of teens reported being victims of physical violence and 10% had experienced sexual violence from a romantic partner in the past year (Vagi, Olsen, Basile, & Vivolo-Kantor, 2015). Given the many adolescents who experience abusive dating relationships in high school, some as early as middle school, prevention efforts must begin early on (Mulford & Blachman-Demner, 2013), helping students to develop the skills needed to form and maintain healthy, nonviolent romantic relationships (CDC, 2012).

Emotional Abuse through Microaggressions

Microaggression refers to the verbal, behavioral, and environmental indignities that convey subtle or blatant denigrating messages (Nadal, 2010; Sue et al., 2007). Research on microaggressions emerged within social and counseling psychology, with educational studies conducted primarily in colleges and universities (e.g., Minikel-Lacocque, 2013; Woodford, Howell, Kulick, & Silverschanz, 2012), and few studies of K–12 students (Allen, 2010). For minority students, microaggressions are a pervasive, wide-ranging problem in school. About 65% of sexual minority teens reported hearing derogatory comments (e.g., "faggot"); 74% often heard "gay" used negatively in school (Kosciw, Greytak, Palmer, & Boesen, 2014). Microaggressions experienced by racial and ethnic minority K–12 students can be blatant, such as receiving harsher or more punitive consequences than peers of other races (Lewis, Butler, Bonner, & Joubert, 2010), or subtle, such as teachers' unwillingness to learn a student's name (Kohli & Solorzano, 2012) or reinforcement of English dominance in the school system (Huber, 2011). School efforts to eliminate microaggression and the biases that underlie them are clearly needed.

Violence toward Educators

Studies of school violence typically focus on student-to-student victimization, with less attention given to violence directed at school staff in U.S. schools (e.g., Reddy et al., 2013), especially as compared with studies conducted in other countries (e.g., Chen & Astor, 2008). Violence against teachers can range from disrespectful behaviors to intimidation, threats, theft, property damage, and physical assault (Espelage, Anderman, et al., 2013). Robers and colleagues (2015) found that 10% of elementary teachers and 9% of high school teachers in the United States were threatened with physical harm by a student in 2011–2012, with higher rates in public than private schools. Although student verbal abuse of teachers decreased from 13% in 1999–2000 to 5% in 2013–2014, over 70% of K–12 teachers reported experiencing at least one type of victimization within the preceding year (Espelage, Anderman, et al., 2013). Such abuse has been associated with mental health symptoms, fear, interpersonal relationship difficulties, impaired work performance, and lower job satisfaction (e.g., Reddy et al., 2013).

Violence against teachers is the result of a complex interaction of student behaviors, teacher practices, classroom management strategies, overall school climate, and violence in the surrounding community (Espelage, Anderman, et al., 2013). To minimize such behavior, Espelage, Anderman, and colleagues (2013) offered several recommendations for schools, including implementation of a three-tiered service delivery prevention model for reducing aggression (i.e., primary, secondary, and tertiary interventions; Walker & Shinn, 2002), use of evidence-based classroom instructional and management strategies; and implementation of social–emotional and behavioral programs that provide students with alternatives to violence and help them acquire the skills needed to manage anger, resolve conflict peacefully, and improve classroom norms and environment. Although preservice teacher training programs in the United States currently provide minimal preparation in these areas (Schonert-Reichl et al., 2015), such efforts have begun to take root, promoted by the Collaborative for Academic, Social, and Emotional Learning (CASEL; *www. casel.org*). Importantly, administrators need to investigate allegations of violence rigorously and address any physical or mental health issues that emerge for teachers who are victimized.

Theoretical Considerations

Owing in part to the long-standing emphasis on deficit models within the field, individual characteristics (e.g., age, sex, psychosocial factors) have been examined extensively in an effort to understand why certain children are more prone to violence or victimization (e.g., Carlyle & Steinman, 2007; Danner & Carmody, 2001). For example, sex differences in physical aggression have been consistently documented (e.g., Archer, 2004; Hyde, 1984). As Jackson Katz depicts in his 2000 film, *Tough Guise,* the vast majority of violence is perpetrated by men and boys, a fact that he attributes to culturally based conceptions of manhood and masculinity (Katz, 1995; see also Way, 2011). Moreover, childhood physical aggression has been found to predict later antisocial behavior in adulthood for boys but not girls (e.g., Broidy et al., 2003). Furthermore, students who display characteristics associated with psychopathology (impulsivity, narcissism, callous–unemotional traits) are more likely to bully others (Fanti & Kimonis, 2012), although such individuals represent a very small portion of the student population. Although individual characteristics clearly contribute to aggressive and violent behavior in youth, they do not fully account for such behavior, leading scholars to consider more complex models.

Developmental Perspectives

Following Bronfenbrenner (1977), scholars have argued for a *social–ecological framework* (e.g., Barboza et al., 2009; Espelage, 2014), viewing school violence as reciprocally shaped by individual, familial, school, peer, community, and societal factors. As neuroscientist Sapolsky (2017) aptly documents, the factors that contribute to negative human behavior are many and varied, both proximal and distal, and not all are easily studied, yet to fully understand their nature and development, one must consider multiple contributing factors.

For decades, *social learning theory* has been the dominant perspective on the development of aggression and violence, with the basic premise that violent and/

or aggressive behaviors are culturally acquired or learned through cycles of rein-forcement and punishment and through modeling. The theory has been especially useful in explaining cycles of violence within the family context (e.g., Patterson, 1982, 1986) and "late onset" models of violence and aggression that reach a peak in adolescence (e.g., Moffitt & Caspi, 2001). Within this literature, a primary focus has been on parenting practices that contribute to the development of aggression and deviant behavior, including harsh and inconsistent parenting, parental negativity, and use of punitive and coercive discipline (e.g., Dishion, Patterson, & Kavanagh, 1992; Patterson, 1986), with more distal correlates such as poverty (e.g., Conger et al., 1992) viewed as factors that limit parent effectiveness. Recent research, however, has begun to broaden our perspective.

First, longitudinal findings have challenged assumptions that physical aggres-sion develops gradually, reaching a peak in adolescence. Instead, Tremblay and colleagues (2000, 2004) have shown that physical aggression emerges in early child-hood, peaks in toddlerhood, and subsequently declines, as most children learn non-violent conflict resolution strategies during primary school. There are, however, a small proportion of youngsters whose physical aggression remains high over time (e.g., Broidy et al., 2003; Tremblay & Nagin, 2005), and whose failure to learn to regulate their aggression is associated with higher rates of delinquency and vio-lence in later life (Tremblay et al., 2004). These findings challenge commonly held beliefs that violence is culturally acquired through social learning, as well as "late onset" theories suggesting that violence in adolescence emerges without a history of aggression in early childhood (Moffitt & Caspi, 2001; Tremblay et al., 1992). Instead of investigating how children "learn" to be aggressive, Tremblay and colleagues (2004) argue that we need to understand the environmental and genetic factors that explain why some children fail to respond to socialization pressures for less aggressive behavior.

Although parent and family socialization has been a major focus to date, a 2002 meta-analysis by Rhee and Waldman examined the relative contributions of genes and environment to antisocial behavior and found that only about 16% of the variance in antisocial behavior is attributable to the "shared environment," with 40% accounted for by genetics and the remaining 43% attributable to the "non-shared environment." This and several other lines of research have contributed to a growing awareness of the role of peers and school context in the socialization of aggression and violent behavior, including studies demonstrating the role of peer deviancy training in which interactions among deviant peers can intensify a youth's own aggression and violence (Dishion, McCord, & Poulin, 1999), shared peer norms that condone violence (e.g., Brendgen, Girard, Vitaro, Dionne, & Boivin, 2013; Huesmann, Guerra, Miller, & Zelli, 1992), and the role of school cli-mate (Konishi, Miyazaki, Hymel, & Waterhouse, 2017) and group dynamics (Hymel, McClure, Miller, Shumka, & Trach, 2015) in youth violence and aggression.

For example, many aggressive children and youth are rejected by the larger peer group (Coie & Dodge, 1998; Newcomb, Bukowski, & Pattee, 1993), leading them to affiliate more with other aggressive peers (Vitaro, Pedersen, & Brendgen, 2007). Such affiliations, in turn, increase the likelihood of aggressive and violent behavior (e.g., Dishion, Véronneau, & Myers, 2010), in part through processes such as deviancy training (Dishion et al., 1999). As well, some aggressive youth hold considerable status among peers (e.g., Rodkin, Farmer, Pearl, & Van Acker, 2000), especially if they possess characteristics that are valued within the group (e.g., attractiveness, athleticism; Vaillancourt & Hymel, 2006). Aggressive behavior among high-status youth enhances perceived acceptability of such behavior. Chang's (2004) *social context model* holds that behaviors that occur frequently within a particular social context are more likely to be seen as acceptable, especially if displayed by high-status individuals, and this effect is particularly strong for deviant behaviors. Similarly, *social information-processing theory* (Fontaine & Dodge, 2006) posits that individual behavior is in part guided by knowledge of group norms, with more reactive aggression evident when such behavior is supported by group norms (Frey, Strong, & Onyewuenyi, 2017). Given such findings, scholars have begun to explore the interplay of family and peer processes in the development and maintenance of aggression. For example, Fosco, Frank, and Dishion (2012) have conducted a series of longitudinal studies examining coercive parenting practices during early adolescence as predictors of later aggression. They argue that family coercive processes serve as "basic training" for use of similar behaviors outside the home and within the peer group (Patterson, De Baryshe, & Ramsey, 1989).

Criminology Theories

Within the criminology literature, several theories have been put forward regarding how both individual and contextual factors contribute to the likelihood of school violence and aggressive behavior. First, Gottfredson and Hirschi's (1990, 2003) *general theory of crime* posits that criminal behavior, defined as using force or fraud to address self-interests, emerges as a result of low self-control plus opportunity. Consistent with this theory, low self-control has been found to be one of the strongest predictors of a variety of criminal and imprudent behaviors in both adults and juveniles (see Pratt & Cullen, 2000). For example, preadolescents with low self-control are found to engage in significantly more delinquency, substance use, and rule breaking than those with greater self-control (Kuhn & Laird, 2013), especially when they had more time unsupervised, had fewer family rules, and had peers who were involved in antisocial behaviors (opportunities). Relatedly, *social control theory* (Booth, Farrell, & Varano, 2008; Gottfredson, 2001; Payne, 2008) posits that individuals with low self-control find it difficult to inhibit gratification and thus act impulsively, making them risk takers who put themselves in situations that elevate the likelihood of violence and victimization. Given the availability of resources and authority, schools are viewed as a major institution for the development of social control in youth (Guo, Roettger, & Cai, 2008).

Moral Cognitions

Contextual factors contribute to aggressive and violent behavior in part through their impact on students' ability to cognitively justify and rationalize the negative behaviors they perpetrate. Among criminologists, *neutralization theory* emerged in the late 1950s (Sykes & Matza, 1957) in an attempt to explain delinquent behavior by exploring the motives embraced by perpetrators for engaging in negative behavior. Sykes and Matza (1957) argued that most individuals who perpetrate violent and criminal behavior do understand right and wrong but utilize a number of cognitive strategies that serve to justify and rationalize their negative behavior, including efforts to deny the extent of injury or their personal responsibility or appeal to higher loyalties. Since the 1950s, the theory has received support from numerous studies of criminal behavior and imprudent behaviors in both adults and youth (see Maruna & Copes, 2005).

More recently, and quite independently, Bandura's (1990; Bandura, Barbaranelli, Caprara, & Pastorelli, 1996) *theory of moral disengagement* emerged within psychology as an extension of social learning theory, initially addressing the question of how soldiers and terrorists are able to engage in serious violent, inhumane behavior yet release themselves from moral self-regulation and self-sanction, without feelings of remorse or guilt. As with neutralization theory, Bandura identified several self-serving cognitive mechanisms through which such negative behavior can be justified, including moral justification (using worthy ends or moral purposes to excuse pernicious means), diffusion of personal responsibility, disregarding or distorting the harmful consequences of one's actions, and blaming the victim (believing the victim deserves his or her suffering).

Moral disengagement or neutralization processes are situated within and learned through social interactions with others, but over time they can develop into habits or dispositions and can occur at both individual and collective levels, contributing to the maintenance of delinquent or negative behavior. Integrating these two theories (and theories of cognitive self-serving biases), Ribeaud and Eisner (2010) found that *moral neutralization* was significantly linked to aggression and delinquent behavior among middle school students. A recent meta-analysis (Gini, Pozzoli, & Hymel, 2014) has also verified that children and youth who engage in aggression and bullying are more likely to morally disengage. It is not yet clear, however, what components of moral disengagement drive the aggression, such as lack of empathy or guilt, or poor regulatory deficits. Still, research to date underscores the need to address self-serving cognitions, as well as behavior, in efforts to reduce school violence.

Addressing School Violence

Given the prevalence of school violence, it is imperative that educational institutions do *something* to address the problem. But what? As the preceding review demonstrates, school violence takes many forms and is a product of multiple factors, both individual, social, and contextual, with a broad range of risk and protective factors identified and several different theoretical arguments regarding causes. Given such complexity, no single solution, program, or practice will effectively eliminate such behavior across schools and youth. A multipronged, multidimensional approach is clearly needed, addressing early risk factors as well as protective and contextual factors. Accordingly, educators have long supported a three-tiered prevention model for reducing aggression (e.g., Walker & Shinn, 2002).

Primary, or targeted, intensive, and individualized, interventions are needed for the small portion of youth who engage in significant and serious forms of violence (Walker & Shinn, 2002). Secondary prevention efforts include selected and/

or small-group interventions for the somewhat larger subset of students who are considered at risk for more serious violence (Walker & Shinn, 2002). In both cases, efforts to address the mental health difficulties that underlie such behavior is a critical preventative focus, especially given evidence that 45% of inmates in U.S. federal prisons and 64% of inmates in local jails have been diagnosed with or receive treatment for mental illness (U.S. Department of Justice, 2004). However, such a focus requires greater availability of mental health services and greater cooperation between schools and local mental health supports, as well as efforts to reduce the stigma of mental illness, a focus increasingly promoted in education and teacher training in Canada (Kutcher, 2015) and the United Kingdom (e.g., Weare, 2010). Schools can play a significant role in the early identification (and referral) of students experiencing mental health difficulties (see Hymel, Starosta, Gill, & Low, 2018). Teachers, with years of experience with hundreds of students, are often the first to recognize students who display such difficulties. Greater emphasis on the nature and treatment of mental illness in both teacher training and professional development would facilitate such efforts. In addition, school psychologists, with their training in assessment, can assist in early identification through universal mental health screening, with a recent pilot program in the United States (Dowdy et al., 2015) demonstrating the utility of such a proactive, school-based effort.

Tertiary prevention efforts are directed to the majority of students through universal programs and practices that (1) help all students to develop social and emotional competencies and alternative, nonviolent approaches to conflict and (2) create school and classroom contexts that foster respect, acceptance, and inclusion of all students and establish social norms for nonviolent behavior. Promoted in the United States by the Collaborative for Academic, Social and Emotional Learning, or CASEL, social–emotional learning emphasizes five broad competencies—self-awareness, self-management, social awareness, relationship skills, and responsible decision making—that serve as "master skills" underlying much of our behavior (Domitrovich, Durlak, Staley, & Weissberg, 2017; Zins, Weissberg, Wang, & Walberg, 2004). These skills are acquired gradually over the school years (Schonert-Reichl & Hymel, 1996) and are increasingly recognized as a foundation for positive social behavior and mental well-being (e.g., Sklad, Diekstra, De Ritter, & Ben, 2012; Weare, 2010). Social–emotional learning programs that address bullying and other forms of aggression draw from the risk and protective framework literature to purposely teach a wide range of skills to prevent conflicts and their escalation. Research over the past decade has demonstrated the positive impact of well-implemented social–emotional learning programs in schools on both social and academic outcomes (e.g., Durlak, Weissberg, Dymnicki, Taylor, & Schellinger, 2011; for reviews, see Domitrovich et al., 2017; Weare, 2010), with a documented benefit–cost ratio of $11 for every $1 spent (Belfield et al., 2015). Particularly relevant to the present chapter is evidence that well-implemented, school-based, social–emotional learning programs aimed at addressing interpersonal conflict and emotion management have succeeded in reducing youth violence, including bullying, fighting, and disruptive behaviors in classrooms (e.g., Espelage, Low, et al., 2013; Wilson & Lipsey, 2007).

Equally important is creating contexts that promote positive behavior, acceptance, and social–emotional competencies, a focus supported by research on school climate. School climate is a multidimensional construct that encompasses the educational structures, values, practices, and relationships that influence student perceptions of their educational experiences (Thapa, Cohen, Guffey, & Higgins-D'Alessandro, 2013), including their feelings of safety, both physical and emotional, and the quality of their relationships with teachers and peers (Cohen, McCabe, Michelli, & Pickeral, 2009). Although school climate is operationalized in different ways across studies, findings consistently show that if students have positive perceptions of their school's climate, they are less likely to engage in aggressive behavior and violence (Espelage, Bosworth, & Simon, 2000; Goldweber, Waasdorp, & Bradshaw, 2013; Totura et al., 2009). In contrast, negative school climates are associated with high rates of bullying behavior (e.g., Gage, Prykanowski, & Larson, 2014; Konishi et al., 2017), encourage aggressive behavior, and discourage reporting of aggression (Bandyopadhyay, Cornell, & Konold, 2009; Espelage, Polanin, & Low, 2014).

In the past two decades, numerous programs have been developed to promote social–emotional competencies and create positive school climates (see *www.selresources.com*). However, many, if not most, of these efforts have not been evaluated empirically, owing in part to the fact that this is a relatively new area of educational focus and to the high cost of conducting well-designed evaluations in educational settings. Nevertheless, such evaluations are sorely needed, and large-scale efforts to identify empirically validated programs have been undertaken by both the University of Colorado's Blueprints initiative (*www.colorado.edu/cspv/blueprints*) and CASEL (*www.casel.org/guide*). Included among those programs that have stood the test of empirical validation are the Committee for Children's Steps to Respect program to address bullying among elementary students (e.g., Brown, Low, Smith, & Haggerty, 2011; Hirschstein & Frey, 2006), and their Second Step program to teach social–emotional skills (Espelage, Low, et al., 2013, 2015; Espelage, Rose, & Polanin, 2015), the RULER program for promoting emotional literacy (e.g., Rivers, Brackett, Reyes, Elbertson, & Salovey, 2013), the Positive Behavioral Supports framework (Sugai & Horner, 2006) with its bullying prevention focus (Ross, Horner, & Higbee, 2009) and its School Wide Positive Behavioral Interventions and Supports program (Waasdorp, Bradshaw, & Leaf, 2012), Creating a Peaceful School Learning Environment (Fonagy, Twemlow, Vernberg, Sacco, & Little, 2005), a K–12 program aimed at creating positive schoolwise climate change, and the SANKOFA Youth Violence Program (Hines, Vega, & Jemmott, 2004), a strength-based, culturally tailored prevention program for African American teens to minimize risk for violence, victimization, and other negative behaviors (alcohol and substance use), to name a few. Many of these programs include direct instruction with youth to help them learn social–emotional skills (e.g., emotional regulation, communication, empathy), training for teachers and staff in managing challenging behaviors, and a focus on promoting positive, supportive schools.

Future Research Directions

School-based interventions to prevent bullying and other forms of interpersonal violence and promote social–emotional skills and prosocial behavior in youth are being developed at a fast rate, but evaluation research lags far behind. Also, many programs are evaluated by the program developers; therefore, these evaluations are not independent. Although such research is critical in guiding educational decisions and policies, once schools become the unit of analysis, costs of research rise substantially, and there is ever-increasing need for statistical tools that allow an evaluation of the complex levels of influence that operate. As one example, at least two meta-analytic studies (Polanin, Espelage, & Pigott, 2012; Ttofi & Farrington, 2011) indicated that antibullying programs *are* effective in reducing aggression and peer victimization and encouraging prosocial behaviors, with greater effects for older (e.g., high school) than younger students, based on analyzing age effects using between-subject analyses (averaging grades of students in each study). Arguing for a within-subjects analysis as more appropriate, Yeager, Fong, Lee, and Espelage (2015) reached the opposite conclusion—that the effectiveness of antibullying interventions drops sharply after grade 7, with evidence of no effects or negative effects. Clearly, more developmental research is needed to determine what works to prevent bullying among older youth and the type of messaging that resonates with this population.

School violence is recognized as a pervasive, multifaceted construct, involving both criminal acts and aggression that can hamper student development and learning and harm the overall climate of a school (Furlong & Morrison, 2000). As such, it is a problem that requires greater attention from educators, policy makers, and researchers. Although research on aggression and youth violence in schools and efforts to address such problems has increased over the past two decades (e.g., with such publications as *Journal of School Violence, Handbook of School Violence* [Jimerson, Nickerson, Mayer, & Furlong, 2012], and special issues on school violence), with documented declines in such behavior, the problem persists (Robers et al., 2015). Our hope is that the present chapter provides a foundational backdrop for further research and practice in this area.

REFERENCES

Allen, Q. (2010). Racial microaggressions: The schooling experiences of Black middle-class males in Arizona's secondary schools. *Journal of African American Males in Education, 1,* 125–143.

Archer, J. (2004) Sex difference in aggression in real-world settings. *Review of General Psychology, 8*(4), 291–322.

Bandura, A. (1990). Mechanisms of moral disengagement. In W. Reich (Ed.), *Origins of terrorism: Psychologies, ideologies, theologies, states of mind.* Cambridge, UK: Cambridge University Press.

Bandura, A., Barbaranelli, C., Caprara, G. V., & Pastorelli, C. (1996). Mechanisms of moral disengagement in the exercise of moral agency. *Journal of Personality and Social Psychology 71,* 364–374.

Bandyopadhyay, S., Cornell, D. G., & Konold, T. R. (2009). Validity of three school climate scales to assess bullying, aggressive attitudes, and help seeking. *School Psychology Review, 38*(3), 338–355.

Barboza, G. E., Schiamberg, L. B., Oehmke, J., Korzeniewski, S. J., Post, L. A., & Heraux, C. G. (2009). Individual characteristics and the multiple contexts of adolescent bullying: An ecological perspective. *Journal of Youth and Adolescence, 38,* 101–121.

Belfield, C., Bowden, B., Klapp, A., Levin, H., Shand, R., & Zander, S. (2015). *The economic value of social and emotional learning.* New York: Center for Benefit-Cost Studies in Education, Teachers College, Columbia University. Retrieved from *http://voicesforservice. org/wp-content/uploads/2016/03/Sep19_Econ_Value_National_Service-2.pdf.*

Benbenishty, R., & Astor, R. (2012). Making the case for an international perspective on school violence: Implications for theory, research, policy, and assessment In S. R. Jimerson, A. B. Nickerson, M. J. Mayer, & M. J. Furlong (Eds.), *Handbook of school violence and school safety* (pp. 15–26). New York: Routledge.

Bernat, D. H., Oakes, J. M., Pettingell, S. L., & Resnick, M. (2012). Risk and direct protective factors for youth violence: Results from the National Longitudinal Study of Adolescent Health. *American Journal of Preventive Medicine, 43*(2), S57–S66.

Booth, J., Farrell, A., & Varano, S. (2008). Social control, serious delinquency, and risky behavior: A gendered analysis. *Crime and Delinquency, 54,* 423–456.

Brandt, N. E., Sidway, E., Dvorsky, M., & Weist, M. D. (2013). Culturally responsive strategies to address youth gangs in schools. In C. S. Clauss-Ehlers, Z. N. Serpell, & M. D. Weist (Eds.), *Handbook of culturally responsive school mental health: Advancing research, training, practice, and policy* (pp. 177–186). New York: Springer.

Brendgen, M., Girard, A., Vitaro, F., Dionne, G., & Boivin, M. (2013). Gene–environment correlation linking aggression and peer victimization: Do classroom behavioral norms matter? *Journal of Abnormal Child Psychology, 43*(1), 19–31.

Broidy, L. M., Nagin, D. S., Tremblay, R. E., Bates, J. E., Browne, B., Dodge, K. A., et al. (2003). Developmental trajectories in childhood disruptive behavior and adolescent delinquency: A six-site, cross-national study. *Developmental Psychology 39*(2), 222–245.

Bronfenbrenner, U. (1977). Toward an experimental ecology of human development. *American Psychologist, 32,* 513–531.

Brown, E. C., Low, S., Smith, B. H., & Haggerty, K. P. (2011). Outcomes from a school-randomized controlled trial of steps to respect: A bullying prevention program. *School Psychology Review, 40*(3), 423–443.

Capaldi, D. M., & Langhinrichsen-Rohling, J. (2012). Informing intimate partner violence prevention efforts: Dyadic, developmental, and contextual considerations. *Prevention Science, 13*(4), 323–328.

Carlyle, K. E., & Steinman, K. (2007). Demographic differences in the prevalence, co-occurrence, and correlates of adolescent bullying at school. *Journal of School Health, 77,* 623–629.

Centers for Disease Control and Prevention. (2012). Sexual violence. Retrieved from *www. cdc.gov/ViolencePrevention/sexualviolence.*

Centers for Disease Control and Prevention. (2016). Teen dating violence. Retrieved from *www.cdc.gov/violenceprevention/intimatepartnerviolence/teen_dating_violence.html.*

Chang, L. (2004). The role of classroom norms in contextualizing the relations of children's social behaviors to peer acceptance. *Developmental Psychology, 40*(5), 691–702.

Charmaraman, L., Jones, A. E., Stein, N., & Espelage, D. L. (2013). Is it bullying or sexual harassment?: Knowledge, attitudes, and professional development experiences of middle school staff. *Journal of School Health, 83,* 438–444.

Chen, J. K., & Astor, R. A. (2008). Students' report of violence against teachers in Taiwanese schools. *Journal of School Violence, 8,* 2–17.

Child Trends Databank. (2014). High school students carrying weapons. Retrieved from *www.childtrends.org/?indicators=high-school-students-carrying-weapons.*

Cohen, J., McCabe, E. M., Michelli, N. M., & Pickeral, T. (2009). School climate: Research, policy, practice, and teacher education. *Teachers College Record, 111,* 180–213.

Coie, J. D., & Dodge, K. A. (1998). Aggression and antisocial behavior. In W. Damon (Series Ed.) & N. Eisenberg (Vol. Ed.), *Handbook of child psychology: Vol. 3. Social, emotional, and personality development* (pp. 779–862). New York: Wiley.

Conger, R. D., Conger, K. J., Elder, G. H., Jr., Lorenz, F. O., Simons, R. L., & Whitbeck, L. B. (1992). A family process model of economic hardship and adjustment of early adolescent boys. *Child Development, 63,* 539–541.

Cook, C. R., Williams, K. R., Guerra, N. G., Kim, T. E., & Sadek, S. (2010). Predictors of bullying and victimization in childhood and adolescence: A meta-analytic investigation. *School Psychology Quarterly, 25,* 65–83.

Cottle, C. C., Lee, R. J., & Heilbrun, K. (2001). The prediction of criminal recidivism in juveniles: A meta-analysis. *Criminal Justice and Behavior, 28*(3), 367–394.

Currie, C., Zanotti, C., Morgan, A., Currie, D., DeLooze, M., Roberts, C., et al. (2012). *Social determinants of health and well-being among young people. Health Behaviour in School-aged Children (HBSC) study: International report from the 2009/2010 survey.* Copenhagen: World Health Organization Regional Office for Europe.

Danner, M. J. E., & Carmody, D. C. (2001). Missing gender in cases of infamous school violence: Investigating research and media explanations. *Justice Quarterly, 18,* 87–114.

Decker, S. H., Melde, C., & Pyrooz, D. C. (2013). What do we know about gangs and gang members and where do we go from here? *Justice Quarterly, 30,* 369–402.

Dishion, T. J., McCord, J., & Poulin, F. (1999). When interventions harm: Peer groups and problem behavior. *American Psychologist, 54,* 755–764.

Dishion, T. J., Patterson, G. R., & Kavanagh, K. (1992). An experimental test of the coercion model: Linking theory, measurement and intervention. In J. McCord & R. Tremblay (Eds.), *The interaction of theory and practice: Experimental studies of interventions* (pp. 252–282). New York: Guilford Press.

Dishion, T. J., Véronneau, M. H., & Myers, M. W. (2010). Cascading peer dynamics underlying the progression from problem behavior to violence in early to late adolescence. *Development and Psychopathology, 22,* 603–619.

Domitrovich, C. E., Durlak, J. A., Staley, K. C., & Weissberg, R. P. (2017). Social–emotional competence: An essential factor for promoting positive adjustment and reducing risk in school children. *Child Development, 88*(2), 408–416.

Dowdy, E., Furlong, M., Raines, T. C., Bovery, B., Kauffman, B., Kamphaus, R. W., et al. (2015). Enhancing school-based mental health services with a preventative and promotive approach to universal screening for complete mental health. *Journal of Educational and Psychological Consultation, 25,* 1–20.

Durlak, J. A., Weissberg, R. P., Dymnicki, A., Taylor, R., & Schellinger, K. (2011).The impact of enhancing students' social and emotional learning: A meta-analysis of school-based universal interventions. *Child Development, 82,* 405–432.

Espelage, D. L. (2014). Ecological theory: Preventing youth bullying, aggression, and victimization. *Theory into Practice, 53,* 257–264.

Espelage, D. L., Anderman, E. M., Brown, V. E., Jones, A., Lane, K. L., McMahon, S. D., et al. (2013). Understanding and preventing violence directed against teachers. *American Psychologist, 68*(2), 75–87.

Espelage, D. L., Basile, K. C., & Hamburger, M. E. (2012). Bullying perpetration and subsequent sexual violence perpetration among middle school students. *Journal of Adolescent Health, 50,* 60–65.

Espelage, D. L., Bosworth, K., & Simon, T. R. (2000). Examining the social context of bullying behaviors in early adolescence. *Journal of Counseling and Development, 78,* 326–333.

Espelage, D. L., & De La Rue, L. (2013). Examining predictors of bullying and sexual violence perpetration among middle school female students. In B. Russell (Ed.), *Perceptions of female offenders: How stereotypes and social norms affect criminal justice responses* (pp. 25–46). New York: Springer.

Espelage, D. L., Low, S., Polanin, J., & Brown, E. (2013). The impact of a middle school program to reduce aggression, victimization, and sexual violence. *Journal of Adolescent Health, 53,* 180–186.

Espelage, D. L., Low, S., Polanin, J., & Brown, E. (2015). Clinical trial of Second Step middle-school program: Impact on aggression and victimization. *Journal of Applied Developmental Psychology, 37,* 52–63.

Espelage, D. L., Polanin, J., & Low, S. (2014). Teacher and staff perceptions of school environment as predictors of student aggression, victimization, and willingness to intervene in bullying situations. *School Psychology Quarterly, 29,* 387–405.

Espelage, D. L., Rose, C. A., & Polanin, J. R. (2015). Social–emotional learning program to reduce bullying, fighting, and victimization among middle school students with disabilities. *Remedial and Special Education, 36,* 299–311.

Espelage, D. L., & Swearer, S. M. (2003). Research on school bullying and victimization: What have we learned and where do we go from here? *School Psychology Review, 32,* 365–383.

Ezeonu, I. (2014). Doing gang research in Canada: Navigating a different kaleidoscope. *Contemporary Justice Review, 17*(1), 4–22.

Fanti, K. A., & Kimonis, E. R. (2012). Bullying and victimization: The role of conduct problems and psychopathic traits. *Journal of Research on Adolescence, 22*(4), 617–631.

Finkelhor, D., Turner, H., Ormrod, R., & Hamby, S. L. (2010). Trends in childhood violence and abuse exposure: Evidence from two national surveys. *Archives of Pediatric Adolescent Medicine, 164,* 238–242.

Fonagy, P., Twemlow, S. W., Vernberg, E., Sacco, F. C., & Little, T. D. (2005). Creating a peaceful school learning environment: The impact of an antibullying program on educational attainment in elementary schools. *Medical Science Monitor, 11*(7), CR317–CR325.

Fontaine, R., & Dodge, K. (2006). Real-time decision making and aggressive behavior in youth: A heuristic model of response evaluation and decision. *Aggressive Behavior, 32,* 604–624.

Forster, M., Grigsby, T. J., Unger, J. B., & Sussman, S. (2015). Associations between gun violence exposure, gang associations, and youth aggression: Implications for prevention and intervention programs. *Journal of Criminology.* Retrieved from *www.hindawi.com/journals/jcrim/2015/963750.*

Fosco, G. M., Frank, J. L., & Dishion, T. J. (2012). Coercion and contagion in family and school environments: Implications for educating and socializing youth. In S. R. Jimerson, A. B. Nickerson, M. J. Mayer, & M. J. Furlong (Eds.), *Handbook of school violence and school safety: International research and practice* (pp. 69–80). New York: Routledge.

Frey, K., Strong, Z., & Onyewuenyi, A. C. (2017). Individual and class norms differentially predict proactive and reactive aggression: A functional analysis. *Journal of Educational Psychology, 109*(2), 178–190.

Furlong, M., & Morrison, G. (2000). The school in school violence: Definitions and facts. *Journal of Emotional and Behavioral Disorders, 8,* 71–82.

Gage, N. A., Prykanowski, D. A., & Larson, A. (2014). School climate and bullying victimization: A latent class growth model analysis. *School Psychology Quarterly, 29*(3), 256–271.

Gini, G., Pozzoli, T., & Hymel, S. (2014). Moral disengagement among children and youth: A meta-analytic review of links to aggressive behavior. *Aggressive Behavior, 40*(1), 56–68.

Gladden, R. M., Vivolo-Kantor, A. M., Hamburger, M. E., & Lumpkin, C. D. (2014). *Bullying surveillance among youths: Uniform definitions for public health and recommended data elements, version 1.0.* Atlanta, GA: National Center for Injury Prevention and Control, Centers for Disease Control and Prevention, and U.S. Department of Education. Retrieved from *https://stacks.cdc.gov/view/cdc/21596.*

Goldweber, A., Waasdorp, T., & Bradshaw, C. (2013). Examining associations between race, urbanicity, and patterns of bullying involvement. *Journal of Youth and Adolescence, 42*, 206–219.

Gottfredson, D. C. (2001). *Schools and delinquency*. Cambridge, UK: Cambridge University Press.

Gottfredson, M. R., & Hirschi, T. (1990). *A general theory of crime*. Stanford, CA: Stanford University Press.

Gottfredson, M. R., & Hirschi, T. (2003). Self-control and opportunity. In C. L. Britt & M. R. Gottfredson (Eds.), *Advances in criminological theory: Vol. 12. Control theories of crime and delinquency* (pp. 5–19). London: Routledge.

Guo, G., Roettger, M. E., & Cai, T. (2008). The integration of genetic propensities into social-control models of delinquency and violence among male youths. *American Sociological Review, 73*, 543–568.

Herrenkohl, T. I., Lee, J., & Hawkins, J. D. (2012). Risk versus direct protective factors and youth violence: Seattle social development project. *American Journal of Preventive Medicine, 43*(2), S41–S56.

Hill, C., & Kearl, H. (2011). *Crossing the line: Sexual harassment at school*. Washington, DC: American Association of University Women. Retrieved from *http://files.eric.ed.gov/fulltext/ED525785.pdf*.

Hines, P. M., Vega, W., & Jemmott, J. (2004). *Final report: A culture based model for youth violence risk-reduction*. Unpublished manuscript.

Hirschstein, M. K., & Frey, K. S. (2006). Promoting behavior and beliefs that reduce bullying: The STEPS TO RESPECT program. In S. R. Jimerson, A. B., Nickerson, M. J. Mayer, & M. J. Furlong (Eds.), *Handbook of school violence and school safety: From research to practice* (pp. 309–324). Mahwah, NJ: Erlbaum.

Howell, J. C., & Lynch, J. (2000, August). Youth gangs in schools. *Juvenile Justice Bulletin: Youth Gang Series*. Retrieved from *www.tampabayschools.org/docs/00/00/05/93/Youth_Gangs_in_Schools.pdf*.

Huber, L. P. (2011). Discourses of racist nativism in California public education: English dominance as racist nativist microaggressions. *Educational Studies, 47*, 379–401.

Huesmann, L. R., Guerra, N. G., Miller, L. S., & Zelli, A. (1992). The role of social norms in the development of aggressive behavior. In A. Fraczek & H. Zumkley (Eds.), *Socialization and aggression* (pp. 139–152). Berlin: Springer.

Hyde, J. S. (1984). How large are gender differences in aggression?: A developmental meta-analysis. *Developmental Psychology, 20*, 722–736.

Hymel, S., McClure, R., Miller, M., Shumka, E., & Trach, J. (2015). Addressing school bullying: Insights from theories of group processes. *Journal of Applied Developmental Psychology, 37*, 16–24.

Hymel, S., Starosta, L., Gill, R., & Low, R. (2018). Challenges in promoting mental well-being and addressing violence through schools. In P. Slee, G. Skzrupiec, & C. Cefai (Eds.), *Child and adolescent well-being and violence prevention in schools* (pp. 3–13). New York: Routledge.

Hymel, S., & Swearer, S. M. (2015). Four decades of research on school bullying: An introduction. *American Psychologist, 70*(4), 300–310.

Jimerson, S. R., Nickerson, A. B., Mayer, M. J., & Furlong, M. J. (Eds.). *Handbook of school violence and school safety*. New York: Routledge.

Jones, L. M., Mitchell, K. J., & Finkelhor, D. (2013). Online harassment in context: Trends from three youth Internet safety surveys (2000, 2005, 2010). *Psychology of Violence, 3*, 53–69.

Juvonen, J., Graham, S., & Shuster, M. A. (2003). Bullying among young adolescents: The strong, the weak, and the troubled. *Pediatrics, 112*, 1231–1237.

Kann, L., Kinchen, S., Shanklin, S. L., Flint, K. H., Hawkins, J., Harris, W. A., et al. (2014).

Youth Risk Behavior Surveillance—United States, 2013. *Morbidity and Mortality Weekly Report, 63*(4), 1–168. Retrieved from *www.cdc.gov/mmwr/pdf/ss/ss6304.pdf.*

Kann, L., McManus, T., Harris, W. A., Shanklin, S. L., Flint, K. H., Hawkins, J., et al. (2016). Youth Risk Behavior Surveillance—United States, 2015. *Morbidity and Mortality Weekly Report: Surveillance Summaries, 65*(6), 1–174. Retrieved from *www.cdc.gov/mmwr/volumes/65/ss/ss6506a1.htm.*

Katz, J. (1995). Reconstructing masculinity in the locker room: The Mentors in Violence Prevention Project. *Harvard Educational Review, 65*(2), 163–175.

Katz, J. (2000). *Tough guise: Violence, media and the crisis of masculinity* [Film]. Northhampton, MA: Media Education Foundation.

Kohli, R., & Solorzano, D. G. (2012). Teachers, please learn our names!: Racial microaggressions and the K–12 classroom. *Race Ethnicity and Education, 15,* 441–462.

Konishi, C., Miyazaki, Y., Hymel, S., & Waterhouse, T. (2017). Investigating associations between school climate and bullying in secondary schools: Multilevel contextual effects modeling *School Psychology International, 38*(3), 240–263.

Kosciw, J. G., Greytak, E. A., Palmer, N. A., & Boesen, M. J. (2014). *The 2013 National School Climate Survey: The experiences of lesbian, gay, bisexual and transgender youth in our nation's schools.* New York: GLSEN. Retrieved from *http://files.eric.ed.gov/fulltext/ED535177.pdf.*

Kuhn, E. S., & Laird, R. D. (2013). Parent and peer restrictions of opportunities attenuate the link between low self-control and antisocial behavior. *Social Development, 22*(4), 813–830.

Kutcher, S. (2015). Mental health and high school curriculum guide: Understanding mental health and mental illness. Retrieved from *http://teenmentalhealth.org/curriculum/wp-content/uploads/2015/06/DRAFT-6-2015-Version-New-Design.compressed.pdf.*

Laub, J., & Lauritsen, J. (1998). The interdependence of school violence with neighborhood and family conditions. In D. Elliott, B. Hamburg, & K. Williams (Eds.), *Violence in American schools: A new perspective* (pp. 127–155). Cambridge, UK: Cambridge University Press.

Lewis, C. W., Butler, B. R., Bonner, F. L., & Joubert, M. (2010). African American male discipline patterns and school district responses resulting impact on academic achievement: Implications for urban educators and policy makers. *Journal of African American Males in Education, 1,* 8–25.

Lösel, F., & Farrington, D. P. (2012). Direct protective and buffering protective factors in the development of youth violence. *American Journal of Preventive Medicine, 43*(2), S8–S23.

Maruna, S., & Copes, H. (2005). What have we learned from five decades of neutralization research? In M. Tonry (Ed.), *Crime and justice: A review of research* (Vol. 32, pp. 221–320). Chicago: University of Chicago Press.

McDougall, P., & Vaillancourt, T. (2015). Long-term adult outcomes of peer victimization in childhood and adolescence: Pathways to adjustment and maladjustment. *American Psychologist, 70*(4), 300–310.

Minikel-Lacocque, J. (2013). Racism, college, and the power of words: Racial microaggressions reconsidered. *American Educational Research Journal, 50,* 432–465.

Moffitt, T., & Caspi, A. (2001). Childhood predictors differentiate life-course persistent and adolescent-limited antisocial pathways among males and females. *Development and Psychopathology 13,* 355–375.

Mulford, C. F., & Blachman-Demner, D. R. (2013). Teen dating violence: Building a research program through collaborative insights. *Violence against Women, 19*(6), 756–770.

Nadal, K. L. (2010). Gender microaggressions: Implications for mental health. In M. A. Paludi (Ed.), *Feminism and women's rights worldwide: Vol. 2. Mental and physical health* (pp. 155–175). Santa Barbara, CA: Praeger.

Nansel, T. R., Overpeck, M., Pilla, R. S., Ruan, W. J., Simons-Morton, B., & Scheidt, P.

(2001). Bullying behaviors among U.S. youth: Prevalence and association with psychosocial adjustment. *Journal of the American Medical Association, 285,* 2094–2100.

National Center for Education Statistics. (2017). *Indicator 2: Incidence of victimization at school and away from school.* Washington, DC: Author. Retrieved from *https://nces.ed.gov/programs/crimeindicators/ind_02.asp.*

Newcomb, A. F., Bukowski, W. M., & Pattee, L. (1993). Children's peer relations: A meta-analytic review of popular, rejected, neglected, controversial and average sociometric status. *Psychological Bulletin, 113,* 99–128.

Olweus, D. (1993). *Bullying at school.* Cambridge, MA: Blackwell.

Patterson, G. R. (1982). *A social learning approach: III. Coercive family process.* Eugene, OR: Castalia.

Patterson, G. R. (1986). Performance models for antisocial boys. *American Psychologist, 41,* 432–444.

Patterson, G. R., DeBaryshe, B., & Ramsey, E. (1989). A developmental perspective on antisocial behaviour. *American Psychologist, 44,* 329–335.

Payne, A. (2008). A multilevel model of the relationships among communal school disorder, student bonding, and delinquency. *Journal of Research in Crime and Delinquency, 45,* 429–455.

Polanin, J., & Espelage, D. L. (2015). Using a meta-analytic technique to assess the impact of treatment intensity measures in a multi-site cluster-randomized trial. *Journal of Behavioral Education, 24,* 133–151.

Polanin, J. R., Espelage, D. L., & Pigott, T. D. (2012). A meta-analysis of school-based bullying prevention program's effects on bystander intervention behavior. *School Psychology Review, 41,* 47–65.

Pratt, T. C., & Cullen, F. T. (2000). The empirical status of Gottfredson and Hirschi's general theory of crime: A meta-analysis. *Criminology, 38*(3), 931–964.

Pyrooz, D. C., & Sweeten, G. (2015). Gang membership between ages 5 and 17 years in the United States. *Journal of Adolescent Health, 56,* 414–419.

Reddy, L. A., Espelage, D., McMahon, S. D., Anderman, E. M., Lane, K. L., Brown, V. E., et al. (2013). Violence against teachers: Case studies from the APA task force. *International Journal of School and Educational Psychology, 1,* 231–245.

Rhee, S., & Waldman, I. D. (2002). Genetic and environmental influences on antisocial behavior: A meta-analysis of twin and adoption studies. *Psychological Bulletin, 128*(3), 490–529.

Ribeaud, D., & Eisner, M. (2010). Are moral disengagement, neutralization techniques, and self-serving cognitive distortions the same?: Developing a unified scale of moral neutralization of aggression. *International Journal of Conflict and Violence, 4*(2), 298–315.

Rinehart, S. J., & Espelage, D. L. (2016). A multilevel analysis of school climate, homophobic name-calling, and sexual harassment victimization/perpetration among middle school youth. *Psychology of Violence, 6,* 213–222.

Rivers, S. E., Brackett, M. A., Reyes, M. R., Elbertson, N. A., & Salovey, P. (2013). Improving the social and emotional climate of classrooms: A clustered randomized controlled trial testing the RULER approach. *Prevention Science, 14*(1), 77–87.

Robers, S., Zhang, A., Morgan, R.E., & Musu-Gillette, L. (2015). *Indicators of School Crime and Safety: 2014* (NCES 2015-072/NCJ 248036). Retrieved from *http://files.eric.ed.gov/fulltext/ED557756.pdf.*

Rodkin, P. C., Farmer, T. W., Pearl, R., & Van Acker, R. (2000). Heterogeneity of popular boys: Antisocial and prosocial configurations. *Developmental Psychology, 36,* 14–24.

Ross, S. W., Horner, R. H., & Higbee, T. (2009). Bully prevention in positive behavior support. *Journal of Applied Behavior Analysis, 42*(4), 747–759.

Sapolsky, R. M. (2017). *Behave: The biology of humans at our best and worst.* New York: Penguin.

Schonert-Reichl, K. A., Hanson-Peterson, J., & Hymel, S. (2015). Social and emotional learning and pre-service teacher education. In J. Durlak, R. Weissberg, C. Domitrovich, & T. Gullotta (Eds.), *Handbook of social and emotional learning: Research and practice* (pp. 406–421). New York: Guilford Press.

Schonert-Reichl, K. A., & Hymel, S. (1996). Promoting social development and acceptance in the elementary classroom. In J. Andrews (Ed.), *Teaching students with diverse needs* (pp. 152–200). Scarborough, ON: Nelson Canada.

Sklad, M., Diekstra, R., De Ritter, M., & Ben, J. (2012). Effectiveness of school-based universal social, emotional, and behavioural programs: Do they enhance students' development in the area of skill, behaviour, and adjustment? *Psychology in the Schools, 49,* 892–909.

Sue, D. W., Capodilupo, C. M., Torino, G. C., Bucceri, J. M., Holder, A. M. B., Nadal, K. L., et al. (2007). Racial microaggressions in everyday life: Implications for clinical practice. *American Psychologist, 62,* 271–286.

Sugai, G., & Horner, R. R. (2006). A promising approach for expanding and sustaining school-wide positive behavior support. *School Psychology Review, 35*(2), 245–259.

Sykes, G., & Matza, D. (1957). Techniques of neutralization: A theory of delinquency. *American Sociological Review, 22,* 664–670.

Thapa, A., Cohen, J., Guffey, S., & Higgins-D'Alessandro, A. (2013). A review of school climate research. *Review of Educational Research, 83,* 357–385.

Totura, C. M. W., MacKinnon-Lewis, C., Gesten, E. L., Gadd, R., Divine, K. P., Dunham, S., et al. (2009). Bullying and victimization among boys and girls in middle school: The influence of perceived family and schools contexts. *Journal of Early Adolescence, 29,* 571–609.

Tremblay, R. E. (2000). The development of aggressive behavior during childhood: What have we learned in the past century? *International Journal of Behavioral Development, 24,* 129–141.

Tremblay, R. E., Masse, B., Perron, D., LeBlanc, M., Schwartzman, A., & Ledingham, J. (1992). Early disruptive behavior, poor school achievement, delinquent behavior, and delinquent personality: Longitudinal analyses. *Journal of Consulting and Clinical Psychology, 60*(1), 64–72.

Tremblay, R. E., & Nagin, D. S. (2005). Developmental origins of physical aggression in humans. In R. E. Tremblay, W. W. Hartup, & J. Archer (Eds.), *Developmental origins of aggression* (pp. 83–106). New York: Guilford Press.

Tremblay, R. E., Nagin, D. S., Séguin, J. R., Zoccolillo, M., Zelazo, P. D., Boivin, M., et al. (2004). Physical aggression during early childhood: Trajectories and predictors. *Pediatrics, 114*(1), e43–e50.

Ttofi, M., & Farrington, D. P. (2011). Effectiveness of school based programs to reduce bullying: A systematic and meta-analytic review. *Journal of Experimental Criminology, 7,* 27–56.

U.S. Department of Education, Office for Civil Rights. (2010, October). Dear colleague letter: Harassment and bullying. Retrieved from *www2.Ed.gov/about/offices/list/ocr/letters/colleague-201010.html.*

U.S. Department of Justice. (2004). Survey of inmates in state and federal correctional facilities. Retrieved from *www.nimh.nih.gov/health/statistics/prevalence/inmate-mental-health.shtml.*

Vagi, K. J., Olsen, E. O. M., Basile, K. C., & Vivolo-Kantor, A. M. (2015). Teen dating violence (physical and sexual) among US high school students: Findings from the 2013 National Youth Risk Behavior Survey. *JAMA Pediatrics, 169*(5), 474–482.

Vaillancourt, T., & Hymel, S. (2006). Aggression and social status: The moderating roles of sex and peer-valued characteristics. *Aggressive Behavior, 32*(4), 396–408.

Vaillancourt, T., Trinh, V., McDougall, P., Duku, E., Cunningham, L., Cunningham, C., et al. (2010). Optimizing population screening of bullying in school-aged children. *Journal of School Violence, 9*, 233–250.

Vitaro, F., Pedersen, S., & Brendgen, M. (2007). Children's disruptiveness, peer rejection, friends' deviancy, and delinquent behaviors: A process-oriented approach. *Development and Psychopathology, 19*(2), 433–453.

Waasdorp, T. E., Bradshaw, C. P., & Leaf, P. J. (2012). The impact of schoolwide positive behavioral interventions and supports on bullying and peer rejection: A randomized controlled effectiveness trial. *Archives of Pediatrics and Adolescent Medicine, 166*(2), 149–156.

Walker, H. M., & Shinn, M. R. (2002). Structuring school-based interventions to achieve integrated primary, secondary, and tertiary prevention goals for safe and effective schools. In M. R. Shinn, G. Stoner, & H. M. Walker (Eds.), *Interventions for academic and behavior problems: Preventive and remedial approaches* (pp. 1–26). Silver Spring, MD: National Association of School Psychologists.

Way, N. (2011). *Deep secrets*. Cambridge, MA: Harvard University Press.

Weare, K. (2010). Mental health and social and emotional learning: Evidence, principles, tensions and balances. *Advances in School Mental Health Promotion, 3*, 5–17.

Wilson, S. J., & Lipsey, M. W. (2007). School-based interventions for aggressive and disruptive behavior: Update of a meta-analysis. *American Journal of Preventive Medicine, 33*(2), S130–S143.

Woodford, M. R., Howell, M. L., Kulick, A., & Silverschanz, P. (2012). "That's so gay": Heterosexual male undergraduates and the perpetuation of sexual orientation microaggressions on campus. *Journal of Interpersonal Violence, 28*, 416–435.

World Health Organization. (2015). Youth violence: The health sector role in prevention and response. Retrieved from *www.bocsar.nsw.gov.au/Documents/BB/bb50.pdf.*

Yeager, D. S., Fong, C. J., Lee, H. Y., & Espelage, D. L. (2015). Declines in efficacy of anti-bullying programs among older adolescents: Theory and a three-level meta-analysis. *Journal of Applied Developmental Psychology, 37*, 36–51.

Yun, I., & Hwang, E. (2011). A study of occasional and intensive weapon carrying among adolescents using a nationally representative sample. *Youth Violence and Juvenile Justice, 9*, 366–382.

Zhang, A., Musu-Gillette, L., & Oudekerk, B. A. (2016). *Indicators of school crime and safety: 2015* (NCES 2016-079/NCJ 249758). Washington, DC: National Center for Education Statistics.

Zins, J. E., Weissberg, R. P., Wang, M. C., & Walberg, H. J. (2004). *Building academic success on social and emotional learning: What does the research say?* New York: Teachers College Press.

CHAPTER 19

International Perspectives on Bullying Prevention

CHRISTINA SALMIVALLI

Brief Introduction

Children and young people spend a considerable share of their waking time at school. Thus it is no wonder that conflicts and aggressive encounters take place in the school context. In the early 1970s, a specific type of aggression among peers at school emerged in the scientific literature—now known as *bullying* in the English-speaking world.

Being bullied was originally defined by Olweus (1978) as *being exposed, repeatedly and over time, to negative actions on the part of one or more other students* within the context of a power imbalance. Three elements are usually considered the defining characteristics of bullying: (1) intent to harm (which is characteristic of all aggressive behavior), (2) a power differential between the targeted child and the perpetrator, and (3) repetition over time. In other languages and cultures, there are concepts referring to the same, or a very similar, phenomenon, such as *ijime* (Japan), or *wang-ta* (South Korea).

The importance of preventing bullying can be understood in light of its severe and sometimes long-lasting consequences. Targeted students suffer from numerous adjustment problems (Cook, Williams, Guerra, Kim, & Sadek, 2010; Hawker & Boulton, 2000). Childhood victimization is a unique predictor of depression and other mental health problems in adulthood, whereas bullying behavior is predictive of later criminal offending (Farrington, Ttofi, & Lösel, 2011; Klomek, Sourander, & Elonheimo, 2015; Lereya, Copeland, Costello, & Wolke, 2015; Ttofi, Farrington, Lösel, & Loeber, 2011). There is evidence that just witnessing bullying bears negative consequences for the bystanders (Rivers, Poteat, Noret, & Ashurst, 2009).

Therefore, research on bullying and its effective prevention has enormous societal relevance, in addition to its scientific value.

This chapter focuses on bullying as a global phenomenon and different approaches taken to address the problem, from national regulatory frameworks (e.g., legislation) to school-based prevention programs and, finally, measures taken to intervene in ongoing bullying. Evidence concerning the effectiveness of different approaches is reviewed, and future directions for research and practice are discussed.

Main Issues

Bullying: A Universal Phenomenon

Systematic research on bullying was initiated by Dan Olweus (1978, 1993), first in Sweden and later on in Norway, inspiring researchers in other European countries, as well as in Australia, Canada, and the United States. Quite independently from research in Western countries, research on bullying had emerged in Japan as early as in the 1980s, where the phenomenon was known as *ijime* (Morita, 1985; Morita & Kiyonaga, 1986). Soon after, both media and researchers in South Korea started paying attention to what was first called *Korean ijime*—and later on *wang-ta* (Kwak & Lee, 2016, pp. 93–94). During the 1990s the Western and Eastern research traditions came together, with increasing mutual influence and collaboration. In the rest of Asia (apart from Japan and South Korea), as well as in Latin America and Africa, societal and academic attention to bullying has risen more recently. Bullying is now acknowledged as a serious global problem (Richardson & Hiu, 2016), influencing the lives of millions of children and youth.

Prevalence

Due to varying definitions and measurement instruments across studies and surveys, the prevalence of young people targeted by bullies or bullying others is not easy to determine. Caution is needed when making country comparisons, especially when relying on data from separate, individual studies done in different countries. Variation that is attributed to country differences can in fact be due to different measurement instruments or different samples that are not necessarily representative of the countries compared. However, there are several large-scale surveys that provide data on the prevalence of students involved in bullying across countries, utilizing identical definition and measurement of bullying, along with large samples of students from comparable age groups.

Based on such international surveys, it seems clear that between-country differences in the prevalence of bullying exist. Recently, Smith, Robinson, and Marchi (2016) suggested caution in interpreting these data. They compared data from four large international surveys: the Trends in International Mathematics and Science Study (TIMSS), Health Behavior in School-Aged Children (HBSC), Global School Health Survey (GSHS), and EU Kids Online Survey (*www.eukidsonline.net*) that all have questions on being bullied. They found only a low agreement between the different datasets concerning victim prevalence rates across countries.

Richardson and Hiu (2016), however, developed a method by which they were able to produce valid estimates of "relative bullying risk" across countries in order to do a proper global comparison on rates of students bullied by their peers. Their study was based on data from 53 countries and six international surveys: TIMSS (2011), HBSC (2001/2002), and GSHS (2003–2014) surveys, Children's Worlds Report (2015), and data from the Second Regional Comparative and Explanatory Study (SERCE) by the Latin American Laboratory for Assessment of the Quality of Education (LLECE) in 2008 and the Third Regional Comparative and Explanatory Study (TERCE) by LLECE in 2015.

The resulting Global Map of Relative Bullying Risk (Figure 19.1) shows that, according to most recent survey data, Canada, the western side of South America, parts of Eastern Europe, the Middle East–Northern Africa region, and islands in the Pacific have the highest relative risk. Countries in Western Europe, the United States, eastern parts of South America, much of the Middle East and North Africa, Australia, Japan, and Mongolia belong to the medium-risk category. Low-risk countries can be found in Northern Europe, Southeast Asia, and Russia, as well as Kazakhstan, South Korea, and Thailand, along with a few countries in Central and South America.

Overall, it can be concluded that bullying is not infrequent in any country in which it has been studied. The prevalence of elementary school students repeatedly victimized by their peers at school varies between 7% and almost 50% across studies and surveys. Part of the variation is probably due to country differences, but the prevalence rates also depend on the definition and measurement of bullying, the age groups studied, and other sample differences. If, for instance, the sample in one country involves high-socioeconomic-status (SES) urban schools and in another country consists of low-SES rural schools, differences in prevalence rates can hardly be attributed to country differences alone.

Cultural Similarities and Differences

It has been discussed whether concepts such as *bullying, ijime,* and *wang-ta* refer to identical phenomena or whether they cover experiences including cultural differences. There seem to be many similarities across cultures, beginning with the defining characteristics of bullying and *ijime.* Morita (1985; see Morita, Soeda, Soeda, & Taki, 1999) originally defined *ijime* as "a type of aggressive behavior by which someone who holds a dominant position in a group-interaction process, by intentional or collective acts, causes mental and/or physical suffering to another inside a group" (p. 320). Thus both bullying and *ijime* have been defined as including intentional harmful acts in the context of a power imbalance.

Empirical studies done in different cultures (see, e.g., Smith et al., 1999) show that these behaviors or experiences take many forms (e.g., physical, verbal, social/relational, online attacks), among which the most common is verbal abuse, such as name calling and public ridicule. Males are more frequent perpetrators as well as targets. Developmental changes are similar across countries: The rates of students

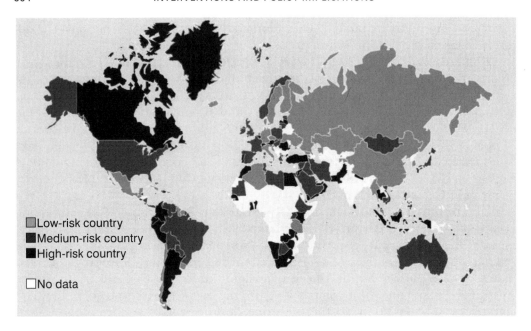

FIGURE 18.1. Global map of relative bullying risk. From Richardson and Hiu (2016). Copyright ©
2016 United Nations. Reprinted by permission.

being targeted decrease by age, whereas the rates of perpetrators increase during
and after preadolescent years. Finally, the correlates of being targeted are similar
across cultures, including, for instance, low self-esteem, depression, anxiety, loneliness, and suicidal ideation.

When it comes to possible differences, both *ijime* and *wang-ta* have been discussed as involving severe social exclusion from the majority of or from all classmates as their key constituent (Sittichai & Smith, 2015; Yoon, Bauman, Choi, &
Hutchinson, 2011). Morita and colleagues (1999, p. 311) pointed out that *ijime* is
conceptualized as an in-group phenomenon, and the reference to mental suffering
comes before the reference to physical suffering in its definition. Thus *ijime* has
predominantly been understood as group-based nonphysical violence, such as the
majority of or all classmates turning against the victim and excluding him or her,
whereas research on bullying started with a clear focus on direct aggression (Salmivalli & Peets, 2009).

Sittichai and Smith (2015) argued that a more collectivistic culture (which both
Japan and South Korea represent) may imply a greater possibility of concerted whole-
group (e.g., whole-class) norms emerging—sometimes leading to severe whole-class
aggression and shunning of a victim. Smith (2016) found support for these assumptions by comparing the relative rates of social exclusion (as part of all bullying) as
well as the ratio of bullies to victims in collectivistic and individualistic cultures;
both were higher in collectivistic cultures. However, bullying was also overall more
prevalent in collectivistic cultures, which was contrary to Smith's expectations.

Besides individualism–collectivism, Smith (2016) tested hypotheses regarding two other dimensions of cultural values (Hofstede, 1980) and bullying: These were masculinity–femininity and uncertainty avoidance. Contrary to expectations, he did not find more sexist/sexual bullying or a greater male–female difference in bully rates in more masculine cultures with highly distinct gender roles. However, as hypothesized, he found a greater male–female difference in victim rates in such cultures. Finally, contrary to expectations, high uncertainty avoidance (the extent to which people feel threatened by ambiguous or unknown situations) was unrelated to bias bullying, referring to bullying based on ethnicity, religion, or physical appearance.

The findings are interesting, although controversial, as some of them supported the hypotheses, whereas others did not. The results may be confounded by factors such as differences in regulative frameworks related to bullying, income inequality differences, differences in educational systems, or overall prevention and intervention work done across countries. For instance, more individualistic, as compared with collectivistic, cultures have antibullying laws and policies in place (Smith, 2016). The role of income inequality is interesting but so far controversial. Elgar and colleagues found students more likely to report bullying others in countries with more unequal distribution of income in one study (Elgar, Craig, Boycec, Morgan, & Vella-Zarb, 2009), but not in another (Elgar et al., 2015).

At this point, the knowledge base on cultural differences in bullying does not enable making recommendations concerning culture-specific bullying prevention. Victimization and bullying, as well as their risk factors and mechanisms, actually look quite similar across countries and cultures. However, normative beliefs related to aggressive and violent behavior (e.g., attitudes concerning corporal punishment of children), the level of violence in the society, awareness of bullying being a serious problem with negative consequences, or teacher education vary across cultures; such factors might have on impact on where to begin with prevention work.

Theoretical Considerations

Theory of Change

Thinking of any systematic approach or program to reduce bullying, there should be an explicated *theory of change*, stating which elements in the approach or program are expected to lead to a reduction of bullying (program theory) and through which mechanisms (conceptual theory). Thus the development of the specific contents or actions involved in a prevention program should be rooted in a program theory. This theory can be further elaborated and developed by empirically testing the unique and interactive effects of different program components, or actions taken. The conceptual theory is about the mechanisms of bullying that are targeted and are expected to lead to the change. The conceptual theory can be tested by examining whether the hypothesized mediators of program effects lead to the desired outcome: decrease in bullying.

Current Understanding of the Nature of Bullying

How we understand bullying (especially the factors responsible for its emergence and maintenance) is the basis for the development of approaches to reduce it—it guides the theory of change. It is a common view that factors influencing bullying can be sought at various systemic levels (society, community, school, classroom, peer clique, family, individual child characteristics). Inspired by Bronfenbrenner's (1979) writings, Espelage and Swearer (2010) have emphasized this thinking in the field of bullying.

Most empirical work on bullying focuses on the classroom, peer clique, and/or individual levels. Less research has been done on school-level factors, and almost no studies have considered factors that might affect the level of bullying in a country or culture (for exceptions, see Elgar et al., 2009, 2015; Smith, 2016).

Although school-level factors have received attention, there is little agreement about the characteristics of schools that make them more or less resistant to bullying (see review by Saarento, Garandeau, & Salmivalli, 2015). Demographic factors such as school size do not seem to make a difference (although some studies find an increased risk for being bullied in larger schools; see Bowes et al., 2009). Although a positive school climate is negatively associated with bullying (Cook et al., 2010), the direction of the effect is unknown.

At the classroom level, classroom norms, the level of hierarchy in classrooms, and teacher responses and characteristics have been found to be associated with bullying. Classroom norms can be reflected in the behaviors of students when witnessing bullying. As the reactions of peers in such situations provide direct feedback to the bullies, they have important implications for the emergence and maintenance of bullying. The frequency of bullying perpetration is indeed higher in classrooms in which reinforcing the bullies' behavior is common and defending the victimized classmates is rare, implying that bullying is socially rewarded (Salmivalli, Voeten, & Poskiparta, 2011). Classroom norms that fuel bullying can also be indicated by low levels of antibullying attitudes and by positive expectations regarding the social outcomes of bullying behavior at the classroom level.

Classroom hierarchy is associated with bullying behavior: There is more bullying in hierarchical classrooms, in which peer status (such as popularity) or power (who typically decides about things) are centered upon a few individuals rather than evenly distributed. Over time, classroom hierarchy leads to increases in bullying over time, rather than bullying leading to more hierarchy (Garandeau, Lee, & Salmivalli, 2014). A nonhierarchical classroom, on the other hand, is not a good soil in which bullying can flourish.

Finally, teacher attitudes toward bullying are associated with the level of bullying problems in a classroom. A study examining the mediators of the KiVa[1] antibullying program (Saarento, Boulton, & Salmivalli, 2015) found that changes in student perceptions of their teachers' bullying-related attitudes mediated program effects. During the year when the KiVa program was implemented, students started to perceive their teachers' attitudes as more disapproving of bullying, and consequently their bullying behavior decreased. This evidences the importance of

---

[1]KiVa = *Kiusaamista Vastaan,* which means "against bullying." The KiVa antibullying program was developed in the University of Turku, Finland, by Salmivalli's team.

teachers' communicating their disapproval of bullying to students (for a discussion on the role of teachers, see also Troop-Gordon, 2015).

The views regarding individual characteristics leading to bullying behavior are somewhat controversial. Some theoretical accounts view bullies as individuals who lack social skills and have low self-esteem, deficiencies in social information-processing, low social standing in the peer group, and other adjustment problems. Others view bullying as functional, adaptive behavior associated with benefits. Empirical studies have not always succeeded in clarifying this issue, partly due to the failure to acknowledge the heterogeneity of young people engaging in bullying. Some of them are victimized themselves (so-called bully/victims), whereas others can be considered "pure" (nonvictimized) bullies. Bully/victims are a distinct, albeit a rather small group of children. They are highly rejected by their peers and show both externalizing and internalizing problems, being more maladjusted than pure bullies.

Bullying behavior used to be seen as associated with a low self-esteem. Although negative self-related cognitions are related to bullying, they do not predict a greater likelihood of being a pure bully (Cook et al., 2010). In contrast, recent evidence suggests that narcissism, or a sense of grandiosity and entitlement, as well as callous–unemotional traits (characterized by lack of empathy and guilt; see Frick & Matlasz, Chapter 2, this volume) are associated with bullying (e.g., Fanti & Kimonis, 2012; Viding, Simmonds, Petrides, & Frederickson, 2009). The belief that bullies are socially incompetent was challenged by Sutton, Smith, and Swettenham (1999), who found that 7- to 10-year-old bullies were skilled in understanding of others' cognitions and emotions. Many (pure) bullies seem to be bistrategic controllers who successfully use both prosocial and coercive strategies to get what they want (Olthof, Goossens, Vermande, Aleva, & van der Meulen, 2011; Reijntjes, Vermande, Olthof, & Goossens, 2018). Bullies value dominance (Olthof et al., 2011; Sijtsema, Veenstra, Lindenberg, & Salmivalli, 2009), and even if they are not personally liked by many classmates, they may be perceived as popular, powerful, and "cool" among their peers (Caravita, Di Blasio, & Salmivalli, 2009; Reijntjes et al., 2013). Moreover, they are often central members of their peer networks and have friends. Underlining the heterogeneity of perpetrators of bullying, Peeters, Cillessen, and Scholte (2010) identified three subtypes of bullies: popular–socially intelligent, popular moderate, and unpopular–less socially intelligent; the last group might represent bully/victims, who are also targeted themselves.

The characteristics of children who end up as victimized can be understood in the light of the bullies' characteristics and goals: Children who are unassertive and insecure may elicit aggression-encouraging cognitions in potential bullies, or make themselves suitable targets for a peer aiming for status and power. Victimization is indeed associated with internalizing problems such as depression, anxiety, and low self-esteem (Cook et al., 2010; Hawker & Boulton, 2000), as well as interpersonal difficulties such as peer rejection, having few or no friends, and negative friendship quality (Cook et al., 2010; Hawker & Boulton, 2000). Also, children with externalizing problems and low levels of prosocial behavior are more likely to be victimized (Card & Hodges, 2008). Children with internalizing or externalizing problems are more likely to become victimized if they also face interpersonal difficulties (Hodges, Malone, & Perry, 1997). By choosing victims who are submissive, insecure about themselves, physically weak, and/or rejected by the peer group, bullies can signal their power to the rest of the group without having to be afraid of confrontation or losing affection of other peers (Veenstra, Lindenberg, Munniksma, & Dijkstra, 2010).

Regarding family influence, bullies tend to perceive their parents as authoritarian, punitive, and unsupportive (Baldry & Farrington, 2000) and their families as incohesive (Bowers, Smith, & Binney, 1994). In a meta-analysis by Cook and colleagues (2010), however, family factors were weakly related to bullying. Although some children who are victimized by peers are also abused in other contexts, including their homes, several studies have found that victims view their home environments as rather positive but overprotective. Overprotection is more strongly related to being a pure victim, whereas abuse/neglect in the family is associated with the bully/victim status (Lereya, Samara, & Wolke, 2013).

It is important to realize that whether individual risk factors for bullying or victimization actually lead to such behaviors or experiences may depend on the context (e.g., Brendgen, Girard, Vitaro, Dionne, & Boivin, 2013; Kärnä, Voeten, Poskiparta, & Salmivalli, 2010). What is a vulnerability in one classroom may not be a vulnerability in another classroom. Kärnä and colleagues (2010) found that social anxiety was most strongly associated with victimization in classrooms in which reinforcing the bully was normative, that is, occurring at high levels. The same can be assumed to apply at the level of schools, communities, and even countries: The greater the tolerance of bullying (or lack of openly communicated disapproval of bullying), the more likely it is that risk factors for bullying or victimization actually lead to such behaviors or experiences.

Prejudice-related bullying, such as bullying against sexual or ethnic minorities, may have its specific contextual predictors, such as attitudes and tolerance toward minorities in a given context. Hatzenbuehler, Duncan, and Johnson (2015) found that the rate of sexual minority youth experiencing relational and electronic bullying was higher in neighborhoods with higher LGBT assault hate crime rates, whereas there was no association between LGBT assault hate crimes and bullying among heterosexual youths.

In summary, many individual-level risk factors for bullying and victimization have been identified, and they seem to be similar rather than different in different parts of the world where bullying has so far been studied. However, norms in a given context play a part in the actualization of the risk. Thus knowing an individual risk factor does not imply that we should target that individual characteristic in our interventions—influencing the context (e.g., increasing tolerance, challenging bystanders to respond differently when witnessing bullying) may be an easier and a more effective strategy. Of course, sometimes it is the only ethical strategy: Some individual risk factors cannot be changed (nor should one even attempt to change them), as is the case with prejudice-based bullying.

Methods of Prevention and Intervention

National Strategies or Frameworks/Legislation

As awareness of the prevalence and negative consequences of bullying has increased, numerous countries have launched nationwide frameworks and/or legislation to address the problem. Norway's national campaign in 1983, launched by the Ministry of Education and led by Dan Olweus, was the first of its kind in the world. By the mid-1990s, both Swedish and Norwegian parliaments had passed school laws requiring schools to develop intervention programs or policies against bullying. Later on, mainly during the 21st century, similar laws have come to force in numerous countries. Antibullying legislation is not limited to Western and/or high-income countries; similar laws exist, for instance, in Japan, the Philippines, Peru, and Mexico.

Typically, the legislation makes it mandatory for schools to have a policy, or an action plan, against bullying. The Education Act in the United Kingdom, for instance, places a duty on all state schools to have a policy including measures to prevent all forms of bullying among pupils. The Dutch Social Safety in Schools Act, commonly called the Anti-Bullying Act, makes it mandatory for school boards to ensure social safety in their schools. Since 2015, the act includes the obligation for school boards to implement a social safety policy and to assign someone the tasks of (1) coordinating the policy on bullying and acting as a point of contact and (2) monitoring the social safety of pupils in a way that provides an up-to-date and representative picture. In the United States, all 50 states have adopted antibullying laws (Rivara & Menestrel, 2016). The first of these laws was passed in 1999, partly in response to the Columbine shootings, and the last ones quite recently (Hatzenbuehler, Schwab-Reese, et al., 2015).

The legislation usually leaves it to the schools to decide on the contents of their antibullying policies. In some countries, departments of education have introduced national frameworks, or recommendations concerning elements the school policies should include. For instance, it may be recommended that a policy clearly define bullying, that it contain elements of prevention as well as intervening in ongoing bullying, or that the policy and its effects be monitored and evaluated. In the United States, the Department of Education has established a framework for antibullying laws, with recommended elements that should be included (Hatzenbuehler, Schwab-Reese, et al., 2015). In Australia, the National Safe Schools Framework, established in 2003, includes 11 guiding principles to assist schools in developing safe and supportive environments (Cross et al., 2011). Austria has a national strategy for violence prevention (Spiel & Strohmeier, 2011).

Besides regulative frameworks, some governments have provided resources for the development and/or implementation of antibullying programs. During the two "manifesto" (against bullying) periods in Norway, the government supported schools in implementing two antibullying programs (Olweus Bullying Prevention Program [OBPP] and ZERO; see Roland, 2011). In Finland, the Ministry of Education provided resources for the development, evaluation, and rollout of a national antibullying program, KiVa (Salmivalli, Kärnä, & Poskiparta, 2010).

At the national level, nongovernment organizations (NGOs) provide guidelines, recommendations, and resources to address bullying in several countries. A great example of nationwide collaboration is PrevNet in Canada, an umbrella network of 122 researchers and 62 national youth-serving organizations. It provides education, training, and research on bullying, working as a national network for knowledge mobilization to influence policy and promote change (Pepler & Craig, 2011).

School-Based Prevention and Intervention

As it is obligatory for students to come to school every day, the responsibility of the education provider in securing a safe environment for them is substantial. Schools have a moral, and often legal, responsibility to address bullying. There are good reasons to believe that school is the context in which bullying can most (cost-) effectively be addressed, as prevention efforts can be targeted at whole cohorts of children. Furthermore, research has shown that risk factors for bullying are not only characteristics of individual children; certain classroom, teacher, and school characteristics may inhibit or fuel bullying problems (for a review, see Saarento, Garandeau, & Salmivalli, 2015). Peer-group dynamics, as well as teacher responses, can best be influenced within the school system. Thus numerous school-based programs have been developed to prevent bullying and intervene in it. Some of them are proactive, or preventive, and mainly aim at inhibiting the emergence of bullying. Such programs are targeted at all students rather than specific at-risk individuals. Other programs, or approaches, are reactive, aiming to stop ongoing bullying. Programs may also combine both proactive and reactive strategies.

Proactive Strategies/Prevention

Many school-based preventive programs are manualized, including curriculum work with children and youth. The core contents are typically delivered by teachers, although whole-school approach and the commitment of all adults in the school is emphasized in many programs. Programs include various strategies to deliver their key messages (e.g., learning-by-doing exercises, classroom rules) via different media (e.g., short films, online games), as well as strategies involving parents.

Bullying prevention approaches can focus on bullying specifically, or they can be more general programs to reduce aggression or to enhance social–emotional learning. There is an ongoing debate on whether bullying is best prevented with bullying-focused or more general programs. Social–emotional learning involves "the systematic development of a core set of social and emotional skills that help children more effectively handle life challenges and thrive in both their learning and their social environments" (Ragozzino & Utne O'Brien, 2009, p. 3; see Smith & Low, 2013), and the targeted skills typically include emotion regulation, empathy, self-awareness, motivation, and social competence (e.g., Kimber, Sandell, & Bremberg, 2008). As aggression in general is known to be associated with deficits in these areas, it has been assumed that bullying behavior might be reduced by enhancing social–emotional skills.

The strongest argument *against* relying solely on social–emotional learning programs in bullying prevention stems from the findings reported since the late 1990s, suggesting that bullying is *not* necessarily related to social skill deficits. Instead, school bullies can be socially intelligent, able to regulate their emotions as well as behaviors, and can have a well-developed theory of mind (Kaukiainen et al., 1999; Sutton et al., 1999). If this is the case, why would improvement in such competences lead to reduced levels of bullying? It is known, for instance, that children who bully to obtain status and power (i.e., who are proactively aggressive) rarely respond to empathy training (Viding, McCrory, Blakemore, & Frederickson, 2011), a common component of bullying interventions.

In favor of social–emotional learning programs, it could be argued that they prevent bullying by helping potential targets to make friends, join groups, or cope better with bullying. Or such programs might empower bystanders to respond constructively when they see bullying happening. For instance, enhancing bystanders' empathy toward vulnerable peers might lead them to provide support for class- or schoolmates targeted by bullying. Oftentimes, however, the mechanisms by which social–emotional learning programs are expected to exert influence on bullying (by influencing whom, and in what way; theory of change) are not well specified.

Even more general than social–emotional learning programs are programs designed to improve "school climate" generally; they, too, are sometimes referred to as bullying prevention programs. Although prevalent bullying problems tend to co-occur with students' negative perceptions of the classroom (or school) climate (Cook et al., 2010), the causal direction of the association is not clear. In other words, it is not clear whether climate becomes more positive when there is no or little bullying or whether a positive classroom climate actually prevents bullying from emerging. A positive climate and social–emotional learning are without doubt hoped-for things. However, programs that focus more directly on factors known to contribute to the emergence and maintenance of bullying problems are more likely to have an influence on such factors. For instance, providing constructive yet low-risk strategies for bystanders witnessing bullying to enhance their support of targeted, vulnerable peers rather than rewarding bullying behaviors has been found to affect bystander intentions as well as behaviors and, consequently, the frequency of bullying in classrooms (Saarento, Boulton, & Salmivalli, 2015).

Besides adult-led programs, different peer support schemes aiming to prevent bullying have been advocated and researched in the United Kingdom (e.g., Naylor & Cowie, 1999), but versions of such schemes have also raised interest in Japan (Kanetsuna & Toda, 2016). In Finland, there is a long tradition for a peer support scheme, established already in the 1970s by a nongovernmental organization, the Mannerheim League for Child Welfare (*www.mll.fi/tietoa-mllsta/welcome-manner-heim-league-child-welfare/mll-peer-support-scheme/*).

Reactive Strategies/Intervening in Bullying

Besides proactive activities designed to prevent bullying from happening, there are various school-based approaches to tackle bullying once it is occurring. Such approaches usually include direct work with the student(s) who have bullied others. Sometimes the targeted student is involved in the discussions, sometimes he or she is met with separately to gain information of what has happened and/or to provide support. Two basic distinctions can be made with respect to reactive strategies. The first is whether the approach taken is confrontational (telling the student that the bullying behavior has come to attention at school, is not acceptable, and needs to stop; perhaps the student is also sanctioned) or nonconfrontational (sharing the concern of the targeted students' situation with the bullies and trying to come up with a solution). There are, however, also approaches that fall somewhere between confrontational and nonconfrontational, such as the restorative approach.

The other distinction lies in the extent to which the approach emphasizes adult intervention versus utilizing peers (e.g., peer mediation, peer supporters, or bully tribunals).

The confrontational approach has been advocated especially by Olweus (1993), who suggests having "serious discussions" with the bullies, demanding that they change their behavior. The nonconfrontational approach stems from the *method of shared concern* introduced by Pikas (1989; for an update, see Rigby, 2011) and the *no blame approach* by Maines and Robinson (1992), an approach that has recently been replaced by the so-called *support-group method* in the United Kingdom.

In the support-group method, a form of nonconfrontational approach, the practitioner gathers a group of peers (including the ones who have been bullying but also noninvolved students who could offer support for the victim) to a meeting to share knowledge of the distress of the targeted child. The responsibility of each one of the group members is emphasized, and they are asked to state publicly what they are prepared to do to improve the situation.

There is no strong evidence of either the confrontational or nonconfrontational method being clearly superior to the other (for details, see the section "The Effectiveness of School-Based Interventions," later in the chapter). Teachers do have their preferences, however. Based on existing evidence, it seems that teachers as well as school counselors in many European countries and in North America prefer to use confrontational rather than nonconfrontational approaches when working with bullies. Burger and colleagues (Burger, Strohmeier, Spröber, Bauman, & Rigby, 2015) presented a hypothetical bullying scenario and a questionnaire of possible responses to 625 teachers in Austria and South Germany. As many as 82% of the teachers preferred a confrontational approach, such as demanding obedience to authority and focusing on externally forced control. Similarly, in surveys done in the United States (Bauman, Rigby, & Hoppa, 2008), Canada (Power-Elliott & Harris, 2012), and England (Thompson & Smith, 2011), teachers as well as counselors were highly likely to endorse confrontational strategies.

The largest pool of data so far on school personnel's preferred strategies has been collected in Finland in the context of annual surveys of schools implementing the KiVa antibullying program. Now that the program is in nationwide use (since 2009), the school personnel (more specifically, school-based KiVa teams tackling the cases of bullying) have been instructed to choose between confrontational and nonconfrontational approaches; they are provided guidelines for both. Only about one-quarter of the schools' KiVa teams are systematically using one of the two, and a vast majority of them (83.5%) have chosen the confrontational approach, whereas 16.5% use the nonconfrontational approach. The remaining schools switch between the two approaches depending on the case (33.9%), use some kind of "mixed" approach (34.3%), or say they do not know which strategy they are using (8.6%). These numbers are from the 2015 survey, but they have been largely similar across the years.

The restorative approach falls somewhere between the confrontational and nonconfrontational methods. This approach comes close to conflict mediation, and it can be done by adult or peer mediators who listen to the views of both parties and help negotiate a solution and perhaps how the bullying students might compensate for the harm they have caused.

Central Research Findings

··

Do National Strategies or Regulative Frameworks Make a Difference?

State-level antibullying legislation has become increasingly common, but its potential in influencing the rates of bullying remains an understudied topic—and a very challenging one. As legislation comes to force at a certain point in time, its effects can readily be mixed with the effects of some other changes taking place in the society, rather than the regulations themselves.

In a recent study (Hatzenbuehler, Schwab-Reese, et al., 2015), the authors used data from 25 U.S. states to examine whether the varying proportions of students being bullied (and cyberbullied) could be explained by antibullying legislation at the state level. The authors used a U.S. Department of Education (DOE) report from 2011, in which the extent to which state antibullying laws adhered to the recommendations provided by DOE were reviewed (Stuart-Cassel, Bell, & Springer, 2011).

Compliance with the DOE recommendations varied considerably across states. The state laws were coded with respect to 16 items (*yes/no*) assigned to four broader categories (one sample item from each category provided in parenthesis): definitions (e.g., prohibited behaviors defined as bullying), district policy development and review (e.g., requirements for districts to develop and implement local policies), district policy components and mandated procedures (e.g., procedures for investigating bullying incidents), and additional components (e.g., procedures for communicating the policy to students, parents, and school staff). Each state law could have a score between 0 and 16, depending on the number of recommended elements included.

The rates of students being bullied ranged between 14.1 and 26.7% (12.3–19.6% for cyberbullying). Students in states in which legislation complied with one or more DOE recommendations (in comparison with states that complied with none of them) had odds reduced by 24% (95% confidence interval [CI]: 15–32%) of being bullied and odds reduced by 20% (95% CI: 9–29%) of being cyberbullied. However, no dose–outcome association was found; a higher overall score was not related to lower rates of being bullied. Within each of the four subscales, having at least one recommended component included in state legislation reduced the students' odds of being bullied, but including a higher number of components did not provide greater protection than having only one. Thus the study findings do not allow the conclusion that better compliance with DOE recommendations is related to less bullying at the state level. Rather, they point to the direction that *complete ignorance of the recommended best practice recommendations is associated with a higher risk*.

A further analysis on individual components indicated that the presence of three components in state legislation was associated with a lower risk of both being bullied and being cyberbullied: statement of scope, description of prohibited behaviors, and requirements for districts to develop and implement local policies. This was an interesting finding that calls for further research, including mediational analyses, as suggested by the authors.

In the study by Bauman, Rigby, and Hoppa (2008), 735 U.S. school teachers and counselors (at least one from each state) responded to an online survey regarding their responses to a hypothetical bullying scenario. The participants whose schools had an antibullying policy were less likely to ignore the incident and more likely to enlist other adults to help address the case than those without a policy. These findings suggest that having an antibullying policy in place is associated with school personnel's greater likelihood of reacting when bullying comes to their attention.

The Effectiveness of School-Based Interventions

So far, evaluation studies (and, consequently, meta-analyses) mainly look at the effects of whole-school programs rather than at actions taken in specific cases of bullying. Thus we know much more about the effectiveness of prevention strategies than actual intervention approaches to stop ongoing bullying. One likely reason for this discrepancy is the need to start with a large sample of classrooms and/or schools in order to have enough bullying cases handled to enable making conclusions about the relative effectiveness of different methods tested.

Most research on the effectiveness of bullying prevention programs comes from Western high-income countries, and, therefore, it is not self-evident that the findings can be generalized to other countries and cultures. The well-known meta-analysis by Ttofi and Farrington (2011) included 44 programs; more than half of them (25) were evaluated in Europe, about one-third (15) in North America, and a few in Australia or New Zealand. Since then, new studies have been published on evaluations done in China (Ju, Shuqiong, & Wenxin, 2009), Hong Kong (Wong, Cheng, Ngan, & Ma, 2011), Turkey (Şahin, 2012), and Romania (Trip et al., 2015). Also, the KiVa antibullying program is currently being evaluated in Chile (Gaete et al., 2017). Much more research is needed, however, to systematically compare program effects across countries and diverse cultures.

In their meta-analysis, Ttofi and Farrington (2011) concluded that whole-school bullying prevention programs are often effective, reaching an average decrease of 20–23% for bullying others and of 17–20% for being bullied. The effects vary considerably across programs, but they are also affected by research designs. More specifically, weaker effects are found when programs are evaluated with more stringent designs, such as randomized controlled trials. It should be noted that some programs do *not* lead to positive outcomes, some have never been evaluated, and some have been evaluated so poorly that no conclusions can be drawn regarding their effects. A systematic review by Evans, Fraser, and Cotter (2014) reported that up to 45% of the studies showed no program effects on bullying perpetration and about 30% showed no program effects on victimization. Which school-based approaches work best, and what exactly are the effective elements of programs, are urgent questions.

The effective ingredients of the reviewed bullying prevention programs were investigated by Ttofi and Farrington (2011). Their conclusion, based on between-programs evaluation, was that the intensity (such as number of hours) and duration (number of days/months) of intervention programs is related to their effectiveness. This suggests that programs need to be long-lasting and intensive in order to have the desired effects. Apart from the intensity and duration, the authors identified two elements that were typical of the most effective programs: They included parent training or parent meetings and disciplinary methods. The disciplinary methods referred to a confrontational approach: sanctions within a warm framework, rather than a zero-tolerance approach or harsh punishments. On the other hand, there is evidence (Garandeau, Poskiparta, & Salmivalli, 2014) that in the context of a whole-school program (in this case, the KiVa antibullying program), nonconfrontational discussions challenging the bullies to think how they could help the situation of their classmate (the targeted child) can be equally effective, in some cases even more effective than a direct confrontation. This is discussed in more detail below.

The mobilization of bystanders, or the silent majority witnessing bullying, has been suggested to be one key to success. First, research findings have clearly demonstrated how peer witnesses' responses are crucial for inhibiting or fueling bullying (see Salmivalli, 2010). Even when there are students with individual characteristics that increase the risk for bullying others or being bullied by others, peer-group responses and norms have an influence on whether this risk becomes a reality. Second, some of the highly effective programs rely on enhancing bystanders' awareness, empathy, and self-efficacy to support victimized peers, instead of reinforcing the bullies' behavior (Kärnä et al., 2011). Importantly, it has been shown that changes in peer responses mediate the effects of the KiVa program on bullying (Saarento, Boulton, & Salmivalli, 2015).

Although the inclusion of the element "work with peers" was not found to strengthen the effects of antibullying programs in the analysis by Ttofi and Farrington (2011), it should be noted that in their coding, work with peers was defined as "formal engagement of peers in tackling bullying" and included the utilization of formally assigned peer mediators, or peer supporters. Thus awareness-raising about the role of *all* peers and formulation of rules for bystander intervention in classrooms was not coded as "work with peers" in their study. On a theoretical as well as an empirical basis, that kind of approach is highly recommended (Salmivalli, 2010), whereas formal peer helpers intervening in ongoing bullying has, on the basis of current evidence, little effect.

There is variation between schools and between individual teachers in how they implement prevention programs. Even programs that were designed to be intensive can be implemented more or less intensively, depending on the resources and commitment on the part of schools. Also, schools and teachers might adapt the programs and even change some critical parts—in other words, not implement the programs as they were designed to be implemented. There is evidence that better implementation fidelity is associated with better outcomes (larger reductions in students' experiences of being bullied; Haataja, Boulton, Voeten, & Salmivalli, 2014).

There are many fewer studies on the effectiveness of reactive strategies, or intervening in ongoing, specific cases of bullying, than on the effects of school-based programs. Some studies are based on teachers' satisfaction with a given approach (e.g., Smith, Howard, & Thompson, 2007)—but this tells little or nothing about the actual effects obtained. In other studies, children are asked very general questions about whether teachers took (some kind of) action and whether that was helpful in making the bullying stop (Fekkes, Pijpers, & Verloove-Vanhorick, 2005; Smith & Shu, 2000). The findings have shown that interventions by teachers do not ensure that the situation of the victim will improve.

In a study of 2,308 early adolescents in England (Smith & Shu, 2000), students reported that bullying had stopped for 27% of the victims and decreased for 29% of them when teachers tried to take action. As many as 28% of victims reported no change in their situations, and for 16 % bullying got worse. Quite similarly, a survey of 2,766 Dutch children (Fekkes et al., 2005) indicated that, after teacher intervention, bullying decreased for 49% of the victims, remained the same for 34%, and got worse for 17%. In both of these studies, it is not clear what the teachers actually did and why their actions were not more successful.

In the context of the evaluation of the KiVa antibullying program in Finland, the effects of adult intervention were investigated in a sample of 339 victimized students whose cases came to attention of school personnel and were addressed by school-based KiVa teams (Garandeau, Poskiparta, & Salmivalli, 2014). The students were from grade levels 1–9, with students from 7 to 15 years of age. In the follow-up meeting with the KiVa team (about 2 weeks after the intervention), as many as 78.2 % of the students said bullying had stopped completely, and 19.5% said it had decreased. The situation had not changed for 2.1% of the students. Only one student (0.3%) stated that bullying got worse after adult intervention. These are very high success rates (improvement for 98% of victims), but they may be partly explained by the short time lag between the intervention and the follow-up. It is also conceivable that some students felt it was socially desirable to tell the KiVa team members that their intervention had been helpful when asked in a face-to-face discussion. Furthermore, the success might be related to the fact that the interventions were carried out in the context of a wider school-based prevention program and that the KiVa teams were following a clear procedure rather than "trying to do something."

During the nationwide implementation of the KiVa antibullying program (since 2009), we have continued collecting data on the effects of the KiVa team interventions. In the latest online survey in 2016, altogether 73% (in primary school grades 1–6, 78%) of students who had been in a KiVa team discussion because they had been bullied and 82% (in primary grades, 91%) of students who had been in a discussion because they had bullied someone said the intervention made was helpful (making bullying stop or decrease). The data involve almost 10,000 victimized students and almost 7,000 students who had bullied others.

Importantly, we have investigated the relative effectiveness of utilizing a confrontational versus a nonconfrontational approach with the bullies, both in the randomized controlled evaluation of KiVa and during the nationwide implementation of the program. In the former study (Garandeau, Poskiparta, & Salmivalli, 2014), we randomly assigned the intervention schools into two conditions: Half of the schools were instructed and trained to use a confrontational approach, whereas the other half were instructed and trained to use a nonconfrontational approach in discussions with students who had been doing the bullying. The findings showed no overall difference in the effectiveness of the confrontational and nonconfrontational approaches. However, some factors moderated their relative effectiveness. First, the confrontational approach was more successful than the nonconfrontational one among secondary school grades 7–9 (but among primary grade students, the approaches were equally effective). As adolescent perpetrators are likely to be conscious of the harm they are causing to the peers they are targeting, attempts at raising their empathy may be less effective than direct confrontation. Second, the nonconfrontational approach was more effective when bullying had been going on for a long time. A potential explanation is that in cases of long-term bullying, confrontational strategies have probably already been tried with no success. As a final note, it should be pointed out that both approaches worked well and the above moderator effects were not large.

In another study with the same sample drawn from the randomized controlled evaluation of KiVa (Garandeau, Vartio, Poskiparta, & Salmivalli, 2016), the independent variable was not the approach the school's KiVa team was instructed to use; rather, it was how the approach was perceived by the individual student ("the bully") who was invited to meet the KiVa team members. The outcome variable was the bullies' self-reported intention to change their behavior. Right after the intervention, the bullies reported in an anonymous questionnaire the extent to which they perceived the KiVa team members trying to enhance their empathy and make them understand how bad a peer was feeling versus blaming them for their unacceptable behavior. The students' intention to change their behavior as a result of the discussion (reported in the same anonymous questionnaire) was equally strongly predicted from perceived empathy arousal and condemning the bullying behavior, also suggesting that the approach (as perceived by the student) does not make much of a difference.

Finally, the data collected during 7 years of nationwide dissemination of the KiVa program provide no evidence of one approach (confrontational vs. nonconfrontational) being superior to the other. What seems to be relevant is organizing systematic follow-ups for each case, handled by adults. In schools in which follow-up meetings were organized after each case, the students who were involved because they had been bullied, students who were involved because they had bullied others, and KiVa team members effectuating the discussions perceived the meetings to be more effective than did students and team members from schools in which follow-ups were not organized at all or were only organized in some cases.

In the United Kingdom, Thompson and Smith (2011) also concluded, based on teacher reports as well as student outcome data, that disciplinary methods are no more successful than either restorative or nonpunitive approaches; in their study, nonpunitive approaches included both the support-group method and the Pikas (1989) method of shared concern.

The effects of the support-group method as such have rarely been examined. Many teachers and local authorities in England, where this method is widely implemented, reported being satisfied with it (Smith et al., 2007). In the context of evaluating the KiVa antibullying program in the Netherlands, the Dutch KiVa teams were instructed to use the support-group approach. It was found (van der Ploeg, Steglich, & Veenstra, 2016) that among the 38 victims for whom a support-group intervention was organized, bullying had stopped or decreased for 84% but remained the same for 16%, according to victim reports in the follow-up meeting. At the end of the school year, however, the situation looked worse. Based on the targeted students' baseline and posttest (at the end of the school year) responses in the online questionnaire, it was concluded that bullying had stopped or decreased for 60.5% but remained the same for 7.9% and increased for 31.6%. These numbers were no better (perhaps slightly worse) than among the students for whom no support group had been organized. However, defending actions received from classmates had clearly increased for students whose cases had been handled in a support group.

Peer mediation and other peer-support schemes, such as peer mentoring, peer counseling, and befriending interventions, have mostly been studied in terms of students' and school personnel's perceptions regarding their benefits and drawbacks (e.g., Naylor & Cowie, 1999) rather than testing their effects on actual bullying behavior or experienced victimization.

Implications

In several countries, it is legally required that schools have antibullying policies. This obligation is desirable, although the effects of introducing such state-level policies have not been much studied. Legislation is likely to be beneficial in signaling that bullying is a serious issue that needs to be tackled and in empowering the administrators and educators to act.

Antibullying legislation typically does not specify what kinds of policies or programs schools should adopt or develop. Also, recommendations provided by national frameworks are often at a very general level. It is therefore challenging for schools to decide what concrete actions their policies should include. Some schools may end up developing very general policies, such as stating in their documents that they "do not accept any bullying" or that they "intervene immediately in incidents of bullying." This provides little guidance for individual teachers or other school personnel in *what* they actually should do to prevent bullying or *how* to intervene in it. Other schools may adopt or develop more concrete strategies that have, however, not been evaluated.

Whole-school programs to prevent bullying are often successful. Their effects do vary, however; some programs show consistent positive effects, whereas others have little or no evidence of effectiveness. So far, there is little evidence of the most effective ingredients of whole-school programs. Involving parents seems to strengthen the effects, as well as the use of disciplinary practices with bullies. Recent evidence suggests, however, that the effectiveness of disciplinary, confrontational practices might be dependent on context, such as school level (primary or secondary), the chronicity of bullying, and the type of disciplinary practice. Raising awareness among students about the role the whole group plays in maintaining bullying and enhancing antibullying norms and responses within classrooms is crucial. It is also highly important that teachers clearly communicate their antibullying attitudes to students.

Apart from their contents, the programs need to be long-lasting and intensive in order to have the desired effects. This conclusion has implications for designing programs but also for their implementation. Even programs that were designed to be intensive can be implemented more or less intensively, depending on the motivation, resources, and commitment on the part of schools and teachers.

When it comes to reactive approaches, or tackling bullying cases that have emerged, student reports indicate that adult interventions often do not work. Overall, when school personnel try to do something to help the situation, their actions are often not perceived as helpful by the students. When they have clear guidelines and training, the likelihood of success is much higher. There are few empirical studies comparing different reactive strategies. So far, there is no evidence of the confrontational approach with bullies working better than the nonconfrontational one. Organizing a follow-up meeting to ascertain that the bullying has stopped seems more important than choice of approach (confrontational vs. nonconfrontational).

Schools should be provided with more guidance regarding most effective practices and programs. Hutchings (2012) pointed out that "home-grown" programs are only justified if they are evaluated with high-quality research designs, if program designers have time to develop the necessary fidelity tools (e.g., manuals), and if there is no existing evidence-based program that addresses the needs of the specific target population. Accordingly, Ttofi and Farrington (2011) suggested a system of accrediting effective antibullying programs in order to ensure that programs adopted by schools contain elements that have been proved to be effective in high-quality evaluations.

Future Directions

There is already a lot we know about counteracting bullying. The urgent and so far unanswered questions in bullying prevention/intervention research are often summarized as "What Works Where, When, for Whom, and Why."

Whole-school programs are often complex. They consist of various components targeted at different levels of influence (individual students, parents, classrooms, whole schools) with a variety of methods (student lessons, videos, meetings). The different components are typically evaluated in combination, that is, they are implemented together, rather than separately. Consequently, the contribution of each individual component to the overall effects of a given program is unknown. It is possible that a program reaches optimal effects when all its components are used together, but it is also conceivable that some components are responsible for the outcomes, whereas others contribute little or nothing.

Asking "what works" means testing our *program theory* and whether it has scientific value in moving the understanding of bullying forward. From the practical, public health perspective, it is necessary to assess interventions regarding their cost-effectiveness. If some components are not effective or only minimally effective, they should be replaced with more intensive implementation of the more effective components already included in the program. Equally important is to put the hypothesized mechanisms of antibullying programs to test, or testing the *conceptual theory* of a given prevention/intervention approach—asking "why it works." It is not enough to know that a given program happens to result in reduction of bullying; we must understand what the underlying mechanism is.

So far very little is known about cultural aspects moderating intervention impact (e.g., whether a particular prevention/intervention approach fits a given culture especially well). Most bullying prevention programs have only been evaluated in their country of origin or have failed to produce equally positive findings in other countries when compared with the original evaluation (Ttofi & Farrington,

2011). It is not clear why this is the case—more research is clearly needed. Testing an evidence-based intervention in a new context, it is advisable to begin with the original program contents (with only surface adaptations in materials). If large adaptations are made right away, it is unclear whether the (possible) differential impact is due to the different program content or the new cultural context. It should be remembered that variability in impact across contexts might also be caused by other factors, such as variation in implementation quality or teachers' attitudes toward the program, including perceived cultural suitability. Studies evaluating prevention approaches and programs in different countries should measure these aspects as well.

Finally, apart from program effects in short-term trials, more information is needed on the sustainability of the effects in the long run, especially during wide dissemination, "scaling up" the programs. It is also crucial to understand how schools can best be supported in their implementation efforts to make them sustainable. We need theoretically grounded intervention models with explicated theories of change and rigorous testing of those theories.

REFERENCES

Baldry, A. C., & Farrington, D. P. (2000). Bullies and delinquents: Personal characteristics and parental styles. *Journal of Community and Applied Social Psychology, 10,* 17–31.

Bauman, S., Rigby, K., & Hoppa, K. (2008). U.S. teachers' and school counsellors' strategies for handling school bullying incidents. *Educational Psychology, 28,* 837–856.

Bowers, L., Smith, P. K., & Binney, V. (1994). Perceived family relationships of bullies, victims and bully/victims in middle childhood. *Journal of Social and Personal Relationships, 11*(2), 215–232.

Bowes, L., Arseneault, L., Maughan, B., Taylor, A., Caspi, A., & Moffitt, T. (2009). School, neighborhood, and family factors are associated with children's bullying involvement: A nationally representative longitudinal study. *Journal of the American Academy of Child and Adolescent Psychiatry, 48*(5), 545–553.

Brendgen, M., Girard, A., Vitaro, F., Dionne, G., & Boivin, M. (2013). Do peer group norms moderate the expression of genetic risk for aggression? *Journal of Criminal Justice, 41,* 324–330.

Bronfenbrenner, U. (1979). *The ecology of human development: Experiments by nature and design.* Cambridge. MA: Harvard University Press.

Burger, C., Strohmeier, D., Spröber, N., Bauman, S., & Rigby, K. (2015). How teachers respond to school bullying: An examination of self-reported intervention strategy use, moderator effects, and concurrent use of multiple strategies. *Teaching and Teacher Education, 51,* 191–202.

Caravita, S., Di Blasio, P., & Salmivalli, C. (2009). Unique and interactive effects of empathy and social status on involvement in bullying. *Social Development, 18,* 140–163.

Card, N. A., & Hodges, E. V. E. (2008). Peer victimization among schoolchildren: Correlations, causes, consequences, and considerations in assessment and intervention. *School Psychology Quarterly, 23,* 451–461.

Cook, C., Williams, K. R., Guerra, N. G., Kim, T., & Sadek, S. (2010). Predictors of childhood bullying and victimization: A meta-analytic review. *School Psychology Quarterly, 25,* 65–83.

Cross, D., Epstein, M., Hearn, L., Slee, P., Shaw, T., & Monks, H. (2011). National Safe Schools Framework: Policy and practice to reduce bullying in Australian schools. *International Journal of Behavioral Development, 35,* 398–404.

Elgar, F., Craig, W., Boycec, W., Morgan, A., & Vella-Zarb, R. (2009). Income inequality and school bullying: Multilevel study of adolescents in 37 countries. *Journal of Adolescent Health, 45,* 351–359.

Elgar, F., McKinnon, B., Walsh, S., Freeman, J., Donnelly, P., de Matos, M., et al. (2015). Structural determinants of youth bullying and fighting in 79 countries. *Journal of Adolescent Health, 57,* 643–650.

Espelage, D. L., & Swearer, S. M. (2010). A social–ecological model for bullying prevention and intervention: Understanding the impact of adults in the social ecology of youngsters. In S. R. Jimerson, S. M. Swearer, & D. L. Espelage (Eds.), *Handbook of bullying in schools: An international perspective* (pp. 61–72). New York: Routledge.

Evans, C., Fraser, M., & Cotter, K. (2014). The effectiveness of school-based bullying prevention programs: A systematic review. *Aggression and Violent Behavior, 19,* 532–544.

Fanti, K., & Kimonis, E. (2012). Bullying and victimization: The role of conduct problems and psychopathic traits. *Journal of Research on Adolescence, 22,* 617–631.

Farrington, D., Ttofi, M., & Lösel, F. (2011). School bullying and later criminal offending. *Criminal Behavior and Mental Health, 21,* 77–79.

Fekkes, M., Pijpers, F., & Verloove-Vanhorick, S. (2005). Bullying: Who does what, when and where?: Involvement of children, teachers and parents in bullying behavior. *Health Education Research, 20,* 81–91.

Gaete, J., Valenzuela, D., Rojas-Barahona, C., Valenzuela, E., Araya, R., & Salmivalli, C. (2017). KiVa anti-bullying program in primary schools in Chile, with and without the digital game component: The study protocol for a cluster randomized controlled trial. *Trials, 18*(1), 75.

Garandeau, C., Lee, I., & Salmivalli, C. (2014). Inequality matters: Classroom status hierarchy and adolescents' bullying. *Journal for Youth and Adolescence, 43,* 1123–1133.

Garandeau, C., Poskiparta, E., & Salmivalli, C. (2014). Tackling acute cases of bullying: Comparison of two methods in the context of the KiVa antibullying program. *Journal of Abnormal Child Psychology, 42,* 981–991.

Garandeau, C., Vartio, A., Poskiparta, E., & Salmivalli, C. (2016). School bullies' intention to change behavior following adult interventions: Effects of perceived blaming and empathy arousal. *Prevention Science, 17,* 1034–1043.

Haataja, A., Boulton, A., Voeten, M., & Salmivalli, C. (2014). KiVa antibullying curriculum and outcome: Does fidelity matter? *Journal of School Psychology, 52,* 479–493.

Hatzenbuehler, M., Duncan, D., & Johnson, R. (2015). Neighborhood-level LGBT hate crimes and bullying among sexual minority youths: A geospatial analysis. *Violence and Victims, 30,* 663–675.

Hatzenbuehler, M., Schwab-Reese, L., Ranapurwala, S., Hertz, M., & Ramirez, M. (2015). Associations between antibullying policies and bullying in 25 states. *JAMA Pediatrics, 169*(10), e152411.

Hawker, D., & Boulton, M. (2000). Twenty years' research on peer victimization and psychosocial maladjustment: A meta-analytic review of cross-sectional studies. *Journal of Child Psychology and Psychiatry and Allied Disciplines, 41,* 441–455.

Hodges, E. V. E., Malone, M., & Perry, D. (1997). Individual risk and social risk as interacting determinants of victimization in the peer group. *Developmental Psychology, 33,* 1032–1039.

Hofstede, G. (1980). *Culture's consequences: International differences in work-related values.* Beverly Hills, CA: SAGE.

Hutchings, J. (2012). From ABA to SPR: 30 years of developing evidence based services for the treatment and prevention of conduct disorder in Wales. *Journal of Children's Services, 7,* 101–112.

Ju, Y., Shuqiong, W., & Wenxin, Z. (2009). Intervention research on school bullying in primary schools. *Frontiers of Education in China, 4,* 111–122.

Kanetsuna, T., & Toda, Y. (2016). Actions against ijime and net-ijime in Japan. In P. K. Smith, K. Kwak, & Y. Toda (Eds.), *School bullying in different cultures: Eastern and Western perspectives* (pp. 334–349). Cambridge, UK: Cambridge University Press.

Kärnä, A., Voeten, M., Little, T., Poskiparta, E., Kaljonen, A., & Salmivalli, C. (2011). A large-scale evaluation of the KiVa anti-bullying program: Grades 4–6. *Child Development, 82,* 311–330.

Kärnä, A., Voeten, M., Poskiparta, E., & Salmivalli, C. (2010). Vulnerable children in varying classroom contexts: Bystanders' behaviors moderate the effects of risk factors on victimization. *Merrill–Palmer Quarterly, 56,* 261–282.

Kaukiainen, A., Björkqvist, K., Lagerspetz, K., Österman, K., Salmivalli, C., Rothberg, S., et al. (1999). The relationships between social intelligence, empathy, and three types of aggression. *Aggressive Behavior, 25,* 81–89.

Kimber, B., Sandell, R., & Bremberg, S. (2008). Social and emotional training in Swedish schools for the promotion of mental health: An effectiveness study of 5 years of intervention. *Health Education Research, 23,* 931–940.

Klomek, A., Sourander, A., & Elonheimo, H. (2015). Bullying by peers in childhood and effects on psychopathology, suicidality, and criminality in adulthood. *Lancet Psychiatry, 2,* 930–941.

Kwak, K., & Lee, S. (2016). The Korean research tradition on wang-ta. In P. K. Smith, K. Kwak, & Y. Toda (Eds.), *School bullying in different cultures: Eastern and Western perspectives* (pp. 93–112). Cambridge, UK: Cambridge University Press.

Lereya, S., Copeland, W., Costello, E., & Wolke, D. (2015). Adult mental health consequences of peer bullying and maltreatment in childhood: Two cohorts in two countries. *Lancet Psychiatry, 2,* 524–531.

Lereya, S., Samara, M., & Wolke, D. (2013). Parenting behavior and the risk of becoming a victim and a bully/victim: A meta-analysis study. *Child Abuse and Neglect, 37,* 1091–1108.

Maines, B., & Robinson, G. (1992). *No blame approach: A support group method for dealing with bullying.* Bristol, UK: Lame Duck.

Morita, Y. (1985). *Sociological study on the structure of bullying group.* Osaka, Japan: Osaka City University, Department of Sociology.

Morita, Y., & Kiyonaga, K. (1986). *Ijime: Kyousitsu no yamai [Ijime: The disease of the classroom].* Tokyo: Kaneko Shobo.

Morita, Y., Soeda, H., Soeda, K., & Taki, M. (1999). Japan. In P. K. Smith, Y. Morita, J. Junger-Tas, D. Olweus, R. Catalano, & P. Slee (Eds.), *The nature of school bullying: A cross-national perspective* (pp. 309–323). London: Routledge.

Naylor, P., & Cowie, H. (1999). The effectiveness of peer support systems in challenging school bullying: The perspectives and experiences of teachers and pupils. *Journal of Adolescence, 22,* 467–479.

Olthof, T., Goossens, F., Vermande, M., Aleva, L., & van der Meulen, M. (2011). Bullying as strategic behavior: Relations with desired and acquired dominance in the peer group. *Journal of School Psychology, 49*(3), 339–359.

Olweus, D. (1978). *Aggression in schools: Bullies and whipping boys.* Washington, DC: Hemisphere.

Olweus, D. (1993). *Bullying at school: What we know and what we can do.* New York: Wiley-Blackwell.

Peeters, M., Cillessen, A., & Scholte, R. (2010). Clueless or powerful?: Identifying subtypes of bullies in adolescence. *Journal of Youth and Adolescence, 39,* 1041–1052.

Pepler, D., & Craig, W. (2011). Promoting relationships and eliminating violence in Canada. *International Journal of Behavioral Development, 35,* 389–397.

Pikas, A. (1989). The common concern method for the treatment of mobbing. In E. Roland & E. Munthe (Eds.), *Bullying: An international perspective.* London: Fulton.

Power-Elliott, M., & Harris, G. (2012). Guidance counsellor strategies for handling bullying. *British Journal of Guidance and Counselling, 40,* 83–98.

Ragozzino, K., & Utne O'Brien, M. (2009). Social and emotional learning and bullying prevention [Issue brief]. Retrieved from *http://casel.org/downloads/ 2009_bullyingbrief.pdf.*

Reijntjes, A., Vermande, M., Olthof, T., Goossens, F., van de Schoot, R., Aleva, L., et al. (2013). Costs and benefits of bullying in the context of the peer group: A three wave longitudinal analysis. *Journal of Abnormal Child Psychology, 41,* 1217–1229.

Reijntjes, A., Vermande, M., Olthof, T., Goossens, F., Vink, G., Aleva, L., et al. (2018). Differences between resource control types revisited: A short term longitudinal study. *Social Development, 27,* 187–200.

Richardson, D., & Hiu, C. F. (2016). Global data on the bullying of school-aged children. In *Ending the torment: Tackling bullying from the schoolyard to cyberspace.* New York: United Nations Special Representative of the Secretary-General on Violence against Children. Retrieved from *http://srsg.violenceagainstchildren.org/sites/default/files/2016/End%20bullying/bullyingreport.pdf.*

Rigby, K. (2011). *The method of shared concern: A positive approach to bullying in schools.* Victoria, Australia: ACER Press.

Rivara, F., & Menestrel, S. (2016). *Preventing bullying through science, policy and practice.* Washington, DC: National Academies Press.

Rivers, I., Poteat, V., Noret, N., & Ashurst, N. (2009). Observing bullying at school: The mental health implications of witness status. *School Psychology Quarterly, 24,* 211–223.

Roland, E. (2011). The broken curve: Effects of the Norwegian manifesto against bullying. *International Journal of Behavioral Development, 35,* 383–388.

Saarento, S., Boulton, A., & Salmivalli, C. (2015). Reducing bullying and victimization: Student- and classroom-level mechanisms of change. *Journal of Abnormal Child Psychology, 43,* 61–76.

Saarento, S., Garandeau, C., & Salmivalli, C. (2015). Classroom- and school-level contributions to bullying and victimization: A review. *Journal of Community and Applied Social Psychology, 25,* 204–218.

Şahin, M. (2012). An investigation into the efficiency of empathy training program on preventing bullying in primary schools. *Children and Youth Services Review, 34,* 1325–1330.

Salmivalli, C. (2010). Bullying and the peer group: A review. *Aggression and Violent Behavior, 15,* 112–120.

Salmivalli, C., Kärnä, A., & Poskiparta, E. (2010). Development, evaluation, and diffusion of a national anti-bullying program, KiVa. In B. Doll, W. Pfohl, & J. Yoon (Eds.), *Handbook of youth prevention science* (pp. 240–254). New York: Routledge.

Salmivalli, C., & Peets, K. (2009). Bullies, victims, and bully–victim relationships. In K. H. Rubin, W. M. Bukowski, & B. Laursen (Eds.), *Handbook of peer interactions, relationships, and groups* (pp. 322–340). New York: Guilford Press.

Salmivalli, C., Voeten, M., & Poskiparta, E. (2011). Bystanders matter: Associations between defending, reinforcing, and the frequency of bullying in classrooms. *Journal of Clinical Child and Adolescent Psychology, 40,* 668–676.

Sijtsema, J., Veenstra, R., Lindenberg, S., & Salmivalli, C. (2009). Empirical test of bullies' status goals: Assessing direct goals, aggression, and prestige. *Aggressive Behavior, 35,* 57–67.

Sittichai, R., & Smith, P. K. (2015). Bullying in South-East Asian countries: A review. *Aggression and Violent Behavior, 23,* 22–35.

Smith, B., & Low, S. (2013). The role of social–emotional learning in bullying prevention efforts. *Theory into Practice, 52,* 280–287.

Smith, P. K. (2016, July). *Investigating and understanding cross-national differences in bullying.* Paper presented at the International Congress of Psychology, Yokohama, Japan.

Smith, P. K., Howard, S., & Thompson, F. (2007). Use of the support group method to tackle bullying, and an evaluation from schools and local authorities in England. *Pastoral Care in Education, 25,* 4–13.

Smith, P. K., Morita, Y., Junger-Tas, J., Olweus, D., Catalano, R., & Slee, P. (1999). *The nature of school bullying: A cross-national perspective.* London: Routledge.

Smith, P. K., Robinson, S., & Marchi, B. (2016). Cross-national data on victims of bullying: What is really being measured? *International Journal of Developmental Science, 10,* 9–19.

Smith, P. K., & Shu, S. (2000).What good schools can do about bullying: Findings from a survey in English schools after a decade of research and action. *Childhood, 7,* 193–212.

Spiel, C., & Strohmeier, D. (2011). National strategy for violence prevention in the Austrian public school system: Development and implementation. *International Journal of Behavioral Development, 35,* 383–388.

Stuart-Cassel, V., Bell, A., & Springer, F. (2011). *Analysis of state bullying laws and policies.* Washington, DC: U.S. Department of Education.

Sutton, J., Smith, P. K., & Swettenham, J. (1999). Social cognition and bullying: Social inadequacy or skilled manipulation? *British Journal of Developmental Psychology, 17,* 435–450.

Thompson, F., & Smith, P. K. (2011). *The use and effectiveness of anti-bullying strategies in schools* (Research Brief DFE-RR098). London: Goldsmiths, University of London.

Trip, S., Bora, C., Sipos-Gug, S., Tocai, I., Gradinger, P., Yanagida, T., et al. (2015). Bullying prevention in schools by targeting cognitions, emotions, and behavior: Evaluating the effectiveness of the REBE-ViSC program. *Journal of Counseling Psychology, 62*(4), 732–740.

Troop-Gordon, W. (2015). The role of the classroom teacher in the lives of children victimized by peers. *Child Development Perspectives, 9,* 55–60.

Ttofi, M., & Farrington, D. (2011). Effectiveness of school-based programs to reduce bullying: A systematic and meta-analytic review. *Journal of Experimental Criminology, 7,* 27–56.

Ttofi, M., Farrington, D., Lösel, F., & Loeber, R. (2011). Do the victims of school bullies tend to become depressed later in life?: A systematic review and meta-analysis of longitudinal studies. *Journal of Aggression, Conflict, and Peace Research, 3,* 63–73.

van der Ploeg, R., Steglich, C., & Veenstra, R. (2016). The support group approach in the Dutch KiVa anti-bullying programme: Effects on victimisation, defending and well-being at school. *Educational Research, 58,* 221–236.

Veenstra, R., Lindenberg, S., Munniksma, A., & Dijkstra, J. K. (2010). The complex relation between bullying, victimization, acceptance, and rejection: Giving special attention to status, affection, and sex differences. *Child Development, 81,* 480–486.

Viding, E., McCrory, E. J., Blakemore, S. J., & Frederickson, N. (2011). Behavioural problems and bullying at school: Can cognitive neuroscience shed new light on an old problem? *Trends in Cognitive Sciences, 15*(7), 289–291.

Viding, E., Simmonds, E., Petrides, K., & Frederickson, N. (2009). The contribution of callous–emotional traits and conduct problems to bullying in early adolescence. *Journal of Child Psychology and Psychiatry, 50,* 471–481.

Wong, D. S. W., Cheng, C. H. K., Ngan, R. M. H., & Ma, S. K. (2011). Program effectiveness of a restorative whole-school approach for tackling school bullying in Hong Kong. *International Journal of Offender Therapy and Comparative Criminology, 55*(6), 846–862.

Yoon, J., Bauman, S., Choi, T., & Hutchinson, A. (2011). How South Korean teachers handle an incident of school bullying. *School Psychology International, 32,* 312–329.

CHAPTER 20

Can Positive Youth Development Programs Prevent Youth Violence?

The Role of Regulation of Action and Positive Social Engagement

NANCY G. GUERRA

Brief Introduction

Positive youth development (PYD) and youth violence prevention programs (YVP) share a common focus on the individual and ecological determinants of healthy and problematic outcomes and the interplay between young people and the multiple contexts they navigate. They both emphasize a set of skills and opportunities that promote health and well-being and prevent or reduce risk among young people, whether labeled *assets* within the PYD framework or *promotive* and/or *protective factors* within a YVP framework. In this sense, it would seem both logical and feasible that PYD programs should have great preventive potential across a range of problematic outcomes, including youth violence. However, typically they have been presented as somewhat different and incompatible approaches: PYD programs involve all youth independent of potential risk for violence and other problems, whereas YVP programs target specific risk and protective factors associated with youth violence and often involve subgroups of youth most at risk. Consequently, very little effort has gone into looking at the impact or potential impact of PYD programs on outcomes such as youth violence.

Before we even ask *whether* PYD programs can be effective in preventing youth violence, perhaps it is more useful to ask *how* (i.e., what are the most important mechanisms of change) and *for whom* these programs might operate to both promote healthy development and simultaneously prevent violence. This could provide a template for designing PYD programs if the intent is to influence violence, as well as for looking at ongoing programs in terms of their supports for these mechanisms of impact. As Bonell and colleagues (2015, p. 3) note, "What is needed is a theory of change defining what PYD interventions involve and the intended causal mechanisms via which they are intended to reduce (substance use and) violence." Identifying these causal mechanisms also might allow us to assess the potential for impact of structured PYD programs on other problem behaviors, given that these behaviors tend to co-occur (Catalano, Hawkins, Berglund, Pollard, & Arthur, 2002). This approach is consistent with calls to expand PYD and prevention programs for youth beyond a focus on a single problem behavior to develop comprehensive and integrated strategies that promote healthy development and prevent a broad range of problems, including violence, substance use, early school leaving, and high-risk sexual behavior (Guerra & Bradshaw, 2008).

Toward this end, this chapter highlights common features across both models that can expand the reach of PYD programs, potentially to include prevention of violence and other problem behaviors. Two general mechanisms associated with key developmental tasks of adolescence are emphasized that can frame and shape intervention targets: *regulation of action* and *positive social engagement*. These mechanisms include a range of skills linked to healthy adolescent development and prevention of problem behaviors such as aggression and violence. Examples of these skills are emotion regulation, coping, decision making, and empathy. As discussed, these skills can be taught directly through structured interventions or learned indirectly within the context of youth serving agencies and extracurricular activities. Still, broad-based PYD programs, particularly those that are not targeted to youth and communities most at risk, may not sufficiently address the multitude of risk factors involved in more serious youth violence, including the presence of gangs, availability of weapons, and social norms supporting violence. To the extent that violence prevention is a specific programmatic focus for PYD interventions, these factors also must be acknowledged and addressed simultaneously.

General Background

Positive youth development is a broad term that includes a range of activities and interventions designed to help youth thrive. The overall goal of these strengths-based programs and practices is to promote supportive contexts and to build strengths in young people, generally between the ages of 12 and 18, in order to help them become competent, productive, healthy, and happy adults. PYD programs are not designed specifically to prevent youth problem behaviors, and typically focus on all youth rather than identified or at-risk youth. In fact, they became popular in the 1990s in the United States, in part, as a reaction to prevention programs focused on at-risk youth, what goes wrong instead of what goes right, and youth as problems to be solved. Proponents of a strengths-based approach argued that such a focus detracted from our ability to treat young people as individuals with problems, challenges, hopes, and dreams (Roth, Brooks-Gunn, & Galen, 1997). The mantra "problem-free is not fully prepared" signaled a shift in policy and practice to incorporate more holistic notions of youth that did not emphasize risk reduction but rather healthy development (Pittman, 1991).

On the other hand, youth violence has been and is a significant public health concern in the United States and worldwide that has serious consequences for perpetrators, victims, and society as a whole. The term *youth violence* includes behaviors considered aggressive, such as verbal insults and getting into fights, as well as more serious behavior, such as gang violence and homicide (Centers for Disease Control and Prevention, 2016). As youth violence rates increased dramatically in the 1990s, targeted prevention and intervention programs proliferated alongside PYD programs. Many programs, particularly those for younger adolescents in middle school, focused on prevention of aggressive behaviors such as bullying and fighting. Building on longitudinal studies of risk and protective factors, programs were designed to reduce risk factors and/or enhance protective factors (Tolan & Guerra, 1994). Protective factors were conceptualized as individual and contextual attributes that "buffered" the effects of risk factors and mitigated or reduced the likelihood of aggression and/or violence, consistent with a resilience framework (Masten, Best, & Garmezy, 1990). However, just as attributes can have protective effects that mitigate risk for aggression, they also can have promotive effects that can prevent aggression independent of risk (Zimmerman et al., 2013).

To a certain extent, PYD and risk prevention models historically have been portrayed as separate paradigms representing opposite ends of a continuum (Small & Memmo, 2004), although in more recent years efforts have been made to utilize integrative approaches (Guerra & Bradshaw, 2008). Still, in everyday settings, schools and communities have tended to organize around either a risk-protective factor model such as Communities That Care (Catalano, Haggerty, & Hawkins, 2014) or a PYD approach such as the Search Institute's 40-Asset model (Benson, 1997). Yet it is clear that we need to embrace and support the strengths of all youth while simultaneously addressing very real problems that interfere with development for some youth and have negative consequences for others. It also is clear that many of the individual and contextual attributes targeted by PYD programs can be protective or promotive factors to prevent youth violence. Although promoting healthy youth development is not targeted directly toward reducing risk, it is likely to decrease a range of problem behaviors, including youth violence. Additionally, both PYD and prevention programs emphasize the interaction of intrapersonal and ecological mechanisms on adolescent development and the importance of intervening to enhance individual skills and optimize contextual supports and opportunities (Schwartz, Pantin, Coatsworth, & Szapocznik, 2007).

Theoretical Considerations and Key Empirical Findings

PYD Framework

The primary focus of PYD is to promote healthy youth development. As applied in the field, it includes a host of programs characterized by an asset-building or strengths-based orientation. These include skill building, mentoring, promoting healthy relationships, creating positive environments, expanding after-school programs, increasing opportunities for engagement, and youth empowerment (Benson, 1997). What links these activities together is a unifying philosophy rather than a focus on a specific set of skills, contextual attributes, or opportunities. This philosophy is based on the assumption that helping youth meet key developmental tasks and achieve their full potential will not only help them do well but also prevent them from experiencing problems, that youth should be partners in this programming, and that communities must provide a comprehensive set of supports and opportunities for youth to succeed (Hughes & Curnan, 2000; Pittman, 1991). Some of these programs may be developed specifically to enhance positive development through funding initiatives or community action, whereas others may be common youth programs (such as sports or music) that have been identified as potentially contributing to PYD but not designed specifically for that purpose.

Perhaps the most well-known and widely implemented PYD program is the Search Institute's 40-Asset model (Benson, 1997). This program focuses on 20 internal and 20 external assets that support healthy development. These include assets ranging from family love and support to participating in organized youth programs to caring about school to knowing how to plan and make decisions and other interpersonal competencies. Although this program has been widely implemented in the United States and worldwide and there is a developmental literature linking many of these assets to lower levels of problem behaviors, empirical studies have not examined the effectiveness of this approach on preventing youth violence. In part, the reason is that the program includes almost anything that could be beneficial to youth, and communities select the particular assets they want to focus on, rendering evaluation of the approach as a whole problematic.

Indeed, the lack of specificity in PYD programming and implementation makes it difficult to test whether PYD broadly construed is effective in preventing youth violence. A central issue in examining the effectiveness of PYD programs on youth violence is that almost any program that emphasizes positive development can be framed as a PYD intervention. At best, we can label programs as PYD if they meet some criteria for focusing on skills, resources, and assets and consider evaluations that have examined the impact of these programs on youth violence. Using this strategy, there are a small number of individual programs to consider. Also, a few systematic reviews and meta-analyses have examined impact across studies.

PYD and Violence Prevention

The Blueprints for Violence Prevention project (*www.blueprintsprograms.com*) cites two PYD programs as model programs for YVP based on empirical studies: Life Skills Training and Positive Action. Life Skills Training, a classroom-based universal program for adolescents ages 12–14, has demonstrated significant reductions in behaviors such as high-frequency fighting and delinquency following intervention (Botvin, Griffin, & Nichols, 2006). Positive Action is a school-based program that includes classroom lessons and schoolwide climate change activities for students in elementary and middle school. A randomized study found that middle-school children (approximately ages 12–13) self-reported lower rates of bullying and violence perpetration following participation (Guo et al., 2015).

Another program that fits within the PYD framework is the 4-H model. The 4-H program provides youth with a range of engagement opportunities in schools and after school with the goal of developing citizenship, leadership, and responsibility. It is the largest PYD organization in the United States, with over 90,000 clubs and 6.5 million members (*www.4-h.org*). A recent evaluation report examined the effects of 4-H participation on more than 4,000 youth. Findings showed that youth who were consistently involved in 4-H for at least 1 year between the ages of 10 and 14 were significantly less likely than comparison youth in other programs to self-report engaging in bullying behaviors (Lerner et al., 2005).

Looking across multiple studies, Catalano, Berglund, Ryan, Lonczak, and Hawkins (2004) systematically reviewed 25 programs that targeted at least one asset or strength associated with PYD and had at least one behavioral outcome for children and youth. The majority of programs were for younger children, and programs for adolescents focused on a range of behavioral outcomes, including substance use, teenage pregnancy, and aggression or violence. Of all the programs reviewed, only two PYD programs were discussed that measured and significantly reduced aggressive behaviors such as fighting (Adolescent Transitions and Responding in Peaceful and Positive Ways), although most all PYD programs had a positive impact on reducing some type of problem behavior. Indeed, it may be that other PYD programs had an impact on aggression and violence, but these outcomes were not measured.

A few recent reviews have looked specifically at the effects of PYD interventions on serious problem behaviors, including substance abuse and youth violence, among a broader age range of youth, with relatively little support for sustained effects. For example, in a meta-analysis of three PYD programs that evaluated violence outcomes, Melendez-Torres and colleagues (2016) marginally significant effects immediately postintervention, but no significant effects across time points. The three programs they reviewed were Big Brothers Big Sisters (BBBS), Quantum Opportunity Project (QOP), and the National Guard Youth Challenge Program (NGYCP), the only PYD programs they were able to locate with published outcome evaluations looking at youth violence. BBBS is a mentoring program in which adult mentors are matched with youth between the ages of 10 and 16 who generally live in risky settings (e.g., single-parent family, low income). QOP is delivered in high schools with dropout rates greater than 40% and promotes a range of youth assets, including cultural awareness, academic achievement, and community service, in order to increase bonding to schools and communities. NGYCP is a military-style boot camp for teenagers ages 16–18 who are not in school, not working, and not in the correctional system. The intervention included life skills education, work preparation, and completion of secondary education. Although these were considered as PYD programs because they focus on general skill building and supports, it is noteworthy that each of these programs were targeted to at-risk youth.

Cid (2017) conducted a systematic review of the effects on aggression and violence of after-school programs for children and youth in Latin America. His review focused on broad programs designed to provide opportunities for participation and engagement for all youth, such as youth sports programs, open schools, and youth orchestras. Across 14 studies he found some positive effects on preventing aggression, particularly among the higher-risk children and youth. For example, Aleman and colleagues (2017) reported on a randomized trial of the El Sistema youth orchestra in Venezuela. The program emphasizes social interactions through group instruction and group performances. After 1 year of participation, young adolescent boys with higher violence exposure showed reductions in aggressive behavior compared with their counterparts in the control condition.

As these studies illustrate, at this juncture it is not possible to say that PYD programs do or do not have a clear and significant impact on the prevention of youth violence. In part, this is due to the small number of studies specifically targeting PYD and measuring violence outcomes. It also is due to the broad range of programs that can be considered PYD, the variation in targeted groups (e.g., younger vs. older adolescents; all youth vs. high-risk youth), and the lack of proposed mechanisms of impact and related assessments to determine whether PYD programs reduce risk for aggression and violence.

Implications and Future Directions

Challenges Linking PYD to YVP

PYD programs span a range of activities designed to promote healthy development, with considerable variation as to what healthy development means and how best to achieve it. As discussed previously, one of the most widely disseminated approaches, the Search Institute's 40-Asset model (Benson, 1997), provides a listing of internal and external assets that range from skills to activities to beliefs. The notion is that the more assets the better, and assets are not prioritized or ranked for importance. This approach also rests on an implicit assumption that all assets are amenable to change, but that it is up to communities to select the assets they think are most important and to provide youth with diverse opportunities to develop them. In some sense, the simplicity of this approach has been both a strength and a weakness. All communities can focus on at least some of the assets, but little is provided in terms of the significance of different assets across different individuals and in different contexts, cultural and community variations, and differential amenability to change through structured programs.

A more focused approach by Lerner and colleagues, the 5C's, highlights five core competencies that youth need to thrive: competence, confidence, connections, character, and caring (Lerner et al., 2005). Competence reflects social, academic, health, and vocational skills. Confidence includes an internal sense of self-worth and self-efficacy. Connections describes positive bonds between youth, other people, and supportive institutions. Character includes a sense of right and wrong and respect for societal institutions. Caring includes sympathy and prosocial orientations. Although the list consists of five essential competencies, when defined, they also include a broad range of skills, beliefs, and social supports. Both the 40-Asset model and the 5C's provide a framework for describing characteristics of positive youth development, but they still are too broad to provide a sufficient framework for a theory of change that specifies mechanisms by which PYD programs can prevent youth violence.

What would be the key targets for PYD programs if an important goal were to prevent or reduce youth violence? Stated otherwise, what characteristics of healthy youth and the contexts they grow up in (that can be enhanced through specific programs) are most likely to prevent them from engaging in violence? Taken further, is there a core set of skills and opportunities than can protect youth from violence and, potentially, other problem behaviors? Building on a PYD model, how can we best promote these skills and opportunities?

It would be helpful if PYD programs could articulate clearly a theory of causal process contributing to health and well-being, highlighting individual developmental and contextual mechanisms with a direct impact on preventing aggression and youth violence and how these can be developed. With such a theory of change it would be possible to assess potential mediators, what contributes to change in these mediators, whether change in these mediators predicts reductions in aggressive and violent behavior, and whether changes are moderated by other factors such as gender, age, and socioeconomic status. Until we are able to develop and utilize this type of framework, we are left to patch together some potential best bets for intervention, looking at both the PYD literature and developmental and prevention studies of youth violence.

Core Components Linking PYD to YVP

Looking at the core components of PYD programs across multiple programs juxtaposed with the literature on risk protection for aggression and violence, what are the most prominent individual skills, attitudes, and beliefs for programming? Several scholars have suggested that a key mechanism by which PYD programs can prevent or reduce aggression is through a set of individual skills labeled *intentional self-regulation* (Bonell et al., 2015; Busseri & Rose-Krasnor, 2009; Schwartz et al., 2007). This includes "intentionality" or assessment of current skills, selecting goals that reflect important life purposes, optimizing activities to pursue these goals, and compensating or redirecting to other activities if one's goals are not achieved (Lerner, Lerner, von Eye, Bowers, & Lewin-Bizan, 2011).

This skill set seems to be most closely aligned with the concept of personal agency or control over one's life. Although this is an intuitively appealing concept, the link between this general type of self-directedness and youth violence has not been studied systematically. There have been some studies looking specifically at agency for enacting aggressive versus prosocial responses. More aggressive youth appear to be more confident in their ability to enact aggressive responses (Crick & Dodge, 1994), whereas youth who are more confident in their ability to enact prosocial responses are less likely to enact aggressive responses (Ludwig & Pittman, 1999).

As this illustrates, a larger issue is that PYD programs tend to invoke broad definitions of skills and competencies (such as intentional self-regulation), whereas the risk literature focuses on specific subsets often linked directly to aggression (such as self-efficacy for aggressive and prosocial behavior). Just as it is not possible to expect that building self-efficacy for prosocial behavior will translate into a broader sense of self-direction and purpose, it is unlikely that broad training in intentional self-regulation will translate to changes in self-efficacy for aggression or prosocial behavior. Indeed, when considering the effects of broadly defined "social competence" building interventions on problem behaviors, including aggression, the effects are weak, particularly for self-reported outcomes (Najaka, Gottfredson, & Wilson, 2001).

Yet an integrated model of PYD and risk prevention must be articulated at a relatively broad yet simultaneously focused level to incorporate a range of assets and strengths that are linked to prevention of aggressive behavior and youth violence and also promote thriving and well-being. Articulating one or two general concepts that can include a broader set of core skills that bridge risk prevention and PYD and that can reasonably be targeted in focused interventions and everyday youth programs would have the potential to support a useful framework that integrates both approaches.

Given the potential utility of this approach, there have been many calls for an integrated model (Catalano et al., 2002; Schwartz et al., 2007; Small & Memmo, 2004). Still, relatively few articulated frameworks exist. Developing this type of framework is challenging for several reasons. First, it is critical to identify the most developmentally relevant skills for adolescents that can help all youth thrive. Second, these skills must be empirically linked to risk for or protection from problem behaviors, including youth violence, and aligned with the risk and protection literature. Third, these skills must be organized into one or two general concepts that provide an overarching direction across different types of programs and settings, with some flexibility in which skills might be targeted. Fourth, skills must be malleable either through direct instruction or through structured supports and opportunities across different contexts. Fifth, it would be advantageous if the general concepts and core skills were associated with multiple problem behaviors rather than just aggression and violence. Finally, if there is a specific focus on preventing youth violence, an integrated approach also must make clear both how core skills can be made most relevant to violence prevention and what is not addressed through this comprehensive framework (e.g., community norms about violence, availability of firearms, presence of gangs).

Guerra and Bradshaw (2008) convened a group of developmental psychologists and prevention researchers to review the literature and identify a set of core competencies aligned with both PYD and prevention approaches that could be applied to a range of youth problem behaviors. They proposed five core competencies: (1) positive sense of self, including self-awareness, agency, and self-esteem; (2) self-control, including delay of gratification and impulse control; (3) decision-making skills; (4) a moral system of belief; and (5) prosocial connectedness, including engagement, attachment, and a sense of belonging. Although these competencies are interconnected—for instance, higher self-control leads to better decision making—each has been studied in its own right and has been linked to one or more problem behaviors (e.g., violence, substance abuse, early school leaving, high-risk sexual behavior).

Sullivan, Farrell, Bettencourt, and Helms (2008) reviewed the literature linking these core competencies to childhood aggression and youth violence. Because of the prominence of social information-processing (SIP) models of aggression and their relevance to prevention programs, they situated the core competencies within the SIP framework. The SIP model highlights the role of decision-making skills and the relevance of the other skills to effective decision making. For example, as they note, core beliefs about the acceptability of aggressive responses and the harm caused (moral system of belief) will influence the solutions that youth generate, their evaluation of consequences, and the solution they select.

In order to provide a more parsimonious framework for skill building consistent with the developmental and prevention literature, Modecki, Zimmer-Gembeck, and Guerra (2017) identified a subset of three skills that fall within the general concept of *regulation of action*: emotion regulation, coping, and decision making. These skills represent a key challenge of adolescence often described within the frameworks of executive function (EF) or executive control (EC). As recent advances in our understanding of adolescent brain development point out, the prefrontal cortex and its underpinning neural systems continue to develop during adolescence and into early adulthood. As teenagers become more autonomous, their decision workload increases, making EC skills even more critical (Luciana, 2013). To navigate daily life challenges and avoid risk behaviors, they must be able to regulate emotional arousal, cope with normative and sometimes extreme stressors, and make good decisions that are consistent with present and future goals. Youth who engage in aggression and other risk behaviors place even greater demands on their executive systems because their heightened emotional reactivity can trigger internal stress and they tend to seek out novel situations that increase the cognitive processing workload.

These three skills are consistent with the developmental tasks of adolescence but focus primarily on the self. What is missing for a more comprehensive framework is a complement to regulation of action that emphasizes what Guerra and Bradshaw (2008) called *moral system of belief* and *social connectedness*. As a general concept, this reflects *positive social engagement*. This is consistent with the skills of connections, character, and caring from the 5C's (Lerner et al., 2005). This category of other-directed skills is particularly important in preventing aggression and violence, given the generally negative relation between aggression/violence and social problem solving and relationship skills (Crick & Dodge, 1999), empathy and concern for others (Pardini, Lochman, & Frick, 2003), and bonding to conventional social institutions such as schools, neighborhoods, and communities (Najaka et al., 2001).

This brief review of potential core skills for PYD and prevention can be summarized as follows. There have been several attempts to list assets and skills youth need for healthy development and prevention of problem behaviors, including aggression and violence. Some lists are quite broad, some lists are shorter but relatively generic, and other lists identify specific skills linked to both competence and prevention. Rather than propose yet another list of assets or skills, a review of the literature suggests that two general concepts can guide and integrate PYD and prevention programming: (1) regulation of action and (2) positive social engagement.

Regulation of action promotes self-directed behavior, emotion regulation, coping, and decision-making skills that facilitate key developmental tasks such as developing a coherent identity, learning how to navigate greater autonomy, and developing longer-term future goals. These skills can also prevent some types of aggression and violence. For example, emotion regulation is important for anger management and likely to lead to reductions in reactive aggression. SIP models of aggression have articulated clearly with strong empirical support how different steps in the decision-making and problem-solving processes can increase or decrease the likelihood of aggressive responding (Crick & Dodge, 1994).

Positive social engagement emphasizes the role of healthy relationships, social skills, and strong bonds with prosocial peers and institutions. As young people break away from their families and establish their autonomy and identities, they develop new social attachments. They continue to develop and refine skills such as empathy and getting along with others and develop relationships that can be healthy or unhealthy. Their lives are intertwined with multiple peer groups, including classmates, friends, romantic partners, siblings, and a virtual online world. They navigate an increasingly large array of institutions and settings, including schools, youth groups, work environments, and communities. Healthy development hinges on learning the skills and having opportunities to invest, engage, and belong. In the same vein, the lack of positive role models and peer groups, and particularly when they are replaced by negative influences such as gangs, can contribute to higher levels of aggression and violence (Farrell et al., 2008; Guerra & Bradshaw, 2008).

An advantage of building an integrated framework around two general concepts is that these concepts can both drive programming and provide a model by which to evaluate the impact of a range of programs and opportunities on PYD, violence prevention, and prevention of other problem behaviors. Specific skills within each general concept can be articulated based on local needs, culture, availability of resources, and whether or not a prevention target has been identified. As an example, a PYD program in a high-violence community that wanted to simultaneously influence violence prevention might devote considerable resources toward building emotion regulation and impulse control. On the other hand, a program with a substance abuse prevention focus might emphasize teaching skills for resisting negative peer pressure.

Implications for Prevention and Promotion

Developing regulation of action and positive social engagement requires both skills and opportunities—there are individual and ecological determinants of outcomes. Skills can be built via direct instruction in classroom or small-group lessons. They can be built through a range of everyday youth programs such as arts, music, mentoring, and service learning in the community. Organizational features of contexts, such as a positive school climate where youth feel supported and connected, also facilitate skill building and healthy development. Finally, organizations and settings provide opportunities not only to learn skills but also to practice these skills regularly.

The majority of direct skill-building programs have been implemented with younger children, typically in school settings, with relatively few programs for adolescents, particularly during the high school years (Williamson, Modecki, & Guerra, 2015). As discussed earlier, Life Skills Training (Botvin et al., 2006) is one of the more rigorous and carefully evaluated skill-building programs with evidence of short- and long-term effectiveness on aggression prevention for young adolescents (ages 12–14). Many of the skills targeted in this universal program clearly reflect regulation of action and positive social engagement. In a more extreme population, the 10-lesson Viewpoints taught decision-making skills to incarcerated youth, leading to short-term reductions in aggressive and externalizing behaviors (Guerra & Slaby, 1990). An adaptation of this program, the 30-lesson Positive Life Changes, expanded on the components of decision making to include a stronger emphasis on goal setting, coping with failure, empathy, and life planning. In a pilot study with youth who had been expelled from high school, Williamson, Dierkhising, and Guerra (2013) reported increased skills and reductions in aggressions for participants compared with matched controls.

On the other hand, youth regularly participate in a range of activities in schools, communities, and other settings. Indeed, many PYD programs are part of young people's regular activities, such as sports, music, civic engagement, and even work. These activities indirectly foster skills such as strategic thinking, decision making, emotion regulation, and initiative. As Aleman and colleagues (2017) found in a large-scale randomized controlled trial of the El Sistema youth orchestra of Venezuela, these programs indirectly influence skills such as self-regulation and empathy through structured experiences.

Rather than selecting a subset of skills and designing programs accordingly, it is possible and plausible to look at a range of youth service and youth engagement activities to identify how they might contribute to building skills linked to regulation of action and prosocial engagement. For example, programs such as BBBS provide adult guidance for youth between the ages of 10 and 16 who generally have few positive role models. Programs such as this provide opportunities for modeling positive behaviors and learning a range of life skills. By looking at these types of programs and identifying potential mechanisms of impact on PYD and prevention, evaluations can focus on whether these specific skills are affected and, if so, whether changes in specific skills promote reductions in aggression, violence, or other problem behaviors (Schwartz et al., 2007).

Two issues are worth mentioning. First, most PYD programs and many skill-building programs are population-based for all youth in a given setting. In some sense, PYD is predicated on all youth thriving, a premise that runs counter to a risk-focused approach targeting identified youth. Yet aggression and violence are very skewed, with a smaller subset of youth at the tail of the distribution. More seriously aggressive and violent youth may have other needs not addressed by PYD programs, such as a host of adverse childhood experiences and early trauma that would need to be considered in a prevention strategy. Stated otherwise, it is unlikely that broad PYD programs delivered without considering community, family, or individual risk would be effective for the more seriously violent youth. As an illustration, Fredricks and Eccles (2005) found that adolescent risk (defined as association with antisocial peers) affected the relation of extracurricular activities to positive and negative behavioral outcomes. At the very least, it would make sense to offer PYD programs, particularly those that enhance opportunities and provide meaningful role models, in more resource-poor communities, where these opportunities may be scarce. In this sense, PYD can target risk at the population level and still be consistent with PYD principles, similar to the programs included in the review by Melendez-Torres and colleagues (2016).

Second, because PYD targets a large number of developmental assets, and because risk prevention programs target a range of risk and protective factors across settings, little has been learned about the relative importance or prioritization of different assets and/or risk factors. There is a general understanding that more assets/protective factors and fewer risk factors are better, but there is little empirical evidence to help prioritize targets for PYD and prevention programming. The general consensus has been to develop multicomponent, multicontext programs targeting the broadest range of assets/protective factors and risk factors possible. Yet in some settings the need can be overwhelming; for instance, in areas where schools are underresourced, where families struggle to make ends meet, where few opportunities for productive engagement exist for youth, and where violence is an everyday feature of community life. This speaks to the need to understand fully the specific needs in a particular community and to prioritize/sequence types of interventions, starting with those that are most easily implemented and sustainable.

Conclusions

Rather than being seen as opposite ends of a continuum, PYD promotion and risk prevention programs have considerable overlap. They both focus on building assets or protective factors that also reduce risk. They emphasize individual and ecological determinants of outcomes and the interplay between individuals and contexts (Tolan & Guerra, 1994). In some sense, the primary outcomes of PYD interventions (increased skills and competencies) often are intervening processes targeted by YVP programs. On the other hand, although PYD programs target increased competencies as a primary outcome, they also acknowledge the importance of prevention of youth problems as a secondary outcome.

PYD promotion and risk prevention programs also have some noteworthy differences. Although skills and assets are important in aggression prevention, aggression is caused by a multiplicity of individual and contextual factors beyond skills and assets. For example, features of communities such as presence of gangs, availability of weapons, street lighting, public spaces, and mechanisms of informal social control have bearing on serious youth violence but are not addressed by a PYD framework (Kumar et al., 2017).

Perhaps the best strategy moving forward is to recognize broadly the importance of an asset-building model, particularly in settings in which opportunities for PYD are scarce, and how it can be adapted to focus on problem behaviors of most concern. In this chapter, the focus was on how to adapt PYD programs to maximize their impact on YVP. As discussed, a focus on two general categories of developmental skills, regulation of action and positive social engagement, can provide an overarching framework for PYD programs that can maximize their potential to prevent or reduce aggression and violence. This strategy can be augmented by targeted risk prevention programs that address risk factors beyond a PYD model, particularly if the focus is on serious youth violence and its multiple individual and contextual determinants.

REFERENCES

Aleman, X., Duryea, S., Guerra, N. G., McEwan, P., Munoz, R., Stampini, M., et al. (2017). The effects of musical training on child development: A randomized trial of El Sistema in Venezuela. *Prevention Science, 18*(7), 865–878.

Benson, P. (1997). *All kids are our kids: What communities must do to raise caring and responsible children and adolescents.* Minneapolis, MN: Search Institute.

Bonell, C., Hinds, K., Dickson, K., Thomas, J., Fletcher, A., Murphy, S., et al. (2015). What is positive youth development and how might it reduce substance use and violence?: A systematic review and synthesis of the theoretical literature. *BMC Public Health, 16,* 1–16.

Botvin, G. J., Griffin, K. W., & Nichols, T. R. (2006). Preventing youth violence and delinquency through a universal school-based prevention approach. *Prevention Science, 7,* 403–408.

Busseri, M. A., & Rose-Krasnor, L. (2009). Breadth and intensity: Salient, separable, and developmentally significant dimensions of structured youth activity involvement. *British Journal of Developmental Psychology, 27,* 907–933.

Catalano, R. F., Berglund, M. L., Ryan, J. A. M., Lonczak, H. S., & Hawkins, J. D. (2004). Positive youth development in the United States: Research findings on evaluations of positive youth development programs. *Annals of the American Academy of Political and Social Science, 591,* 98–124.

Catalano, R. F., Haggerty, K. P., & Hawkins, J. D. (2014). *Research brief.* Seattle, WA: Social Development Research Group.

Catalano, R. F., Hawkins, J. D., Berglund, M. L., Pollard, J. A., & Arthur, M. W. (2002). Prevention science and positive youth development: Competitive or cooperative frameworks? *Journal of Adolescent Health, 31,* 230–239.

Centers for Disease Control and Prevention. (2016). Youth violence data sheet. Retrieved from *www.cdc.gov/violenceprevention/pdf/yv-datasheet.pdf.*

Cid, A. (2017). Interventions using regular activities to engage high-risk school-age youth: A review of after-school programs in Latin America and the Caribbean. *Prevention Science, 18,* 879–886.

Crick, N. R., & Dodge, K. A. (1994). A review and reformulation of social information: Processing mechanisms in children's social adjustment. *Psychological Bulletin, 115,* 74–101.

Farrell, A. D., Erwin, E. H., Bettencourt, A., Mays, S., Vulin-Reynolds, M., Sullivan, T., et al. (2008). Individual factors influence effective nonviolent behavior and fighting in peer siuations: A qualitative study with urban African American adolescents. *Journal of Clincial Child and Adolescent Psychology, 37,* 397–411.

Fredricks, J. A., & Eccles, J. S. (2005). Developmental benefits of extracurricular involvement: Do peer characteristics mediate the link between activities and youth outcomes? *Journal of Youth and Adolescence, 34,* 507–520.

Guerra, N. G., & Bradshaw, C. P. (2008, Winter). Linking the prevention of problem behaviors and positive youth development: Core competencies to prevent problem behaviors and promote positive youth development. *New Directions for Child and Adolescent Development, 122,* 1–17.

Guerra, N. G., & Slaby, R. G. (1990). Cognitive mediators of aggression in adolescent offenders: II. Intervention. *Developmental Psychology, 26,* 269–277.

Guo, S., Wu, Q., Smokowski, P. R., Bacallao, M., Evans, C. B. R., & Cotter, K. L. (2015). A longitudinal evaluation of the Positive Action program in a low-income, racially diverse, rural county: Effects on self-esteem, school hassles, aggression, and internalizing symptoms. *Journal of Youth and Adolescence, 44,* 2337–2358.

Hughes, D., & Curnan, S. (2000). Community youth development: A framework for action. *Community Youth Developmental Journal, 1,* 9–13.

Kumar, A. K. S., Stern, V., Rubrahmanian, R., Sherr, L., Burton, P., Guerra, N., et al. (2017). Ending violence in childhood: A global imperative. *Psychology, Health and Medicine, 22*(Suppl. 1), 1–16.

Lerner, R. M., Lerner, J. V., Almerigi, J., Theokas, C., Phelps, E., Gestsdottir, S., et al. (2005). Positive youth development, participation in community youth development programs, and community contributions of fifth-grade adolescents: Findings from the first wave of the 4-H Study of Positive Youth Development. *Journal of Early Adolescence, 25*(1), 17–71.

Lerner, R. M., Lerner, J. V., von Eye, A., Bowers, E. P., & Lewin-Bizan, S. (2011). Individual and contextual bases of thriving in adolescence: A view of the issues. *Journal of Adolescence, 34,* 1107–1114.

Luciana, M. (2013). Adolescent brain development in normality and psychopathology. *Development and Psychopathology, 25,* 1325–1345.

Ludwig, K. B., & Pittman, J. F. (1999). Adolescent prosocial values and self-efficacy in relation to delinquency, risky sexual behavior, and drug use. *Youth and Society, 30,* 461–482.

Masten, A. S., Best, K. M., & Garmezy. N. (1990). Resilience and development: Contributions from the study of children who overcome adversity. *Developmental Psychopathology, 2,* 425–444.

Melendez-Torres, G. J., Dickson, K., Fletcher, A., Thomas, J., Hinds, K., Cambell, R., et al. (2016). Positive youth development programmes to reduce substance use in young people: Systematic review. *International Journal of Drug Policy, 36,* 95–103.

Modecki, K., Zimmer-Gembeck, M., & Guerra, N. G. (2017). Emotional regulation, coping and decision-making: Three linked skills for preventing externalizing problems in adolescence. *Child Development, 88,* 417–426.

Najaka, S. S., Gottfredson, D. C., & Wilson, D. B. (2001). A meta-analytic inquiry into the relationship between selected risk factors and problem behavior. *Prevention Science, 2,* 257–271.

Pardini, D. A., Lochman, J. E., & Frick, P. J. (2003). Callous/unemotional traits and social–cognitive processes in adjudicated youths. *Journal of the American Academy of Child and Adolescent Psychiatry, 42,* 364–371.

Pittman, K. J. (1991). *Promoting youth development: Strengthening the role of youth-serving and community organizations.* Washington, DC: Center for Youth Development and Policy Research.

Roth, J., Brooks-Gunn, J., & Galen, B. (1997). *Promoting healthy adolescence: Youth development frameworks and programs.* Princeton, NJ: Robert Wood Johnson Foundation.

Schwartz, S. J., Pantin, H., Coatsworth, J. D., & Szapocznik, J. (2007). Addressing the challenges and opportunities for today's youth: Towards an integrative model and its implications for research and intervention. *Journal of Primary Prevention, 28*(2), 117–144.

Small, S., & Memmo, M. (2004). Contemporary models of youth development and problem prevention: Towards an integration of terms, concepts, and models. *Family Relations, 53,* 3–11.

Sullivan, T. N., Farrell, A. D., Bettencourt, A. F., & Helms, S. W. (2008, Winter). Core competencies and the prevention of youth violence. *New Directions for Child and Adolescent Development, 122,* 33–46.

Tolan, P. T., & Guerra, N. G. (1994). *What works in reducing youth violence: A critical review of the field.* Boulder: University of Colorado, Center for the Study and Prevention of Violence.

Williamson, A. A., Dierkhising, C. B., & Guerra, N. G. (2013). Brief report: Piloting the Positive Life Changes (PLC) program for at-risk adolescents. *Journal of Adolescence, 36,* 623–628.

Williamson, A. A., Modecki, K. L., & Guerra, N. G. (2015). Social–emotional learning programs in high school. In J. A. Durlak, C. E. Domitrovich, R. P. Weissberg, & T. P. Gullota (Eds.), *Handbook of social and emotional learning: Research and practice* (pp. 181–196). New York: Guilford Press.

Zimmerman, M., Stoddard, S. A., Eisman, A. B., Caldwell, C. H., Aiyer, S. M., & Miller, A. (2013). Adolescent resilience: Promotive factors that inform prevention. *Child Development Perspectives, 7*(4).

CHAPTER 21

Challenges and Priorities
for Researchers

KENNETH H. RUBIN and TINA MALTI

Challenges and Priorities for Researchers

Aggression in childhood and adolescence remains one of the most challenging mental health concerns in contemporary society. All too often, the consequences of aggression and violence for the perpetrator, target, and society at large are serious, costly, and even irreparable (see Malti & Averdijk, 2017). The chapters that appear in this *Handbook* have provided comprehensive reviews of the foundations and trajectories of aggression, as well as its biological, dispositional, social (social-interactional, -cognitive, -relational, -group), and contextual antecedents. The chapters have also contributed to our understanding of state-of-the-art treatment programs, approaches, and models that aim to prevent and reduce aggressive behaviors in childhood and adolescence.

Since the turn of the new millennium, the study of child and adolescent aggression has moved forward in remarkable ways. Among the more notable contributions have been programmatic studies of (1) the genetic underpinnings of aggression; (2) differences in the forms and functions of aggressive behavior in youth; (3) risk and protective factors that may contribute to principles of equifinality and multifinality vis-à-vis trajectories of aggression; (4) programs designed to prevent or intervene with *en-face* or online bullying and victimization; and (5) novel procedures designed to treat those who have been identified as aggressive at home, school, and in their neighborhoods. There have been strong efforts to move from theory to research to treatment to policy. In short, we have learned a good deal in a relatively brief amount of time, and much of this new knowledge has been described in this *Handbook*. Nevertheless, despite the conclusions that we can draw from the given foundational research, several gaps remain that will need to be addressed in the future.

In this chapter, we provide a succinct discussion of the challenges that remain for researchers and practitioners who focus on the development and treatment of aggression in children and adolescents. We review both the progress made and the extant shortcomings in contemporary research on the proximal and distal contributors to the development and treatment of aggression in youth, and we conclude by identifying key priorities that we believe will help to advance our current understanding of the emergence, development, and treatment of aggression in childhood and adolescence.

Future Directions for Research on Foundations, Trajectories, and Antecedents of Aggression in Childhood and Adolescence

Foundational research on aggression in childhood and adolescence has revealed the impact of genetic predispositions, biopsychosocial factors, as well as individual cognitive, affective, and motivational characteristics that may accompany or affect the display of aggressive behavior in youth. Recent theoretical and methodological advancements speak to the role of gene–environment interactions in the emergence of aggression and distinct trajectories thereof. Research on behavior genetics and psychophysiology has informed our understanding of the antecedents of aggression. There is increasing evidence that epigenetic mechanisms may play an important role in explaining the gene–environment interactions that enhance aggression. Given evidence for gene–environment interactions on aggression trajectories (see Brendgen, Vitaro, & Boivin, Chapter 4, this volume), future research is warranted to assess the causal nature of this association in the genesis and development of aggression in its different forms and functions. Robust evidence suggests that early environmental experiences in diverse contexts, such as abuse and neglect in the family, or exposure to trauma and victimization in peer relationships, can alter biological markers, which may in turn influence the demonstration of aggressive behavior in one form or another. Thus, future work that integrates measures of epigenetic mechanisms with twin designs may help generate new information about heritable and environmental influences on the development and stability of aggression in childhood and adolescence (see Brendgen et al., Chapter 4, this volume; van Dongen et al., 2016). Such research may also allow us to better understand how neurobiological systems mediate and may moderate contextual effects on aggression (e.g., van Goozen, Fairchild, Snoek, & Harold, 2007).

Similarly, research on the interactions among different psychophysiological systems, contextual factors, and the affective, cognitive, and behavioral correlates of agonistic behavior may extend our current knowledge on the emergence and pathways of direct and indirect forms of aggression (Branje & Koot, Chapter 5, this volume; Malti, Zhang, Myatt, Peplak, & Acland, in press). It should be noted that for the most part, the extant research on the associations among physiology, social–emotional development, and aggression has often relied on single autonomic nervous system (ANS) measures and analytic procedures that fail to capture experiences as they unfold in real time (Kahle & Hastings, 2015). Promising directions for future research should explore latent statistical approaches that can model dynamic ANS responses by linking them to interindividual differences in aggressive behavior (Colasante, Zuffianò, Haley, & Malti, in press).

Much progress has also been made in classifying aggressive behaviors, identifying associated cognitions and emotional processes, and distinguishing pathways of aggression and its various subtypes. For example, subgroups of children are increasingly being identified on the basis of the presence of unique intrapersonal social–emotional profiles, such as callous and unemotional traits (Frick & Matlasz, Chapter 2, this volume; Frick, Ray, Thornton, & Kahn, 2014); low levels of other-oriented emotional responses, such as sympathy (Zuffianò, Colasante, Buchmann, & Malti, 2017); and/or the lack of the expression of guilt (Colasante & Malti, 2017; Malti, 2016; Malti & Krettenauer, 2013; see Malti & Song, Chapter 7, and Malti, Colasante, & Jambon, Chapter 11, this volume). Moving forward, studies utilizing longitudinal designs extending from the early childhood years to the period of adolescence are needed to fully explore (1) how various subtypes of aggression develop, (2) the risk and protective factors that distinguish them, and (3) when in development potential triggers matter the most (Moffit, 1993; see Frick & Matlasz, Chapter 2; Ostrov, Perry, & Blakely-McCure, Chapter 3; and Malti et al., Chapter 11, this volume).

Research on the psychological antecedents of aggression in childhood and adolescence has included a focus on such temperamental/dispositional dimensions as emotion reactivity and regulation, as well as on social-cognitive and social–emotional processes. Further exploration of the relations among neurological processes, emotional reactivity and regulation, and the processing of incoming social information may well enhance our understanding of mechanisms that may account for individual differences in the enactment of varying forms of aggressive behavior in childhood and adolescence (see Moore, Hubbard, & Bookhout, Chapter 6, this volume; Portnov et al., 2014).

Another new and relevant perspective involves understanding how children process conflicting environmental cues, and how this attention allocation is associated with emotional and behavioral development (Dys, Zuffianò, Orsanska, Zaazou, & Malti, 2018; Malti, Dys, Colasante, & Peplak, 2018; see Lansford, Chapter 8, and Malti & Song, Chapter 7, this volume). For instance, do children who proactively aggress spend more time attending to self-serving environmental cues (e.g., a stolen treat) than to other-oriented cues (e.g., a victim's facial expression)? To date, attending to self-oriented over other-oriented cues has been linked to a focus on selfish interests and other-oriented emotions (e.g., empathy–sympathy) in response to transgressing (Dys et al., 2018), but has not yet been tested in relation to aggression in childhood and adolescence. Thus, further empirical research on possible *mechanisms* underlying emotion–aggression and cognition–aggression links across development, such as attention allocation, can extend our current knowledge of the causes and situational triggers of aggressive behaviors in youth. Such research would involve the application of multilevel analyses of developmental and moment-to-moment dynamics in affective and cognitive processes associated with aggression, as well as the study of connections among neural, affective, and behavioral variability.

A related promising direction for future research includes the joint investigation of distinct emotional experiences, such as empathy, guilt, and anger, as well as their regulatory correlates, in the emergence and development of aggression. More broadly, research on *universal* affective and social-cognitive mechanisms that may facilitate the emergence and development of aggression is warranted (Eisner & Malti, 2015). For example, research on the social-cognitive and regulatory anteced-ents of aggression has had a long tradition in developmental science. A direction for future research would be to advance our understanding of universal factors that may *prevent* aggressive behavior. For example, although exposure to violence and child abuse is linked to social-cognitive biases and low regulatory capacities, which in turn can facilitate the expression of aggressive behavior, not all children develop these high-risk social-cognitive, social–emotional, and behavioral profiles. Thus, identification of unique markers and universal mechanisms that help inhibit aggression is essential for theoretical advancement, assessment development, and the refinement of intervention approaches and techniques.

In summary, research on the foundations, trajectories, and individual ante-cedents of aggression in childhood and adolescence has made substantial progress since the turn of the 21st century. Further narrowing of *who* aggresses (e.g., children with low guilt, high psychophysiological arousal, and/or high callous–unemotional traits; see Frick & Matlasz, Chapter 2, and Malti & Song, Chapter 7, this volume); *when* they aggress (e.g., affective and social-cognitive markers, genetic risks, psy-chophysiological correlates, and/or temperamental characteristics; see Brendgen et al., Chapter 4; Branje & Koot, Chapter 5; Malti & Song, Chapter 7; Lansford, Chapter 8; and Moore et al., Chapter 6, this volume); and *why* aggression increases or decreases over time will generate greater knowledge on how to prevent behaviors that are harmful to others. This research will benefit from the systematic utiliza-tion of long-term longitudinal designs, multimethod approaches, and an increased specificity in measuring the various subtypes of aggression (see Ostrov, Perry, & Blakely-McClure, Chapter 3, this volume). Together, each of these topics suggest future directions for research on causes, antecedents, and pathways of aggression, integrating biological and psychological dynamics across time and various levels of analysis.

Future Directions for Research on Aggression in Context

Part II of the *Handbook* has focused on contemporary research on the socialization contexts that contribute to the development of child and adolescent aggression. Much progress has been made in our understanding of the influences of peer inter-actions, peer and family relationships, social networks, and cyberspace on aggres-sive behavior in youth (see Bukowski & Vitaro, Chapter 10; Salmivalli, Chapter 19; Raby & Roisman, Chapter 9; Sijtsma & Ojanen, Chapter 12; and Underwood & Bauman, Chapter 13, this volume; see also Rubin, Bukowski, & Bowker, 2015). Mov-ing forward, we propose a significant focus on the roles of *context* (e.g., exposure to family adversity, poverty, neighborhood violence, cultural norms, social network dynamics, and levels of social inequality; see Leventhal, Dupéré, & Elliott, Chap-ter 14; Underwood & Bauman, Chapter 13; and Sijtsema & Ojanen, Chapter 12, this volume); *group membership* (e.g., members of a minority group or deviant peer group; see Bukowski & Vitaro, Chapter 10, and Sijtsema & Ojanen, Chapter 12, this volume); and *timing* (e.g., duration and intensity of exposure to family adversity; see Raby & Roisman, Chapter 9, this volume) on the development of aggression.

Over several decades, much information has been accumulated about how selection of and affiliation with deviant friends, peer groups, and social networks can enhance a child's propensity to engage in aggressive acts (Dishion, Andrews, & Crosby, 1995; Dishion, McCord, & Poulin, 1999; see Bukowski & Vitaro, Chapter 10, and Sijtsma & Ojnanen, Chapter 12, this volume), yet peer group processes are complex, and certainly not every aggressive child or adolescent has deviant friends or is involved in an aggressive subgroup of peers. While it is clear that the principle of homophily "drives" youth toward others who share similar behavioral proclivities (Rubin et al., 2015), it is also the case that becoming aggressive in the peer group depends on a variety of factors, and there is a need to study the moderators and mediators and selection processes to fully understand this similarity (Killen & Malti, 2015; Veenstra, Lindenberg, Munniksma, & Dijkstra, 2010; see Sijtsma & Ojnanen, Chapter 12, this volume).

Similar to research on the influence of peer relations, there has been substantial advancement in our understanding of parental and family contributions to aggression. For example, numerous studies, with rigorous designs, have provided strong support for the notion of a causal role of insensitive and coercive parenting in the development and maintenance of aggressive behaviors in childhood and adolescence (see Raby & Roisman, Chapter 9, this volume). Nevertheless, many gaps remain to be addressed. For example, additional information is required to fully understand the impact of early childhood experiences in the family context on aggression trajectories into the adulthood years (again see Raby & Roisman, Chapter 9, this volume), including the study of the influence of siblings in the development of agonistic behavior in childhood and adolescence.

Another suggested future direction is the simultaneous examination of multiple, contextual influences (e.g., peers, parents, social media) on agonistic behavior and their long-term effects on developmental trajectories of aggression. Thus, we once again emphasize the need for longitudinal research across diverse populations. Relatedly, research on how *different types* of peer and parent–child interactions and relationships, within and across various cultural and ethnic groups, may differentially affect the development and trajectories of different forms of aggressive behavior is warranted (see Bukowski & Vitaro, Chapter 10, and Malti et al., Chapter 11, this volume).

In addition to the investigation of joint context effects on aggression and its subtypes from early childhood into adulthood, research on the biological and psychological *moderators* and *mediators* of context effects on aggression is needed (see the chapters in Part I of the *Handbook*). For instance, important questions that remain to be addressed pertain to how children's heritable characteristics moderate the link between peer affiliation–rejection and aggression (see Bukowski & Vitaro, Chapter 10, this volume); the roles that social-cognitive processes play in the associations among dyadic and group relationships and the demonstration of aggressive behavior (e.g., Burgess, Wojslawowicz, Rubin, Rose-Krasnor, & Booth-LaForce, 2006); and how physiological reactivity and regulation influence the relations among anger, sympathy, and aggression (see Malti & Song, Chapter 7, and Malti et al., Chapter 11, this volume). There is also a need to further examine the interactions between family processes and individual dispositional characteristics (e.g., emotion reactivity and regulation, sympathetic and parasympathetic nervous system activity) as they predict aggressive tendencies in youth (e.g., Wagner, Hastings, & Rubin, in press).

Various chapters in the *Handbook* have indicated that theories and empirical accounts of the development of aggressive behavior within a social-ecological framework have made substantial contributions to our understanding of aggression during the first two decades of life (Bronfenbrenner, 1977; Hinde, 1987; see Malti & Rubin, Chapter 1, and Leventhal et al., Chapter 14, this volume). Importantly, such frameworks increasingly incorporate indicators of social inequality, such as access to economic, social, and cultural resources, in their theorizing on the causes and correlates of aggression in youth. In the future, such theoretical accounts will likely benefit from the integration of various levels of analyses and a focus on the identification of mechanisms through which social inequality transmits to aggressive outcomes during different developmental periods. For instance, modernization involves processes of rapid and radical social change (Silbereisen & Chen, 2010), which has often been shown to be accompanied by high rates of youth unemployment, economic deprivation, and low social security (Durkheim, 1968). In addition, we are currently facing a child refugee and migrant crisis; large numbers of children and adolescents across the globe are either directly or indirectly affected by the consequences of war. Such youth are witnessing extreme violence in their experiences of marginalization and replacement (UNICEF, 2017). Undoubtedly, exposure to severe adversity creates unprecedented numbers of children affected by trauma and mental health challenges (e.g., Garbarino, 2008; Henrich & Shahar, 2013). The disintegration of the collective normative order, experiences of serious and prolonged trauma, and the alienation of those who lose access to modernization can create internalized feelings of humiliation and vulnerability, as well as anger directed toward potential opponents in an ever-increasing competition for perceived scarce resources (Edelstein, 2005; Hinde & Rotblat, 2003). Obviously, not all pathways to stable problem behaviors are characterized by fragile identities, but this pattern is important because it is likely associated with a lifelong, persistent pattern of aggression and violence. Thus, an integration of individual characteristics (e.g., emotional experiences associated with experiences of social change and competition) and factors at the macrolevel (e.g., poverty and discrimination) is likely to extend current theorizing on the role of social experiences, opportunities, and structural constraints in aggression and violence (see Leventhal et al., Chapter 14, this volume; Piketty, 2014).

In summary, research on children's and adolescents' aggression *in context* has demonstrated the powerful influence of peer relationships, family dynamics, and conditions in the larger social environment on the expression of aggressive behavior among youth. It has also shown how societal inequality—such as poverty, constrained access to opportunities and resources, and exposure to extreme adversity—can influence the emergence of aggression and subsequently perpetuate and maintain agonistic attitudes and behavior. Future work at the intersections of environmental, genetic, epigenetic, and environmental analyses is likely to generate new knowledge on the foundations and pathways of aggression in childhood and adolescence. In addition, the application of multilevel analyses of developmental and moment-to-moment dynamics in affective and cognitive processes associated with aggression provides promising venues for future work in the area of childhood and adolescent aggression. Joint investigations of macro- and microlevel factors that affect variations in aggression during different periods of development are likely to elucidate further when and why aggression emerges. This is likely to deepen and transcend contemporary research on aggression.

Future Directions for Research on Interventions and Policy Implications

There has been a substantial increase in research on the prevention and treatment of aggression since the turn of the 21st century. Profound knowledge regarding the questions of what works, for whom, and when treatment should be introduced has been generated. The translation of basic developmental theory and research into clinical usage has provided insights into the question of *why* certain approaches and practices work. Future work needs to continue this trend and test the underlying theories and causal mechanisms of the intervention approach. This research will not only address the "*why* it works" question but will also increase quality of treatment by ensuring that underlying mechanism(s) are addressed. An increased understanding of the mediators and moderators of treatment effects and processes that facilitate positive change and decrease aggression can in turn help target the developmental needs of every child within and across diverse groups (Costello, 2016; Malti, Chaparro, Zuffianò, & Colasante, 2016; Weisz et al., 2017; see Salmivalli, Chapter 19, this volume).

A related future direction is the study of protective factors and group-level risk factors in the development of prevention and intervention programs. While there is an understanding that a focus on protective factors can help reduce aggression and associated behavioral risks in children and adolescents, additional empirical evidence is warranted to answer how target factors in interventions can (and should) be prioritized (see Guerra, Chapter 20, this volume). Increasingly, researchers have emphasized the need to develop theoretically sound screening and assessment tools to identify protective factors and dimensions of social–emotional development. This trend came in response to a narrow focus on risk factors, mental health challenges, and problem avoidance. Strengths-focused screens and assessment tools can guide the selection and implementation of approaches that target the needs of children and serve them in better ways. Further, although researchers have developed a variety of tools and standardized assessments to examine the extent to which youth demonstrate varieties of aggressive inclinations and behaviors, new trends reveal that it is also important to assess indicators of peer, family, and neighborhood group processes, such as victimization and exposure to violence, to enable a stronger prediction of aggression and crisis (Leuschner et al., 2017; Yablon, 2017). Moving forward, attempts to map children's social–emotional development and strengths are required and must be integrated with risk-focused approaches to assessment. There is also a need to make systematic use of the above diagnostic information in intervention planning and implementation, and to identify the best course of action based on the needs and contextual conditions in which a child is immersed (see Malti, Zuffianò, & Cheung, Chapter 15, this volume). Clearly, the effectiveness of a treatment approach depends largely on the congruency between the needs of the child and the target of the intervention strategies. Treatment effectiveness is also related to the extent of whether and how the timing of risky and beneficial experiences (e.g., bullying in early childhood; having a close, prosocial friend in middle childhood) are considered in treatment planning (Costello, 2016).

In addition to efforts to integrate assessments into intervention planning, additional implementation research is warranted to understand *why* it is that particular approaches and strategies work (see Stormshak & Garbacz, Chapter 17, this volume). These efforts will provide basic information pertaining to how widely various treatment approaches are effective within and across developmental periods as well as within and across diverse populations (Metz & Bartley, 2012; Malti, Noam, Beelmann, & Sommer, 2016). This includes not only efforts to reduce defragmentation of services but also the need to provide practitioners and clinicians with better training opportunities to equip them with the necessary skills and resources to implement practices with rigor (see Lochman, Boxmeyer, Andrade, & Muratori, Chapter 16, and Stormshak & Garbacz, Chapter 17, this volume). Ultimately, these are the necessary steps required to allow us to address the question of how to improve entire service systems and reduce a lack of coordination among settings, which is necessary for sustainable impact (Ghate, 2016; see Lindstrom Johnson, Low, & Bradshaw, Chapter 22, this volume).

Finally, a seminal topic for future research is the adaptation of intervention programs that have demonstrated efficacy, including asking questions regarding whether and how to adapt content and structure of intervention approaches at the level of the individual child, as well as the program (Malti et al., 2016). Earlier in this chapter, we discussed the need to identify protective factors and developmental characteristics of each child to inform intervention practice and to create truly developmentally appropriate treatments (see Malti et al., 2016). Additional research concerning the match between given interventions and the particular needs of each child or adolescent can maximize effectiveness and possibly reduce the duration and intensity of the intervention (see Malti et al., Chapter 15; Hymel & Espelage, Chapter 18; and Guerra, Chapter 20, this volume). This suggestion also applies to research on the effectiveness of integrated interventions (e.g., cognitive-behavioral therapy and mindfulness) targeting various developmental challenges faced by severely aggressive children (see Lochman et al., Chapter 16, this volume). In addition, modifications to evidence-based intervention programs and strategies are likely necessary to create a better fit given particular contextual features and cultural strengths (Beelmann, Malti, Noam, & Sommer, in press; Wessells, 2009; see Lindstrom Johnson et al., Chapter 22, this volume).

Conclusions

In this chapter, we have described several strengths and priority areas for researchers who study the foundations, trajectories, and individual and contextual features associated with aggression. We have also suggested future directions pertaining to prevention and treatment, including how to prevent and treat the emotions, thoughts, interactions, and relationships that appear to accompany and predict upward developmental spirals of aggressive behavior. These topics have been thoroughly described throughout this handbook.

The chapters in the *Handbook* highlight issues and suggest solutions to several challenges in the current field. It is clear that there known risk and protective factors at the biological, individual, and contextual levels that contribute to the emergence of aggression, its development, and its persistence. What we know less about is how the interplay of factors at different levels of analysis (i.e., biological, individual, contextual) affects aggression during different developmental periods and across time, suggesting that a joint investigation of these critical factors may advance the field and enhance our understanding of why aggression evolves and/or changes within an individual. Clearly, this integrated analysis would greatly benefit from rigorous longitudinal designs and the study of diverse populations to enhance long-term predictability and generalizability of findings.

Similarly, effective approaches to prevent and treat aggression have recently been developed for various contexts and age ranges. Moving forward, those who are involved in the day-to-day treatment of aggressive youth will benefit from focusing on the identification of mechanisms that underlie treatment effects. It will also be essential to study how to tailor intervention services to the strengths and developmental needs of children across and within ages. Relatedly, we urge researchers to explore how strengths-based screening and assessment tools may be more systematically integrated into the design, implementation, and evaluation of intervention approaches that have been shown to be effective. What is now needed is a broad investigation of the highly debated question of how to adapt evidence-based intervention programs to various contexts—a time-sensitive aim that may help further clarify what works on a larger scale and across diverse populations of children and adolescents. Finally, additional research on how to coordinate among settings and sectors can facilitate more integrated and effective services. Taken together, focusing on these priority areas in future research is likely to innovate, deepen, and broaden contemporary theorizing and research on aggression in childhood and adolescence.

ACKNOWLEDGMENTS

The writing of this chapter was supported in part by a Canadian Institutes of Health Research Foundation scheme grant awarded to Tina Malti (No. FDN-148389) and by a National Institute of Mental Health grant to Kenneth H. Rubin (No. R01 MH 103253).

REFERENCES

Beelmann, A., Malti, T., Noam, G., & Sommer, S. (in press). Methodological and conceptual innovations: Current status and future directions for prevention science and intervention research. *Prevention Science*.

Bronfenbrenner, U. (1977). Toward an experimental ecology of human development. *American Psychologist, 32*(7), 513–531.

Bukowski, W. M., Laursen, B., & Rubin, K. H. (Eds.). (2018). *Handbook of peer interactions, relationships, and groups* (2nd ed.). New York: Guilford Press.

Burgess, K. B., Wojslawowicz, J. C., Rubin, K. H., Rose-Krasnor, L., & Booth-LaForce, C. (2006). Social information processing and coping styles of shy/withdrawn and aggressive children: Does friendship matter? *Child Development, 77,* 371–383.

Colasante, T., & Malti, T. (2017). Resting heart rate, guilt, and sympathy: A developmental psychophysiological study of physical aggression. *Psychophysiology, 54*(11), 1770–1781.

Colasante, T., Zuffianò, A., Haley, D., & Malti, T. (in press). Children's autonomic nervous system activity while transgressing: Relations to guilt feelings and aggression. *Developmental Psychology.*

Costello, J. (2016). Early detection and prevention of mental health problems: Developmental epidemiology and systems of support. *Journal of Clinical Child and Adolescent Psychology, 45*(6), 710–717.

Dishion, T. J., Andrews, D. W., & Crosby, L. (1995). Antisocial boys and their friends in early adolescence: Relationship characteristics, quality and interactional process. *Child Development, 66,* 139–151.

Dishion, T. J., McCord , J., & Poulin, F. (1999). When interventions harm: Peer groups and problem behavior. *American Psychologist, 54,* 755–764.

Durkheim, E. (1968). *The division of labor in society.* New York: Free Press.

Dys, S. P., Zuffianò, A., Orsanska, V., Zaazou, N., & Malti, T. (2018). *Children's attention allocation is associated with their kind and selfish emotions.* Manuscript under review.

Edelstein, W. (2005). The rise of right-wing culture in German youth: The effects of social transformation, identity construction, and context. In D. B. Pillemer & S. H. White (Eds.), *Developmental psychology and social change* (pp. 314–351). Cambridge, UK: Cambridge University Press.

Eisner, M. P., & Malti, T. (2015). Aggressive and violent behavior. In M. E. Lamb (Vol. Ed.) & R. M. Lerner (Series Ed.), *Handbook of child psychology and developmental science: Vol. 3. Socioemotional processes* (pp. 794–841). New York: Wiley.

Frick, P. J., Ray, J. V., Thornton, J. C., & Kahn, R. E. (2014). Can callous–unemotional traits enhance the understanding, diagnosis, and treatment of serious conduct problems in children and adolescents?: A comprehensive review. *Psychological Bulletin, 140,* 1–57.

Garbarino, J. (2008). *Children and the dark side of human experience: Confronting global realities and rethinking child development.* New York: Springer.

Ghate, D. (2016). From program to systems: Deploying implementation science and practice for sustained real world effectiveness in services for children and families. *Journal of Clinical Child and Adolescent Psychology, 45*(6), 812–826.

Henrich, C. C., & Shahar, G. (2013). Effects of exposure to rocket attacks on adolescent distress and violence: A 4-year longitudinal study. *Journal of the American Academy of Child and Adolescent Psychiatry, 52,* 619–627.

Hinde, R. A. (1987). *Individuals, relationships and culture.* Cambridge, UK: Cambridge University Press.

Hinde, R. A., & Rotblat, J. (2003). *War no more: Eliminating conflict in the nuclear age.* London: Pluto Press.

Kahle, S. S., & Hastings, P. D. (2015). The neurobiology and physiology of emotions: A developmental perspective. In R. A. Scott, S. M. Kosslyn, & N. Pinkerton (Eds.), *Emerging trends in the social and behavioral sciences: An interdisciplinary, searchable, and linkable resource* (pp. 1–15). Hoboken, NJ: Wiley.

Killen, M., & Malti, T. (2015). Moral judgments and emotions in contexts of peer exclusion and victimization. *Advances in Child Development and Behavior, 48,* 249–276.

Leuschner, V., Fiedler, N., Schultze, M., Ahlig, N., Goebel, K., Sommer, F., et al. (2017).

Prevention of targeted school violence by responding to students' psychosocial crises: The NETWASS program. *Child Development, 88*(1), 68–82.

Malti, T. (2016). Toward an integrated clinical-developmental model of guilt. *Developmental Review, 39,* 16–36.

Malti, T., & Averdijk, M. (Eds.). (2017). Severe youth violence: Developmental perspectives [Special section]. *Child Development, 88*(1), 5–82.

Malti, T., Chaparro, M. P., Zuffianò, A., & Colasante, T. (2016). School-based interventions to promote empathy-related responding in children and adolescents: A developmental analysis. *Journal of Clinical Child and Adolescent Psychology, 45*(6), 718–731.

Malti, T., Dys, S. P., Colasante, T., & Peplak, J. (2018). Emotions and morality: New developmental perspectives. In C. Helwig (Vol. Ed.) & M. Harris (Series Ed.), *Current issues in developmental psychology: New perspectives on moral development* (pp. 55–72). New York: Psychology Press.

Malti, T., & Krettenauer, T. (2013). The relation of moral emotion attributions to prosocial and antisocial behavior: A meta-analysis. *Child Development, 84*(2), 397–412.

Malti, T., Noam, G. G., Beelmann, A., & Sommer, S. (2016). Toward dynamic adaptation of psychological interventions for child and adolescent development and mental health. *Journal of Clinical Child and Adolescent Psychology, 45*(6), 827–836.

Malti, T., Zhang, L., Myatt, E., Peplak, J., & Acland, E. (in press). Emotions in contexts of conflict and morality: Developmental perspectives. In V. LoBue, K. Perez-Edgar, & K. Buss (Eds.), *Handbook of emotional development.* New York: Springer.

Metz, A., & Bartley, L. (2012). Active implementation frameworks for program success: How to use implementation science to improve outcomes for children. *Zero to Three Journal, 32*(4), 11–18.

Moffitt, T. E. (1993). Adolescence-limited and life-course persistent antisocial behavior: A developmental taxonomy. *Psychological Review, 100*(4), 674–701.

Piketty, T. (2014). *Capital in the twenty-first century.* Cambridge, MA: Harvard University Press.

Portnoy, J., Raine, A., Chen, F. R., Pardini, D., Loeber, R., & Jennings, J. R. (2014). Heart rate and antisocial behavior: The mediating role of impulsive sensation seeking. *Criminology: An Interdisciplinary Journal, 52,* 292–311.

Rubin, K. H., Bukowski, W., & Bowker, J. (2015). Children in peer groups. In M. Bornstein & T. Leventhal (Vol. Eds.) & R. M. Lerner (Series Ed.), *Handbook of child psychology and developmental science: Vol. 4. Ecological settings and processes* (pp. 175–222). New York: Wiley.

Silbereisen, R. K., & Chen, X. (Eds.). (2010). *Social change and human development.* London: SAGE.

UNICEF. (2017, May 3). A child is a child: Protecting children on the move from violence, abuse and exploitation. Retrieved from *www.unicef.org/publications/index_95956.html.*

van Dongen, J., Nivard, M. G., Willemen, G., Hottenga, J. J., Heimer, Q., Dolan, C. V., et al. (2016). Genetic and environmental influences interact with age and sex in shaping the human methylome. *Nature Communications, 7,* 11115.

van Goozen, S. H., Fairchild, G., Snoek, H., & Harold, G. T. (2007). The evidence for a neurobiological model of childhood antisocial behavior. *Psychological Bulletin, 133,* 149–182.

Veenstra, R., Lindenberg, S., Munniksma, A., & Dijkstra, J. K. (2010). The complex relation between bullying, victimization, acceptance, and rejection: Giving special attention to status, affection, and sex differences. *Child Development, 81*(2), 480–486.

Wagner, N. J., Hastings, P. D., & Rubin, K. H. (in press). Callous–unemotional features and autonomic functioning in toddlerhood interact to predict externalizing behaviors in preschool. *Journal of Abnormal Child Psychology.*

Weisz, J. R., Kuppens, S., Ng, M. Y., Eckshtain, D., Ugueto, A. M., Vaughn-Coaxum, R., et al. (2017). What five decades of research tells us about the effects of youth psychological therapy: A multilevel meta-analysis and implications for science and practice. *American Psychologist, 72*(2), 79–117.

Wessells, M. (2009). Do no harm: Toward contextually appropriate psychosocial support in international emergencies. *American Psychologist, 64*(8), 842–854.

Yablon, Y. B. (2017). Students' reports of severe violence in school as a tool for early detection and prevention. *Child Development, 88*(1), 55–67.

Zuffianò, A., Colasante, T., Buchmann, M., & Malti, T. (2017). The co-development of sympathy and overt aggression from childhood to early adolescence. *Developmental Psychology. 54*(1), 98–110.

CHAPTER 22

Challenges and Priorities
for Practitioners and Policymakers

SARAH LINDSTROM JOHNSON, SABINA LOW,
and CATHERINE P. BRADSHAW

Brief Introduction

Multiple stakeholders are invested in reducing aggression due to the negative health and developmental consequences for children and adolescents, as well as the social and economic burden for society as a whole (Connor, 2002; Piquero, Farrington, Nagin, & Moffitt, 2010). Although some of these stakeholders are researchers, the vast majority come in contact with aggression through their roles in health care, social services, education, criminal justice, public health, or even as parents. Given the broad reach of youth aggression, there are multiple opportunities for practitioners and policymakers to play a role in prevention and intervention; however, there can also be some challenges that hinder progress in this area.

This chapter considers some of the key priorities in the study of prevention of and intervention for aggression, with a particular focus on practitioners and policymakers. Given the bidirectional relationship between practice and policy (Giddens & Pierson, 1998), we consider macro- or cross-cutting challenges and priorities that are relevant to both groups and their interaction. Grounded in Gibbon's (2008) exchange model of knowledge building, which highlights the critical role of application in furthering knowledge production, we build on the previous chapter's focus on challenges and priorities for researchers. Additionally, we apply a conceptual use lens and identify some of the complex and indirect ways that research can influence practice and policy (Nutley, Walter, & Davies, 2007; Weisz et al., 2005). We conclude by identifying areas of research that should be addressed to advance practice and policy and to help bridge the gap.

Integration of the Issues and Coordination of the Solutions

••

Given the vast number of varying stakeholders, such a diverse group will likely face a myriad of challenges and priorities in their aggression prevention and intervention efforts. In fact, depending on the focus of the practitioner of policymaker, even the use of the term *aggression* versus *violence* might differ. This subtle difference has important implications, as it divides a diverse group of youth aggression or violence stakeholders and provides somewhat of a background about the solutions that these groups promote. In this chapter, we utilize the term *aggression* insofar as it is a broader category of behaviors than *violence* (which is limited to use of physical force; see Krahé, 2013, for operational distinctions). We outline a common framework to conceptualize the varying stakeholder groups' unique barriers and challenges. Specifically, we focus on two issues: (1) applying the principles of multifinality and equifinality in aggression prevention/intervention and (2) developing a coordinated and effective delivery system.

Practitioners and policymakers are exposed to the variability that exists in antecedents to aggression (Eisner & Malti, 2015). This can be a major impediment, as it makes it more difficult to predict occurrences and to identity a solution to the problem. Likewise, they are also exposed to often co-occurring "diagnoses," including conduct disorder, delinquency, drug use, and school difficulties (Farrington, 2009). Thus, through their interactions with individuals and communities, practitioners and policymakers are exposed to the principles of equifinality and multifinality. *Equifinality* refers to an understanding that multiple different pathways can lead to the same outcome (see Gatzke-Kopp, Greenberg, Fortunato, & Coccia, 2012, for an example dealing with aggression), whereas *multifinality* suggests that common processes can lead to diverse outcomes (Cicchetti & Rogosch, 1996). Diversity in outcomes, in particular, suggests significant variability in how youth respond to risk factors and infers that developmental risks are not fate (i.e., fixed). Rather, such diversity implies a greater need to identify features of resilience and a broader class of assets that promote positive adaptation (Curtis & Cicchetti, 2003; Masten, 2007). This makes it a particularly helpful framework to draw upon in this chapter, as promoting resilience and positive adaptation is an important focus of most practitioners and policymakers.

The challenges and priorities of practitioners and policymakers span a continuum of prevention and intervention efforts, including universal prevention, which tries to prevent a disease or injury before it occurs; selective prevention/intervention, which focuses on reducing the impact of a disease or injury and returning individuals to health; and indicated prevention/intervention, which aims to soften the impact of an ongoing illness or injury (National Research Council & Institute of Medicine, 2009). It should be noted that applying a prevention framework to aggression represents a relatively recent societal shift. Violence (as a subtype) was once deemed solely the jurisdiction of criminal justice (Dahlberg & Mercy, 2009). Although most would applaud this change, as it allows for a broader solution set, it has also meant that diverse disciplines are now seeing their roles in the prevention of aggression (e.g., schools and bullying). This, then, necessitates a coordination of effort. The National Research Council and Institute of Medicine (2009) Committee on the Prevention of Mental Disorders and Substance Abuse among Children, Youth, and Young Adults suggested as one of its primary recommendations the need to "develop a coordinated and effective delivery system" (p. 371). The report noted both difficulties in coordinating care across different service sectors and barriers to implementation in certain "advantageous" settings, such as day care, schools, and primary medical care, that serve (access) large populations.

Challenges That Arise Due to Principles of Multifinality and Equifinality

Building on the work of Gendreau and Archer (2005), Figure 22.1 summarizes the multiple different types of aggression and their antecedents. We emphasize those factors that could potentially be modifiable and put less emphasis on biological factors (i.e., genetic background or neurocognitive or physiological differences) and events that are tangential to the domain of prevention broadly defined (i.e., war, poverty). We also highlight the different programmatic and policy efforts that are meant to address aggression and violence across the life course. Our effort is not meant to be exhaustive, but illustrative of the following challenges.

Challenge 1: *Aggression is closely related to other risk behaviors, but each is addressed by its own programs, educational and clinical approaches, and policies.*

As depicted in the center of Figure 22.1, there are different types of aggression and risk behaviors that exist upon a continuum and share definitional features, as well as behavioral manifestations. For example:

- School violence researchers study aggression that happens in schools, mainly peer victimization and bullying, which can take many forms (e.g., verbal, physical, relational). Disentangling peer victimization and bullying is difficult; in fact, the recent National Academies of Sciences, Engineering, and Medicine (2016) report, *Preventing Bullying through Science, Policy, and Practice,* cites, as one of its main recommendations, the need for a consistent definition of bullying. Researchers are beginning to study bullying perpetration from a developmental framework, trying to understand, for example, relations with teen dating violence (Debnam, Waasdorp, & Bradshaw, 2016). Additional work has found bullying perpetration to be a mediator between family violence and teen dating violence (Espelage, Anderson, Low, & De La Rue, in press), supporting an intergenerational transmission of violence.

- Externalizing behaviors consist of disruptive, hyperactive, and aggressive behaviors (Hinshaw, 1987). Although aggression is a type of externalizing behavior, research has suggested that it may be meaningfully different, attributable more to individual factors than contextual factors (Burt, 2009). An example of an individual factor is genetics; the expression of serotonin transporter 5HTT has been linked with aggression and conduct disorder (Cadoret et al., 2003; Haberstick, Smolen, & Hewitt, 2006). Conduct disorder is a mental health disorder diagnosed by the presence of repeated violations of social norms. The prevalence of conduct disorder

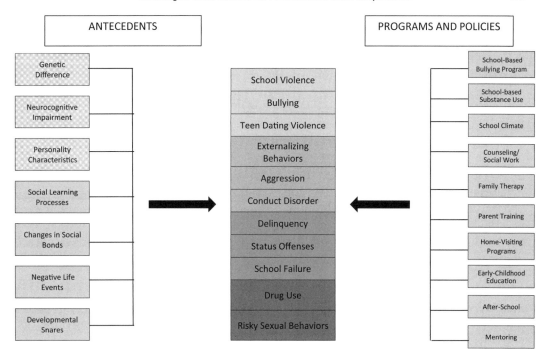

FIGURE 22.1. Multifinality and equifinality exist in aggression-related causes and solutions.

and the related oppositional defiance disorder has been found to be stable across countries (Canino, Polanczyk, Bauermeister, Rohde, & Frick, 2010), suggesting that national differences in rates of aggression and violence may be strongly influenced by contextual differences.

   • Aggression can be classified as overt antisocial behavior, which is distinguished from covert antisocial behavior and authority conflicts (Farrington, 2009). The latter two often lead to delinquency or status offenses (e.g., special category of delinquent acts that are only against the law for minors). Studies have shown that youth who engage in violent crime are also likely to engage in delinquency (i.e., theft) and status offenses (i.e., alcohol use; Van Lier, Vitaro, Barker, Koot, & Tremblay, 2009). Low IQ and low school achievement have been shown to be predictors of aggression, conduct disorder, and delinquency (Moffitt, 1993), but involvement in these behaviors also can have a negative impact on educational success through poor academic engagement or missed instructional time (Bierman et al., 2013).

   • Although adolescent substance use is fairly normative, early use of substances and substance abuse have been associated with aggression, high school dropout, and young adult unemployment (Green & Ensminger, 2006; Schulenberg & Maggs, 2002). School failure has also been related to an increased likelihood of substance use, particularly if the student is involved in aggressive behaviors (Dishion, Patterson, Stoolmiller, & Skinner, 1991). Likewise, although sexual initiation is normative

during adolescence, risky sex (i.e., not using contraception or having multiple partners) and sexual violence have been related to use of substances (Ritchwood, Ford,
DeCoster, Sutton, & Lochman, 2015).

   The above is just a cursory overview of what is known about the connections
between aggression and violence, mental health disorders, criminal involvement,
academic success, and drug abuse. The majority of this work has taken a variable-
centered approach, that is, it investigated the likelihood of involvement in one of
these behaviors given another behavior (Laursen & Hoff, 2006). Of course, this is
not how practitioners experience the overlap between these behaviors. Practitioners interact with a youth who has a conduct disorder and a substance use problem
or a youth who is engaged in bullying and not doing well in school. Researchers are
just beginning to understand the increased risk associated with comorbid conditions. Capaldi and Stoolmiller (1999) found the effects of conduct problems and
depression to be additive, but not interactive. Potentially important extensions of
this work will involve the use of person-centered approaches, such as latent class/
profile analysis (Lanza & Rhoades, 2013), which seeks to find groups of individuals
that share similar characteristics and identify differential outcomes of these groups
(Laursen & Hoff, 2006). This approach has been used to identify subgroups of
bullying victimization (Bradshaw, Waasdrop, & O'Brennan, 2013), substance use
(Cleveland, Collins, Lanza, Greenberg, & Feinberg, 2010), and violence exposure
(Ballard et al., 2015) and differences in relative functioning. Such approaches yield
greater translational significance and, as such, can help bridge the gap between
research and policy/practice (Nutley et al., 2007; Weisz et al., 2005). As can be
seen by the previous examples, more work is needed to examine patterns across
different types of risk and protective factors and understand differential effects on
aggression and related behaviors. Additionally, more research is needed to understand developmental cascades of behavior, both to support early intervention and
to identify the most likely comorbid conditions (Masten & Cicchetti, 2010). For
example, the presence of anxiety symptoms and reactive behavior may indicate
risk for comorbid anxiety and conduct disorder or oppositional defiant disorder
(Bubier & Drabick, 2009). Many of the aggressive, violence, and risk behaviors in
Figure 22.1 debut or become more prevalent in adolescence, further supporting the
need for research identifying early risk factors.
   Although there has been an increase in the development and dissemination
of evidence-based aggression prevention programs (Aarons, Hurlburt, & Horwitz,
2011), the majority of these programs focus on one particular outcome (e.g., Blueprints for Healthy Youth Development [*www.colorado.edu/cspv/blueprints*] or the
Substance Abuse and Mental Health Services Administration's National Registry of
Evidence-Based Programs and Practices [*www.samhsa.gov/nrepp*]), often neglecting
shared risk factors and behaviors. Part of the difficulty is that the majority of programs were designed to address a specific outcome, and therefore they only assess
effects related to that outcome. For example, many of the randomized controlled
trials on violence and aggression prevention do not provide evidence that allow
an understanding of the effects on bullying behaviors (Bradshaw, 2015). A recent
meta-analysis was only able to identify 44 interventions aimed at addressing two
adolescent risk behaviors, and most focused on use of multiple substances (Hale,

Fitzgerald-Yau, & Viner, 2014). This is most likely the result of applying a treatment model in which there is an identified problem, rather than a prevention model in which the focus is on supporting adaptive development and resilience, perhaps with youth who have known risk factors (Catalano, Berglund, Ryan, Lonczak, & Hawkins, 2002).

Policymakers likewise have a difficult time and seem to take a reactionary, siloed approach to addressing aggression, violence, and related risk behaviors (Hale & Viner, 2012). Programs implemented are often based on political or social pressure, anecdotes, or general perceptions of what works (Latessa, Cullen, & Gendreau, 2002). And due to fiscal constraints, often the "new" program is often funded through cuts in other programs (Fagan, 2013). Two evidence-based models for assisting communities in identifying social program priorities and adopting appropriate evidence-based interventions exist: Communities That Care (Hawkins, Catalano, & Arthur, 2002) and Promoting School–Community–University Partnerships to Enhance Resilience (PROSPER; Spoth, Greenberg, Bierman, & Redmond, 2004). These models encourage stakeholder investment, data-based decision making, and implementation monitoring and have demonstrated effects on multiple outcomes, including substance use, delinquency, and conduct problem behaviors. Positive Behavioral Interventions and Supports (PBIS; Sugai & Horner, 2009) is a similar framework that operates at the school level. These models address the problem of redundant programming by trying to coordinate the efforts of organizations around focal issues. Optimal impact of such interventions is, however, highly dependent on various contextual factors, such as school climate, administrator leadership, and staff buy-in (Domitrovich et al., 2010).

Challenge 2: *There are common antecedents to aggression, suggesting the importance of programs and policies that comprehensively support youth development.*

Theories of crime can be grouped into two main developmental theories and lend themselves to an analogous framework for aggression (Nagin & Paternoster, 2000). Population heterogeneity includes factors such as genetic differences, neurocognitive differences as a result of early life adversity, or highly stable personality characteristics such as psychopathy or callous–unemotional traits. Although these are certainly relevant for practitioners and policymakers, particularly to the extent that interventions can be put into place to prevent their occurrence or mitigate their influence on behavior, the state-dependence theories represent more malleable social interventions. Specifically, Eisner and Malti (2015) described four major causal mechanisms: social learning processes, stability and change in social bonds (i.e., prosocial and antisocial), strains and negative life events, and developmental snares (e.g., drug addiction, imprisonment, teenage pregnancy, interrupted education). Social learning processes are thought to explain the connection between socioeconomic status and aggression, with children being socialized toward attitudes and beliefs that may be protective in the immediate environment but carry risk (Chen, 2004). Similarly, Malti, Averdijk, Ribeaud, Rotenberg, and Eisner (2013) found that youth who are involved in aggression throughout childhood tended to be of a lower social class and exhibit low trust and trustworthiness. Perceptions of neighborhood collective efficacy have been related to parental socialization concerning violence (Lindstrom Johnson, Finigan, Bradshaw, Haynie, & Cheng, 2011), whereas exposure to neighborhood violence (i.e., a strain) has been associated with impulsive behavior and depression (Lambert, Nylund-Gibson, Copeland-Linder, & Ialongo, 2010). Moreover, developmental snares have been shown to increase the likelihood of maintaining aggressive behavior across the life course (McGee et al., 2015).

Taking the perspective of Link and Phelan (1995), this amounts to focusing more on the social causes of disease and less on the proximal causes. As Eisner and Malti (2015) state, "Many risk factors associated with aggression are in themselves widely held to be undesirable conditions that reduce the welfare and well-being of individuals at all stages of the life course, meaning that efforts to eliminate or reduce them are desirable" (p. 798). In fact, practitioners and policymakers are often more interested in promoting positive youth outcomes than focusing on risk behaviors (Fagan, 2013; Hall, Simon, Lee, & Mercy, 2012; see Guerra, Chapter 20, this volume). Broadly, practitioners are invested in supporting the development of competencies or promoting resiliency and policymakers in ameliorating negative conditions and providing supports for adaptive/healthy development. This perspective supports exploring why individuals do not engage in violence in the first place and the investigation of what have been termed promotive factors. A novel series of studies led by the Centers for Disease Control and Prevention's Division of Violence Prevention aimed to identify common risk, protection (buffering from negative outcomes in the context of risk), and promotive factors for aggression across four large longitudinal studies (Hall et al., 2012). Using common data analytic techniques, Hall and colleagues (2012) concluded that 18% of individual and contextual factors could be classified as promotive effects, that is, something that prevented involvement in aggression. The majority of promotive factors were educationally related items, such as high educational aspirations and school attachment, and peer behaviors, such as low peer deviancy and high peer prosocial behavior.

These promotive factors validate the implementation of programs and policies that focus on the social and environmental factors that affect the successful completion of developmental tasks (Catalano et al., 2002). In fact, many of the evidence-based programs and policies (Aos, Phipps, Barnoski, & Lieb, 2001; *www.blueprintsprograms.com*) listed on the right side of Figure 22.1 take a positive youth development approach toward preventing youth involvement in aggression. A review of the literature identified 161 programs that aimed to support youth development, of which 71 had appropriate evaluations and 25 showed positive effects on youth behavioral outcomes (Catalano et al., 2002). The effective programs addressed multiple youth competencies, had a structured curriculum, were delivered over a longer period of time and with a focus on fidelity, and had rigorous evaluations. For example, the Middle School Second Step program (Committee for Children; *www.cfchildren.org*) integrates adolescent brain development, social psychology, and the risk and protective factors framework to build the life skills necessary to be successful in and outside of school. Such cross-disciplinary, strengths-based programs have potential to address the various concerns of stakeholders (e.g., substance use, bullying, teen dating violence) while maximizing efficiency and cost.

Unfortunately, system and agency priorities often hinder the implementation of positive youth development programs. Commonly assessed outcomes measured in the varying disciplines, such as test scores in education or health and safety of incarcerated juveniles in criminal justice, do not align with a focus on fundamental causes or a positive youth development approach (Greenberg et al., 2003; Greenwood, 2008). Part of this is due to a dearth of research on how preventative interventions address outcomes of primary interest to practitioners and policymakers. For example, a review of the literature identified that only one-third of studies of school-based mental health interventions addressed educational outcomes (Hoagwood et al., 2007). This is an artifact of the siloed system of research and practice funding, which focuses either on improving educational outcomes or on improving health outcomes.

Challenges to Creating Effective Delivery Systems

Challenge 1: *Lack of coordination between settings does not allow for the "blanketing" of services.*

As can be seen in the bottom of Figure 22.2, interventions to prevent or reduce aggression occur in multiple different settings, including educational, medical, home, and community. The recent National Academies of Sciences, Engineering, and Medicine (2016) report, *Preventing Bullying,* found that all universal violence prevention efforts, that is, efforts focused on preventing aggression in the entire population regardless of risk, occurred in the school setting. The school context has also been the focus of policies on bullying, with many states requiring professional development or school-based programming related to bullying (Child Trends, 2015; U.S. Department of Education, 2011). Although this may make sense, as schools have large numbers of students reinforcing attitudes and norms about aggressive behaviors, there is concern that violence prevention programming in education may represent an unfunded and poorly monitored mandate (Sheras & Bradshaw, 2016; Srabstein, Berkman, & Pyntikova, 2008). Additionally, the perceived ownership of the issue by schools may make other venues, such as primary care practitioners, less likely to engage in discussions about violence prevention (Lindstrom Johnson, Bradshaw, Cheng, & Wright, 2017).

Selected or indicated interventions, that is, programs for students at risk for or currently displaying aggression, all involved the family (National Academies of Sciences, Engineering, & Medicine, 2016). However, most also included at least one other setting, often a medical or community setting. Catalano and colleagues (2002) reviewed positive youth development programs and found that two-thirds of effective programs operated in multiple contexts. Without a high level of cooperation between sectors (i.e., schoolteachers, after-school programs, and professional community service providers), there is concern that the burden of coordination falls on the family, and the effectiveness of the intervention might decrease (Dodge & Mandel, 2012).

To remove this burden and facilitate coordination, services are often colocated, mostly with noneducational services being placed in schools. One example

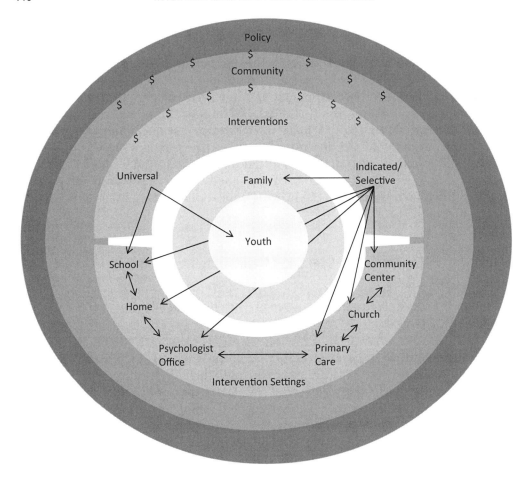

FIGURE 22.2. Challenges to effective delivery systems include the need for coordination and an understanding of cost.

of this practice is school-based health centers. Having health suites in schools has been thought of as a way to reduce disparities in access to care and to increase the percentage of youth who receive primary and preventative services (Parasuraman & Shi, 2014). School-based health center use has also been related to improved school connectedness and attendance, which can be related to improvements in grade-point average (Strolin-Goltzman, Sisselman, Melekis, & Auerbach, 2014; Walker, Kerns, Lyon, Bruns, & Cosgrove, 2010). Unfortunately, the school-based health center often operates in isolation from the school. New models are going beyond colocation to coordination. For example, the Family Check-Up has been integrated with PBIS (Stormshak et al., 2011). Following the tiered approach to intervention outline in PBIS, the model included the establishment of a family resource center for the provision of feedback about child behavior in school, as well as resources and three sessions of motivational interviewing (e.g., the Family Check-Up). Another novel example of colocation of services is the Healthy Futures intervention that provided career counseling in a pediatric primary care clinic (Lindstrom Johnson, Jones, & Cheng, 2015). Unfortunately, these interventions are often difficult to implement with fidelity and to sustain with high fidelity, as they require a common understanding of the problem and solution. They also require the dedication of resources and often are the first initiatives cut when budgets are tight (Glisson & Schoenwald, 2005).

Challenge 2: *Little attention is paid to the costs of prevention relative to its benefits.*

Most research focuses on understanding the benefits of interventions with little attention to the costs. Part of this a "distaste" for the notion that the decision about which services to provide to youth and families is in part dictated by cost; however, limited resources make understanding which programs and policies yield better returns an important consideration in decision making (Aos et al., 2001). In a seminal book on decision making, Rivlin (1971) identified four critical elements: (1) defining the problem, (2) figuring out who would be helped and by how much, (3) systematically comparing the benefits and costs of different possible programs, and (4) figuring out how to produce more effective social programs. In current prevention efforts, the third element often presents a challenge, as individuals designing and implementing programs often do not have the resources, knowledge, or skills to effectively estimate the costs of an intervention (National Research Council & Institute of Medicine, 2009). Current best practices in assessing cost go beyond a focus simply on the budget and require an understanding of all the resources needed to conduct an intervention (i.e., ingredients method; Levin & McEwan, 2001). In order to address this lack of data, funders are beginning to suggest a cost aim as a component of grant applications (National Research Council & Institute of Medicine, 2009). This is an important component of sustainability; as can be seen at the top of Figure 22.2, the majority of costs for intervention or policy are borne by the community.

Consideration of the cost of the elements required to implement interventions requires a focus on implementation fidelity and sustainability. Most of the effects of programs are determined from carefully controlled trials (i.e., effectiveness designs) and represent best-case scenarios with high levels of funding and supervision. Oftentimes these conditions do not exist when an intervention is scaled up, and, due to this, intervention effects may be less strong (Dodge & Mandel, 2012). One key concern is staff training, with most youth-serving organizations needing extensive and ongoing training to ensure the implementation of evidence-based programs with fidelity (Mihalic & Irwin, 2003) . Such training is not always available from program developers or is costly, particularly in light of frequent staff turnover. An additional concern related to scaling up an intervention is the extent of the intervention that is needed in order to be maximally effective. From a cost perspective, an economy of scale suggests that each additional person served will cost less; similarly, public health principles support the notion of a tipping point for benefits. Some work has suggested this point to be 60% in order to produce socially significant benefits. This is difficult and requires external supports for change, policies to enable effective practice, and practice–policy communication (Fixsen, Blasé, Metz, & Van Dyke, 2013).

Additionally challenging to capture are the "costs" of the benefits derived from the intervention. Oftentimes long-term outcomes (such as graduation, incarceration, disability [including mental health], and mortality) are not assessed and have to be extrapolated from known associations in the literature. This situation provides uncertainty in the data and can result in widely differing results (Foster, Dodge, & Jones, 2003). Fortunately, studies comparing costs and benefits of youth prevention programs suggest that, because the negative outcomes (i.e., delinquency or dropping out) are so costly, only a few events have to be averted for a program to have a positive cost–benefit ratio (Aos et al., 2001). Prevention programs face an additional challenge, as the primary cost-saving benefits are not actualized until far into the future. For example, although interventions in the school setting to promote behavioral management are aimed to improve classroom behavior and academics, the true cost-saving mechanism is the reduction in criminal activity that will not be actualized until adolescence or, more likely, adulthood. This means two things: First, the intervention will incur a cost to society before (in many cases, well before) the benefit is realized; and, second, the cost will be incurred by a different system than that which realizes the benefit. This has important implications for the sustainability of preventative interventions.

Conclusions

This chapter identified four main challenges and priorities for practitioners and policymakers:

1. Aggression is closely related to other risk behaviors, with shared risk and protective factors, but each is addressed by its own programs, approaches/ strategies, and policies.
2. There are shared antecedents to aggression (and related risk factors), suggesting that societal-level investment in programs and policies that comprehensively support positive youth development may be optimally efficient and effective.
3. Lack of coordination between settings does not allow for the "blanketing" of services.
4. Little attention is paid to the costs of prevention relative to its benefits.

In identifying these main challenges, we drew upon the principles of multifinality and equifinality, as well as considerations from the field of implementation science. Together, this research highlights the importance of these issues and suggests some possible solutions for the field going forward. It is clear that there are now interventions that work to prevent youth involvement in aggression and related risk behaviors. Additionally, much is known about the supports that are needed to implement programs with fidelity and to get results (Domitrovich et al., 2008). What is now needed is a shift from thinking about individual outcomes to a focus on common supports. Such a shift may require reconsideration of the allocation of resources and coordination of services to improve implementation. It also may require modifications to evidence-based programs and strategies to make them more efficiently and feasibly fit with the goals of various delivery systems (Malti, Noam, Beelmann, & Sommer, 2016). Only in this way will we create a society focused on promoting and improving youth outcomes, rather than the traditional reactive approach to ameliorating illness.

We also want to highlight the existence of resources from varying stakeholder groups' professional organizations in order to further both work in youth aggression and violence prevention and opportunities to begin to address the aforementioned priorities and challenges.

- The National Conference of State Legislatures (*www.ncsl.org*) provides support to its members around outcomes such as youth violence and dropout prevention.

- The American Psychological Association (*www.apa.org*) has a division focused on peace, conflict, and violence, but also has divisions that address the care of individuals exposed to violence (i.e., trauma psychology) or exhibiting aggression (i.e., school psychology).

- The National Association for Social Workers (*www.naswdc.org*) has a special practice section focused on social and economic justice and peace, as well as sections dedicated to children, adolescents, and young adults.

- The National Education Association (*www.nea.org*) focuses on the specific issues of bullying and school safety.

- The American Public Health Association (*www.apha.org*) has a section of members focused on injury control and emergency health services and school health education and services.

- The Community Oriented Policing Services Office of the U.S. Department of Justice (*https://cops.usdoj.gov*) provides materials related to child and youth safety and healing communities.

- The World Health Organization (*www.who.int/violence_injury_prevention/violence/en*) provides information about the epidemiology of violence across countries and has a Global Partnership to End Violence against Children.

- The World Bank (*www.worldbank.org/en/topic/fragilityconflictviolence*) has resources that explore the important connection between poverty and conflict and violence.

REFERENCES

Aarons, G. A., Hurlburt, M., & Horwitz, S. M. (2011). Advancing a conceptual model of evidence-based practice implementation in public service sectors. *Administration and Policy in Mental Health and Mental Health Services Research, 38*(1), 4–23.

Aos, S., Phipps, P., Barnoski, R., & Lieb, R. (2001). *The comparative costs and benefits of programs to reduce crime* (Version 4.0) (Document No. 01-05-1201). Olympia: Washington State Institute for Public Policy.

Ballard, E. D., Van Eck, K., Musci, R. J., Hart, S. R., Storr, C. L., Breslau, N., et al. (2015). Latent classes of childhood trauma exposure predict the development of behavioral health outcomes in adolescence and young adulthood. *Psychological Medicine, 45*(15), 3305–3316.

Bierman, K. L., Coie, J., Dodge, K., Greenberg, M., Lochman, J., McMohan, R., et al. (2013). School outcomes of aggressive–disruptive children: Prediction from kindergarten risk factors and impact of the fast track prevention program. *Aggressive Behavior, 39*(2), 114–130.

Bradshaw, C. P. (2015). Translating research to practice in bullying prevention. *American Psychologist, 70*(4), 322–332.

Bradshaw, C. P., Waasdorp, T. E., & O'Brennan, L. M. (2013). A latent class approach to examining forms of peer victimization. *Journal of Educational Psychology, 105*(3), 839–849.

Bubier, J. L., & Drabick, D. A. G. (2009). Co-occurring anxiety and disruptive behavior disorders: The roles of anxious symptoms, reactive aggression, and shared risk processes. *Clinical Psychology Review, 29*(7), 658–669.

Burt, S. A. (2009). Are there meaningful etiological differences within antisocial behavior?: Results of a meta-analysis. *Clinical Psychology Review, 29*(2), 163–178.

Cadoret, R. J., Langbehn, D., Caspers, K., Troughton, E. P., Yucuis, R., Sandhu, H. K., et al. (2003). Associations of the serotonin transporter promoter polymorphism with aggressivity, attention deficit, and conduct disorder in an adoptee population. *Comprehensive Psychiatry, 44*(2), 88–101.

Canino, G., Polanczyk, G., Bauermeister, J. J., Rohde, L. A., & Frick, P. J. (2010). Does the prevalence of CD and ODD vary across cultures? *Social Psychiatry and Psychiatric Epidemiology, 45*(7), 695–704.

Capaldi, D. M., & Stoolmiller, M. (1999). Co-occurrence of conduct problems and depressive symptoms in early adolescent boys: III. Prediction to young-adult adjustment. *Development and Psychopathology, 11*(1), 59–84.

Catalano, R. F., Berglund, M. L., Ryan, J. A. M., Lonczak, H. S., & Hawkins, J. D. (2002). Positive youth development in the United States: Research findings on evaluations of positive youth development programs. *Prevention and Treatment, 5*(1).

Chen, E. (2004). Why socioeconomic status affects the health of children: A psychosocial perspective. *Current Directions in Psychological Science, 13*(3), 112–115.

Child Trends. (2015) All 50 states now have a bullying law: Now what? Retrieved from *www.childtrends.org/all-50-states-now-have-a-bullying-law-now-what*.

Cicchetti, D., & Rogosch, F. A. (1996). Equifinality and multifinality in developmental psychopathology. *Development and Psychopathology, 8*(4), 597–600.

Cleveland, M. J., Collins, L. M., Lanza, S. T., Greenberg, M. T., & Feinberg, M. E. (2010). Does individual risk moderate the effect of contextual-level protective factors?: A latent class analysis of substance use. *Journal of Prevention and Intervention in the Community, 38*(3), 213–228.

Connor, D. F. (2002). *Aggression and antisocial behavior in children and adolescents: Research and treatment.* New York: Guilford Press.

Curtis, W. J., & Cicchetti, D. (2003). Moving research on resilience into the 21st century: Theoretical and methodological considerations in examining the biological contributors to resilience. *Development and Psychopathology, 15*(3), 773–810.

Dahlberg, L. L., & Mercy, J. A. (2009). History of violence as a public health issue. *AMA Virtual Mentor, 11*(2), 167–172.

Debnam, K. J., Waasdorp, T. E., & Bradshaw, C. P. (2016). Examining the contemporaneous occurrence of bullying and teen dating violence victimization. *School Psychology Quarterly, 31*(1), 76–90.

Dishion, T. J., Patterson, G. R., Stoolmiller, M., & Skinner, M. L. (1991). Family, school, and behavioral antecedents to early adolescent involvement with antisocial peers. *Developmental Psychology, 27*(1), 172–180.

Dodge, K. A., & Mandel, A. D. (2012). Building evidence for evidence-based policy making. *Criminology and Public Policy, 11*(3), 525–534.

Domitrovich, C. E., Bradshaw, C. P., Poduska, J., Hoagwood, K., Buckley, J., Olin, S., et al. (2008). Maximizing the implementation quality of evidence-based preventive interventions in schools: A conceptual framework. *Advances in School Mental Health Promotion: Training and Practice, Research and Policy, 1*(3), 6–28.

Eisner, M. P., & Malti, T. (2015). Aggressive and violent behavior. In R. M. Lerner (Ed.-in-Chief) & M. E. Lamb (Vol. Ed.), *Handbook of child psychology and developmental science: Vol. 3. Socioemotional processes* (7th ed., pp. 794–841). Hoboken, NJ: Wiley.

Espelage, D. L., Anderson, C. A., Low, S., & De La Rue, L. (in press). Longitudinal associations among bullying, sexual, and dating violence from early to late adolescence: Role of family violence, anger, and delinquency. *Developmental Psychology.*

Fagan, A. A. (2013). Enhancing the quality of stakeholder assessments of evidence-based prevention programs. *Criminology and Public Policy, 12*(2), 333–341.

Farrington, D. P. (2009). Conduct disorder, aggression and delinquency. In R. M. Lerner & L. Steinberg (Eds.), *Handbook of adolescent psychology* (3rd ed., Vol. 3, pp. 683–722). Hoboken, NJ, Wiley.

Fixsen, D., Blasé, K., Metz, A., & Van Dyke, M. (2013). Statewide implementation of evidence-based programs. *Exceptional Children, 79*(2), 213–230.

Foster, E. M., Dodge, K. A., & Jones, D. (2003). Issues in the economic evaluation of prevention programs. *Applied Developmental Science, 7*(2), 76–86.

Gatzke-Kopp, L. M., Greenberg, M. T., Fortunato, C. K., & Coccia, M. A. (2012). Aggression as an equifinal outcome of distinct neurocognitive and neuroaffective processes. *Development and Psychopathology, 24*(3), 985–1002.

Gendreau, P. L., & Archer, J. (2005). Subtypes of aggression in humans and animals. In R. E. Tremblay, W. W. Hartup, & J. Archer (Eds.), *Developmental origins of aggression* (pp. 25–46). New York: Guilford Press.

Gibbons, M. (2008, June 10). Why is knowledge translation important?: Grounding the conversation. *Focus* (Technical Brief No. 21). Retrieved from *http://ktdrr.org/ktlibrary/articles_pubs/ncddrwork/focus/focus21/Focus21.pdf.*

Giddens, A., & Pierson, C. (1998). *Conversations with Anthony Giddens: Making sense of modernity.* Redwood City, CA: Stanford University Press.

Glisson, C., & Schoenwald, S. K. (2005). The ARC organizational and community intervention strategy for implementing evidence-based children's mental health treatments. *Mental Health Services Research, 7*(4), 243–259.

Green, K. M., & Ensminger, M. E. (2006). Adult social behavioral effects of heavy adolescent marijuana use among African Americans. *Developmental Psychology, 42*(6), 1168–1178.

Greenberg, M. T., Weissberg, R. P., O'Brien, M. U., Zins, J. E., Fredericks, L., Resnik, H., et al. (2003). Enhancing school-based prevention and youth development through coordinated social, emotional, and academic learning. *American Psychologist, 58*(6–7), 466–474.

Greenwood, P. (2008). Prevention and intervention programs for juvenile offenders. *The Future of Children, 18*(2), 185–210.

Haberstick, B. C., Smolen, A., & Hewitt, J. K. (2006). Family-based association test of the 5HTTLPR and aggressive behavior in a general population sample of children. *Biological Psychiatry, 59*(9), 836–843.

Hale, D. R., Fitzgerald-Yau, N., & Viner, R. M. (2014). A systematic review of effective interventions for reducing multiple health risk behaviors in adolescence. *American Journal of Public Health, 104*(5), e19–e41.

Hale, D. R., & Viner, R. M. (2012). Policy responses to multiple risk behaviours in adolescents. *Journal of Public Health, 34*(Suppl. 1), i11–i19.

Hall, J. E., Simon, T. R., Lee, R. D., & Mercy, J. A. (2012). Implications of direct protective factors for public health research and prevention strategies to reduce youth violence. *American Journal of Preventive Medicine, 43*(2), S76–S83.

Hawkins, J. D., Catalano, R. F., & Arthur, M. W. (2002). Promoting science-based prevention in communities. *Addictive Behaviors, 27*(6), 951–976.

Hinshaw, S. P. (1987). On the distinction between attentional deficits/hyperactivity and conduct problems/aggression in child psychopathology. *Psychological Bulletin, 101*(3), 443–463.

Hoagwood, K. E., Olin, S., Kerker, B. D., Kratochwill, T. R., Crowe, M., & Saka, N. (2007). Empirically based school interventions targeted at academic and mental health functioning. *Journal of Emotional and Behavioral Disorders, 15*(2), 66–92.

Krahé, B. (2013). *The social psychology of aggression.* New York: Psychology Press.

Lambert, S. F., Nylund-Gibson, K., Copeland-Linder, N., & Ialongo, N. S. (2010). Patterns of community violence exposure during adolescence. *American Journal of Community Psychology, 46*(3), 289–302.

Lanza, S. T., & Rhoades, B. L. (2013). Latent class analysis: An alternative perspective on subgroup analysis in prevention and treatment. *Prevention Science, 14*(2), 157–168.

Latessa, E. J., Cullen, F. T., & Gendreau, P. (2002). Beyond correctional quackery: Professionalism and the possibility of effective treatment. *Federal Probation, 66*(2), 43–49.

Laursen, B., & Hoff, E. (2006). Person-centered and variable-centered approaches to longitudinal data. *Merrill–Palmer Quarterly, 52*(3), 377–389.

Levin, H. M., & McEwan, P. J. (2001). *Cost-effectiveness analysis: Methods and applications* (2nd ed.). Thousand Oaks, CA: SAGE.

Lindstrom Johnson, S., Bradshaw, C. P., Cheng, T., & Wright, J. (2017). The role of physicians and other health providers in bullying prevention. In C. Bradshaw (Ed.), *Handbook on bullying prevention: A life course perspective* (pp. 261–268). Washington, DC: NASW Press.

Lindstrom Johnson, S. R., Finigan, N. M., Bradshaw, C. P., Haynie, D. L., & Cheng, T. L. (2011). Examining the link between neighborhood context and parental messages to their adolescent children about violence. *Journal of Adolescent Health, 49*(1), 58–63.

Lindstrom Johnson, S., Jones, V., & Cheng, T. L. (2015). Promoting "healthy futures" to reduce risk behaviors in urban youth: A randomized controlled trial. *American Journal of Community Psychology, 56*(1), 36–45.

Link, B. G., & Phelan, J. (1995). Social conditions as fundamental causes of disease. *Journal of Health and Social Behavior, 35,* 80–94.

Malti, T., Averdijk, M., Ribeaud, D., Rotenberg, K. J., & Eisner, M. P. (2013). "Do you trust him?": Children's trust beliefs and developmental trajectories of aggressive behavior in an ethnically diverse sample. *Journal of Abnormal Child Psychology, 41*(3), 445–456.

Malti, T., Noam, G. G., Beelmann, A., & Sommer, S. (2016). Toward dynamic adaptation of psychological interventions for child and adolescent development and mental health. *Journal of Clinical Child and Adolescent Psychology, 45*(6), 827–836.

Masten, A. S. (2007). Resilience in developing systems: Progress and promise as the fourth wave rises. *Development and Psychopathology, 19*(3), 921–930.

Masten, A. S., & Cicchetti, D. (2010). Developmental cascades. *Development and Psychopathology, 22*(3), 491–495.

McGee, T. R., Hayatbakhsh, M. R., Bor, W., Aird, R. L., Dean, A. J., & Najman, J. M. (2015). The impact of snares on the continuity of adolescent-onset antisocial behavior: A test of Moffitt's development taxonomy. *Australian and New Zealand Journal of Criminology, 48*(3), 345–366.

Mihalic, S. F., & Irwin, K. (2003). Blueprints for violence prevention: From research to real-world settings—factors influencing the successful replication of model programs. *Youth Violence and Juvenile Justice, 1*(4), 307–329.

Moffitt, T. E. (1993). Adolescence-limited and life-course-persistent antisocial behavior: A developmental taxonomy. *Psychological Review, 100*(4), 674–701.

Nagin, D., & Paternoster, R. (2000). Population heterogeneity and state dependence: State of the evidence and directions for future research. *Journal of Quantitative Criminology, 16*(2), 117–144.

National Academies of Sciences, Engineering, & Medicine. (2016). *Preventing bullying through science, policy, and practice.* Washington, DC: National Academies Press.

National Research Council & Institute of Medicine. (2009). *Preventing mental, emotional, and behavioral disorders among young people: Progress and possibilities.* Washington, DC: National Academies Press.

Nutley, S. M., Walter, I., & Davies, H. T. (2007). *Using evidence: How research can inform public services.* Bristol, UK: University of Bristol, Policy Press.

Parasuraman, S. R., & Shi, L. (2014). The role of school-based health centers in increasing universal and targeted delivery of primary and preventive care among adolescents. *Journal of School Health, 84*(8), 524–532.

Piquero, A. R., Farrington, D. P., Nagin, D. S., & Moffitt, T. E. (2010). Trajectories of offending and their relation to life failure in late middle age: Findings from the Cambridge Study in Delinquent Development. *Journal of Research in Crime and Delinquency, 47*(2), 151–173.

Ritchwood, T. D., Ford, H., DeCoster, J., Sutton, M., & Lochman, J. E. (2015). Risky sexual behavior and substance use among adolescents: A meta-analysis. *Children and Youth Services Review, 52,* 74–88.

Rivlin, A. M. (1971). *Systematic thinking for social action.* Washington, DC: Brookings Institution.

Schulenberg, J. E., & Maggs, J. L. (2002). A developmental perspective on alcohol use and heavy drinking during adolescence and the transition to young adulthood. *Journal of Studies on Alcohol, March*(Suppl. 14), 54–70.

Sheras, P. L., & Bradshaw, C. P. (2016). Fostering policies that enhance positive school environment. *Theory into Practice, 55*(2), 129–135.

Spoth, R., Greenberg, M., Bierman, K., & Redmond, C. (2004). PROSPER community–university partnership model for public education systems: Capacity-building for evidence-based, competence-building prevention. *Prevention Science, 5*(1), 31–39.

Srabstein, J. C., Berkman, B. E., & Pyntikova, E. (2008). Antibullying legislation: A public health perspective. *Journal of Adolescent Health, 42*(1), 11–20.

Stormshak, E. A., Connell, A. M., Véronneau, M., Myers, M. W., Dishion, T. J., Kavanagh, K., et al. (2011). An ecological approach to promoting early adolescent mental health and social adaptation: Family-centered intervention in public middle schools. *Child Development, 82*(1), 209–225.

Strolin-Goltzman, J., Sisselman, A., Melekis, K., & Auerbach, C. (2014). Understanding the relationship between school-based health center use, school connection, and academic performance. *Health and Social Work, 39*(2), 83–91.

Sugai, G., & Horner, R. H. (2009). Responsiveness-to-intervention and school-wide positive behavior supports: Integration of multi-tiered system approaches. *Exceptionality, 17*(4), 223–237.

U.S. Department of Education, Office of Planning, Evaluation and Policy Development, Policy and Program Studies Service. (2011). Analysis of state bullying laws and policies. Retrieved from *http://files.eric.ed.gov/fulltext/ED527524.pdf.*

Van Lier, P. A. C., Vitaro, F., Barker, E. D., Koot, H. M., & Tremblay, R. (2009). Developmental links between trajectories of physical violence, vandalism, theft, and alcohol–drug use from childhood to adolescence. *Journal of Abnormal Child Psychology, 37*(4), 481–492.

Walker, S. C., Kerns, S. E. U., Lyon, A. R., Bruns, E. J., & Cosgrove, T. J. (2010). Impact of school-based health center use on academic outcomes. *Journal of Adolescent Health, 46*(3), 251–257.

Weisz, J. R., Sandler, I. N., Durlak, J. A., & Anton, B. S. (2005). Promoting and protecting youth mental health through evidence-based prevention and treatment. *American Psychologist, 60*(6), 628–648.

Author Index

Aarons, G. A., 436
Aber, J. L., 238, 280, 341
Aboud, F. E., 233
Achenbach, T. M., 25, 269, 304, 305, 306, 347
Ackerman, B. P., 341
Acland, E., 421
Adams, E., 130, 132, 218
Adams, E. A., 272
Adams, R., 191, 199, 200
Adluru, N., 115
Aguilar, B., 51, 52
Ahadi, S. A., 111
Ahn, H., 235, 238, 256
Ahn, H.-J., 238
Ainsworth, M. D. S., 6, 170
Ajzen, I., 252, 260
Akbas, S., 303
Akee, R. K., 281
Aksan, N., 130
Alakortes, J., 301, 310
Alavi, N., 259
Alegria, A. A., 179
Aleman, X., 410, 416
Aleva, E. A., 217
Aleva, L., 387
Alink, L. A., 131, 135
Alink, L. R. A., 87, 89, 95, 97, 175, 179
Allen, Q., 365
Allport, G. W., 43
Almas, A., 300
Almeida, D., 348
Ames, A., 53
Amodio, D. M., 159
Anastasio, J., 287
Anastassiou-Hadjicharalambous, X., 95
Anderman, C., 298
Anderman, E. M., 365, 366
Andershed, A.-K., 71
Anderson, C. A., 47, 146, 150, 158, 434
Anderson, E., 276
Anderson, S., 286

Andrade, B. F., 318, 320, 427
Andrews, D. W., 152, 424
Ang, P. M., 350
Ang, R. P., 259
Angold, A., 21, 25, 135, 279, 281, 282
Aos, S., 438, 441, 442
Aoyama, I., 255
Applegate, B., 27
Appleyard, K., 43
Archer, J., 43, 154, 366, 434
Ardila-Rey, A., 219
Aricak, O. T., 257
Armstrong, K., 34
Arnold, K. D., 250
Arsène, M., 256
Arseneault, L., 69
Arsenio, W. F., 12, 46, 111, 115, 128, 130, 131, 132, 133, 134, 135, 136, 147, 149, 150, 212, 214, 216, 217, 218, 220
Arthur, M. W., 306, 407, 437
Asarnow, J. R., 148
Ashurst, N., 381
Asscher, J. J., 329
Assink, M., 52
Astor, R. A., 219, 360, 365
Aucoin, K. J., 33, 117
Auerbach, C., 440
August, G. J., 242
Aunola, K., 203
Averdijk, M., 4, 420, 437
Axas, N., 259
Axelrod, J. L., 199
Azar, S. T., 151
Azrael, D., 275
Azria-Evans, M. R., 200
Azurmendi, A., 96

B

Bachorowski, J., 148
Bae, N. Y., 305
Baglioni, A. J., 306
Bagwell, C. L., 191, 200, 203, 232, 237

Baibarazova, E., 93
Bajgar, J., 322
Baker, E., 93
Baker, L. A., 68, 69, 70
Bakermans-Kranenburg, M. J., 173, 174
Baldry, A. C., 256, 388
Ball, C., 215
Ball, C. L., 222
Ballard, E. D., 436
Bandura, A., 7, 62, 150, 170, 233, 253, 369
Bandyopadhyay, S., 371
Banerjee, R., 176
Banny, A. M., 53, 192
Barbaranelli, C., 7, 369
Barber, B. K., 172, 176
Barboza, G. E., 366
Barden, R. C., 214
Bariola, E., 346
Barker, E. D., 25, 27, 69, 74, 85, 111, 113, 114, 115, 132, 203, 435
Barker, G. J., 108
Barkin, S. H., 273, 280
Barkoukis, V., 252, 260
Barlett, C. P., 257
Barliñska, J., 260
Barnoski, R., 438
Baron, L., 155
Barret, K. C., 133
Barrig, P. S., 111
Barry, C. T., 30, 108
Barry, R. A., 130, 180
Barry, T., 135, 222
Bartel, P., 33
Bartels, M., 26
Barth, J. M., 193
Bartley, L., 427
Baruch, G., 329
Basile, K. C., 363, 365
Baskin-Sommers, A. R., 33
Bass, D., 326
Bastiaensens, S., 257
Basto-Pereira, M., 175

449

Subject Index

Note. f or *t* following a page number indicates a figure or a table.